THE 21st CENTURY MAN

Publisher's Legal Disclaimer

This book presents a wide range of opinions about a variety of topics related to health and wellbeing, including certain ideas, treatments, and procedures that may be hazardous or illegal if undertaken without proper medical supervision. These opinions reflect the research and ideas of the author or those whose ideas the author presents, but are not intended to substitute for the services of a trained healthcare practitioner. Consult with your healthcare practitioner before engaging in any drug, diet, or exercise regimen. The author and the publisher disclaim responsibility for any adverse effects resulting directly or indirectly from the information contained in this book.

Author's Disclaimer

Humans are complex beings. A drug that works on 90% of men does not work on 10% of men. I put my heart and soul into assembling an exceptional panel of experts to provide the most up-to-date recommendations available. Medical science is constantly updating information. This book reflects that state of the art when it was published. Future editions will reflect the evolution of medical research.

My advice is to be an active participant in your medical care and partner with physicians and other medical professionals, as well as your family, to take the best possible care of yourself.

This book was written to address the common challenges that all men face. Individual issues of race, color, religion, culture, ethnicity, gender, and sexual orientation are intentionally not addressed in this book. I have no expertise or advanced training in these subjects. We did our best to avoid making controversial statements about any of these issues.

— Judson Brandeis, MD

THE 21st CENTURY MAN

Advice from 50 top doctors and men's health experts
so you can feel great, look good, and have better sex

by

Judson Brandeis, MD
and More Than 50 Colleagues

AFFIRM SCIENCE, INC.
San Ramon, California

[Hardback]
ISBN 13: 978-1-7373796-0-7

[E-Book]
ISBN 13: 978-1-7373796-1-4

Library of Congress Number: *forthcoming*

Managing & Developmental Editor:
Nancy Faass

Book Design & Production:
Mark Weiman [Regent Press]

MANUFACTURED IN THE U.S.A.
AFFIRM Science, Inc.
100 Park Place Suite 140
San Ramon, CA 94583
www.TheTwentyFirstCenturyMan.com

Overview of the Contents

Contents

PART 5. EXERCISE

PART 6. ADDICTIONS

PART 14. LEAVING A LEGACY

Introduction

I take care of men. I've been a urologist for almost 25 years and have seen thousands of men as patients, many of whom have shared with me their most personal thoughts and feelings. I've followed many of the men in my practice for 15 to 20 years and have witnessed the slow physical decline that is inevitable with age. Over that time, I, too, have aged. I've lost most of my hair, a portion of my muscle mass, and some of my libido. I've grown love handles, ear hair, and nose hair, and like most men in midlife, my prostate is starting to enlarge. Yet many of my patients have had it far worse than I have.

At the age of 50, I discovered the use of shockwave therapy for erectile dysfunction, which then led to an interest and sub-specialization in sexual medicine for men. Sitting down and talking openly and honestly with hundreds of men who had, to varying degrees, lost their sexual function helped me understand that if men don't feel good or feel like they look good, their interest in sex and their enjoyment of life declines. Since this revelation first dawned on me, I've focused my practice on male rejuvenation: helping men to feel better, look better, and have better physical intimacy.

Having seen hundreds of men over the past three years who had lost the capacity for sexual intimacy and delved deep into their psyches and their physical limitations, I identified a pattern. As a rule, men take pride in being capable and selfless. They give of themselves freely and willingly to their spouses, children, community, and career. They happily provide extra effort, time, money, or support without expecting anything in return. However, at a certain point, usually between age 45 and 65, the vitality of youth begins to fade. These self-sacrificing men lose the energy they once had given so freely to others. They become the ones who need help but, having trained everyone around them to take from them, they don't know how to ask for help from others.

These generous men begin to put on weight, lose their hair, become grumpy and exhausted, shed their muscle mass, and lose their enthusiasm for life. When I ask them what they do for fun—for themselves—there's usually an awkward silence. Twenty years before, they would have easily come up with a laundry list of favorite hobbies and activities. But now, all they can think of are the things that their wives or children enjoy.

As a physician, I exist in the conventional medicine realm and the communities that serve functional medicine, aesthetic medicine, and lifestyle biohackers.

In 2020, I wrote a chapter for the Large Urology Group Practice Association Textbook and gave a course at their annual meeting. But I also ran the Sexual Medicine Section at The Aesthetic Show, podcasted with biohackers Dr. Drew and Ben Greenfield, and traveled the country promoting Emsculpt (electromagnetic therapy to build muscle and reduce fat). In addition, I saw patients at BrandeisMD (my sexual medicine practice) and ran clinical trials on shockwave therapy for erectile dysfunction (ED) and for Peyronie's disease, platelet-rich plasma for penile elongation, Emsella for improving orgasms, and a transdermal supplement to enhance penile blood flow. I try to incorporate the best of all the fields of medicine into my approach to treatment.

When I created the male rejuvenation center at BrandeisMD, I added a number of new technologies. Many of these technologies were already being used extensively in women's health and aesthetics, but some were brand new, and some were specific to men. Once I began training physicians in sexual medicine, I became interested in creating a male rejuvenation summit to showcase these technologies. At the same time, I began to consider a book that would help men over 40 understand the options available to them, to help them maintain the glow and vitality of youth.

I decided to utilize three basic pillars of health to organize the subject—feeling good, looking good, and having great sex. Then I evaluated each pillar from the top down and tried to think of everything that a man in midlife could do to slow or reverse the inevitable decline that age brings to all of us. In the process, I engaged experts in the field to help identify the bad habits that all of us fall into and suggest biohacks, techniques, or routines that we can utilize to stay vital and potent as we age.

I hope that you find this book engaging and useful. I genuinely care about my patients. I meticulously research all of the technologies that I bring to BrandeisMD, and I try them all out on myself. Only then do I offer them to my patients. The best of these treatments include shockwave therapy and P-shots for ED, platelet-rich protein (PRP) for hair growth, Dysport for wrinkles, facial lasers to improve skin, Emsculpt for muscle building, Emsella for sexual enhancement, vasectomy, and numerous others. I have field-tested many of the things that I discuss in this book, as I hope you will.

How to Use This Book

Approach *The 21st Century Man* as you would a world-class buffet, like Bacchanal at Caesar's Palace, which was recently voted the best in Las Vegas. Everyone starts with a plate and utensils, but not everyone chooses the same dishes. Some start with salads, move on to the main course, and finally go back for dessert, while others select their meal randomly. Some eat only their favorite foods, and others take advantage of the huge selection to sample new delicacies they've never tried before.

I created and wrote *The 21st Century Man* to help men feel great, look good, and have better physical intimacy. This is a buffet of world-class information written by extraordinary professionals. The book's plate and utensils are the introduction and first chapter "The Hero's Journey," which addresses the life path that we all walk. I see them as essential, as is "Smart Ways to Reduce Your Health Risks," because it talks about the conditions that cause premature death, so that you can work on preventing those disease processes.

After you finish this introduction, I recommend that you browse the table of contents just as you'd browse the buffet at Caesar's. Start with the chapters that are most relevant to you. But don't be afraid to explore topics that you might have heard of, but don't know anything about, that you might be worried about, or even those that you find a little embarrassing.

The book is organized in 14 sections, each focused on a different topic, with reader-friendly information drawn from a variety of medical specialists.

Part 1. The Journey. Heroes come in all different shapes, sizes, colors, religions, ethnicities, orientations, and nationalities. In this book we address what is common to the male experience rather than what is specific to any particular ethnicity or orientation. All men embark on a hero's journey, in a sense. How far you get is determined by your commitment to maximizing your potential and living your best life. Eventually every hero must confront dragons. In terms of health, chapter 2, on reducing your health risks, offers insight on the nature of those dragons for most of us. Since we all need someone to watch our back at times, we've included suggestions on how to enlist your partner and your doctor as allies on your journey.

Part 2. Preventive Maintenance. Here we review the most common causes of premature death for men, including fresh insight into the causes of these disorders and offering new approaches to treatment. Select the chapters that you feel are relevant to your current situation, factoring in environmental exposures where you live and work, as well as the genetic risks reflected in your family history.

Part 3. Advice from Specialists. This section features physicians who are top in their field. Here too, I would initially read the chapters that most relate to your current health. As the years go by, some of the other chapters may become more relevant to you.

Part 4. Food. We have taken the macro-to-micro approach to understanding food and nutrition. Fad diets come and go, but the underlying principles of nutrition are the same. I would suggest that since everyone eats, understanding the basic principles of food is essential to your health. Tragically, poor diet has surpassed smoking as the primary underlying cause of poor health. We have included a range of practical strategies that will enable you to rediscover the pleasure of delicious, healthy food.

Part 5. Exercise. Exercise is helpful in so many ways, but as we age, it becomes more difficult to exercise without injury. Will Workman, the team orthopedist for the Oakland A's, has written an essential chapter on pleasurable low-impact exercise, as well as key nutrients and herbs that reduce inflammation. This useful information is intended to reduce your risk of hip, knee, or shoulder replacement. Stretching, yoga, Emsculpt and working with a trainer are important tools for the aging athlete. In my case, only by using Emsculpt have I been able to stay in shape during the challenges of the past two years.

Part 6. Addictions. Many of us fall into bad habits during the highs and lows of life. Tobacco, alcohol, cocaine, marijuana overuse, and other addictions cause trillions of dollars of economic damage and emotional pain. The purpose of this section is not to shame you but rather to help you understand the dynamics underlying these destructive behaviors so that you can make informed decisions. We offer glimpses from the research of emerging strategies to reduce the impact of these disorders.

Part 7. Looking Good. Looking good is more important to men than many of us would like to admit. We all shave and use shampoo and maybe even conditioner multiple times every week, but how do these products actually work? Aesthetic medicine focuses on women, but men benefit as much or more from hair removal, hair replacement, neurotoxins like Dysport and Botox, fat reduction, and cosmetic surgery procedures. Excellent dental health and a radiant smile are also definitely essential to our presentation. Given the competitive job market, these resources become more essential as we enter midlife and beyond.

Part 8. Making Life Fun. Having fun reduces stress and gives meaning to life. Music and sports can bring us together. Imagination and design provide opportunities to use your creativity, enhancing your personal contentment.

Part 9. Mental Health. Socrates famously said, "an unexamined life is not worth living." Addressing mental health is critical to the enjoyment of life and worth. Work-life balance is something that almost every man I know struggles with, and the loss of this balance results in the anxiety and depression rampant in our age. Sadly, this has led to alcohol and opioid abuse and suicide rates that have ultimately reduced longevity for men in the United States. Here you'll also find insight on coping with depression and anxiety, and on increasing your quality of life.

Part 10. Relationship Skills. "Happy wife, happy life" is not just a cute slogan; the quality of our relationships impact the enjoyment and productivity of our existence. Finding the right partner, deepening your communication with them, and growing together are critical to fulfillment. Being a father for the right reasons and growing in that role can be a rewarding aspect of becoming a man. Another crucial milestone in a heterosexual relationship is menopause. Understanding menopause with empathy can lead to the golden years, but ignorance (and/or lack of empathy) will result in misery and possibly divorce. This section also includes clever pearls of wisdom from a seasoned family law attorney.

Part 11. Sexual Healing. There are several forms of meaningful intimacy, but physical intimacy deeply connects us with our partner and allows us to share feeling and pleasure in a unique way. For most couples, penetrative intercourse is an essential part of physical intimacy. Sadly, as men age, maintaining an erection adequate for intercourse becomes challenging. "Sexual Healing" provides leading-edge information about supplements, medications, and rejuvenative technologies that can be instrumental in restoring intimacy. I have included both low-tech and high-tech strategies that support male sexual health and efficacy. You will definitely want to read the final chapter in this section, intimate-wellness expert Susan Bratton's chapter on how to please a woman.

Part 12. Sexual Medicine. "Optimizing Testosterone," by Gary Donovitz, founder of BioTE, anchors the section on men's health, followed by my chapter on the prostate. These are essential reading, as these two issues eventually affect every man. We'll also provide insight on sexually transmitted infections and Peyronie's disease. Essentials on circumcision, vasectomies, and reversing vasectomies and national expert Dr. Philip Werthman on fertility complete part 12.

Part 13. Navigating Healthcare. I looked everywhere for a synopsis on health insurance, but we decided to write it when I was unable to find one. The result is a comprehensive summary of health insurance that makes this bewildering topic comprehensible. Equally important are how to find a good doctor and how to make the most of your limited time with your healthcare provider.

Part 14. Leaving a Legacy. As a urology resident, I appreciated Dr. Bernard Churchill's unique ability to explain difficult concepts and integrate knowledge. It was an honor to invite him to contribute a chapter, and he has wisely explored the effects of gratitude on health. Brian Banmiller, who has spent his life interviewing presidents and business leaders, offers first-hand knowledge on inspiration. "The heart that gives is the heart that gathers" is the legacy that Larry Bienati creates every day.

Until chapter 101, I intentionally omitted the details of my life from the book. However, at the ripe age of 50, I began my own hero's journey. Mark Twain once said, "The two most important days in your life are the day you are *born*, and the day you *find out why*." In this chapter, I reveal my own story. We all have problems and suffer hardship at some point in our lives. What matters most is how we deal with it. My sincere hope is that this book inspires you to live your best life and to leave a legacy for the next generation.

The author and volume editor. Judson Brandeis, MD has been voted top urologist in the San Francisco Bay Area for eight years in a row. A graduate of Brown University and Vanderbilt University School of Medicine, with Urologic Surgery residency at UCLA and a post-doc fellowship at Harvard, today he specializes in the emerging field of sexual health and medicine. Dr. Brandeis's practice focuses on the issues that people are too embarrassed to discuss, a source of untold suffering, from erectile dysfunction and premature ejaculation to prostate cancer. The book addresses each of these issues and many others, with candor, tact, and expertise.

PART 1
THE JOURNEY

Chapter 1
The Hero's Journey
Judson Brandeis, MD, Urologist

The privilege of a lifetime is being who you are.
— Joseph Campbell

What is the journey of life for a man?

Each of us is born with individual gifts and walks a unique life path of hardship and opportunity. With mindfulness and determination, we all have the chance to become the hero of our own story. Some men start early in their quest for fame and fortune. Others are late bloomers.

Although Darwin was just 22 when he began the voyages that informed his life's work, he was 50 years old before he published *On the Origin of the Species* in 1859, the theory for which he is best known today. Or Sam Walton, who opened his first Walmart at age 44, and Bill Wilson who turned his life around and co-founded Alcoholics Anonymous at age 40. Central to success in life is the ability to adapt to new circumstances and to keep learning. At the age of 51, after almost a decade as chief of urology at a major Bay Area

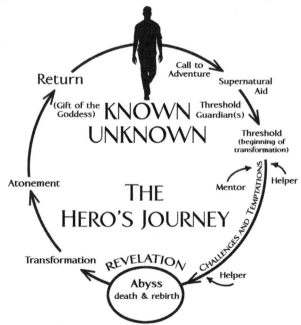

Figure 1.1. Steps in the Hero's Journey, based on the work of Joseph Campbell.

hospital and head of a successful urology practice, I left hospital medicine to focus on men's sexual health and rejuvenative medicine. The transition wasn't easy, but it brought creativity and drive back into my professional life at an age when many men are looking to coast or slowly wind things down.

Heroes come in all shapes and sizes, and motivations. Hollywood heroes like James Bond and Rambo are fearless and run toward danger. The movies glorify these men, but the real stories are more complex. Many are reluctant heroes, ordinary people who find themselves faced with an extraordinary challenge. Think of John McCain, a navy pilot, who after being shot down spent six years in the Vietnamese POW camps but refused early release in solidarity with his fellow prisoners. Or Jackie Robinson, born into a family of sharecroppers in rural Georgia, who braved death threats to break the color barrier in the all-white Major Leagues.

Life circumstances pushed these men into extreme situations that they faced with self-doubt and trepidation. Many heroes wish someone else would handle the task for them, but they rise to the occasion in the end. Often men in these situations aren't comfortable with their role as heroes, but they understand that this is their life path and grow into the role. The inner struggle for the unwilling hero is his desire to return to normal, but this is an impossible dream. Our hero is no longer the same innocent boy who began the journey to manhood.

MILESTONES IN THE JOURNEY

One source of insight into the hero's journey is the work of Joseph Campbell, who spent his life studying the epic stories of world cultures and exploring their underlying meaning. The hero's journey in mythology is a process of personal transformation, from an inexperienced boy into a mature man of wisdom. It is helpful to understand how this process unfolds in Campbell's model.

The departure. Every boy is born into a culture with traditions and beliefs. His life begins at home, where he understands his surroundings, people, and traditions. There is comfort in knowing the world in which he lives. He takes for granted that this is the way that things are supposed to be. Yet to achieve manhood, he must put aside security and challenge conventions and himself to create a new reality and identity. To accomplish that, he must leave the comfort of the familiar, so the initial phase of the hero's journey is the departure.

Think about the place where you were born and raised and how far you have journeyed since then. For some of your friends, the comfort of home prevented them from achieving their full potential when opportunities arose. The high school quarterback and prom queen may never leave town to test their abilities at the next level. Some men would rather be a big fish in a small pond, but in doing so, they miss the chance to reach their true potential.

The call to action. Other men refuse the call to action out of a sense of duty or obligation to family or friends, due to the fear of failure, or the lack of internal motivation. A hero's journey must come from within, although frequently, a mentor facilitates the quest for independence and achievement. This guide could be a wise parent, an athletic coach, a teacher, or a religious figure. Think about a pivotal figure in your life who inspired you to trust yourself and your instincts. Sadly, many men shrink back from the call to action and live mediocre lives, wondering what could have been. Fortunately, at any age, you can do something truly remarkable. Consider the life of Nelson Mandela. After serving 27 years of a life sentence, the South African government released him from prison at the age of 71. At 75, he became the first black president, in a fully representative, multiracial South Africa.

As George Eliot wrote,
"It's never too late to be what you might have been."

Astronaut John Glenn joined the NASA space program at 37 (just shy of the program's cut-off of age 40) to become the first American to orbit the earth and the third American in space. At the age of 43, he joined the U.S. Senate, where he served for 24 years.

Point of no return. Once a man leaves the familiarity of home, he becomes more deeply committed to the journey, and at some point, there's no turning back. Houdini, for example, knew from a young age that he wanted to be a magician, despite his parent's objections. He ran away from home by hopping a freight train, eventually ending up in New York City, where he had to panhandle on the streets to eat. He went on to achieve astonishing success. Elon Musk made $180 million when he sold his stake in PayPal in 2002. Musk then invested all his time and money in SpaceX, Tesla, and Solar City. By 2008, he had completely run out of money and found himself in divorce court. His total commitment to the realization of his innovations enabled Musk to succeed beyond his wildest dreams.

Forging a new identity. As the journey begins, the hero entirely separates from his known world. One crucial aspect of the quest is to discover and then forge a new identity. Although he reveals his willingness to undergo a change, he soon encounters danger or setbacks that test his will and skills. Our hero realizes that he no longer has the safety net of his previous life and must fend for himself. Early setbacks, followed by success, give him the confidence to move forward. In 1919, Walt Disney was fired from one of his first animation jobs at the *Kansas City Star* because his editor felt he "lacked imagination and had no good ideas." Disney later acquired Laugh-O-Gram animation studios, which he drove into bankruptcy. These early failures gave no hint of his colossal vision and the success Disney achieved later in life.

A multitude of trials. As the quest deepens, the hero moves toward initiation. The first step is the road of trials, a series of tests the hero must undergo to begin the transformation. Often it appears that the hero will fail these tests. The odds are against him. Frequently a mentor or higher power helps our hero with advice or gifts. In the Greek epic *The Odyssey*, Odysseus encounters a multitude of trials, including Lotus Eaters (addiction), Cyclops (monsters), the Laestrygonians (cannibals), Circe (sorcery), the Underworld (life in hell), Sirens (enchantment or delusion), Calypso (seduction), Scylla and Charybdis (confrontation with massive danger, forcing the choice between the lesser of two evils), and finally Helios and Poseidon (conflict with God). These dangers are all metaphors for different aspects of human reality. Along the journey, temptations of the flesh and of material wealth may lead a man to abandon or stray from the quest. Who can forget how Robin Givens distracted "Iron Mike" Tyson or how sex and drugs destroyed so many rock-and-roll legends? Imagine the fantastic music Jimi Hendrix, Jim Morrison, and Kurt Cobain could have made had their lives had not been cut short.

Saboteurs. Friends and family may have positive intentions, but they can also derail a quest and hinder a man's development. Men on a hero's journey are often called selfish, unrealistic, or crazy. Your ability to identify obstructions on your path and align with supporters is critical to your mission's success. Because few people complete their hero's journey to mature adulthood, most people will unconsciously attempt to sabotage your journey.

The live-or-die moment. The next step in the journey is entering the dragon's lair: consider, for example, the bravery of the American soldiers landing on the beach in Normandy. The live-or-die moment of the journey is often accompanied by despair when everything seems to be lost. At this critical juncture, our hero gains access to a previously unavailable part of himself – one last breath of energy, strength, or creativity to defeat the overwhelming forces he must confront. The hero must call on inner power that he does not know he possesses. Audie Murphy was one of the most decorated soldiers in World War II. In December 1945, the Allied generals ordered Murphy and his unit to hold against a German counterattack. After the Germans hit the M10 tank destroyer, causing it to burst into flames, Murphy ordered his troops to fall back. Alone, he covered their retreat and held off the Germans by mounting the burning tank's .50 caliber machine gun and calling in artillery strikes. His position was attacked on three sides by six tanks and waves of infantry. Wounded and out of ammunition, he returned to his company, refused medical treatment, and organized a successful counterattack. For an hour, the Germans tried every available weapon to eliminate 2nd Lieutenant Murphy, but he held his position.

Transformation. In the end, our hero overcomes his greatest adversary and achieves the objective that he set out to complete. The successful completion of the quest brings money, power, love, and fame. However, these actual treasures become secondary to the personal transformation that has occurred. Edward Aikau was a champion surfer from Hawaii, but he is best known as the first lifeguard on the island of Oahu, where he saved more than 500 lives. Eddie would brave waves that often reached 30 feet or more when no one else would go out. Instead of enjoying the accolades of being a champion athlete, Eddie chose the thankless job of a lifeguard.

The long road home. After the climax of the quest comes the long passage home carrying the riches earned during the struggles. Dangers and roadblocks clutter the path back. During the return journey, our hero must deal with whatever mental baggage remains from his upbringing and life that may present itself later as weakness. Before the final homecoming, there are often more unforeseen obstacles to overcome. This ultimate test of our hero's fortitude further defines and deepens his mental and emotional growth. The strength he has built during the quest enables him to overcome this final obstacle.

Lewis and Clark reached the Pacific Ocean in November 1805. In March 1806, the weary explorers headed for home and St. Louis. They retrieved their horses and crossed the Bitterroot Mountains. On the return trip, the expedition separated into two parties in Idaho to explore the country more thoroughly. During that time, Blackfoot warriors attacked Lewis's company. To make matters worse, Lewis was wounded in a hunting accident. Lewis and Clark reached the end of their 8,000-mile journey in St. Louis on September 23, 1806.

(Not every quest is successful. The massive effort can make or break a man.)

Tragically, Lewis committed suicide several years later at the age of 35. On the other hand, Clark became one of the leading officials in the West and an advisor to many American presidents.

Ironically, when our hero returns, he finds that he no longer fits into the world that he once knew. His worldview and capabilities have expanded far beyond the world he left. Unfortunately, this has become a significant issue in the United States as many Afghanistan and Iraq war veterans have had real difficulties fitting back into civilian life. It has also been the reality of many Vietnam vets and has probably been true of soldiers returning from war throughout history.

What's the point of all of this? I believe that we are born on this earth with a purpose and a Hero's Journey waiting for all of us. Unfortunately, most of us never reach our true potential. We are too comfortable or too afraid to change, or we stumble and fall while battling the dragon and do not have the persistence to keep fighting. For those who succeed, it comes down to determination. Do you have the drive to do what you know is right? This book is intended as a resource for men on how to live a better, healthier life, written by national experts in their respective fields. Our website will provide additional resources for you to live your best life. Many of the most effective interventions are free and simply require personal commitment and determination. I wish you all the best on your own journey, and I hope that you inspire and mentor the next generation of heroes.

THE HERO'S JOURNEY: IMMIGRATION

The immigrant's journey is often synonymous with the hero's path. This assumption has been true since the First Peoples began migrating out of Africa 60,000 years ago and is still true today. Here is one such story:

Rajesh was born in Judwadli, a little farming town in Southwest India, where his parents owned a small cotton and peanut farm. There was no electricity or indoor plumbing. He remembers taking a lantern to the outhouse at night and finding a cobra in the toilet. Life wasn't easy: his mother passed away when he was young, and his father favored his older brother. Fortunately, the local schoolteachers noticed his aptitude for math and encouraged him to go to a better school in the neighboring town. His father and grandparents wanted him to take over the family farm and discouraged him from continuing his education. Even though his parents were illiterate, he was able to go to boarding school, studied hard, and got top scores on the national math and science exams so that he could attend university. His family tried to drag him back to the farm by cutting off the few rupees that paid for his board. At that point, Rajesh had no source of support but his own drive. He remembers those times now at age 85: "Whatever hurdle comes in, you face it."

After graduating from the university, he found employment in India in the public works system for a year but learned from friends of opportunities in America. He began dreaming of going to the U.S. and was one of the only students in his class to pass the engineering certification exam. To gain admission to an American college, he had to travel to Bombay to apply for a scholarship to the engineering school at the University of Kansas.

"Only eight dollars in your pocket when you leave for the U.S." Rajesh recalled. He took a steamboat to New York and was 30 days at sea.

"It is a blow to the mind when you land in New York. I had never seen an escalator or neon lights. You get depressed because you feel so backward, and they seem so advanced. I did not even know how to turn on the faucet."

Although he had tuition paid for a year, he washed dishes at night to support himself in Kansas. He sought out a church charity to get an overcoat for the cold Kansas weather and rented a basement room in a house with three other students. Rajesh drove a used car he purchased for $30. During college, he started designing and building bridges with a structural engineering *company in Kansas City. One day, he received a letter from his friend Mahendra Kardani, telling him about the beautiful weather and the beaches in California.*

In 1966 Rajesh drove his VW bug to Los Angeles, stayed at the YMCA, and found a job with CalTrans in downtown LA, building the California highway system and designing overpasses.

Secure in his job, he went back to India determined to find a beautiful bride. Their courtship and honeymoon lasted three days. In the ensuing years in Los Angeles, they had two beautiful children, while Rajesh designed and built his own house. During economic downturns, he was able to purchase properties, so he and his wife were able to send both their children to dental school to become professionals.

When asked about moments of doubt on arriving in a new country without a safety net, Rajesh replied, "I believed I could do anything. I never looked at the negative. Failure was never an option—there was never a possibility of failure."

Things were going well until 1994, when Rajesh's heart failed. He went to the Emergency Room at Kaiser one afternoon with chest pain and a cough. Given his accent and quiet nature, he could not adequately explain his symptoms and was sent home with cough medicine. Three days later, he returned to the hospital near death. He barely survived a six-vessel bypass. A large part of his heart had died, and at that point, his heart function was 30% of normal.

Determined to see his children married and to have grandchildren one day, Rajesh changed his eating habits and took up yoga, walking, and meditation. However, two years after his heart surgery, he began having difficulty walking and experienced pain in his legs. His physician diagnosed problems with the veins in his legs. Within a year, he was nearly paralyzed, and an MRI showed severe impingement of the nerves in his back. He underwent a six-hour spine operation, but it took a full year for Rajesh to walk normally again.

Rajesh and his wife had both worked for CalTrans for almost 40 years and retired with full pensions. He enjoyed his children's weddings and the birth of six grandchildren, who are now all teenagers. Rajesh still walks every day, does yoga, and mediates. Angiograms of his heart show collateral blood vessel growth and no new blockages. He is still able to count cards when he plays blackjack and tells clever stories to his grandchildren (who include my four children).

> **Not every hero plays major league sports, flies a fighter plane, or plays guitar in front of thousands of screaming fans. In fact, most heroes are quietly thriving in your neighborhood. They are also working to inspire and prepare the next generation of men to take the sacred hero's journey of their age.**

Chapter 2
Smart Ways to Reduce Your Health Risks
Judson Brandeis, MD, Urologist
& Michael Abassian, MPH, Researcher

I'm not afraid of death, I just don't want to be there when it happens.
— Woody Allen

The goal of this chapter is to inform you of your risks and offer you practical strategies for reducing those risks. There are so many things that can be done to materially improve the quality of your life. Here is what you need to know to take better care of yourself.

OUR DOUBLED LIFESPAN

The good news: You will probably live to 76. The average life expectancy for men in the United States reflects a gain of about 40 years over the last 150 years, when male lifespan averaged 35 years of age. Major advances in medicine and public health have extended and improved our lives and increased our lifespan spectacularly.

The bad news: We're losing ground. For the first time in 150 years, longevity is declining for American males. In middle age, for example, white males are dying at such a high rate, they are statistically increasing the death rate for all middle-aged males as a group. This chapter and the demographic trends it describes are the call to action that *The 21st Century Man* seeks to address.

Protect yourself by knowing your risks. There's an old saying: "If you'd have known better, you'd have done better." (It's remarkable, the number of people who don't know what's wrong with living on fast food.) So this content is intended to support you in rethinking coping strategies that may have become bad habits....

CUTTING YOUR RISKS IN HALF

Taking a closer look at the numbers, heart disease and cancer are responsible for almost half (46%) of deaths in men, so reducing just those two risks essentially cuts your risks in half. There is a surprising amount of similarity in the underlying causes of heart disease and cancer. If you develop a healthy diet, stay physically active, and avoid tobacco, that will also reduce your health risks by about half.

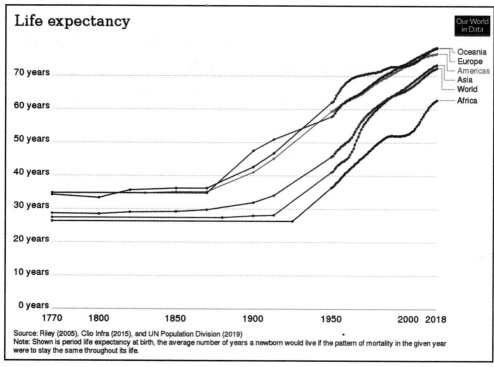

Figure 2.1. Increased life expectancy reflecting the development of public health and antimicrobial therapy. (Max Rosner, Martin School, Oxford, U.K.).

Progress in reducing the risk of heart disease. Heart disease is significantly preventable. Study after study has shown that modifiable risk factors make a tremendous difference in the quality of life and life expectancy in terms of risk of heart disease. A prospective cohort analysis funded by the National Institutes of Health (NIH) has shown that:

- Smoking cessation can reduce the risk of heart disease by about 40% *within five years*—almost cutting the risk in half.

- Exercise in your 40s is crucial to heart health, whether or not you exercised in your 20s or 30s. Statistics show major decreases in heart disease for individuals who exercise, even those who begin exercising in midlife.

- Exercise can also reduce cancer risk. Individuals who start exercising past their 40s can still reduce cancer mortality.

Cardio risk—24.2% of fatalities. Cardiovascular disease encompasses a range of conditions that affect the heart and blood vessels, including myocardial infarctions (heart attack), aneurysms, stroke, and heart failure.

Heart disease is responsible for one in every four male deaths,
causing 350,000 male deaths in the United States in 2017 alone.

What is particularly concerning is that half of the men who die from coronary heart disease have no warning: no signs or symptoms to give them a heads up. We can be at risk of heart disease and not be aware of our vulnerability if we lack the symptoms. For this reason, cardiovascular risk assessment is now an important part of routine annual checkups.

Cancer risks—21.9% of fatalities. Cancer continues to be a leading cause of death for men from 40 to 80 years of age and beyond, with about 900,000 men diagnosed with cancer annually, and 320,000 men lost to some form of the disease in 2019 alone. More than 40% of men will be diagnosed with cancer at some time during their life—almost one in two. The risk of cancer rises dramatically when we reach 50. The chance of a cancer diagnosis:

- From birth to 50 years of age is just over 3%.
- Risk from 50 to 59 years of age is 6%.
- For 60 to 69-year-old men, risk rises to 13%.
- For men 70 and over, risk is about 32%.

The most common newly diagnosed cancers involve the lungs, prostate, and digestive tract, reflecting the effects of smoking and poor diet.

CONDITION	NUMBER	PERCENT
Heart disease	659,041	23%
Cancer	599,601	21%
Accidents-unintentional injury	173,040	6%
Chronic respiratory diseases	156,979	5%
Stroke-cerebrovascular diseases	150,005	5%
Alzheimer's disease	121,499	4%
Diabetes	87,647	3%
Kidney disease	51,565	2%
Influenza and pneumonia	49,783	2%
Suicide	47,511	2%

Figure 2.2. Estimated deaths from all causes in males, U.S., 2019.

In terms of prostate cancer, tracking the PSA (prostate-specific antigen) after the age of 50 can lead to early intervention before malignancy in the prostate spreads. Overall death rates from cancer in men have been declining since the early 1990s. (Death dates that are declining in prostate, myeloma, and bladder cancers are due to changes in environmental and behavioral risk factors and better screening, detection, and treatment.)

WHAT MAKES A DIFFERENCE?

Knowing the factors that increase the risk of common, fatal cancers can empower you to make life-saving changes. You'll also want to look for patterns within your family and put greatest emphasis on likely genetic risks factors. Issues to address when reducing cancer risk include smoking cessation, reducing excess body weight, eating nutritiously, and getting enough physical activity.

Many men are physically active when they are young, and then stop exercising later in life and never pick it up again. Surprisingly, their health risks are far worse than the risks of those who begin exercising later in life and continue to do so.

Chronic illness. The United States is in the midst of a significant demographic shift that began in the twentieth century. By 2030, all the baby boomers will have reached the age of 65, and approximately 20% of the United States population will be of retirement age. We will be a society with more chronic diseases, given the rates of heart disease and cancer as we age. Chronic respiratory disease, liver disease, cirrhosis, and diabetes are also on the increase, with impact on quality of life. Chronic conditions such as diabetes can feel overwhelming and can be difficult to reverse.

It's important to remind yourself that you have the power
to make significant changes in your health risks.

Diabetes and sexual vitality. Diabetes directly accounts for more than 46,000 male deaths each year. Men make up about 65% of all type 1 diabetes cases. Type 2 diabetes prevalence increases with age:

- 10% of those ages 45-54
- 20% of those 55-64
- 23% of men 65 and older.

These numbers show the impact of diabetes across our population. On a human level, symptoms suggest that diabetes (and prediabetes) impairs quality of life in ways unique to men, reflected in low testosterone, decreased sex drive, erectile dysfunction, and impotence.

A proactive approach. We cannot control the effects of culture, education, or poverty on our health when we're young. However, in adulthood, we can understand the benefit of being proactive. What's more, we can choose to move step-by-step toward our health goals. We can have the greatest impact on our risks of heart disease by:

- Quitting tobacco
- Addressing nutrition, weight gain (especially around the waistline), high blood pressure (hypertension), and body mass index (which all have the same underlying nutritional causes)

- Becoming physical active
- Moderating alcohol use (seven drinks a week or less is the recent finding, associated with lower risk of obesity).

Five-year survival rates for the most common cancers in men range considerably, with prostate cancer having an overall survival rate of about 98%. In comparison, the five-year overall survival rate of pancreatic cancer is just over a depressing 9%.

Guys, Check in with Your Doctor . . . .

In the United States and globally, men are generally not good at utilizing primary care services. Qualities associated with masculinity in our culture such as self-sufficiency, independence, and strength are reflected in unwillingness to seek care.

Many men don't bother to get checkups, which is sobering.

Why bother? By optimizing your lifestyle, you can cut your risk of stroke by 80%. And blood tests are now available that will screen for several types of cancer (often before symptoms develop). The point here is that screening is worth the effort—it could save your life.

There is strength in taking action to reduce our risks. And if we are struggling, we need to become proactive about our health, scheduling that long overdue appointment with our primary care provider. We owe that to ourselves.

(For healthy approaches to weight loss, please see chapters 31 to 36; for realistic strategies to get back in shape, see chapters 37 to 43; and for effective ways to reduce a tobacco habit, see chapters 44 and 45.)

KEY TAKE AWAYS

- The leading causes of death for 40- to 80-year-old men are heart disease and cancer.
- The most important risk factor you need to avoid is smoking, which contributes to virtually all types of cancer, including lung, protate, and colorectal cancer.
- Make an absolute commitment of a healthy diet that includes fresh fruits and vegetables, and work toward a moderate to vigorous level of physical activity.
- Access to good quality health insurance, obtained for most Americans through employment, is a powerful predictor of positive health outcomes.

For additional references and resources, please see www.TheTwentyFirstCenturyMan.com.

Chapter 3
What Women Need to Know About Men's Health
Men's Health Network
& HealthyMen.org

More than half of premature deaths among men are preventable,
but you can't prevent a problem if you don't know it exists.
— Armin Brott

Although guys clearly like being self-reliant, there's a good chance that without some gentle pushing from you, he may not get that annual check-up or have that worrisome symptom looked at. *So it may be up to you.* More than half of premature deaths among men are preventable. By educating yourself about potential male health problems and passing that information on to the men you love, you may be able to save his life.

On average, men are less healthy and have a shorter life expectancy than women. In part, they don't take care of themselves as well as women do. They are also less likely to have health insurance, more likely to work in a dangerous occupation, and often don't seek medical attention when they need it. Men are more likely to engage in unhealthy behaviors, and less likely than women to adopt preventive health measures. Unfortunately, most of these issues, especially the ones having to do with sex or masculinity, are difficult for men to talk about.

Men die younger than women—and in greater numbers—of heart disease, cancer, diabetes, stroke, and numerous other diseases. In 1920, women outlived men by an average of one year. Today, that difference is more than five years.

HEALTH PROBLEMS SPECIFIC TO MEN

Throughout the book we'll discuss the main health issues that men face. Each chapter focuses on a single health issue or group of related conditions. We'll talk about the factors that increase risk, how to recognize symptoms, and offer practical insights on prevention, diagnostic testing, and early interventions.

Low testosterone. Testosterone is the most important of men's hormones. Millions of older men suffer from testosterone deficiency, which, if left untreated for too long, is linked with long-term health problems such as loss of muscle mass, bone loss (osteoporosis), low sex drive, erectile dysfunction, and difficulty with concentration and focus.

Erectile dysfunction/impotence. Erectile dysfunction (ED) is the inability of a man to achieve or maintain an erection sufficient for his sexual needs or the needs of his partner. Although ED becomes more common with age, men of any age can suffer from it—and most guys experience this problem at some point in their life. Frequently, erectile problems are caused by an underlying health problem such as diabetes, clogged arteries, or high blood pressure. Unfortunately, most men refuse to discuss ED with either their partners or healthcare providers. As a result, men feel embarrassed, and women feel that their man no longer finds them attractive.

Prostate problems. Located in the pelvis, this walnut-sized gland produces semen and naturally enlarges as men age. Potential problems include prostate infection (prostatitis) and enlargement, called BPH (benign prostatic hyperplasia), which can cause difficult or painful urination.

Prostate cancer. Prostate cancer is a concern for men 50 and older, and for high-risk men 40 and older. Those at highest risk include African-Americans, men with a family history of prostate cancer, and men exposed to Agent Orange, all of whom should be screened yearly. Caught early, this disease is often treatable.

Testicular cancer. Cancer of the testicles is the most common cancer in men ages 15 to 35. Although it can't be prevented, thanks to improved treatments and diagnostics, testicular cancer, like prostate cancer, has a very high cure rate if caught early.

PRACTICING PREVENTION

Some of the most effective things you can do for your man (and yourself, for that matter), are to support his health by encouraging:

- Healthy, fresh food
- Regular exercise
- Quitting smoking
- Self-exams
- Periodic screenings and checkups.

These simple steps can drastically reduce the chances that he will succumb to four of the ten leading causes of death: heart disease, cancer, stroke, and diabetes.

Screening to Rule Out Serious Conditions

One of the most important steps you can take is to get the men in your life into the habit of getting regular medical checkups. Here are several health maintenance milestones recommended by leading health organizations:

Men in their 20s:

- Testicular self-exam every month
- Blood pressure check every year
- A complete physical every three years
- Screening for cancers of the thyroid, testicles, lymph nodes, mouth, and skin every three years
- Cholesterol test for total, LDL, and HDL (the good kind) every three years

Men in their 30s & 40s, all of the above, plus:

- A complete physical every two years

Beginning in a man's 40s, all of the above, plus annual screenings:

- A baseline prostate-specific antigen (PSA) test and digital rectal exam (DRE) at age 40. These screenings should be repeated every year if the man is in a high-risk group. Other men should consult with their healthcare provider about whether they need an annual exam.
- Cancer tests every year
- A stool test (for colon and rectal cancers) every year

Starting at age 50, all of the above, plus:

- A prostate-specific antigen (PSA) and digital rectal exam (DRE) test every year
- A sigmoidoscopy or colonoscopy (for colon cancers) every three to four years or as recommended by your healthcare provider

Sources: American Cancer Society, American Heart Association, Men's Health Network

Finding a physician. If he doesn't have a family physician or can't afford one, look for health fairs, free or low-cost clinics, and free screening events in the area. Research health coverage available through an employer, government (federal, state, county, or city), fraternal organization, or place of worship, for example. (See www.MensHealthNetwork.org.)

Screening: Self-exams. Somewhere along the line we got the idea that self-exams have to be done by ourselves. Nothing could be further from the truth. There's no reason why your man can't help you with your breast exams or you with his testicular exams. Checking each other out can serve several purposes. First, it will double the chances that his (and your) exams get done regularly and thoroughly. Also don't forget about his back. Women get most skin cancers in places where they can more easily be spotted, on their hands and face and below the dress line. Men get most of theirs on their backs, where they're a lot harder to see.

RECOGNIZING SYMPTOMS

When the warning light flashes on the car dashboard, most men usually take the car to the shop. Yet when they sense warning signs of a health issue, most men don't take notice. This may be one of the reasons that men die younger than women.

Here are a few warning signs you should be on the lookout for:

Changes in health status. Persistent backaches, changes in the color of urine or stool, obvious changes in warts or moles, unusual lumps, recurrent chest pains or headaches, bleeding that won't stop, a nagging cough, unexplained weight loss, and extreme fatigue can all be symptoms of serious health problems.

Changes in bowel or bladder habits. This can be an indication of prostate or bladder problems. And blood in the urine is a common indicator of kidney problems. Does he get up five times a night to go to the bathroom? That could be a symptom of an enlarged prostate, a common condition among men as they get older.

Depression. Although women may be more likely to attempt suicide, men are four times more likely to succeed. Because men are reluctant to ask for help and often try to hide their depression, you may recognize the symptoms sooner than he does. These could include acting overly anxious, having trouble sleeping, complaining of feeling sad or "empty" or helpless, engaging in unusually risky or reckless behavior, anger, overwork, or losing interest in hobbies or other pleasurable activities (including sex).

Osteoporosis. Although usually considered a women's disease, osteoporosis affects men too and is generally under-diagnosed in men. This disease, which causes the bones to become fragile and more likely to break, can lead to permanent disability or death.

Breast cancer. Men have breast tissue too, and hundreds of men die of breast cancer each year. Men often confuse their symptoms with a sports or work injury, and because they're less likely to recognize or report symptoms, they're usually diagnosed only after the disease has spread.

Erectile dysfunction. Most of the time, erectile problems are caused by an underlying health problem, such as diabetes, clogged arteries, or high blood pressure. Research shows that this is particularly true of younger men.

If you want to make love and he says he has a headache, pay attention—it might be something far more serious.

KNOW WHEN TO CALL THE PROFESSIONALS

If you identify a symptom, get your man to the doctor immediately—and don't take no for an answer!

**Courtesy of the Men's Health Network, Health Education and Advocacy
www.MensHealthNetwork.org.
and HealthyMen.org.
For additional references and resources,
please see www.TheTwentyFirstCenturyMan.com.**

Chapter 4
Building a Relationship with Your Doctor
Judson Brandeis, MD, Urologist
& Armin Brott, Medical Writer

The good physician treats the disease.
The great physician treats the patient who has the disease.
— William Osler

Since men don't go to the doctor often enough and most causes of illness, infirmity, and premature death are preventable, having a relationship with a medical provider is an important part of keeping yourself healthy. When we use the term medical provider, or primary care provider, we are including nurse practitioners and other clinicians who provide primary care.

PARTNERS IN HEALTH

There are no two ways about it: we men sometimes don't take very good care of ourselves. Far too many of us don't ever see a doctor unless there's something seriously wrong or unless our partner makes the appointment for us. Men are half as likely to visit a doctor for a checkup as women are, and there are over 7 million American men who haven't seen a doctor in over 10 years. And even when we do go to the doctor, we often don't feel comfortable talking about our health.

Women make at least twice as many preventive care visits as men.

So why don't we take better care of ourselves? Part of the reason is the way we're brought up. As little boys, we're taught not to cry, not to complain, and not to show any signs of weakness. We ignore our aches and pains and play through our injuries. In our 20s, we think we're indestructible and see going to the doctor as a waste of time and money. In our 30s, we're too busy with our career and family to go. By the time we're in our 40s we don't go because we're afraid of what we'll find out, or we don't want to have a rectal exam (who does?).

Being tough may have some advantages. But it's also killing us. One recent study found that two-thirds of men wouldn't even go to the doctor if they were experiencing chest pain or shortness of breath—two of the big early warning signs of a heart attack. Most life-threatening illnesses, including heart disease, cancer, and diabetes, can be treated or cured if they're caught early.

MAKING A CHOICE

So here's the deal. If you can't remember the last time you had a complete physical, pick up the phone and make an appointment. (You wouldn't let ten years go between oil changes, would you?) If something is hurting or just doesn't seem right, call. Even if you're feeling great, call anyway. The time to see your doctor isn't when you're hooked up to life support. It's now, when you're feeling healthy.

Unfortunately, finding a good primary care physician isn't as easy as it should be. Your insurance coverage may limit your choices, and if you don't have insurance, cost can be a big factor. But starting and maintaining a long-lasting relationship with a good doctor is critical.

So how do you find a doctor? If you have medical coverage, start by checking the list of "preferred providers" (doctors covered by your insurance). Then ask friends or co-workers for recommendations. If you're in good health, you can probably go with a general practitioner. But if you know you have a particular problem, try to choose a specialist in that area as your primary care doctor.

The next step is to interview a few candidates and check their references. One way to do that is by calling the American Board of Medical Specialties at 1-866-275-2267 or visit their website, www.abms.org.

If you don't have health insurance, consider exploring free or low-cost healthcare, prescription drug assistance, and discounted drug programs such as www.goodrx.com. You can find information on a number of programs, as well as Medicare, Medicaid, and clinical trials at www.healthclinicsonline.com.

THE PARTNERSHIP

Actually, you're not just looking for a doctor, you're looking for a healthcare partner. And just as with any partner, you need a partnership agreement. Here's how it works:

It's your responsibility to give your doctor the information he or she needs to do his or her job. That means paying attention to your body and how you feel, being aware of unusual changes or aches and pains that don't go away, finding out as much as you can about the health of other members of your family, and honestly answering questions. If you're not honest, your doctor won't be able to help you as much as if you were honest.

It's the doctor's responsibility to use all the information you give him or her to help you stay healthy when you are, and to help you to get well when you're not.

It's your responsibility to follow the doctor's recommendations. That means making the lifestyle changes he or she suggests, taking medication according to the directions, keeping follow-up appointments, and seeing specialists when required.

DEEPENING YOUR COMMUNICATION

The basics. Unfortunately, men don't see their healthcare providers as often as women do. And if they do make a visit, they tend not to ask the questions they need to be asking. So once you've made your appointment to see your healthcare provider, make sure you get answers to the following broad questions:

- What is my risk of developing a cardiovascular condition?

- What is my blood pressure?

- What are my cholesterol levels (the HDL and LDL)?

- Am I at risk for developing diabetes?

- How much should I exercise?

- What's the best way to quit smoking?

- How much alcohol is okay for me to drink every day?

- Could any of the medications I regularly take increase my risk of developing cardiovascular problems?

Coping with a diagnosis. Bring a friend or a medical advocate with you, particularly if your symptoms or diagnosis are serious or if you've been feeling poorly. Record your doctor's responses in your phone or in an audio recorder.

- What is my diagnosis?

- How serious is my condition?

- What is the underlying cause of my condition?

- What could have an adverse effect on my condition?

- What are my treatment options?

- What are the benefits of the medications you have prescribed for me?

- If you have another health condition, ask how you can best manage these conditions together?

A Doctor's Perspective: Making the Most of Your Visit

Have you ever left the doctor's office wishing you had more time? Wondering if your doctor really listened to you or understood your symptoms? Would you like the inside scoop on how to maximize your time at the doctor's office? Lean in and I'll tell you.

First, understand where your doctor is coming from. Doctors haven't received a raise from Medicare in 20 years. In addition, the reporting requirements from Medicare and the time required to document care in the electronic medical record have forced physicians to spend more and more time on paperwork. In order to pay the bills, doctors have to see more patients in a day. This translates into appointments that are fifteen minutes or less. If you spend this time talking to your doctor about the weather or your pet cat, you're wasting valuable time. To maximize your visit, you need to stay focused on why you're there.

Be clear about the purpose of your visit. So when you make your appointment, explain clearly why you've come to see the doctor and make sure that your doctor accepts your insurance (actually, you can save a few minutes by asking about insurance before you make your appointment).

Come to the appointment prepared. You don't want your doctor to spend time asking obvious questions that you already know they're going to ask. Prepare that information for them in advance of your visit. I love it when patients hand me their notes. I use my voice dictation system to quickly summarize the pertinent findings, and then move on to the second- and third-level questions that allow me to form a diagnosis and treatment plan.

If this is a visit to a new physician, write out your medical history. The website at HIVE80.com has a form that you can use for this purpose. In order for your doctor to do their job, you must be honest. Be sure to include:

- Any medical issues and prior diagnoses
- Surgeries
- A list of your medications and supplements
- Allergies
- Your family's medical history
- Any personal history of smoking, drinking, or drugs
- Bring any earlier records from other physicians that you have seen for similar issues, and any lab tests, X-rays, or other studies.

Bring a description of your symptoms. Write a detailed list of your symptoms and when they started. For example, "The pain in my lower back started 5 days ago when I lifted a sofa. At first, the pain was a 10 out of 10 pain but now it's 5 out of 10. The pain radiates down my left leg, and I haven't been able to go to work or even drive. It's worse when I stand and better when I lie on my right side. I've taken Advil with some relief, and also use an ice pack."

Bring an advocate. It's OK to take notes or even to record the appointment so that you can remember what the doctor said. It's also fine to bring a family member, a friend, or a medical advocate who can help you to remember key information. Sometimes patients will even call a family member to listen in. Make sure your family member knows about the appointment in advance. Once time I spoke to my patient's son while he was taking a shower.

Ask for clarification. Never be embarrassed to ask for more information. Sometimes doctors use medical terminology that's unfamiliar, but it's important that you understand what your physician is recommending and why.

Get copies of your records at each visit. We encourage you to keep detailed records of your medical care. So always ask for a copy of the results of any test the doctor orders for you. Today most tests are available as a PDF, which makes it easier to save, organize, and find your records. Be an advocate for yourself. Your doctor takes care of thousands of patients. It is hard for them to remember all the details for every patient.

- Ask your doctor to explain any test results to you.
- Request a copy of your test results for your files (either a photocopy or a digital version).
- Before you leave, be sure you understand what needs to happen next.
- Do you need any further diagnostic tests?
- When will you get the results?
- If you have just received a diagnosis, what are your treatment options? And write down the answers!
- If you have been given a prescription for a new medication, do you understand how and when the medication should be taken?
- Are there any side-effects you should watch for?
- How will you know if the medication is working?
- What happens if you miss a dose?

You can also ask whether your doctor recommends any specific reading materials or websites about your condition. Ask the doctor for written information on any medication, procedure, or test that you'll be undergoing.

Find out the best way to contact your doctor, If you have any other questions or problems, who's the best person to contact, day or night? Is there a secure email address or phone number that you can call? Personally, I have an email address that I respond to every day.

Be sure to answer your healthcare provider's questions honestly and completely. This is no time to be shy or to be keeping secrets. Even the smallest details could make the difference between life and death. Here are some additional questions you should ask your provider:

- What changes do I need to make in my lifestyle, including diet modification and physical activity level?
- Will I still be able to work?
- Can I still have sex?
- Are there any complementary therapies that might help me feel better—would I benefit from seeing a nutritionist, an acupuncturist, or a chiropractor?
- What other lifestyle changes could improve my symptoms?
- What are the most important signs that I'm getting worse or at risk of a flare?
- What are the key symptoms I should monitor to stay on top of my situation?
- At what point do I call you or the nurse-on-call?
- What symptoms indicate that it's time to call an ambulance or go to the emergency room?
- How often should I come in for monitoring, screening, and checkups?

Remember: Always ask questions whenever you don't understand something. When it comes to your health, there's no such thing as a stupid question. It could make the difference between an unhealthy life and a healthy one.

For the work of Dr. Judson Brandeis, please see: www.BrandeisMD.com. Information on the work of Armin Brott is available at: www.MrDad.com. Additional references and resources can be accessed at: www.TheTwentyFirstCenturyMan.com & www.HIVE80.com.

PART 2
PREVENTIVE MAINTENANCE
Introduction
Judson Brandeis, MD

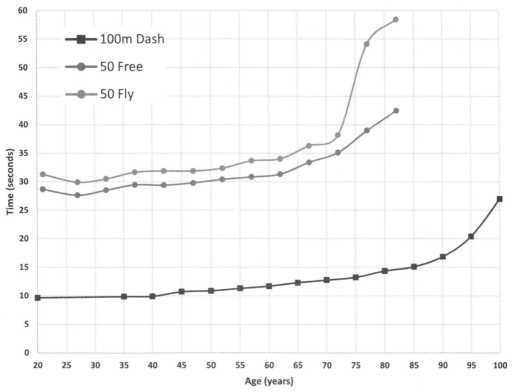

Figure, Part 2. The effects of aging on performance reflected in 100 meter sprint world records (World Masters Athletics) and 50 meter freestyle and butterfly qualifying times (U.S. Masters Swimming).

It is up to us to take charge of our health. In the same way that preventive maintenance can extend the life of your car thousands of extra miles, managing your physical, mental, and emotional health can prevent a great many of the conditions and injuries that lead to poor performance and illness. Unfortunately, lack of health education, dangerous work environments, and unhealthy lifestyles have caused a steady deterioration of the well-being of American men. The goal is to manage your health in a way that avoids health issues or catches them while they are still minor problems.

The best place to start is to know the likely causes of death and disability, and then work to prevent the most common of those causes.

#1—Heart disease. The number one cause of fatalities among American men, cardiovascular disorders include high blood pressure, heart attacks, strokes, and aneurysms. According to the American Heart Association, more than one in three adult men has some form of cardiovascular disease.

#2—Cancer. This is an umbrella term that describes malignant growths that can form in almost any living tissue in the body. The diagnosis and treatment vary widely. Tragically, cancer is now outpacing heart disease as the leading scourge among American men. This is a case in which "clean living" really can make a difference, improving your quality of life and reducing your cancer risk.

#3—Accidental injuries. The third leading cause of premature death, injuries that lead to death or disability are to some degree preventable through caution, preparation, and protection. Men frequently throw caution to the wind with disastrous consequences. Yet one simple effort, such as wearing safety glasses or protective gloves, could prevent a life-changing injury. Forewarned is forearmed.

#4—Chronic respiratory diseases. COPD, emphysema, and lung cancer are preventable by avoiding tobacco abuse and protecting yourself from occupational hazards like asbestos, silica, and sawdust, as well as common household contaminants such as harmful chemicals and toxic mold.

#5—Stroke. Any loss of brain tissue (essentially brain injury) has devastating consequences for quality of life. Stroke and Alzheimer's have a greater impact than almost any other form of disability. It is vital that you know the risk factors for these conditions, the most important aspects of prevention, and signs of impending trouble.

#6—Alzheimer's disease. In less than 20 years, Alzheimer's disease has doubled and joined the top ten causes of premature death. The aging population is fueling an "Alzheimer's Tsunami" for which we all are poorly prepared. The good news is that a growing body of research makes it clear that caught early enough, cognitive impairment can be reversed.

#7—Type 2 diabetes. Untreated, diabetes leads to nerve and kidney damage, heart disease, stroke, blindness, and erectile dysfunction. Simple interventions like weight management, exercise, and reduction in sugar consumption and processed food can dramatically reduce the risk of Type 2 diabetes.

#8—Infectious diseases. The serious contagious conditions of our time include influenza, COVID-19, HIV, and pneumonia, which are often preventable through vaccinations, limiting exposure, and early intervention.

#9—Kidney disease. This is an under-appreciated disorder that can erode quality of life. Although we can replace the function of the kidney with dialysis or transplantation, kidney disease still results in significant morbidity and mortality. Impaired kidney function is often an aspect of complex chronic disease (CCD), reflected in the association with both heart disease and diabetes.

#10—Mental health disorders. Poorly managed stress can lead to depression and stress-related physical issues, as well as self-harm. These conditions are tragic for both the individual and for their family and friends. Although more complex genetic mental disorders are beyond the scope of this book, useful information is included on anxiety and depression.

Life is busy, and sometimes we need crutches or short cuts. In the end, we often pay the price for poor decisions. The information contained in this section is not exhaustive, but will give you the what-to-do and why-to-do-it for prevention and early intervention in a number of the major causes of misery, illness, and premature death in men.

Chapter 5
Strengthening Your Heart
Joel Kahn, MD, FAAC, Cardiologist

The problem with heart disease is that the first symptom is often fatal.
— Michael Phelps

On September 23, Victoria received a phone call that her husband of 23 years and father of her two children had died suddenly at age 46. He had been playing hockey with his friends when he collapsed, and resuscitation was unsuccessful. Dean had been a successful computer executive in Silicon Valley. His death came without warning, without known health risks, and without a family history of early heart disease. Dean had recently had his annual physical and was in excellent health. He was not overweight, did not smoke, and was physically active (a runner, mountain bike rider, hockey player, and skier). He had normal blood pressure and cholesterol levels. An autopsy revealed a life-ending level of plaque that had blocked one of his heart arteries. On the day that Dean died, the cholesterol plaque in his heart ruptured without any warning signs or symptoms. The sudden heart attack and fatal heart rhythm that occurred had been building up for years, choking off the circulation to his heart muscle. How can this possibly happen with all the advancements in medical technology? The purpose of this chapter is to make sure it never happens to you.

Almost 400 years ago, English physician Thomas Sydenham wrote that "a man is as old as his arteries." Optimized men believe that "you are as *young* as your arteries." Arteries are muscular pipes that supply nutrients to your heart, brain, and pelvis by contracting and pushing blood forward. All your organs, even teeth, and bones, require blood circulation to be healthy. If you lined up all the blood vessels in a man's body, they would circle the earth twice, so blood delivery to all 50,000 miles of vessels is a daunting task. Understanding how your arteries work and how to identify, prevent, and reverse damage and aging to arteries is fundamental to living a long and healthy life, including a life of continued sexual function.

HEALTHY ARTERIES AND A HEALTHY LIFE

A health goal, perhaps the number one goal that men should have, is to maintain healthy "endothelium." Every artery in the body has an inner lining that is only one cell layer thick. This protective layer, the endothelium, lines every blood vessel like wallpaper. It is estimated if the endothelium were removed and stretched out, it would cover eight tennis courts in surface area, making it one of the largest organs in the male body.

The discovery of the role of the endothelium led to the Nobel Prize in Medicine in 1998. Three scientists received the coveted prize for their findings: that when endothelial cells of arteries are healthy, they produce nitric oxide (NO), a gas that enables arteries to relax, dilating the vessels and allowing more blood to flow to the organs. As a result, blood pressure remains healthy, and arteries are clean and resistant to plaque and blood clots (the cause of most heart attacks and strokes).

In terms of sexual health, penile erections require clean arteries and nitric oxide-mediated dilation of the penile arteries. Many factors may prevent nitric oxide production and lead to aging arteries. This process is termed endothelial dysfunction (ED) and will be discussed in detail. It is coincidental but also meaningful that the same abbreviation, ED, is used to denote erectile dysfunction, a disease of impaired endothelium.

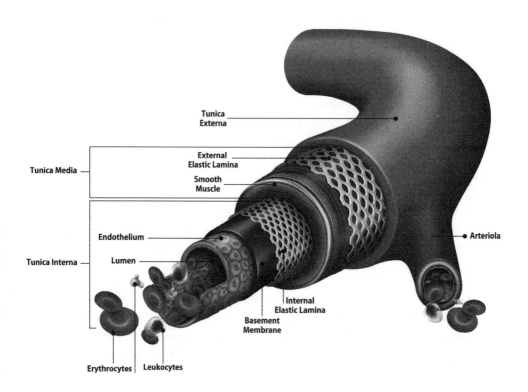

Figure 5.1. Artery structure showing the endothelium.

Maintaining Your Endothelium

You have probably heard a million times that eating fruits and vegetables can improve your health. Yet less than 2% of American men get enough fruit and vegetables daily. Diet is a significant factor in the health of the endothelium, in nitric oxide production, and in the maintenance of healthier, younger arteries. Other important influences on endothelial health include smoking, high blood pressure, high blood cholesterol, high blood sugar, and a sedentary lifestyle.

The Standard American Diet (abbreviated as SAD) is high in processed foods packed with chemicals like hormones and antibiotics, unhealthy fats, and excess sugar and salt. Diets emphasizing "plant-powered" and rainbow-colored foods, being naturally low in animal-sourced fats while also being rich in minerals, vitamins, and other nutrients, support endothelial health and young arteries. If you want to make more nitric oxide and have healthier arteries, eat beets and beans, not beef; eat greens, not grease; and grab an apple, not a donut.

Erectile Dysfunction—A Powerful Predictor of Aging Arteries

Erectile dysfunction is a powerful predictor of future cardiovascular events like heart attacks and even heart death, years before there are any detectable signs of endothelial aging. In an example cited by the Mayo Clinic, if a man lives in Olmsted County, Minnesota, and experiences erectile dysfunction between the ages of 40 to 49, there is up to a 50-fold higher risk of having new heart events compared to men the same age without ED. Rarely in medicine is there ever a risk factor this powerful.

AVOIDING SILENT HEART DISEASE

At age 50, a healthcare provider will recommend a colonoscopy to search for silent colon lesions. Women schedule mammograms even though they have no complaints. Yet, men are rarely screened for damaged arteries with unhealthy endothelium that cause unnecessary heart attacks, bypass operations, stents, and even tragic deaths.

Cardiologists agree that a man with erectile dysfunction should have an extensive cardiovascular evaluation. Sadly, this is rarely recommended, even though a comprehensive statement from the NIH for providers regarding this issue has been available for over a decade.

The concept that heart disease and early endothelial damage can be identified and prevented is not new. More than 60 years ago, Harvard Medical School professor Paul Dudley White, MD, challenged the medical system to provide better preventive care for cardiovascular health. White declared that "A heart attack after age 80 is an act of God, before age 80 it is a failure of medicine." Dr. White was caring for President Eisenhower after the president's massive heart attack in 1955. So, what can you do today to know the actual age of your arteries and heart?

Step 1: Get a coronary artery calcium scan (CACS). A coronary artery calcium scan (CACS) is a CT scan of the heart. This simple exam lasts less than a minute, uses no dye or needles, has very low radiation exposure (equivalent to a mammogram), and costs $75 to $125 at most hospitals. This evaluation is the only way to actually see heart arteries in a painless and simple manner. Weakened arteries and endothelium supplying the heart become calcified like a bone, a condition that is never healthy, yet very easy to detect and quantify. The ideal result of a CACS score is zero, indicating young heart arteries with a long-term risk of a future heart attack that is very low. Even a slight elevation in the CACS above zero raises the chance of a heart attack in the future. For those with a stent, heart bypass surgery, a known heart blockage, or a history of heart attack, the CACS is not necessary, since the diagnosis of aged heart arteries is already known. Your healthcare provider needs to order the CACS test.

Step 2: Request advanced lab tests. The same standard lab studies done during a physical exam in the 1980s are performed today as if there have been no advances. Ask your healthcare provider to order the following additional tests on your next visit as they are widely available.

- **Advanced cholesterol panel.** Rather than the "calculated" LDL cholesterol level found on routine panels (lab work that can be subject to serious inaccuracies), an advanced cholesterol panel directly measures the LDL-cholesterol and adds the number and size of this risk factor for aging arteries. These tests are widely available and relatively inexpensive.

- **hs-CRP.** The high sensitivity C-Reactive Protein (hs-CRP) is a blood test patented by Harvard Medical School to measure inflammation or the "fire" that results from an irritated immune system. The higher the hs-CRP, the greater the risk of aging arteries and damaged endothelium. It also predicts future heart attacks, strokes, and even conditions such as cancer and dementia.

- **Lipoprotein (a).** This is a genetic form of cholesterol that's elevated in about 25% of the public. It's rarely utilized even though hundreds of research studies indicate that if it's elevated, the risk of heart attack, stroke, or heart valve disease can be quite high. This marker has been found to run high in many families with generations of heart disease and strokes. It is measured in all labs and requires a lab requisition slip from your provider.

- **Homocysteine.** Homocysteine is an amino acid produced by a process called methylation, and homocysteine can injure arteries when elevated. It may be due to a genetic defect in a gene called MTHFR, which is easily measured. Elevated homocysteine can be reduced safely and easily with a B-complex vitamin, so it is worth requesting this lab test.

- **ADMA level.** It is now possible to directly measure the health of the endothelium in a lab test called an ADMA level. The higher the ADMA level, the lower the nitric oxide production and the more ED is present. When we heal our ED, the ADMA level drops as nitric oxide production is boosted.

Step 3: Do not leave an emergency room (ER) visit without a complete evaluation. If by some misfortune in you end up in an ER with chest discomfort, a blackout spell, shortness of breath, or racing heartbeats, please, DON'T GO HOME without a thorough evaluation for aging arteries.

- **Serial cardiac enzymes.** Ask the medical team for "serial" cardiac enzymes that are repeated two or three times, even if you need to stay a few extra hours.

- **Repeat electrocardiogram (ECG).** Ask for a repeat electrocardiogram (ECG) to compare to the one performed within the first few minutes of arrival.

- **Coronary CT angiogram (CCTA).** The definitive test of aging arteries. Many ERs offer a coronary CT angiogram (CCTA), which is by far the most accurate way to be sure your arteries are clean and free of the damaged endothelium and blockage. Ask for a definitive test of aging arteries before you are discharged.

Aging arteries are reversible. The training in medical school has been that the aging of arteries progresses from minor "streaks" in youth, to visible plaques in young adulthood, and finally to complicated plaques and major problems in our 40s and beyond. This conventional wisdom is simply not the case.

EFFECTIVE INTERVENTIONS

Modern science has shown that the reversal of arterial aging is now possible.

Statin cholesterol medication. A recent study looked at a database of 13,644 patients evaluated over nine years for heart artery disease by coronary artery calcium scanning (CACS). The group was also analyzed as to whether they were on statin medications like Lipitor and Crestor. The findings indicated that when the CACS was abnormal (over 100), being treated with a statin was associated with a lower risk of adverse outcomes.

On the other hand, patients with a CACS score below 100 rarely need these prescription medications.

Plant-based nutrition. Dr. Dean Ornish demonstrated the reversibility of damaged heart arteries in the 1990s. He prescribed a plant-based diet without added fats to patients with proven heart blockages. He also recommended walking, social support, and stress management to help their hearts. He demonstrated that the patients who adhered to his lifestyle program felt better and showed reductions in the narrowing of their arteries over the next five years. The Ornish Lifestyle program was recognized by Medicare in 2010 for reimbursement as a therapy for coronary artery disease to promote heart disease reversal. Another similar program, based out of the Pritikin Longevity Center in southern Florida, also received the same Medicare designation in 2010.

Aged garlic. Although all whole plant foods contribute to heart disease reversal, special mention is earned by a few. The ability of garlic to lower blood pressure, cholesterol, and blood clotting has been recognized for some time. There have been a surprising number of studies testing the ability of aged garlic extract to halt heart disease progression. For example, in a study published in early 2016 that used baseline and follow-up CT angiograms of heart arteries, aged garlic extract reduced areas of plaque in heart arteries at the one-year follow-up. In addition to the sulfur content of garlic, onions also provide a source of sulfur in the diet that may be crucial for maintaining optimal amounts of antioxidants.

Pomegranate. Pomegranate juice and seeds have powerful antioxidant properties. In studies of mice, pomegranates were found to reduce atherosclerosis, although translating animal research to human health can be misleading. In humans at risk for coronary artery (CAD), pomegranates can reduce evidence of arterial damage. In a three-year study, pomegranate juice reduced the degree of narrowing in carotid arteries of five study subjects.

Chelation therapy. Over 60 years ago, data surfaced suggesting that chelation therapy using EDTA could reverse heart artery disease. It took many decades until the Trial to Assess Chelation Therapy (TACT) was published in 2013. This research demonstrated an improvement in outcomes after a heart attack by providing intravenous EDTA chelation therapy. The TACT trial showed a substantial reduction in cardiovascular disease events and all-cause mortality in the subgroup of patients with diabetes. An interesting oral supplement containing EDTA and additional agents has been shown to lower the calcification of coronary arteries in peer-reviewed data.

PROMISING NUTRACEUTICAL THERAPIES

Additional promising therapies for the reversal of atherosclerosis using nutraceutical therapies have appeared:

Nattokinase. In a recently published randomized study from China, 76 patients with carotid atherosclerosis were treated with either *nattokinase* (NK) 6,000 FU or simvastatin 20 mg. Reversal of atherosclerosis over 26 weeks was profound with nattokinase, and plaque volume fell by 37%.

Bergamot citrus. Another agent, bergamot citrus from southern Italy, was studied in patients with aging arteries over six months. The results showed a stunning decrease in a measure of carotid artery aging called the CIMT from 1.2 cm to 0.9 cm, which indicates more youthful arteries.

Vitamin E. This nutrient has eight different forms that have been identified to date. Four of them are classified as *tocotrienols*. In a study of 50 patients with carotid disease, 25 received a source of tocotrienol from palm plants. Over 18 months of therapy, 7 of the 25 patients treated with the vitamin E preparation experienced plaque regression. No one in the control group regressed, and ten untreated patients in the control group progressed to higher levels of harmful plaque.

Pycnogenol. A promising combination therapy of pycnogenol and *Centella asiatica* has been reported to promote the reversal of carotid atherosclerosis. A randomized study followed 391 patients with ultrasound measurements of plaque for more than four years. The progression of plaque over time was least in the patients treated with the combination nutraceutical. There was a reduction in the number of angina episodes and heart attacks in that treated cohort. A more recent study with the same combination treatment reported a drop in the degree of calcification in heart arteries over one year.

Green algae extracts. Recently a study of green algae extracts in a capsule given twice a day for two months was examined in terms of impact on carotid plaque using MRI to assess the arteries. The preliminary findings of this ongoing study in China indicate significant decreases of 50% or more in this measure of disease.

A LIFESTYLE PLAN FOR YOUNG ARTERIES

Ample data from around the world indicate that a lifelong commitment to a healthy lifestyle can prevent aging of the endothelium, clogged arteries, heart attacks, strokes, and erectile dysfunction.

The addition of advanced testing, medications, and supplements can lower the risk of aging arteries by 85% or more.

This stunning statement should motivate all men to strive for a young spirit, a young body, and youthful arteries. The scientific studies indicate that if men will simply avoid smoking, walk or exercise 30 minutes a day, strive to maintain a waistline well below 40 inches, eat over 5 servings of fruits and vegetables a day, plan on 7 hours of sleep at night, and limit alcohol to 1-2 drinks a day maximal, their risk of heart disease can be reduced dramatically.

It is not acceptable for anyone to suffer from silent aging of arteries, heart attacks, strokes, or early death. No one should suffer the fate of 46-year-old Dean, whom we introduced in this chapter. His widow Victoria has subsequently dedicated her life to educating men about the risks underlying cardiovascular disease and the benefits of early diagnostic testing. This chapter outlines a proven method for the prevention, early detection, and reversal of damaged endothelium and arteries.

Do not wait. The earlier in life you institute a plan to monitor and maintain healthy arteries, the higher are the odds that you will live a long life with vitality, health, and freedom from adverse events and the need for medical intervention. There is tremendous hope that even with significant disease, the advances in nutrition, chelation, and nutraceutical therapies can improve the quality and quantity of life.

BOOKS

Joel K. Kahn, MD. *The Plant-Based Solution: America's Healthy Heart Doc's Plan to Power Your Health.* Louisville, CO: Sounds True, 2018.

Joel Kahn, MD. *Your Whole Heart Solution (What You Can Do to Prevent and Reverse Heart Disease Now).* New York, NY: Reader's Digest, 2014.

For additional information on heart health and the work of Dr. Kahn, please see www.DrJoelKahn.com.

Chapter 6
Reducing Your Risk of Heart Disease
Men's Health Network
& HealthyMen.org

You change your life by changing your heart.
— Max Lucado

Every year almost half a million men die of cardiovascular disease (CVD). These disorders are also a major cause of disability and decrease the quality of life for millions. Because CVD interferes with the heart's ability to pump blood through the body, it can limit the ability to work, to maintain an active life, and even to have sex.

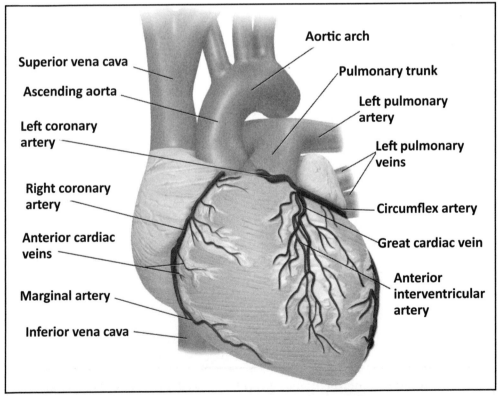

Figure 6.1. Coronary circulation (anterior). Image of the heart and the massive arteries that provide every cell in the body with oxygen and nutrients.

VITAL RISK FACTORS

The most significant risks for cardiovascular disease are smoking (smokers suffer heart attacks on average ten years younger than non-smokers do) and having had a previous heart attack.

Lifestyle and habits:

- Smoking (which more than doubles the risk of heart disease)
- Being overweight
- Having a sweet tooth and/or favoring comfort foods like pasta
- Little or no exercise
- Under too much stress at work and/or at home
- More than two alcoholic beverages every day
- Use of over-the-counter medicines that contain caffeine or other stimulants
- Recreational drugs, particularly stimulants such as cocaine or amphetamines

Underlying health issues:

- Existing heart disease
- High blood pressure
- Diabetes. More than 80% of people with diabetes die of some form of cardio-vascular disorder.
- Obesity (waist size above 40 inches)
- High cholesterol
- Gum disease. Research suggests that there may be a connection between gum disease and increased risk for heart disease and stroke. So be sure to brush your teeth twice a day, floss, and see your dentist regularly. Using chewing gum after a meal can also be helpful.
- Prescription medications that affect blood pressure such as Ritalin and other drugs for attention deficit disorder, as well as steroids, migraine medications, and oral decongestants used to manage allergy symptoms

Givens:

- Age. Once men reach the age of 45, the risk of developing cardiovascular disease doubles each decade.

- Being male. Take care of yourself. Men suffer heart attacks ten years earlier in life than women.

- Genetics. Your risk of having CVD is higher if an immediate family member (father, mother, brother, sister) developed a heart condition or high blood pressure before the age of 55.

- High-risk heritage. African Americans, Hispanic peoples, Native Americans, Ha-waiians, and some Asian Americans have higher risk for heart problems.

Naturally, there is nothing you can do to change your age, family history, or ethnic background. If any of the above risk factors apply to you, you'll want to take prevention seriously. It turns out there is plenty you can do to reduce your risks.

CARDIOVASCULAR CONDITIONS

HIGH BLOOD PRESSURE / HYPERTENSION

Blood pressure is a measurement of the pressure of your blood against the walls of the blood vessels throughout your body. The higher the pressure, the harder your heart has to work to do its job. It's perfectly normal for your blood pressure to rise and fall throughout the day. For example, if you exercise or get into an argument, your blood pressure will go up. But after you've had a chance to catch your breath or calm down, it should return to normal.

Unfortunately, at least a quarter of American men have blood pressure that stays high all the time—and that's a problem. This extra pressure puts a strain on the heart and blood vessels. It increases the risk of damage to the heart, eyes, kidneys, and other organs, raising the risk of having a heart attack or a stroke. The good news is that high blood pressure can usually be treated easily and safely. The bad news is that because high blood pressure has no apparent symptoms, millions of people have high blood pressure without knowing it, which is why it's often called "the silent killer."

Diagnosing high blood pressure. Diagnosing high blood pressure is easy—all you have to do is have it checked regularly. However, because men are less likely than women to visit their healthcare provider, they're also less likely to know their blood pressure level. Blood pressure readings are given as two numbers, for example, 110/80 (stated as "one-ten over eighty").

Where to get your blood pressure checked. Some readily available places to get your blood pressure checked besides your doctor's office include large chain drugstores and also local firehouses. (If they're not out on a call, they are often more than happy to help.) User-friendly blood pressure monitors for home use are now widely available and inexpensive.

Systolic blood pressure. When your heart beats, it pushes blood into the aorta (the largest artery in your body). The lining of arteries is composed of highly elastic tissue, so the aorta stretches. The pressure in the artery when it stretches is the systolic blood pressure. The top number (*systolic* blood pressure) is the pressure of the blood flowing through your arteries when your heart beats.

Diastolic blood pressure. When the aorta and the other arteries contract, the blood is pushed further along the vascular tree. Once the artery is finished contracting and relaxes, the pressure inside the artery decreases. The bottom number (*diastolic*) is the pressure of the blood in the arteries *between* beats, when the heart is resting. You also want to know what readings are normal and which ones aren't. Unless your doctor tells you otherwise, use the chart below.

Blood Pressure Category	Systolic Blood Pressure	&/or	Diastolic Blood Pressure
Normal	Below 120	&	Below 80
Elevated	120-129	&	Below 80
Hypertension			
Stage 1	130-139	or	80-89
Stage 2	Higher than 140	or	Higher than 90

Figure 6.2. Measuring blood pressure levels in adults.

CORONARY HEART DISEASE (CHD)

CHD is caused by *atherosclerosis*, which is the gradual buildup of *plaque* inside the arteries. Plaque is made up of cholesterol, fat, and other substances that narrow the arteries and reduce the amount of blood that can flow to your heart and other organs. The real danger occurs when plaque completely blocks an artery or when a piece of it breaks off and causes a clot that stops blood flow. If this happens near the heart, a heart attack occurs. If it happens near the brain, a stroke occurs. (For additional information, see chapter 14, "Minimizing Your Stroke Risk.") The risk factors for CHD are essentially the same as for hypertension.

ANGINA

The most common symptom of CHD is chest pain or discomfort (*angina*). If you have angina, you may feel a sense of heaviness, as if someone were stepping on your heart. You'll feel it under your breastbone or in your neck, arm(s), stomach, or upper back. Angina pain usually happens with physical activity (such as running up stairs or even having sex), strong emotions (especially anger), rapid weather changes, and overeating. In most cases, angina pain lasts only a few minutes and either goes away on its own with rest or after taking a medicine such as nitroglycerin.

> *If you experience any of the above symptoms, do not ignore them—*
> *contact your healthcare provider immediately. The fact that you*
> *experienced symptoms of angina means you are at increased risk of*
> *having a fatal heart attack.*

HEART ATTACK

Men who suffer heart attacks (also termed *acute myocardial infarctions*) are more likely to die of a heart attack than women of the same age. A heart attack occurs when the heart is deprived of oxygen, because blood flow is severely reduced. Like any other living thing, lack of oxygen causes the heart muscle to begin to die. The risk factors for heart attack are similar to those for high blood pressure and coronary heart disease.

> *Tragically, half of the men who die of heart disease were not even*
> *aware that they had a problem. In fact, the most common symptom*
> *of a heart attack is, unfortunately, sudden death.*

The lifestyle approaches to the prevention of heart attack are the same as those for preventing (or at least reducing) the risk of coronary heart disease and high blood pressure. Your doctor may prescribe medication (to lower cholesterol and to control your blood pressure) and may recommend surgery.

A-FIB (ATRIAL FIBRILLATION)

A-Fib is characterized by an irregular heartbeat, a condition described as *arrhythmia*. The arrhythmia may be continuous, or it can come and go.

Some people may have no symptoms at all. Others may notice one or more of the following:

- Racing, irregular heartbeat
- Heart palpitations (feeling as if your heart is skipping a beat, fluttering)
- Chest pain (angina)
- Confusion
- Shortness of breath or weakness, especially when exercising
- Symptoms of going into shock, such as sweating and dizziness or fainting

(For more information, see the section "Hidden Causes of a Stroke: A-Fib" in chapter 14.)"

Symptoms of a Heart Attack

In the movies, heart attacks are often portrayed as painful and dramatic. But in real life, the symptoms are usually more subtle. Below are the most common warning signs of a heart attack.

Chest pain (angina). Angina symptoms include pain or pressure in the center of the chest, as if you're being crushed. Other heart-related symptoms can include a sense of tightness, clinching, crushing, burning, choking, or aching. Angina can also present with shortness of breath, restlessness, rapid heartbeat, dizziness, nausea, and/or fatigue

Sudden pain in either or both arms, the back, shoulder, jaw, or neck. You should be able to tell the difference between this pain and the kind of pain you get when you pull a muscle.

Sudden shortness of breath. Difficulty breathing is a warning sign that something's wrong. Shortness of breath combined with chest or upper body pain is another reason to call 9-1-1 immediately.

Racing heartbeat. You know your body, and you know how your pulse reacts when you exercise, are nervous, or are in a stressful situation. In most cases, your heart rate should slow down quickly after the event. If it doesn't, you may be having a heart attack—especially if you're having chest pain at the same time.

Sudden cold sweats, nausea, or feeling faint. These symptoms, characteristic of shock, can be signs of a heart attack.

When to call the ambulance:

- **If you experience chest pain for more than a minute**
- **If the pain comes on suddenly and is severe enough to double you over**
- **If the pain doesn't go away immediately, once you sit down**

Call 9-1-1 right away. Not sure? Make the call anyway and let the paramedics figure it out.

> **You have the best chance of surviving a heart attack and minimizing damage to your heart if you get treatment within an hour.**

> **The first hour after the onset of heart attack is called "the golden hour." Appropriate action within the first 60 minutes of a heart attack can reverse its effects, in some cases with near-complete recovery.**

CONGESTIVE HEART FAILURE (CHF)

CHF is a gradual reduction of the heart's pumping capacity, a condition that usually starts many years before it is ever noticed and gets progressively worse over time. The heart tries to compensate for lost capacity by getting bigger and by pumping faster. To ensure that the heart and the brain have adequate blood supply (since they're the most critically important organs in the body), blood is diverted away from other less-important organs. At the same time, the body starts retaining fluid, which backs up into the lungs and other areas of the body.

Congestive heart failure is the leading cause of hospitalization in people 65 and older. Over 39 million American men (one in three) suffer from some form of cardiovascular disorder, affecting their heart and blood vessels.

Causes of congestive heart failure. CHF has numerous causes, but the most common ones include:

- Narrowing or blockage of the vessels that supply blood to the heart muscle (see chapter 5, on heart disease.)

- Weakness of the heart

- Heart attacks

- Aging of the heart muscles, so they become weaker and more brittle

- High blood pressure, which can make the muscles in the heart thicken so they don't pump as efficiently and must work harder

- Damaged heart valves, which can allow blood to move through the heart in the wrong direction, resulting in an enlarged heart that does not pump as effectively

- Diseases of the heart muscle itself (*cardiomyopathy*)

- Defects of the heart from birth (*congenital heart defects*)

- Infection of the heart valves (*endocarditis*) or muscle (*myocarditis*).

Major symptoms. Over three million men currently suffer from CHF, and about 350,000 more are diagnosed each year. Be sure to call your doctor right away if any of these warning signs appear:

- Sudden weight gain. Three or more pounds in one day, five or more pounds in one week, or whatever amount your doctor told you to report

- Shortness of breath. A feeling of not getting enough air, even when you are not active

- Increased swelling of your feet, ankles, and legs

- Swelling or pain in the abdomen/stomach area

- Trouble sleeping or waking up short of breath

- Repeated dry cough, especially when you are lying down

- Fatigue, weakness, or tiring very easily

- Confusion or difficulty thinking clearly

- Coughing or wheezing when you are active

- Coughing up pink or bloody mucus

- Dizziness or feeling as if you might pass out

- The need to urinate many times at night

- Loss of appetite

- Low blood pressure

- Faster heartbeat (a racing heart).

LIFESTYLE FACTORS

We used to think that heart disease was caused by a high-fat diet. More recent research has shown that high-carb diets and insulin resistance (associated with prediabetes) are major factors in cardiovascular disease and in risk.

Eat right. Reduce simple carbs and sugars by eating more fresh food, including:

- Fruit, vegetables, nuts, and non-GMO whole grains (all fiber-rich foods that will nourish you and satisfy your hunger).

- For protein, go for lean meats, fish, and beans.

- Avoid highly processed food (almost anything that comes in a box) such as breakfast cereals, pasta, and baked goods.

  (See chapters 31 to 36 for ideas on practical, heart-healthy nutrition.)

Get plenty of exercise. If you have any type of heart disease, seek a recommendation from your doctor about an exercise program.

If you're basically healthy, at least thirty minutes every day is ideal and cuts your risk of developing high blood pressure by 25% to 50%. And remember, it doesn't have to be all at the same time. Walking the dog, going dancing, or doing yard work all count. A minute here, a minute there, and you're up to 30 before you know it.

Quit smoking. If you don't smoke, but you live in a home where someone else does, encourage them to quit.

Watch what you drink. Don't drink more than two caffeinated beverages per day and limit yourself to no more than two alcoholic drinks a day.

Get your blood pressure checked regularly and get regular physical exams. Make sure to tell your healthcare provider about all symptoms—even ones that might not seem like they have anything to do with your heart at all. For example, both erectile problems and depression can be caused by cardiovascular disease.

Relax. Research has shown that petting animals lowers blood pressure (even watching fish in an aquarium can be relaxing). Meditation, walking meditation, yoga, and practices such as tai chi and qigong (in the tradition of martial arts) are also successful in reducing blood pressure.

High Cholesterol

Thirty years ago, we used to think that cholesterol levels in the diet and in the blood were major factors in developing cardiovascular disease. What we didn't know then is that a diet high in sugars and simple carbs plays a major role in raising blood fats to dangerously high levels. At that time, no one made the connection between high fats in the blood and high sugars in the diet.

The good side of cholesterol. Although no one seems to have anything nice to say about cholesterol, the fact is that you literally can't live without it. Cholesterol is essential. It helps build the walls of every cell in your body. Equally important, cholesterol is the raw material from which your hormones are made, including:

- Sex hormones such as testosterone and progesterone

- Stress hormones, including cortisol, adrenaline (also called epinephrine) and nor-adrenaline (norepinephrine)

- Well-being hormones, such as DHEA and pregnenolone.

Understanding your cholesterol levels. Cholesterol testing continues to be a useful tool in determining cardio risk. To measure your cholesterol levels, you'll need a blood test. Your doctor will select which of the different forms of cholesterol he wants to monitor:

- **Total cholesterol**. This is the most common cholesterol test in current practice. It provides a measurement of all the different subfractions of cholesterol grouped together. Ideally, you want your total cholesterol to be less than 200 (200 to 239 is considered moderately high; 240 and above is high).

- **LDL (low-density lipoprotein)**. Often called the "bad" cholesterol, LDL can clog the blood vessels. An LDL score of 100 or less is great, while a score of 130 or more means you're at risk of developing heart disease.

- **HDL (high-density lipoprotein)**. HDL is called the "good" cholesterol, because it actually removes the LDL. A score of 60 or more generally means your heart disease risk is low, while a score of 40 or less may mean your risk is high.

- **Oxidized LDL**. This form of low-density lipoprotein reflects levels of degraded fats in the bloodstream that have been subjected to oxidative stress (the equivalent of rust in our bodies). This critical measure of potential risk or safety is now available through standard laboratories such as LabCorp.

- **Advanced cholesterol testing**. This testing expands on traditional cholesterol tests, increasing the precision of determining cardiovascular risk. These recently developed blood tests (also termed VAP—vertical auto profile) measure the subfractions of cholesterol with a high degree of accuracy. In addition, this information will help your doctor develop an individualized program for you. Repeated testing is also useful in measuring your progress over time.

**Courtesy of the Men's Health Network, Health Education and Advocacy,
www.MensHealthNetwork.org,
and Healthy Men.org,
Also see American Heart Association,
www.heart.org.**

Chapter 7
Preventing Cancer
Ethan Basch, MD, MSc, Medical Oncologist
& Judson Brandeis, MD, Urologist

Cancer can take away all of my physical abilities. It cannot touch my mind, it cannot touch my heart, and it cannot touch my soul.
— Coach Jim Valvano

Half of all the cancer deaths in men are preventable, yet each year, over 300,000 American men die of cancer.

In the U.S., new annual cancer diagnoses are currently estimated at more than 1,735,000 individuals. We all die eventually, but 150,000 American men die earlier than they should each year from a preventable cancer. Despite a similar number of diagnoses of cancer, men are 60% more likely to die from the disease than women. This is one of the reasons why the average life expectancy for women is 81 years, and it's about 76 years for men.

Medical researchers have identified the major preventable causes of cancer in our era. Tobacco use, poor diet, obesity, inactivity, and excessive alcohol intake cause two-thirds of all cancers in the U.S. For those under the age of 85, cancer now outranks cardiovascular disease as the #1 cause of death in the United States.

CANCER	ESTIMATED NEW CASES	ESTIMATED MORTALITY	
Lung	116,300	72,500	
Prostate	191,930	33,330	
Colon	52,340	28,630	
Pancreatic	30,400	24,640	
Liver & Bile Duct	30,170	20,300	
Leukemia	35,470	13,420	
Urinary Bladder	62,100	13,050	
Non-Hodgkin's Lymphoma	42,380	11,460	
Kidney & Renal	45,520	9,860	
Skin Melanoma	60,190	4,610	

Figure 7.1. Estimated new diagnoses and deaths from cancer in males, U.S., 2020.

SOURCES OF EXPOSURE

Primary prevention integrated with early diagnosis and therapy are the most effective ways to reduce the risk of cancer mortality. Cancer is not just one disease. It is an assortment of different diseases with causes that range from infectious agents to behavioral and environmental exposures. Consequently, there is no single solution that will decrease the rate of cancer.

Tobacco-related cancers—30% of cancer deaths in the U.S. Tobacco use is the most preventable cause of cancer and accounts for 21% of worldwide total cancer deaths and 30% of cancer deaths in the U.S.

Approximately one-half of all smokers die of tobacco-related disease, and adult smokers lose an average of 13 years of life as compared to non-smokers.

Tobacco addiction increases the risk of lung cancer 10- to 30-fold over that of non-smokers. Almost 25% of cancer-related deaths are due to lung cancer. Smoking also raises the risk of cancer of the oral cavity, nasal cavity, sinuses, nasopharynx, larynx, esophagus, stomach, colon, pancreas, liver, kidneys, and bladder. Men who quit reduce their risk, even if they have smoked for many years.

Obesity-related cancers—20% of U. S. deaths. For the first time, more people worldwide are overweight than are underweight. Obesity has been estimated to be a major factor in 20% of all cancers. Excess weight is associated with an increased risk of thyroid cancer, esophageal adenocarcinoma, gastric, colorectal, pancreatic, renal, and hepatocellular cancers. Weight loss has been found to decrease the risk of death from cancer.

The diet we eat has a significant effect on the risk of cancers. In 2018, one-third of all cancer deaths were associated with cancers of the digestive tract, particularly the colon, pancreas, and liver. A high intake of red meat has been identified as an increased risk of colon cancer. The risk increases by 17% per 3½ ounces / 100 grams/day of red meat consumption and increases by 18% per every 2 ounces / 50 grams/day of processed meat consumed. The reason for this is not known, although the use of preservatives, additives, and coloring in products such as luncheon meats may be a factor. Charred beef may be a particular risk for cancer development.

Despite an enormous body of research published over the past three decades, the overall contribution of diet and nutrition to cancer is ill-defined. There is evidence that a high intake of fresh fruits and vegetables is associated with a reduction in cancers. Intake of dietary fiber has been shown to reduce the risk of colon cancer.

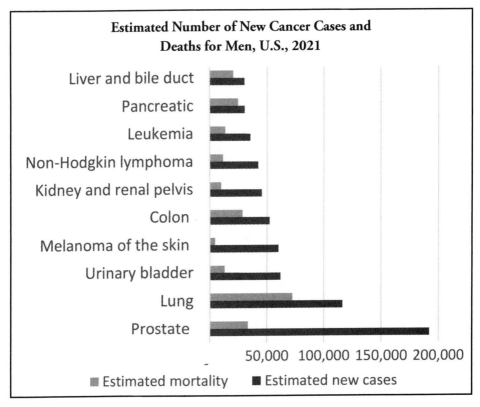

Figure 7.2 New cancers and number of cases per 100,000 American men, 2021.

Several anti-inflammatory herbs have been proposed to have protective effects. Curcumin, which is found in turmeric, resveratrol from red wine and berries, and green tea polyphenols have been recommended for their anti-inflammatory effects. However, evidence of benefits specifically in human cancers is scarce. (Anti-inflammatory herbs alone seem unlikely to prevent cancer. Rather, they may be beneficial in the context of a complete lifestyle program and ongoing medical screening.)

Infectious illness—17% of cancers are due to hepatitis and the human papilloma virus. Infections cause 17% of all new cancers worldwide. Human papillomavirus (HPV) leads to squamous cell cancers of the head and neck, as well as anogenital cancers. Almost all cervical cancer is caused by HPV. Hepatitis B and C can cause liver cancer. HIV causes adult T-cell leukemia, as well as non-Hodgkin's lymphoma. *H. pylori* bacteria are associated with gastrointestinal malignancies, including stomach cancer. The majority of these viruses are spread through contact with infected body fluids or blood, thus offering opportunities for prevention. Vaccinations for hepatitis B and human papillomavirus are beneficial. HPV vaccines are now recommended for children to prevent their lifetime risk of associated cancers.

Lack of exercise—5% of U.S. cancer deaths. A sedentary lifestyle appears to increase cancer risk, and researchers estimate that a lack of activity is associated with 5% of all cancer deaths, especially colon and breast cancer. For men who do not smoke, exercise is one of the most important modifiable risk factors.

Alcohol consumption—3% to 10% of all cancers. Excess alcohol intake increases the risk of multiple cancers, including those of the esophagus, liver, rectum, and breast. The overall risk of cancer has been reported to increase by 6% for every 10 grams/day of alcohol consumed (10 grams is the level of alcohol content in a standard beer, a glass of wine, or a shot of liquor). Worldwide, it is estimated that 3.6% to 10% of cancers are associated with chronic alcohol consumption.

Sun exposure and ultraviolet radiation—3% to 10% of cancer deaths. Every year, U.S. healthcare providers diagnose and treat more than 1 million cases of skin cancer. Most benign basal cell and squamous cell carcinomas are not life-threatening. Still, there are more than 70,000 cases of malignant melanoma in the United States annually. Although a vast majority of skin cancers are curable, there are at least 10,000 deaths a year related to melanoma. Radiation from the sun is the primary cause of both melanoma and nonmelanoma skin cancers. Genetic mutations from ultraviolet radiation interfere with immune function. The total lifetime sun exposure correlates with the risk of squamous cell and basal cell cancers as well as melanoma. Ultraviolet exposure from tanning booths in younger men increases the risk of melanoma by 75%. Simple interventions like limiting exposure, using sunscreen, wearing hats, sunglasses that provide UV protection, and protective clothing reduce the exposure that can lead to malignancy.

Occupational exposures—at least 3% to 6% of cancers worldwide. Occupational carcinogens have been a public health success. Elimination or substantial reduction of exposure to asbestos, aromatic amines (found in tobacco smoke, diesel exhaust, and commercial hair dyes), benzene, and other carcinogens have prevented many thousands of cancer cases. Reducing asbestos use has decreased mesothelioma rates in the United States. However, the list of carcinogens published by NIOSH (the National Institute of Occupational Safety and Health) includes substances in everyday use, such as gasoline, welding fumes, and wood dust, so it is helpful to research exposures associated with your occupation.

SCREENING AND EARLY INTERVENTION

Screening recommendations change over time and may vary in different countries, settings, or populations. Below are some basic guidelines, but screening appropriate for a given person should be discussed and planned with a healthcare provider.

- **Lung cancer.** Some professional societies recommend that for men who have smoked at least one pack a day for 30 years and are between the ages of 55 and 80, it is appropriate to obtain a periodic low-dose CT scan of the lungs to identify lung cancers in their early stages.

- **Colorectal cancer.** It is recommended that men obtain a colonoscopy once every ten years starting at age 50 unless they are at high risk for colorectal cancer, in which case they need to be screened more frequently.

- **Prostate cancer.** Men should be screened for prostate cancer with a PSA every other year between the ages of 50 and 75 unless they are at high risk for prostate cancer, in which case screening starts earlier and is more frequent. However, PSA screening has been a controversial topic, and recommendations have changed several times based on available research.

- **Testicular cancer.** These cancers typically affect men between 15 and 45 but can afflict men up to 55. Monthly self-examination of the testicles for firm lumps or bumps is an easy way to identify the possibility of testicular cancer.

- **Skin cancer.** It is important to monitor yourself for abnormal skin lesions and report them to your physician.

GENETIC SCREENING

Over the coming decade, men will likely see increased use of genetic screening tests to identify risks of cancers and other diseases. There are already well-known genetic syndromes that can be identified. For example, BRCA1 and BRCA2 mutations may increase the risk of multiple cancer types, including breast, ovarian, pancreas, and prostate cancers. For people with multiple close relatives who have had these cancers, a discussion regarding testing with a doctor or genetic counselor may be warranted. Another example is Lynch Syndrome (also called hereditary non-polyposis colorectal cancer), which affects up to 1 in every 300 people. Lynch syndrome substantially increases the risk of colorectal and endometrial cancers but can also increase the risk of multiple other cancer types.

Large-scale studies continue to identify new genetic markers associated with increased risk of cancers. There are several commercially available genetic screening tests, although not all of the genetic variants that can be identified have implications for treatment.

The evolution of cancer detection and treatment will be personalized and high-tech. However, the fact remains that many cancers are preventable with low-tech, low-cost interventions.

General lifestyle recommendations include promoting physical activity; maintaining a healthy weight; eating a diet rich in fresh fruits, vegetables, and whole grains; and minimizing saturated/trans-fats, red meat, and processed meat. Vaccination against HPV reduces the risk of multiple types of cancer. Cancer prevention also means avoiding tobacco, limiting alcohol, protecting against sexually transmitted infections, minimizing sun exposure, and undergoing recommended regular screening for cancers.

PREVENTION AND EARLY DETECTION

According to the American Cancer Society, the approximate lifetime
risk of developing cancer is 1-in-2 for men and 1-in-3 for women.

More than 700,000 men are diagnosed with cancer each year, and nearly 300,000 die of it. Over the course of a lifetime, half of all men will get cancer at least once. Cancer can strike anyone at any age, but the majority of cases happen to people 55 and over.

Tragically, most of these cancers and premature deaths are preventable. At least one-third of cancer deaths are caused by smoking, and another one-third may be caused by poor diet and/or lack of exercise. The two keys to beating cancer are reducing risk and early detection.

Prevention. There are many steps you can take that have been shown to reduce the risk of developing cancer:

- Don't smoke. Smoking causes 90 percent of lung cancers and dramatically increases the risk of cancers of the mouth, kidney, bladder, pancreas, and esophagus.

- Limit your exposure to sunlight. A little bit of exposure will stimulate your body to produce vitamin D, which researchers think may reduce the risk of several cancers. Yet too much can cause skin cancer. Having fair skin or having had severe sunburn in childhood greatly increases the risk of developing skin cancer.

- Eat a low-fat, high-fiber diet with lots of fresh fruits, vegetables, and whole grains. High-fat, low-fiber diets are at least partly responsible for most colorectal cancers. They also increase the risk of pancreatic and bladder cancers.

- Limit foods that are smoked, salted, pickled, or high in nitrates (such as hot dogs and luncheon meats). These foods are associated with an increased risk of stomach cancer.

- Limit your exposure to chemicals such as PVCs (polyvinyl chloride), tar, and creosote, which have been linked to several cancers, including cancers of the liver and skin.

- Spend some time getting to know yourself and your body. See your physician if you notice any significant changes.

- Get screened. These tests are designed to detect certain types of cancer (such as colon, bladder, kidney, testicles, and prostate) in their earliest stages. These cancers can be treated successfully if they are caught early.

(See chapter 90 on prostate cancer for more information on that condition.)

Early detection. You can't detect cancers if you don't know what to look for. Below are a number of symptoms that could be indicators. Many of them could be caused by other conditions, but you should notify your doctor if you notice anything unusual or abnormal.

- Lumps that you can feel through the skin

- Sores that don't heal

- Changes in the size, color, or texture of a wart or mole

- Blood in the urine, stool, or saliva

- A cough, sore throat, hoarseness, or trouble swallowing that won't go away

- Persistent backache

- Unexpected weight loss

- Unexplained pain

- Pressure or tenderness in the chest

- Unusual bleeding

- Chronic nausea or gas

- Fever that lasts more than a few days

MALE BREAST CANCER

Although breast cancer is usually thought of as a women's disease, about 1 percent of breast cancers occur in men. No less a man than Richard Roundtree, who played Shaft in the 1970s movies, has been diagnosed with breast cancer. The most common early symptom is a lump in the breast, usually right underneath the nipple. More advanced symptoms include a bloody discharge from the nipple or a retraction of the nipple. If you notice either of these symptoms or just feel that something isn't right, schedule a medical appointment right away.

*Many men who notice symptoms like these put off going to the doctor
because they believe that a "real man" wouldn't get breast cancer.
That kind of attitude could kill you.*

TESTICULAR CANCER

Testicular cancer is the most common type of cancer in young men ages 15 to 35. Early detection is critical because testicular cancer typically grows quickly and spreads to other parts of the body just a few months after the first symptoms appear. But treated early, it is almost 100 percent curable.

Risk factors. There are several factors that increase men's risk of developing testicular cancer:

- Undescended testicle(s), even if they were brought to normal position as a child

- Family history of testicular cancer

- Being Caucasian. White men are slightly more likely to develop testicular cancer than Hispanics, twice as likely as Asian-Americans, and five to ten times more likely than African-Americans.

KEY TAKE AWAYS

- At least half of all cancers are preventable with simple lifestyle changes.

- Cancer screening can help identify cancer at an early stage when it is most easily treated. Important screenings include chest CT scan in high-risk smokers, colonoscopy, and PSA, as well as self-exam for testicular and skin cancer.

- Genetic testing may help identify syndromes that increase the risk of cancers, particularly for men with close family members who have developed cancer.

**For additional information on the work of Dr. Basch, please see his page
on the website of the University of North Carolina School of Medicine at
https://unclineberger.org/directory/ethan-basch/.
For additional information about cancer, see
The American Cancer Society at cancer.org.**

Testicular Self-Exam

The best way to identify symptoms is to do a simple, three-minute self-exam once a month beginning on your 15th birthday. Here's how to do the exam:

- Get into the shower or a warm bath. Heat causes the scrotal skin to relax, making the exam easier.

- Soap up. Fingers glide over soapy skin, making it easier to concentrate on the texture of the tissue underneath.

- Using both hands, slowly roll each testicle between the thumb and fingers, applying slight pressure. It's completely normal to find that one testicle is slightly larger.

- Try to find hard, pea-sized, painless bumps in the testicles ("balls") themselves.

- Ignore the epididymis. The epididymis is a cord-like structure on the top and back of the testicle that stores and transports the sperm.

- See your doctor promptly if you feel or see anything suspicious. Also, tell your doctor if you experience any pain or a heavy feeling in either testicle. By doing these exams regularly, you'll learn what a normal testicle feels like, and that will make it much easier to know if something changes.

Courtesy of the Men's Health Network, Health Education and Advocacy, Washington, D.C.: www.MensHealthNetwork.org.

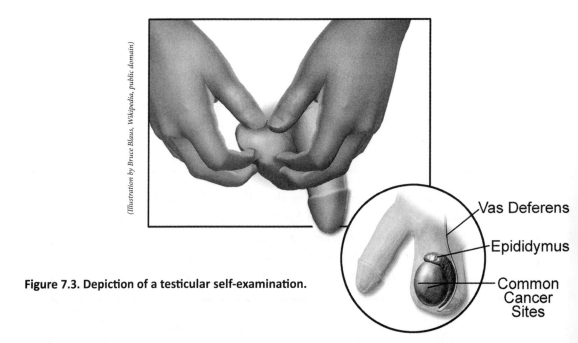

(Illustration by Bruce Blaus, Wikipedia, public domain)

Vas Deferens

Epididymus

Common Cancer Sites

Figure 7.3. Depiction of a testicular self-examination.

Chapter 8

Decoding Your Cancer Genes
Heather Hannon, MSN, RN, ANP-BC, ACGN
Oncology Nurse Practitioner

Health is a function of three things:
1. Luck, 2. Genetics, and 3. Choices in your lifestyle.
— Bill Walton

Larry James was diagnosed with prostate cancer in his late fifties. His cancer had been detected at an early stage, and he underwent successful surgical treatment that rendered him "cancer-free." Larry wasn't overly worried, but his physician expressed concern after reviewing the family history. Larry's mother and maternal grandmother had died of advanced breast cancer. He knew the disease was more common in the women in his family but wasn't sure how this applied to him. Still, he wanted to optimize his health and decided to opt for genetic testing, which involved collecting a small amount of saliva by having him spit into a test tube. Not the most refined approach to obtaining a sample, but it didn't hurt, and it got the job done.

Larry's genetic test results revealed he had inherited a harmful genetic change (a mutation) in the BRCA2 gene, a gene responsible for protecting the body from cancer. His test results indicated he was at increased risk of developing several types of cancer, including male breast cancer, and his doctor immediately sent him for a screening mammogram. Larry was shocked when his mammogram showed early-stage male breast cancer. He credits genetic testing with saving his life, because the test results played a role in detecting his risk and subsequently his breast cancer, before it had reached a more advanced stage. That enabled him to escape the premature deaths of his mother and grandmother.

As a Nurse Practitioner who has provided genetic counseling and testing for more than eight years, I have witnessed firsthand the powerful impact testing can make in the life of an individual such as Mr. James. Genetic testing offers the opportunity to identify individuals who are at the highest risk, enabling them to lower that risk dramatically and by detecting cancer at an earlier stage when outcomes are better. I am especially passionate about the importance of genetic testing because I have worked with far too many men who learn they carry a harmful BRCA gene mutation only after a daughter was diagnosed with breast or ovarian cancer and underwent genetic testing. For these men, finding out after the fact is a heartbreaking experience. They are left wondering perhaps had they known sooner about their genetic mutation, maybe it would have made a difference for their daughters.

Thankfully, inherited genetic mutations that substantially raise disease risk are not common in the general population, and it is unlikely that the average man reading this book harbors a harmful BRCA mutation that is hiding in his DNA. Only about 1 in 400 individuals in the United States has an inherited BRCA gene mutation like Mr. James's (the prevalence is higher, about 1 in 40, among individuals with Ashkenazi Jewish ancestry). But, as with many things in life, genetic risk is not black and white; rather, it exists on a spectrum. The key to unlocking our health is in understanding where we fall on that spectrum and addressing the risks that matter most, depending on whether our risk is hig, low, or somewhere in the middle.

THE NATURE OF GENETIC MATERIAL

Our genetic makeup plays an essential role in our wellbeing. All of our genetic information is stored in our DNA, found in every cell of the body. In a sense, DNA resembles sophisticated computer code that provides commands to make proteins. These proteins are the instructions for traits such as eye color and blood type, as well as the information that enables our cells to carry out the functions that maintain life.

The DNA is made up of four different nucleic acids, referred to as base letters or bases, designated by four letters: A, T, C, and G. The nucleic acids combine in countless ways to form amino acids, the building blocks of protein. When scientists sequence a genome, they "read" the gene to determine the exact order of DNA letter bases (As, Ts, Cs, and Gs) contained in that individual's genetic code.

Genes are small snippets of DNA letter bases that are passed down from our parents. We inherit two copies of every gene (one copy from mom and one from dad) for each trait or function. Frequently a particular attribute or function will be defined by a number of different genes. So there is usually not a single gene for cancer or for allergies, for example, that might enable us to crack the code on disease.

GENETIC EXPRESSION

One might wonder how cells manage to carry out such vastly different functions when they contain the same DNA or set of commands. Gene expression is the process by which the written code in DNA is translated into a useful product, such as a protein. But not all genes, or commands, are expressed at once. Gene expression is tightly regulated so that only specific genes are "turned on" in a cell while others are silenced or "turned off." This explains how heart cells are able to perform different tasks than the cells in our lungs and our brain, even though they share the same DNA. Researchers do not yet fully understand what triggers certain genes to turn off and others to turn on, but it appears that triggers from other cells (including hormones and neurotransmitters) can influence gene expression. Externally, exposure to environmental hazards, nutrition, social conditions, and the aging process itself can help determine which genes are turned on or off.

Although our DNA is around 3 billion bases long, only 1% is made up of genes that make proteins. Researchers used to think that the remaining 99% of our DNA was junk, but it appears these non-protein making regions help regulate the expression of the protein-making genes by turning them on and off.

If you lined up all of your DNA, it would form a strand 6000 miles long! To fit inside a tiny cell, DNA is tightly packaged inside chromosomes. Human beings have 46 chromosomes or 23 pairs. Chromosomes contain thousands of genes. We have around 25,000 genes. Our genes vary in size in terms of the amount of information they contain, from as small as a few hundred DNA base letters to over a million DNA bases.

HOW GENES AFFECT RISK

In most cases, identifying a harmful genetic pattern does not indicate whether an individual will develop a particular condition. Individuals do not inherit a disease—they inherit the *risk* for developing the disease. Our environment and lifestyle mediate our genes, and most diseases result from a combination of factors. Without intervention, we cannot change the genes we are born with, but we have the ability to modify, to some degree, various lifestyle and environmental factors that contribute to disease by engaging in a healthy lifestyle.

The importance of lifestyle and environment in disease prevention should not be underestimated! For example, it is suggested that changes in lifestyle can prevent at least four out of every ten cancer cases. Eating a healthy diet and engaging in regular physical activity can lower heart disease risk by around 50%.

Adopting a healthy lifestyle is a great tool for optimizing health regardless of age or genetic makeup. However, genetic testing gives us the ability to go one step farther and target our unique risks. Additionally, for those patients who are at the highest level of risk, lifestyle and environment may not be enough to protect against disease. Genetic testing, as in the case of Mr. James, helps uncover whether we require more than lifestyle strategies to stay healthy.

Men need to be aware of new guidelines for prostate cancer and genetic testing.

Research indicates that as high as 15% of men with metastatic prostate cancer have a hereditary mutation. And genetic testing is now recommended for *all* men with metastatic prostate cancer, regardless of age. Men with a Gleason score of 7 or higher should talk with their doctors about genetic testing, especially if members of their family have had breast and/or ovarian cancer. For these men, standard detection and treatment strategies may need to be adjusted due to their higher risk level.

THE IMPACT OF GENETIC CHANGES

Understanding genetic changes helps identify a person's level of risk and focuses efforts to address that risk effectively.

Genetic mutations. Specific changes that alter the usual sequence of DNA letter bases that make up a gene are termed genetic mutations. Most gene mutations are not harmful, but rather are part of the evolutionary process. However, a small percentage of genetic mutations alter how a gene functions, resulting in proteins that don't work correctly or are missing entirely. When a genetic mutation affects a protein that plays a critical role in maintaining our well-being, that mutation can increase the risk of a given disease. Sometimes the BRCA1 and BRCA2 genes are referred to as the "breast-cancer" genes. This is a misnomer because all of us have two copies of each of these genes. It is the presence of a mutation in a BRCA gene that raises the risk, not the genes themselves.

Acquired mutations. These mutations occur during a person's lifetime and are present only in specific cells in the body. Researchers estimate that individuals accumulate trillions of new mutations in a typical day, but most of these mutations are not located in areas of DNA that have significant consequences. The accumulation of multiple acquired mutations in a gene that protects against cancer or heart disease has the potential to disrupt normal gene function and contribute to disease risk.

- **Acquired mutations can occur spontaneously** when a mistake is made during cell division. This helps explain why people with no known risk factors can be diagnosed with a severe illness even though they did "everything right."

- **Environmental factors can trigger acquired mutations,** due to air pollution or exposure to radiation, and lifestyle factors like smoking, alcohol, an unhealthy diet, a sedentary lifestyle, etc. We can protect against certain diseases by addressing the lifestyle and environmental factors that trigger acquired mutations and contribute to developing these conditions. Almost 25% to 30% of cancer-related deaths are linked to tobacco use and 30% to 35% are linked to diet. Steps like avoiding smoking and maintaining good nutrition make a difference in protecting against disease.

■ **Hereditary mutations.** Inherited mutations are passed down from a parent and, like other genes, remain throughout life. Inherited mutations are present in every cell in the body (including egg and sperm cells called germ cells; hence they are also referred to as germline mutations).

■ **Hereditary diseases.** Conditions associated with inherited mutations can cause significantly increased disease risk.

■ **One gene or both?** Most hereditary diseases are inherited from just one parent. This has important implications. First, it means that an individual only has to inherit *one* copy of a mutant gene to be at increased risk for the associated hereditary disease. It is possible to inherit a gene for a particular risk from either parent.

■ **Children are at risk too.** When the parent has a dominant hereditary mutation, each child has a 50% chance of inheriting the mutant gene from an affected parent.

Many hereditary mutations raise risk substantially. Lifestyle and environment are still critical tools for lowering risk. But risk associated with hereditary mutations may require additional strategies. Individuals with the highest level of risk may benefit from specialized screening tools and more frequent screening, like annual breast MRI for detecting breast cancer early or specific medications for controlling blood pressure and harmful cholesterol in the case of inherited cardiac disease. Those with the highest risk may also want to consider risk-reducing surgeries, like mastectomy in the case of individuals with a BRCA 1 or 2 gene mutation. In the case of hereditary mutations, it's not just the individual who is at risk, but we also must consider family members.

SNPs—genetic glitches. SNPs (pronounced "snips"), or Single Nucleotide Polymorphisms, are another type of inherited genetic variation. SNPs represent a change in *a single* DNA letter base and are found in stretches of DNA between protein-making genes.

■ Both SNPs and hereditary mutations are inherited, but SNPs are much more common in the population.

■ There are roughly 10 million SNPs in the human genome (and around 400 genetic mutations).

■ Although SNPs have a minimal effect on raising disease risk, inheriting multiple SNPs may combine to increase disease risk to a significant level.

- SNPs may underlie genetic susceptibility to common diseases and have been linked to a range of disorders from addiction to mental illness, high cholesterol to obesity, and from lactose intolerance to inflammatory bowel disease.

The presence of particular SNPs may cause a person to have the same level of risk as an inherited mutation. Specific SNP profiles (such as polygenic risk scores) may warrant targeted screening and prevention tools similar to individuals with a known inherited mutation, such as BRCA genes.

Epigenetic changes. While mutations alter the sequence of DNA bases, epigenetic changes influence disease risk by alternating gene expression. Research concerning epigenetics is ever-evolving, and scientists hope to soon provide better insight into how our environment and lifestyle trigger certain genes to turn on and others to turn off.

Epigenetics reminds us that adopting healthy lifestyle choices can make a difference in optimizing health across our lifetime.

Protective behaviors. Similar to the development of acquired mutations, the following behaviors are believed to protect against adverse epigenetic changes. They include:

- Maintaining a healthy weight

- Getting regular exercise

- Eating a healthy diet, one that is high in fiber and fresh fruits and vegetables with less processed foods and meat

- Using sunscreen and covering up while out in the sun

- Avoiding smoking and tobacco products

- Limiting or avoiding alcohol

- Avoiding exposure to harmful chemicals in the workplace.

EVALUATING WHETHER YOU ARE AT RISK

Recent literature suggests that around 20% of us have an inherited mutation linked to a genetic condition.

Genetic predisposition or susceptibility. These are the terms used to describe someone who has a higher chance of developing a particular disease because of a hereditary mutation. Identifying individuals with a genetic predisposition can result in early detection, intervention, and prevention of disease.

Knowing your family history. The health history of your family remains one of the most valuable tools we have for helping to predict risk. Individuals with several family members or relatives who have a particular condition are often at higher risk for that condition. For example, children of someone with an alcohol abuse disorder are four times more likely to develop problems with alcohol than people in the general population. (Holiday gatherings provide an excellent opportunity to connect with multiple relatives at once and learn more about what conditions "run" in the family.)

Red flags. Look for red flags in your family and personal history that might indicate an inherited genetic condition. Families are likely to share familiar environments and lifestyles, as well as genes. Checklists are a simple tool to help tease out genetic risk. Don't forget to look at both sides of the family. Individuals who are adopted or unsure about family history may benefit from genetic testing and should also talk with their doctor about the results.

Have you or anyone in your family:

- Been diagnosed with a disease at an earlier age than the condition typically occurs?

- Been diagnosed with a rare condition?

- Had multiple family members (on the same side of the family) diagnosed with the same disease?

- Been diagnosed with or had several family members with multiple types of the same disease (i.e., breast and ovarian cancer)?

Resources for calculating cancer risk:

Myriad Genetics—myRisk test. This is a brief, easy-to-use quiz for evaluating hereditary cancer risk that is available online at https://www.hereditarycancerquiz.com/.

Checklist. Hereditary cancer and hereditary heart disease checklists are provided online at www.TheTwentyFirstCenturyMan.com.

Risk models. A person's probability of carrying a specific cancer-related gene mutation can be estimated using a risk model. For example, BOADACIEA, BRCAPRO, and PENNII are different models that estimate the probability that a woman carries a BRCA mutation. The PREMM5 model looks at the probability an individual carries a hereditary mutation associated with Lynch Syndrome (a condition that significantly raises the risk for multiple cancers). About 1 in 200 individuals has Lynch Syndrome, although many do not realize it. This particular model is appropriate for both females and males. Visit https://premm. dfci.harvard.edu/ for more information of the PREMM5 model.

GENETIC TESTING

Genetic testing is a valuable tool to help us learn more about our risk for developing certain conditions and design specific strategies to target that risk. Genetic testing uses a simple blood or saliva sample to look for specific inherited genetic mutations in an individual's DNA that may increase the risk of disease.

Multigene panel testing. These panels are a common type of genetic evaluation that look for mutations in a number of important genes. This type of testing is more efficient than looking at single genes sequentially and provides a more comprehensive picture of risks.

Different options exist for learning more about our genetic makeup and whether the genes we have inherited place us at risk for certain diseases. Two common types of genetic testing utilized for learning more about health risks are direct-to-consumer tests (DTC)s, such as 23andMe and AncestryDNA) and professional genetic testing that looks at genes associated with specific hereditary conditions that can cause harm.

DIRECT-TO-CONSUMER TESTS

What about 23andMe? 23andMe and AncestryDNA are examples of direct-to-consumer genetic tests that can be purchased online and in stores. DTCs have increased in popularity as the cost of testing has fallen. (Of note, the first sequencing of the human genome was completed around 2004 at a cost of $2.7 billion.) Today you can have your entire genome sequenced for $200. DTCs provide information on ancestry and novel traits (such as ice cream flavor preference). Many DTCs are now expanding to provide information about a person's health risks as well, including (but not limited to) conditions such as:

- Parkinson's disease
- Alzheimer's
- Celiac disease
- Gaucher disease type 1
- Early-onset primary dystonia
- Alpha-1 antitrypsin deficiency
- Blood and blood clotting disorders (hereditary hemochromatosis, hereditary thrombophilia, Factor XI deficiency).

Direct-to-consumer tests—benefits and limitations. Proven, research-based recommendations for lowering risk or preventing disease do not exist for some of the genetic changes DTC tests look for. A person can be left with a result that indicates higher risk for developing a serious condition and have no proven way to lower their risk or prevent the disease.

- Results can sometimes be misleading. For example, 23andMe can screen for the three most common BRCA gene mutations, but the test is not FDA approved to look for the remaining 1,000 plus BRCA mutations that can raise cancer risks. An individual may believe they are not at risk when they really are.

- DTC tests usually do not involve a healthcare professional and do not provide guidance regarding whether you are testing for the appropriate genes (the ones you are interested in). Also, DTC tests do not offer counseling concerning what the results mean and the implications of those results.

- Most DTCs use third-party interpretation (TPI) tools (such as Promethease, GED Match, and Livewello) to interpret raw DNA data and convert it into information about health risks. But TPIs don't fall under the same guidelines as other genetic testing types, and ensuring the quality and accuracy of the information obtained through a TPI is difficult.

- Different DTCs and TPIs have varying privacy policies. Remember to ask what steps the lab takes to protect your privacy and how long your sample is kept.

But this does not mean that DTCs don't have a useful role. Benefits of direct-to-consumer testing include:

- A good starting point for talking with your doctor

- Results that can prompt individuals to make substantial lifestyle changes they otherwise might not have considered, had they not had the test

- Accessibility and affordability for most people

- Provision of health-related testing that is not offered through other genetic testing laboratories.

The key to harnessing the information from DTCs is to do your research before undergoing testing. First, consider your reasons for testing and make sure you understand what the test may or may not be able to tell you about your health. Think about how you might feel if you were to receive a concerning result. Most importantly, if you receive a concerning result using a DTC, it is critical to speak with a genetics professional who can confirm the accuracy of the results and discuss the next steps.

PROFESSIONAL GENETIC TESTING

Genetic testing ordered by physicians typically focuses on actionable genes that are associated with defined, evidence-based medical recommendations. These tests focus on genetic expression, so the recommended lifestyle changes, when implemented, have been shown to improve outcomes, including reduced illness and mortality. Genetic testing for conditions like heart disease and cancer offers "actionable results," providing information that doctors and nurses can "act on" in guiding the prevention, detection, and treatment of these conditions. Actionable genes are those with a harmful mutation that could potentially be addressed by medical intervention (some type of treatment supported by evidence of improved outcomes). By way of example:

Cardiovascular disorders. At least 1 in 200 individuals has an inherited form of heart disease that can result in sudden cardiac death. While all of us can benefit from adopting healthy behaviors to enhance heart health, individuals with an inherited form of heart disease most certainly want to consider specific lifestyle interventions, such as engaging in regular exercise and avoiding smoking, alcohol, caffeine, and high-fat foods. Knowing someone has higher cardiac risk also provides a legitimate basis for discussing certain medications to control blood pressure and heart rate and to prevent blood clots. In very high-risk patients, surgery to correct damaged valves or to implant an automatic defibrillator may be warranted. Genetic testing allows us to identify who requires more complex medical intervention.

Cancer risk. About 5% to 10% of all cancers are due to an inherited genetic mutation. These individuals are often at the highest level of risk for cancers. While lifestyle factors are essential in preventing cancer, additional screening and protective strategies are necessary to target the cancer risks caused by an inherited mutation in the BRCA genes or the genes associated with Lynch Syndrome. For example, research has shown that taking a daily aspirin for more than two years reduces the risk of colorectal cancer in patients with Lynch Syndrome. Inherited mutations can place entire families at risk, and family members may also need targeted lifestyle changes and screening earlier and more frequently than the general population.

UNDERSTANDING GENE-RELATED RISKS

There are too many inherited genetic mutations and corresponding syndromes to list individually in this chapter. Your family and personal history serve as a guide for illuminating hereditary conditions and relevant inherited mutations that you might have and do not yet realize. The vital thing to know is that different gene mutations are associated with various risks. Understanding your specific gene-related risks can help you create a personalized plan to optimize your health.

Hereditary mutations vary in the degree to which they influence risk. Some hereditary mutations raise disease risk dramatically, while others have only a modest effect. For example, inheriting a mutation in the MSH2 gene is associated with a 52% to 82% lifetime risk of colorectal cancer, while inheriting a mutation in the PMS2 gene is associated with only a 15% to 20% lifetime risk of colorectal cancer. Depending on the degree of risk a gene mutation confers, we might recommend different or more frequent screening options (e.g., colonoscopy annually vs. every three years). Additionally, hereditary mutations can contribute to the development of multiple conditions. FH gene mutations, for example, can raise the risk for kidney cancer and uterine fibroids in women and managing risks means implementing strategies to address each condition.

- BRCA2 mutations have important implications for men and raise the risk for more than one cancer. Men with a BRCA2 mutation have a higher risk of prostate, male-breast, and pancreatic cancer, as well as melanoma.

- Men with a BRCA2 mutation will want to consider earlier, and more frequent screening for prostate cancer (starting in their early- to mid-40s), annual skin checks with a dermatologist, and annual clinical breast exams.

- Pancreatic cancer is a deadly malignancy because it rarely causes symptoms until it is in an advanced stage (and survival rates for advanced pancreatic cancer is in the single digits). But screening to catch pancreatic cancer early does exist, and research using this approach for those individuals with the highest-risk level is showing promising results.

Early detection can mean the difference between a predicted 80% chance of survival at five years or a 5% survival rate.

EMERGING SCIENCE

Some genetic variants are linked to raising risk for serious conditions, but considerable caution is recommended before testing. The APOE gene is a good example of this, and it is important to discuss this in more detail.

- The APOE gene is responsible for packaging cholesterol and maintaining healthy levels within the body. There are three different versions of the gene: e2, e3, and e4. APOE e3 is the most common version of the gene found in the population.

- Inheriting the APOE e4 version is associated with raising a person's risk for developing Alzheimer's disease.

- People who inherit one copy of APOE e4 have around a 20% to 25% risk of Alzheimer's disease by age 85.

- A person who inherits two copies of APOE e4 has around a 30% to 35% risk of Alzheimer's by age 85. There is speculation that being born with two copies of APOE e4 may also lead to slightly earlier onset of the disease.

Not everyone with two copies of the APOE e4 variant will develop Alzheimer's, and upwards of 50% of patients who develop Alzheimer's are negative for APOE e4. Additionally, there is no proven way to cure Alzheimer's disease, and sometimes finding out one carries the e4 version of the APOE gene can lead to more anxiety, not less. More importantly, this information could cause problems for people trying to obtain long-term care insurance. The impact of this type of testing on children and families is also not as clear.

That said, there are situations in which an individual might wish to consider this test. Researchers believe that changes in the brain occur several years before the first symptoms of Alzheimer's are evident. This indicates a potential window of time one might be able to intervene to protect against the disease. The MIND diet (a combination of the DASH and Mediterranean diets) has been linked to cognitive benefits and is being studied as an effective intervention to prevent or delay Alzheimer's. Additionally, steps such as controlling blood pressure and engaging in regular exercise and certain "brain" training activities have shown promise in preventing and slowing the disease. Thus, test results can serve as a powerful motivator to change or enhance certain lifestyle choices. Anyone with a strong family history of Alzheimer's who is concerned about developing the disease may want to consider adopting a healthy lifestyle. Interventions such as controlling blood pressure, engaging in regular exercise, and eating a healthy diet are beneficial regardless. (For more information on the DASH and Mediterranean diets, see chapter 36.)

BENEFITS AND LIMITATIONS OF TESTING

Understanding the risks and limitations of genetic testing can help you make thoughtful, informed decisions. Genetic testing can help you:

- Find out if you are at increased risk for a certain condition

- Create a personalized screening plan leading to early detection and better outcomes

- Adopt lifestyle strategies known to reduce risks

- Make informed decisions about medical and surgical options for reducing risks

- Protect family members by helping them identify and manage their risks

- Lower anxiety and fear about the risk of developing a specific condition

- Guide decisions about biopsy, surgery, and medications

- Determine follow-up care for a specific disease

- Expand treatment options for advanced diseases, opening doors for targeted therapy, immunotherapy, and clinical trials.

Seeking out a genetics professional. As you can see, there are several essential factors to consider when exploring genetic testing. We recommend seeking a healthcare professional with expertise in genetic counseling and testing to ensure the appropriate test is selected and to understand your results and how they affect you. Licensed Genetic Counselors (LGCs) as well as doctors and Advanced Practice Providers (NPs/PAs) with additional training in genetics are all excellent options.

Limitations of testing. Remember: genetic testing cannot tell us if someone will develop a condition; it can only tell us about risk. Even with the best interventions, we cannot entirely eliminate the risk of developing a disease. Sometimes test results are inconclusive and that can lead to increased anxiety. Learning that you have a higher risk for a disease can also cause worry. In addition, parents can experience guilt if they have passed a harmful mutation on to their child.

What to expect. Genetic testing is typically separated into two counseling visits. At the pre-test visit, the genetics professional will review your history in detail and discuss critical considerations about testing (benefits, limitations, results, insurance issues, etc.) so that you may make an informed decision. Test results can impact entire families, and it is not uncommon for close family members to attend these visits as well. Sometimes people worry that they will lose their health insurance if they test positive for genes that carry high risk.

The Genetic Information Non-Discrimination Act. GINA is a federal law that protects individuals undergoing genetic testing from health insurance discrimination and employment discrimination. GINA does not address long-term disability and life insurance, so speaking to a genetics professional can provide helpful information.

If you decide that genetic testing is a good fit, a DNA sample can be obtained the same day using saliva or blood. Results take two to four weeks and can be rushed in situations in which the findings might alter treatment decisions. During the post-test visit, the genetics professional will review your results and discuss how they will impact you and your family members. Learning the results can trigger a range of emotions. Genetics professionals can clarify misconceptions, connect you with resources, and provide support.

Cost. Most insurance carriers, including Medicare and Medicaid, cover genetic testing, especially if the test results will help guide a person's medical care and/or if there is a reasonable chance that the individual has a hereditary mutation. As science has advanced, the price of testing has come down significantly. The majority of individuals pay approximately $100 or less, out of pocket, for genetic testing. Most labs will also verify the cost before testing, and some offer self-pay options for around $250. A genetics professional will review payment options at the first visit. Multiple safeguards are in place to make sure you do not get a costly bill.

LABORATORIES AND TESTING

A genetic test is valid only if it provides accurate results, and all laboratories and tests are not the same. Federal regulatory standards (called CLIA standards) exist to help control the quality of laboratories and ensure the accuracy of the tests offered. Most genetic tests are over 90% accurate, and some are 99% accurate. A genetics professional can make sure that the appropriate laboratory and test are selected. For the purpose of this chapter, we have highlighted some standard testing options for inherited mutations for adults.

Myriad Genetics—myRisk test. This test is a solid, multigene panel for hereditary cancers. It offers a full selection of genes, covering the important basics without being too broad. Test reports are easy to understand and include helpful educational information and resources. Myriad provides counselors who can answer questions and explain results. The test is limited in that it does not cover genes associated with some of the rarer hereditary cancer syndromes, such as HLRCC.

Ambry Genetics. A variety of multigene panels for cancer, heart disease, and neurological conditions are available from this laboratory. The OvaNext, BreastNext, ProstateNext, etc., provide the option of ordering testing based on cancer type. Their larger panel test, CancerNext Expanded, is a good option when you need to look beyond the usual risks. Ambry recently launched RNAinsight to provide even greater accuracy for re-classifying inconclusive results (which are a natural aspect of all tests). Ambry offers self-pay options for around $250 for most tests, and also has genetic counselors available.

Invitae. This laboratory offers an impressive selection of multigene panel tests as well as single-gene tests, including options for cancer, heart disease, neurological disorders, and rare genetic conditions (such as Ehlers-Danlos Syndrome). Invitae's patient portal is user-friendly and provides patients with updates. The lab offers self-pay options for most tests for around $250 to $300. Invitae communicates with patients through email and text messaging and is not the best fit for patients who do not use the internet or a cell phone.

LabCorp and Quest Diagnostics. Both of these CLIA-certified labs offer a wide array of laboratory testing, including hereditary cancer panels and several tailored panels for inherited forms of heart disease. LabCorp and Quest also offer testing for APOE variants, although Quest offers it under testing for cardiovascular health (remember APOE is involved in packaging cholesterol). Both labs have contracts with numerous insurance companies, and many physicians are familiar with ordering through these labs.

UNDERSTANDING THE RESULTS

A positive result. This means that an inherited genetic mutation was found. The genetics professional will review with you the specific gene-related risks associated with your results.

A negative result. When no genetic mutation is found, the negative result tends to be more complicated than it appears. A negative result does not mean you won't develop a particular condition. Most diseases are not caused by inherited mutations or by single genes. Also, we can only test for what we currently know about. You might be carrying a mutated gene that isn't being tested for currently or has yet to be identified. If you have a strong family history of a disease or a personal medical history with *red flags*, you might still be at risk and would benefit from personalized, risk-reducing strategies.

Sometimes there is conflicting evidence about whether a particular gene or set of genes raises risk. Although this is uncommon, a genetics professional can help make sense of inconclusive test results.

MANAGING RISKS, PROTECTING HEALTH

Whether you are at risk because of a positive test result, a strong family history, or a personal history of a health condition, there are multiple options for managing risk.

Personalized screening. When risk is identified, it is important to follow up with earlier, more frequent screening and specialized types of testing (for example, PSA test starting in your early to mid-40s as opposed to 50 years of age).

Lifestyle changes. Knowing you are at higher risk can motivate you to make healthier choices regarding diet, exercise, etc. If you are at higher risk and you have vowed to make changes but so far without success, consider the insight on genetic risk a call to action. Seek out support. For example, optimize your diet by working with a nutritionist, joining a weight loss program, or seeking a support group. A few medical centers have support groups specifically for individuals with inherited mutations, and online forums such as FORCE (Facing Our Risk of Cancer Empowered) are a great option as well. Sharing your experience with others who understand the emotions and decisions that come from being at higher risk can also empower you to take action.

Prophylactic surgery. Those with the highest risk may choose surgeries to significantly lower their risk (e.g., removing breasts and/or ovaries for BRCA mutation carriers or removing the stomach for CDH1 mutation carriers). Deciding to undergo prophylactic surgery to dramatically lower the risk of disease is a big decision. A genetics professional, together with your physician, can help you better understand your risk level and help you weigh the benefits and limitations of surgical options for disease prevention.

Personalized treatments. Individuals with cardiac risk might benefit from medications to regulate heart rhythm or minimize blood clots; individuals with colorectal cancer risk might benefit from daily aspirin. Targeted drugs called PARP inhibitors exist to treat breast, ovarian, pancreatic, and prostate cancers associated with a BRCA mutation. Immunotherapy checkpoint inhibitors are a valuable tool for patients with germline and/or tumor-acquired mutations in DNA mismatch repair genes.

FUTURE OPTIONS

Genetics is transforming healthcare, and the future possibilities for using information about our genetic makeup to improve our well-being are endless. There are several exciting options on the horizon.

First, SNPs will likely become essential markers for predicting the risk of common but debilitating disorders, such as addiction, diabetes, and mental illness. In terms of breast cancer, polygenic risk scores (using SNPs) are already being investigated for predicting breast cancer risk.

Second, future research will illuminate why specific genes are turned on or off and why certain people with a specific genetic makeup develop a disease while others don't.

Third, clinical trials for cancer now include studies of treatment based on the individual patient's genetic makeup and on the genetic makeup of the tumor, rather than by cancer type. In the future, doctors will sequence your genes to determine the type of treatment that is likely to work best for you.

Down the road, we hope to use gene therapy to introduce a missing gene or fix a mutated one. CRISPR is a scissor-like gene-editing tool that cuts up strands of DNA, altering the sequence of base pairs, and modifying gene function with the potential to someday cure disease. This technology is being applied to sickle cell disease, for example. However, technologies that allow us to modify a person's genetic makeup also raise ethical questions about how to use these technologies.

In the era of personalized medicine, genetic testing is one of the most critical interventions available for protecting your health. There are many test options, and results are not always straightforward. Talking with your doctor or a genetics professional could help you decode your options and focus your efforts on the path to wellness.

BOOKS

Siddhartha Mukherjee, MD. *The Gene: An Intimate History*. New York, NY: Scribner, 2017.

James Watson, PhD. *The Double Helix: A Personal Account of the Discovery of the Structure of DNA*. New York, NY: Touchstone, 2001.

Nessa Carey. *The Epigenetics Revolution: How Modern Biology is Rewriting our Understanding of Genetics, Disease, and Inheritance*. New York, NY: Columbia University Press, 2013.

Clarissa Foster. *Understanding BRCA: Living with the Breast Cancer Gene*. London, UK: Hammersmith Health Books, 2017.

Dina Roth Port. *Previvors: Facing the Breast Cancer Gene and Making Life-Changing Decisions*. New York, NY: Avery, 2010.

Chapter 9
Avoiding Stupid Accidents
Malcolm Johnson, MD, Emergency Medicine
& Michael Abassian, MPH, Researcher

Life is a gamble. You can get hurt. People die in plane crashes and car accidents.
People die every day. It's the same with fighters: some die, some get hurt, some go on.
You just don't let yourself believe it will happen to you.
— Muhammad Ali

One Sunday after watching his favorite football team and having a few beers, Tom notices that the second-story windows of his house are filthy. He is worried that he'll forget to clean them later, so he finds his ladder and extends it to its maximum reach, which ends just below the window he intends to clean. Realizing that the ladder is too short, Tom duct tapes a window cleaning brush to the end of a broomstick. He then climbs up the ladder with the broomstick in one hand and the bucket of water in the other. He stands on the second-to-the-top step of the ladder and places a bucket of water on the top step. With little room to maneuver, Tom attempts to wash the window.

Trying to reach the very top of the window, Tom bumps against the bucket, knocking it off the ladder. Forgetting that he's in an awkward position 20 feet above the ground, he lunges to catch the bucket and realizes at that moment that he's made a big mistake. The ladder shoots out underneath him, and he falls to the ground. He ends up in the emergency room with two broken legs (both femurs) and a nasty bruise (hematoma).

Tom's injuries are so extensive that he has a long recovery period in the hospital and requires months of physical therapy and rehabilitation. He continues to have pain and becomes addicted to pain killers. Even after recovering from his injuries, Tom now faces an addiction problem that will require in-patient substance abuse treatment, and may take months (if not years) to beat.

The *Darwin Award* is a darkly humorous honor awarded to people who have died in "an extraordinarily idiotic manner." Between 1995 and 2014, 89% were men. Research has shown that men are more likely than women to be admitted to the emergency room after accidental injuries, tend to be more prone to traumatic injury due to increased engagement in dangerous activities, and are more likely to die in traffic accidents (which are often caused by risky driving).

The United States spends more than $660 billion every year on medical and work-loss costs due to injury. Nearly $130 billion of annual fatal injury costs are attributable to unintentional injuries alone. Costs related to falls (37% of spending) and transportation injuries (21% of spending) account for the majority of costs in emergency departments, and males account for the majority (78%) of fatal injury costs ($167 billion) as well as the majority (63%) of nonfatal injury costs ($288 billion).

HOW OUR BODIES CHANGE AFTER 40

For insight on how and why men 40 and over suffer traumatic injury, it's important to understand how the human body changes as men age and begin to enter midlife. Oftentimes, middle-aged and older men are caught off guard when an activity that they could easily do as a teenager or young adult has become significantly more difficult.

Bones. As men age, bone thinning (osteoporosis) and loss of bone density (osteopenia) are common. The most frequent causes of bone loss in men are deficiencies in testosterone, calcium, and vitamin D. Osteoporosis can also be caused by many prescription drugs, as well as smoking. Weight-bearing exercise and a nutritional, balanced diet are some of the best ways to combat osteoporosis.

Muscles. As men grow older muscles tend to lose their mass. Muscle loss due to age is known as "sarcopenia." Being proactive about maintaining physical strength as you age is important in minimizing frailty, falls, and injuries due to weakened muscles. The best way to prevent muscle deterioration is to emphasize both strength training and cardiovascular exercise. (You may also want to review chapter 89, "Optimizing Testosterone," on maintaining testosterone levels.)

Cartilage and tendons. Similar to muscle and bone loss, cartilage and tendons can deteriorate and decline in elasticity and strength. A constant regimen of exercise will help combat this deterioration and reduce the risk of injuries.

Vision and hearing. Sensory deficits occur with age and time. If your work involves computer use, vary your tasks and take periodic breaks in order to give your eyes a rest. Position your work area so strong light is to your side, to minimize glare. Do what you can to avoid extremely loud noise. Corrective vision and hearing support can make a huge difference in minimizing the risk of falls and injuries. (See chapters 23 and 24—"Spine Care" and "Protecting Your Vision"—for practical information on protecting these vital senses.)

Mental focus. Cognitive decline can occur gradually over time and increases the risk of injury. To help combat this process, engage in mentally and socially stimulating pursuits as much as possible.

Men and risk. Men tend to play riskier sports, have occupations that involve higher-than-average risk, and engage in more risky behaviors. In the moment, it's easy to overlook the hazards of taking seemingly small risks in your day-to-day life, as well as the potential long-term consequences if you suffer a traumatic injury. Develop the habit of pairing mindfulness with physical activity to sharpen your focus.

STUPID THINGS MEN DO THAT LAND THEM IN THE ER

According to data from the CDC's Web-based Injury Statistics Query and Reporting System (WISQARS), over 5.8 million men suffered nonfatal injuries, and over 80,000 men died from traumatic injuries in 2018. That year, the most common cause of nonfatal injury in men ages 40 to 79 was falls. Other common injuries included accidents involving motor-vehicles, poisoning, cuts and pierces, and overexertion.

ACCIDENTAL INJURIES

In men 40 and older, certain types of injuries have become particularly common. Unintentional injuries were the third leading cause of death in the U.S. in 2019. According to the CDC's WISQARS database, the most common fatal injuries among men over 40 that year were:

- Motor vehicle accidents

- Medication poisoning

- Falls

- Firearms accidents.

Motor accident fatalities. Accidents caused over 80,000 deaths among men over 40 between 2017 and 2018. When it comes to risky behaviors like drinking and driving, there are no tricks or treatments to improve the outcome. Ultimately, it is up to you to consider the wellbeing of yourself and others.

- **Wear your seatbelt.** This is one of the easiest ways to reduce the risk of motor accident fatality; in fact, wearing your seatbelt has been proven to reduce mortality rates by about 50%.

■ **Call a friend, a taxi, or a service like Uber when you've been drinking.** In the United States, once an hour, someone dies in a drunk driving accident. Make a conscious effort to avoid unnecessarily dangerous situations by finding an effective solution to get you home safe and sound.

Falls. Falls are the most common type of accident involving people age 65 and over. A surprising number of falls involve a roof or a ladder. More than 500,000 falls from ladders occur every year, and 97% of those falls occur at home.

Medication poisoning. Drug poisoning caused about 75,000 deaths among men over 40 between 2017 and 2018 alone (almost twice as many as the roughly 36,000 deaths caused by firearms). This number includes opioid overdoses and deaths due to medication (both accidentally used at too high a dosage, as well as fatalities when taken as prescribed). It is believed that medication errors affect more than seven million patients and cost almost $21 billion annually. About 30% of hospitalized patients have at least one error in their medication instructions at discharge.

OCCUPATIONAL INJURIES

Research studies have identified heroic and hypermasculine behaviors in many high-risk male occupations such as mining, farming, construction, firefighting, the military, protective service, and professional sports. Expectations that men must be brave, embrace the normalization of risk, endure discomfort and pain, and be okay with exposure to hazards play a role in traumatic injury.

> *Men in high-risk occupations often experience increased exposure to physical risks associated with mechanical, electrical, or chemical hazards, or violence. Normative expectations of masculinity (also known as "hypermasculinity") encourage men to be physically tough and fearless to the point of carelessness.*

Low-back conditions. Back injuries are now a $50 billion problem in direct medical costs and lost wages. Many people, especially men, develop lower back problems in their 40s. Common conditions that can affect the lower back include slipped discs, disc degeneration, spinal stenosis, and sciatica (a nerve or myofascial condition that causes numbness/discomfort in the hip(s) or leg(s). Deconditioning of the back occurs with age and can be accelerated with improper posture and/or abdominal weight gain. Torn or pulled muscles, ruptured vertebral discs, and spinal nerve compression are among the most painful lower back injuries. Lower back injuries also tend to occur from bending or lifting improperly. Tiger Woods, the renowned golfer with 15 major golf championship wins, has dealt with back injuries multiple times throughout his career and has even had to withdraw from tournaments due to intense back pain.

Hearing injuries. The most common causes of ear-related injuries involve falls, trauma to the head, sports injuries, and loud noise or loud music. Occupational noise exposure is a problem that leads to many ear injuries; the CDC estimates that 22 million individuals (22% of workers) are exposed to potentially damaging noise at work every year. If you need to raise your voice to speak to someone 3 feet away, noise levels might be over 85 decibels, meaning your environment is too loud to be considered safe for your ears. If you notice ringing or humming in your ears when you leave work, that's another sign that your workplace is too loud.

The Hearing Loss Association of America reports that the average person losing hearing waits seven years to seek medical help. This is despite the fact that people with unaided hearing loss earn $20,000 less a year than individuals with intact hearing. What's more, only one in five people who would benefit from a hearing aid actually uses one. (See chapter 25—"Preserving Your Hearing"— for insight on preserving your hearing and how to protect it.)

Eye injuries. More than 2 million eye injuries occur in the United States every year. Most involve everyday household products or occupational settings. This results in an estimated $300 million lost every year in terms of lost productivity, medical treatment, and workers' compensation.

Working at the computer. To minimize eye inflammation:

- Wearing computer glasses reduces the risk of related eye disorders by 90%.

- Position the screen 25 inches away (about an arm's length).

- Take 20-second breaks from work several times an hour to relax your eyes.

- Adjust the lighting and brightness of your screen with bright lighting to the side of your screen, rather than in front or in the back of the screen.

Signs of eye injury. Symptoms that merit your attention include apparent pain or difficulty seeing, having a cut or torn eyelid, one eye moving differently or protruding more than the other, unusual pupil size or shape, blood in the clear part of the eye, or having something in the eye or under the eyelid that cannot be easily removed.

Protective eyewear. Get a pair of snazzy protective goggles that you really like. Around the house, use them in your workshop, when you're mowing or weed whacking, painting, working on your car....

Immediate Care for a Knocked-Out Tooth.

Dental avulsion is a true clinical emergency. If the tooth is intact, a gentle rinse with saline water and immediate reimplantation is the best treatment. A trip to the dentist means placing the tooth in a suitable storage medium. Whole milk is generally available and will suffice. Typically, 20 to 40 minutes is the window of time and, if the tooth is still viable, the timing significantly affects the outcome. A dentist will clean the socket and the tooth and replant the tooth into the socket. Splinting the tooth to the adjacent teeth will stabilize it for a week to ten days, at which point a root canal can be performed. Long-term survival of the tooth depends on the favorable healing of the periodontal ligament. The chance of success is about 50/50 or perhaps greater but worth the effort. *(This information also appears in chapter 53, "A Healthy Smile.")*

ORTHOPEDIC AND DENTAL INJURIES

Knee injuries. Surprisingly, there are more than six million knee injuries a year, the most frequent among all orthopedic disorders. Four major ligaments hold the knee together, connecting the upper and lower leg at the knee joint.

- *The meniscus* is cartilage that provides cushioning between the upper and lower leg within the joint. There are both medial and lateral menisci on each knee and both types of meniscus can be injured, usually due to a significant force being applied to the knee, but also from overuse.

- *Ligament injuries* are often coupled with a meniscus injury since ligaments and the meniscus work together to produce rotation in the knee.

Both occupational and sports injuries can cause ligament or meniscus tears. Many NFL football players, such as Adrian Peterson, J.J. Watt, and Rob Gronkowski, have had ACL and MCL injuries.

Dental injuries. Over five million teeth are knocked out (avulsed) in the United States every year (with associated costs of nearly $500 million in care). Some studies of sports injuries report dental trauma in up to 80% of participants. Rugby tends to have the highest rate of dental damage (22% to 33%), surprisingly higher than basketball (5%) or hockey (5%).

If you play sports or have a job with risk of injury, get a comfortable, well-fitting mouth guard. *(For more on selecting the right one, see chapter 53, "A Healthy Smile.")*

Studies have shown that dental injuries can be reduced by as much as 50% when a mouth guard is worn.

Tennis elbow. These injuries (a.k.a. lateral epicondylitis) affect more than one million people a year. Tennis elbow involves the tendons on the outside of the elbow joint, which weakens grip strength and can cause soreness or burning in the outside of the elbow. This injury usually results from overuse and repetitive movements as in tennis or on the job. However, it can also be caused by trauma from accidents related to skiing, biking, and other sports. Typically, the remedy for tennis elbow is to minimize the repetitive motion that caused the injury, get plenty of rest, and apply ice and take NSAIDs (nonsteroidal anti-inflammatories) as needed.

Stress fractures. Thin, hairline bone fractures are common, because they occur in so many situations—as occupational injuries, in sports injuries, and with aging, osteoporosis, and due to poor nutrition. Stress fractures are caused by impact force on a bone, but also become more likely with repetitive motion and overuse, similar to tennis elbow. Sports that involve a lot of jumping, such as basketball and track and field, or running, such as marathons and triathlons, are more likely to cause stress fractures. For example, the famous Houston Rockets basketball player Yao Ming was forced to end his promising career due to a stress fracture in his foot.

Rotator cuff. Torn rotator cuffs affect an estimated 400,000 to 600,000 people a year. These injuries involve the muscles and tendons that stabilize the shoulder socket joint as the result of traumatic forces and are especially common in men over 40. This is also one of the most frequent injuries associated with extreme sports such as climbing, for example. Well-known athletes who have dealt with rotator cuff injuries include Kobe Bryant, Drew Brees, Ray Lewis, and Paul George.

Calf and ankle injuries. According to the Mayo Clinic, calf muscle injuries are common in men over 40 who are runners. These types of injuries usually heal but can take 12 weeks or more for a man in midlife. Related is the Achilles ligament, which attaches the calf muscle to the back of the heel bone of the foot and allows you to push off with your toes when you run or to stand on your toes. This injury is commonly known as "a weekend warrior injury." These conditions usually develop when people who are out of shape overexert themselves, causing a rupture of the muscles. But even professional athletes have suffered Achilles injuries, including Kevin Durant, David Beckham, and Kobe Bryant.

Sex. Injuries related to sex are more common than most people realize. According to one study, 15% to 22% of Americans admit to experiencing a sex injury. These injuries are embarrassing to talk about because men do not always feel comfortable with sensitive topics relating to their sex lives. (For more information on injuries associated with sex, see chapter 91, "Peyronie's Disease," which is a condition in which scar tissue develops after injury, making penetrative intercourse difficult.)

Spinal cord injury. Fewer than 18,000 new cases of spinal cord injury occur every year. However, cumulatively almost 300,000 people in the U.S. live with these debilitating conditions. Most of these injuries are the result of a car crash (39% of cases) or a fall (31.8% of cases) and can vary in severity.

EXTREME SPORTS

Accidents involving extreme sports are another common reason that men find themselves in the emergency room. According to the CDC, over 60% of sports and recreation injuries involve men.

In 2006, ATVs alone caused almost 150,000 emergency room visits and over 800 deaths. Climbing, an increasingly popular activity that ranges from casual indoor climbing to mountain climbing, can result in rotator cuff tears, dislocations (subluxation), muscle sprains and tears (pulley tears), and tendonitis, all of which can require an ER visit. Mountain biking is associated with injuries ranging from knee and lower back pain (sciatica) to abrasions, lacerations, and broken bones. Surfing causes many fatalities every year primarily due to drowning, and also can cause contusions, head trauma, shoulder strain, and back pain. Other extreme sports are often misunderstood. For example, skydiving, one of the most notorious "bucket list" extreme sports, actually resulted in only 15 fatalities in 2019, most of which involved advanced skydivers performing complex maneuvers rather than first-timers. Skydiving injuries usually occur while landing and can include concussions, fractures, and neck and back injuries.

Similar to skydiving is BASE (Building, Antenna, Span, and Earth) jumping, which is considered to be the most dangerous adventure sport in the world, due to the precision-timing of pulling the chute. The number of current active BASE jumpers in the world is only about 3,000, and most of them are experienced veterans, but the death rate for BASE jumping is still one death per 60 participants, a rate that is about 43 times higher than that of skydiving. The two most popular snow sports, skiing and snowboarding, actually tend to involve less injury than many traditional sports like football or basketball, but can still cause injuries ranging from knee tears and sprains to fractures.

AVOIDING RISKY BEHAVIORS

Clearly, men tend to engage in risky behaviors. One study found that males were more likely than females to cross busy roads when it's risky to do so (interestingly, males were even more likely to cross busy roads at risky times when they were around females). Another study found that men are more likely to engage in hazardous activities such as smoking, alcohol overuse, and unsafe sexual practices. That same study found that men are less likely to engage in health-seeking and health-promoting behaviors, to discuss their health, to attend to serious symptoms, or to address physical pain or mental health issues.

One study found that risk-taking continues in men until about the age of 50. Another study found that head injuries were most common among men aged 35 to 50. According to the CDC, drowning rates and motorcycle accidents among men are highest during the mid-forties, indicating that engaging in risky behavior is far from exclusive to younger men.

ACCIDENT PREVENTION AND SAFETY
Men's Health Network

Accidents are the #1 cause of death in men under age 44 and the third leading cause of death for all American men. Men are far more likely than women to be injured or killed in an accident, largely because men tend to engage in riskier behavior. Here we'll recap the major types of accidents.

Motor Vehicle Crashes. Car crashes are the leading cause of accidental death among men. Men are more likely to be involved in a fatal crash than women. While you can't control what other drivers do, there are a number of steps you can take to reduce accidents:

- Always wear your seatbelt, even on short trips.
- Follow posted speed limits.
- Don't drive after drinking or when you're tired.
- Don't ride with a driver who's intoxicated or exhausted.
- Always wear a helmet when riding a motorcycle, bicycle, or skate board.
- Practice defensive driving. Assume that other drivers may not be alert, so you need to be twice as focused.

Accidental Poisoning. This is the second leading cause of accidental death. Men are more than twice as likely as women to die from poisoning. You should keep the national poison control number (1- 800- 222-1222) in your contacts and programmed into your speed dial. Here's what else you can do to reduce your risk:

(Cont'd from previous page.)

- Install smoke and carbon monoxide detectors in your home. Replace the batteries twice a year.
- Carefully follow the instructions on household cleaning products. Mixing bleach and ammonia, for example, produces a toxic gas.
- If you're using chemicals, be sure you've got plenty of ventilation.
- Take prescription medication exactly as your doctor advised, and follow directions on non-prescription drugs.

Falls. Accidental falls are the leading cause of injury and injury-related death among those over 65.

- Stay active. Physical activity helps preserve your strength and balance.
- Use appropriate lighting. Not being able to see in the dark can lead to tripping and falls.
- Install railings on stairways and next to bathtubs and showers.
- Put non-skid pads underneath rugs and carpets.
- Use ladders safely.
- Starting at age 60, get screened for osteoporosis.

Workplace Accidents. Over 90% of people who die on the job are men. That's largely because men are much more likely than women to work in high-risk jobs, such as construction, mining, hazardous materials, or roofing.

- Take every safety precaution. As appropriate, wear a hard hat; use a seat belt, safety harnesses, mask, and eye protection, and ask for help when you need it.
- Take extra care when handling chemicals. Many are linked with cancer, asthma, and infertility.

Guns. The easiest way to prevent accidental shootings is to not keep firearms in your home. But if you do, be sure to:

- Keep guns unloaded and securely locked.
- Keep ammunition in a secure gun locker.
- Keep guns and ammunition in a gun safe or secure gun locker.
- Be especially careful when cleaning guns—this is when many gun accidents happen.

Courtesy of The Men's Health Network, Washington, DC,
Health Education and Advocacy; www.MensHealthNetwork.org.

For additional sources and references, please see TheTwentyFirstCenturyMan.com.

Chapter 10
Managing Persistent Pain
William Longton, MD, Anesthesiology & Pain Medicine

Behind every beautiful thing, there's some kind of pain.
— Bob Dylan

Chronic pain is one of the most debilitating conditions a man can experience. We can't exercise or sleep or focus, we gain weight, and we can become irritable, if not downright depressed. More than 40 million males are estimated to be affected. Why is this happening?

THE LIFESAVING VALUE OF PAIN

The ability to perceive pain is vital to species survival and protects us by helping us detect injury, initiating the body's response to acute tissue damage. Our longevity is made possible by the ability to heal, restoring traumatized and damaged tissues and calming inflammation. Unfortunately, this ability starts to diminish over time. If this healing capacity is disrupted, that can play a role in the development of chronic tissue degeneration and pain.

PAIN IN AMERICA

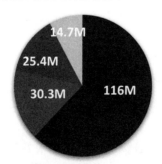

MORE PEOPLE LIVE WITH CHRONIC PAIN THAN CANCER, HEART DISEASE, AND DIABETES COMBINED

More than 30% of Americans are living with some form of chronic or severe pain

■ Chronic pain: 1166M   ■ Diabetes: 30.3M
■ Heart disease: 25.4M   ■ Cancer: 14.7M

Figure 10.1 Pain in America.

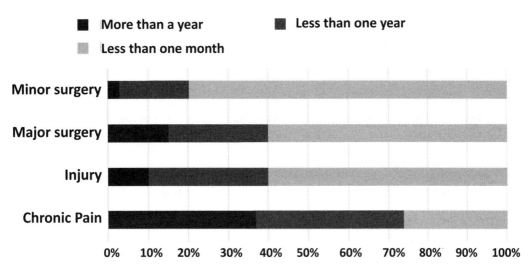

Figure 10.2. Why are Americans taking opioids?

Let's first explore how pain is perceived and how acute pain can progress to chronic pain.

ACUTE PAIN

Sudden, immediate pain is a response to tissue trauma, detected in the tissues by specialized cells (nociceptors) that can identify thermal, pressure, or chemical injury and transmit that information along ascending sensory nerves to the spinal column. These signals travel up the spine to the brain, where that information is processed, resulting in actions such as, "Take your burning foot out of the campfire!"

Pain brain. In the case of repeated trauma, nerve damage, and/or inflammation, the pain pathway can go awry, resulting in increased pain sensitivity, nerve inflammation, and the development of chronic neuropathic pain sometimes referred to as "pain brain."

The importance of an accurate diagnosis. An accurate diagnosis of the cause of the pain is critical because if recognized and diagnosed early on, that can prevent the development of chronic pain. There are multiple targets for the treatment of nociceptive pain, due to physical damage or pathology, such as an injury or arthritis.

Treatment of acute pain. Pain control for acute pain generally involves a series of steps, including:

- Reduction of inflammation with ice and anti-inflammatory medications

- Interruption of pain signals with an anesthetic nerve block or cortisone injections

- Stronger opioid pain medication, used in the short term to mask the pain, temporarily allowing some degree of increased mobility and activity.

Unchecked chronic pain. In these disorders, multiple segments of the pain pathway have become dysfunctional or neuropathic, reflected in:

- Chronically swollen tissue

- Pain receptors that have become hypersensitive to pain

- Nerve endings that preferentially pass along pain signals

- Central/brain processes leading to depression.

The incidence of chronic pain. Pain disorders increase as men age, with 7% of chronic pain sufferers between the ages of 18 and 24, growing to 22% between 45 and 64. From at least 65 on, 27% of the population is afflicted by chronic pain, which is an enormous economic burden costing over $500 billion (2010 U.S.), including direct healthcare costs, lost productivity, and disability programs, as well as an incalculable human cost.

PAIN SYNDROMES

A detailed listing of all the causes of chronic pain and chronic pain syndromes is beyond this chapter's scope. However, we can draw many commonalities from familiar pain syndromes, namely lumbar disc degeneration and osteoarthritis.

DISC PAIN

Nearly everyone experiences some level of lumbar pain from disc degeneration by the age of 40. Initial causes are usually related to repeated strains and overuse. There is emerging evidence that infection may also play a role in the development of lumbar disc degeneration. Aging is also a factor. The lumbar spine has a normal aging process that accelerates as the disc loses cushioning:

- Tears occur in the disc's outer annulus surface with subsequent damage to the inner disc nucleus.

- Ultimately this trauma induces loss of water content from the disc.

- The resiliency and cushioning of the disc is reduced.

- The disc then loses height.

- The vertebra may shift, and inflammation ensues.

- Nerves and spinal joints become inflamed, causing pain and/or spasms.

- Nerve compression can occur, resulting in sciatica and nerve injury.

- As the spine ages further, degenerative arthritis and bone spurs result.

- This narrows the spinal canal, termed spinal stenosis.

- Spinal stenosis can further compress spinal nerves.

Thus the younger man tends to suffer more from disc and vertebra joint inflammatory processes, whereas the older man will suffer more from spinal stenosis.

Lumbar discogenic spinal pain has been found to afflict even the most robust and fit amongst us—astronauts! In space, under zero-gravity conditions, lumbar discs gain height and cause the spine to extend length up to a few centimeters. Astronauts frequently report moderate to severe, dull lower back pain possibly caused by disc expansion in space.

OSTEOARTHRITIS

This is a classic age-related disorder of the joints, a form of chronic degeneration. In osteoarthritis, degradation and loss of joint cartilage are a central feature of wear and tear of the joints. The prevalence of osteoarthritis increases from 10% at age 45 to 30% at age 60 and 50% by the age of 80.

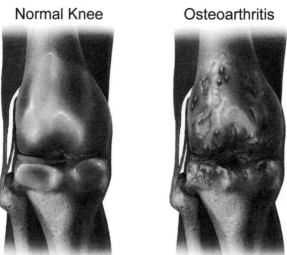

Normal Knee   Osteoarthritis

Figure 10.3 How osteoarthritis deteriorates the joint structure.

Effects of aging. In all degenerative diseases, cell and tissue aging results in age-related loss of the ability to heal and repair cells. Some individuals are able to adapt to biomechanical stress on the knee more successfully than others: think lightweight, long-distance runners with normal knee anatomy. However, other individuals, such as the obese, or those with joint misalignment, will develop a maladaptive response to joint stress resulting in osteo-arthritis. As our bodies age, the basic cell mechanisms that repair injury decline, leading to reduced ability to repair damage, and further destruction of joint tissue. Cigarette smoking, obesity, and disorders such as diabetes accelerate degenerative changes. Stress and depression also play a role.

LIFESTYLE FACTORS

Men need to avoid activities that promote chronic inflammation, which leads to reduced ability to heal injured tissues.

The role of smoking in chronic pain. Cigarette smoking is strongly associated with increased chronic pain, including low-back pain from lumbar disc degeneration. There are numerous harmful effects from components of tobacco smoke on cell functioning. A number of cancer-causing (carcinogenic) toxins are present in cigarette smoke. Less well known is the negative effect of toxins on immune response and tissue regeneration (due to carbon monoxide, nicotine, and other chemical additives). Nicotine and cigarette smoke:

- Weaken discs and joints
- Inhibit cell growth within the disc
- Cause localized constriction of blood vessels surrounding the lumbar disc
- Damage collagen production
- Result in skin wrinkling
- Weaken the outer lining of the disc (the annulus).

Smokers are more likely to have loss of knee joint cartilage than nonsmokers as measured by MRI studies. Increased carbon monoxide from smoking starves the tissue of oxygen to some degree (termed hypoxia), further stressing the health of knee and lumbar joints, which by their nature have relatively limited blood flow.

Obesity as a factor in inflammation. Addressing obesity is key in preventing and treating chronic pain because excess weight contributes to chronic inflammation (increasing pro-inflammatory mediators such as tumor necrosis factor (TNF-alpha)). We know that patients undergoing gastric bypass procedures have a measurable decrease in inflammatory markers within 12 months of surgery.

The link between stress, depression, and inflammation. Both stress and depression are common in people with chronic pain. There is considerable evidence that those with diagnosed depression have higher markers of pro-inflammatory mediators, suggesting a link between depression and inflammation:

- Vagal nerve tone is reduced.

- Reduced tone diminishes opportunities to reduce inflammation.

- This results in increased stress response.

- Stress dials down the relaxation response and slows cell healing.

LIFESTYLE STRATEGIES TO COMBAT CHRONIC PAIN

Exercise. It may seem like common sense to exercise, thereby reducing the risks of cardiovascular disease and obesity, improving metabolism, and strengthening the heart, muscles, and bones. Studies have also shown that as little as 20 minutes a day of exercise can reduce blood levels of pro-inflammatory chemicals (such as TNF-alpha), allowing the body to heal injured tissues more efficiently.

As humans, we breathe up to 20,000 times per day, so we have ample opportunities to perfect this pain-relieving skill. The use of breathing techniques to improve the control and tone of the vagus nerve is a simple technique that can be practiced by anyone.

The practice of mindfulness meditation. Functional MRI studies (which show brain activity in real time) have found that mindfulness meditation rapidly increases the ability to tolerate pain. This has been demonstrated in research studies involving patients with no prior experience with meditation. Imaging studies have shown that meditation improves blood flow to critical brain areas involved in pain processing. Your efforts at meditation can be supported by:

- An app on your phone

- Books or podcasts on meditation

- HeartMath devices and software

- The Headspace app.

Nutrition—the gut-inflammation connection. Recent studies have focused on the role of the gut microbiome (the friendly bacteria in the digestive tract) on osteoarthritis:

- We now have evidence of a genuine relationship between certain gut bacteria and low-grade inflammation in the knee (as well as arthritic knee pain, independent of obesity).

- Studies have also demonstrated significant differences in the bacterial content shared between gut and disc segments.

- Differences are also evident in the spine when comparing normal, degenerative, and herniated lumbar disc segments. This suggests that certain gut flora may be more favorable in minimizing disc inflammation. It also suggests that disc infection may be one possible initiator of lumbar disc disease.

Anti-inflammatory diet. Dietary interventions to manipulate or optimize the gut flora (the microbiome) could play an increased role in inflammation control. This may become more widely utilized in the future as we gain understanding of the complex relationship between the gut microbiome and inflammation.

To reduce levels of inflammation and optimize the microbiome, it's best to have an overall healthy diet. If you're looking for a simple diet that promotes anti-inflammatory foods, consider the Mediterranean diet, which is high in fruits, vegetables, nuts, whole grains, fish, and healthy oils. Include these foods in your menu to reduce inflammation: olive oil, green leafy vegetables, nuts (almonds and walnuts), fatty fish, and fruits such as citrus, berries, and stone fruit, such as cherries and peaches. These fruits and vegetables are rich in natural antioxidants and polyphenols—protective compounds that reduce inflammation.

Coffee, which contains polyphenols and other anti-inflammatory compounds, can also reduce free radicals and protect against inflammation.

Foods to avoid. You will want to find healthy substitutes for refined carbohydrates, fried foods (such as French fries), sodas, red meat, processed meat such as luncheon meat, margarine, and lard.

To optimize the gut flora, eat like the Hadza, a small Tanzanian group of indigenous hunter-gatherers believed to have extremely high levels of microbiome diversity. Their diet consists almost entirely of food they find from foraging, including wild berries, fiber-rich tubers, honey, and various wild game. By modifying the Western diet, it is possible to facilitate a healthier gut microbiome.

Two main factors may be as simple as cutting down on unhealthy fats and eating significantly more fiber-rich foods (such as fresh fruits and vegetables). Additional suggestions to improve the gut microbiome include eating fermented foods such as sauerkraut and miso, taking probiotics, and avoiding the unnecessary use of antibiotics. Healthy lifestyle habits that promote a more diverse gut microbiome include reducing stress, avoiding smoking, getting adequate sleep, and exercising regularly.

CLINICAL STRATEGIES FOR PAIN MANAGEMENT

Common treatments for chronic pain include:

- Medication management

- Exercise

- Non-medication therapies such as spinal manipulation, massage, or acupuncture

- Interventional treatments, including injections

- Minimally invasive surgical treatments.

MEDICATIONS

NSAIDS. Nonsteroidal anti-inflammatories are commonly used to treat acute and chronic inflammation pain, with

- Diclofenac 150 mg/day has been reported in some studies as the most effective NSAID for pain relief for osteoarthritis or rheumatoid arthritis. The studies compared diclofenac with naproxen (1000 mg/day), ibuprofen (2400 mg/day), celecoxib (200 mg/day), or acetaminophen (4000 mg/day). Since side effects include renal and hepatic toxicity and gastrointestinal (GI) bleeding that can be potentially fatal, diclofenac is not available over the counter and physician-directed lab monitoring will be required periodically.

- Over the counter NSAIDS such as 200 mg naproxen 1-2 capsules as needed every 12 hours may be preferable due to naproxen's longer duration of action.

- Topical Voltaren and other topical analgesic agents, including lidocaine, capsaicin, and Traumeel can also be used for smaller areas of pain and inflammation.

Antidepressants and anti-seizure medications. Gabapentin (Neurontin) and pregabalin (Lyrica) are prescribed for neuropathic pain (injury to the nerves from the skin that transmit information to the spinal cord and the brain, usually experienced as a burning sensation). These medications work by reducing nerve transmission along the pain pathway of the central nervous system but can cause side effects of drowsiness.

Topical medications:

- Topical preparations, including lidocaine, NSAIDs, and capsaicin, reduce pain when applied to painful joints or to the lumbar region.

- Diclofenac 1% in a topical formulation can be effective for smaller joints near the skin surface, such as those of the hands, elbows, and knees. Formulated as a gel, there is less systemic uptake, so the risk of toxicity is less when taken at the prescribed dosage.

SUPPLEMENTS AND BOTANICALS

Meta-analysis of nutritional supplements for osteoarthritis (the knee, hip, or hand) reported pain reduction in the short term (less than three months). Clinically significant effects were reported for several supplements:

- L-carnitine (an amino acid)

- Pycnogenol, an extract of passion fruit peeling

- Curcumin and frankincense

- Collagen hydrolysate.

Note that, in the long-term, no supplement was found to have clinically significant effects on pain.

Magnesium deficiency. Insufficient levels of magnesium are often a major contributor to chronic low-grade inflammation, and a magnesium oxide supplement in a 500 mg dose has been shown to reduce inflammatory markers such as IL-6 (interleukin 6). Magnesium supplements have also been shown to improve endurance in magnesium-deficient athletes.

Zinc. This critical mineral appears to support the immune system, while reducing several markers of inflammation.

Curcumin. The key ingredient of turmeric, curcumin has been shown to benefit inflammatory conditions and pain. It is a polyphenol that has antioxidant and anti-inflammatory effects. A typical dose is 400-600 mg, three times daily.

Frankincense. Studies have shown that frankincense (*Boswellia serrata* resin) can reduce both inflammation and pain and is a relatively fast-acting supplement that may help with osteoarthritis pain within as little as five days. The typical dosage is an extract containing 30% to 40% boswellic acids, 300–500 mg doses two to three times per day.

Curcumin and frankincense in combination. Using these two botanicals together increases potency, suggested in studies on patients with knee osteoarthritis. Patients sensitive to the gastrointestinal side effects of NSAIDs may tolerate this supplement combination better and still get meaningful pain relief.

PRESCRIPTION OPIOIDS

The use of opioids to treat chronic non-cancer pain is controversial due to limited evidence of long-term efficacy and the potential risk of serious harm. For patients with chronic non-cancer pain, opioids should only be used when non-opioid therapies have not provided sufficient pain relief, resulting in reduced function and/or compromised quality of life.

In terms of decision-making, the potential benefits of opioid therapy should outweigh potential harms. To minimize the amount of opioids required, opioids should be provided in tandem with nonopioid medication and physical treatments including acupuncture, chiropractic, and physical therapy. Treatment should be accompanied by improved physical functioning.

The use of opioids for pain relief requires additional levels of monitoring to assess medication misuse or abuse. Risk factors for misuse of opioids include a personal or family history of substance use disorder, younger age (less than 45 years of age), more severe pain, and/or co-occurring mental health disorders.

A variety of medications are typically prescribed before a trial of opioids, including NSAIDs, and certain antidepressants (Cymbalta-duloxetine, Elavil-amitriptyline) or anti-seizure medications (Gabapentin, Lyrica-pregabalin) to target neuropathic pain.

For patients who require particularly large doses of opioids, resulting in intolerable side effects such as fatigue or drowsiness, implantable spinal delivery systems that provide intrathecal administration of opioids can be considered. Intrathecal analgesic therapy should be reserved for intractable severe pain with significant impact on quality of life that is resistant to all other appropriate treatments.

Newer opioids that stimulate opioid kappa receptors in peripheral tissue (for example, kappa receptors in knee joints) and do not cross the blood-brain barrier may be more effective and safer than traditional opioid drugs and are currently in development.

WORKING WITH A PAIN-MANAGEMENT PHYSICIAN

Seek out a physician who is fellowship-trained and board-certified in pain medicine. Other credentials relevant to pain medicine include residency training in fields such as anesthesiology, neurology, physical medicine and rehabilitation, family medicine, psychiatry, or radiology.

A qualified pain management physician will be comfortable performing a number of different interventional procedures, including nerve blocks, joint injections, and spinal injections. They will be able to evaluate and treat a variety of acute and chronic pain problems, prescribe or optimize appropriate medications, and refer patients for physical therapy and rehabilitation. No single physician is an expert in every treatment and technique, so a qualified doctor should also know when to refer to other experts and subspecialty physicians.

Preparing for a visit. Patients should be prepared in advance to discuss their medical history and pain symptoms in detail:

- When the pain started

- Where it is located

- The quality, intensity, and timing of the pain

- The radiation pattern, if any

- Aggravating and alleviating factors.

Medical records. The patient should collect relevant imaging studies and have a list of treatments, surgeries, and medications tried thus far. The patient should ask the doctor:

- The diagnosis

- The prognosis

- Appropriate treatment options, starting with the most conservative options.

Assessing the physician's expertise. The patient should make sure that the physician is highly skilled in performing any interventional treatments being offered. The patient should get an understanding of what needs to be done to optimize his health and lifestyle to prevent or minimize further pain episodes.

SPECIFIC INTERVENTIONS

Injecting local anesthetics and cortisone. Injections, applied along nerve pathways, interrupt the pain signal, allow restored mobility, and can "reset" a dysfunctional pain pathway. Spinal injections include epidural and facet joint injections that reduce inflammation around compressed spinal nerves and joints due to herniated discs, vertebral degeneration, or spinal stenosis.

Nerve blocks. These are relatively brief treatments that often take only a few minutes to perform. If specialized x-ray equipment is involved and a number of nerves are being injected, the procedure usually takes 10 to 15 minutes. X-rays are usually taken using a fluoroscope, which creates a live image with different viewing angles. Imaging makes the injection process much safer and faster. Most nerve blocks and injections are not overly painful and can be performed in an office setting with just a local anesthetic. However, some spinal injections are performed at a surgery center with light intravenous sedation combined with local anesthetic for patient comfort.

Pain relief should occur relatively quickly, even before you leave the office, because of the rapid-onset of the local anesthetic. The addition of a steroid is designed to promote a longer-lasting anti-inflammatory effect on inflamed nerves and tissues.

Shockwave therapy. Treatment of greater trochanteric pain syndrome, patellar tendinopathy, and Achilles tendinopathy, as well as plantar fasciitis and calcific tendinopathy of the supraspinatus or Achilles tendon, with ESWL shockwave therapy can provide meaningful pain-relief. This is typically performed by a sports medicine doctor.

Minimally invasive surgical treatments. This type of treatment includes nerve ablation (with radiofrequency energy applied through a small needle) and neurostimulation (using small implanted electrodes to minimize nerve transmission along the pain-pathway without causing weakness). Delivery of imperceptible electrical stimulation pulses at specific frequencies across the spinal cord can inhibit the pain circuitry responsible for the transmission of pain. This stimulation reduces the hyperactivity of neurons implicated in chronic pain. Spinal cord and peripheral nerve stimulation is used in a variety of pain syndromes, including persistent spinal or sciatic pain after failed spinal surgery, persistent nerve pain syndromes such as chronic regional pain syndrome (CRPS), extremity pain from ischemia, post-amputation pain, and other peripheral nerve pain syndromes.

Advancements in spinal neurostimulator technology and algorithms. High-frequency spinal stimulation can be provided at a level that is imperceptible, yet offers substantial pain relief in a variety of chronic nerve pain conditions including peripheral neuropathy and chronic spine and sciatic pain. This type of treatment also includes PRP (platelet rich plasma) injections to facilitate improved local tissue healing and remodeling and to promote nerve axon healing and recovery.

Implanted vagal nerve stimulators. Targeted vagal nerve stimulation (VNS) has been demonstrated to reduce pain. A decrease in severity of a variety of pain conditions has been documented in:

- Pelvic pain

- Visceral pain

- Headaches

- Chronic rheumatoid arthritis pain and inflammation

- Epilepsy

- Depression.

The vagus nerve is the longest of the cranial nerves, extending from the brain to the abdomen. Many important autonomic functions in the brain and the body are affected by vagal function (processes that are usually somewhat beyond our awareness and control). Influencing the vagus nerve can normalize neurotransmitter levels, reduce inflammation levels, and regulate metabolism. While implantable vagus nerve stimulation (VNS) is an emerging technology, there are a number of commercially available non-invasive devices that externally stimulate the vagus nerve at the ear or at the neck. The mechanism of VNS pain relief points to anti-inflammatory effects working in conjunction with both central and peripheral pain pathways.

Radiofrequency energy. This type of treatment creates heat generated by radio waves, which can be directed through small needles to lesion sensory nerves, for example to the knee (genicular nerve ablation). Radiofrequency energy can also be applied to lesion areas of inflammation inside spinal discs and vertebral bodies (intradiscal nerve ablation and basivertebral nerve ablation).

Minimally invasive spinal surgery. Other surgical and radiographic advances have allowed the development of minimally invasive spinal surgery (MISS), which can be performed with 3D CT guidance, using small incisions and specialized techniques to minimize tissue disruption and promote rapid recovery.

SELF-MANAGEMENT OF PAIN

Lumbar pain, typically referred to as "having your back go out," is extremely common. Estimates of the prevalence of low back pain have ranged from 22% to 48%, with surveys that found 26% of respondents reported low back pain lasting at least one day in the last three months. Risk factors associated with back pain complaints include smoking, obesity, age, physically strenuous work, sedentary employment, psychologically strenuous work, workers' compensation insurance, and job dissatisfaction. Psychological risk factors include anxiety, depression, and somatization disorder (stress and emotions expressed through the mind-body connection).

The most common diagnosis is non-specific low back pain. These are conditions in which no specific tissue injury can be diagnosed, but the underlying cause is likely to be a combination of muscle, disc, tendon, and/or ligament strain. The vast majority of patients will recover within two weeks with brief episodes of rest (but avoid bed rest), NSAIDs, and muscle relaxants. If sciatica is present, a short course of oral steroids may be appropriate and may provide relief.

If the pain persists beyond two to four weeks and is not improving, then medical evaluation is needed with possible referral for physical therapy, massage, and chiropractic treatment, as well as a review of imaging studies and pain management referral.

MEN'S PAIN VS. WOMEN'S PAIN

Women appear to have a lower pain tolerance than men and require relatively higher doses of pain medication. A greater percentage of women than men have chronic pain. Common chronic pain conditions that are more frequent in women than men include fibromyalgia, migraines, chronic tension-type headaches, irritable bowel syndrome, TMJ pain, and interstitial cystitis. There is evidence that some genes responsible for pain are coded on the X chromosome, and as men's sex chromosomes are XY and women XX, there is increased pain-enhancing genetic expression in women, who are also more likely to develop chronic neck, shoulder, or back pain after a motor vehicle accident, for example. Additionally, testosterone is thought to be protective against pain.

Pain tolerance is an interesting area of study. The research indicates measured differences in pain tolerance of experimental pain. These differences are apparently related to mutations in proteins responsible for opening sodium channels on nerve endings. Some patients may simply transmit pain signals much more readily than others. On the other end of the spectrum, certain mutations of the sodium channel gene SCN9A, for instance, results in the inability to perceive pain, termed Congenital Insensitivity to Pain (CIP).

In summary, chronic pain is extremely common in men, especially in midlife, and can lead to significant distress and lifestyle limitations. Lifestyle factors that minimize chronic inflammation and promote tissue healing and restoration are key to mitigate the risks of developing or worsening chronic pain. Fortunately, greater understanding of the biology of chronic pain and emerging interventions and surgical technologies are allowing men to combat pain more successfully. Emerging high-tech devices, medications, and lifestyle behavioral therapies focus on reducing chronic cellular inflammation. The continued development of the biology of longevity will hopefully allow for the means to prevent the development of chronic pain in the first place.

At the end of the day, the most common question I get from men is,
When can I play golf again?

**For additional information on pain management
and the work of Dr. Longton, please see
www.painmedicineconsultants.com.**

Chapter 11
Coping with a Chronic Lung Condition
Armin Brott & Nancy Faass,
Medical Writers

Winning is the most important thing in my life, after breathing.
Breathing first, winning next.
— George Steinbrenner

Meeting over coffee, Chris brought me up to date on his struggles with bronchitis, which his doctor says is a type of COPD:

The scariest episode I've had lately happened last month. I was just sitting in the living room watching a movie, and all of a sudden, I couldn't breathe. No warning. Instant. Total. Immobilizing. I was gasping for air. I'm not sure how I called the taxi, because I couldn't really talk. I went downstairs and got in the cab, and it started easing up a little bit.

When I got to the ER, it was terrible. I could walk a little, but I still couldn't talk. Approaching a group of nurses, I was gasping for breath. They understood right away, took me in, laid me down, and gave me oxygen. I was on 100% oxygen for about 15 minutes. The oxygen feels so wonderful after being deprived of it. You don't realize how important it is until it's gone. Your mind clears immediately, it's like the clouds just part, and the sun comes out. I could think again!

Chronic obstructive pulmonary disease (COPD) is a group of disabling lung conditions that interfere with the ability to breathe. COPD impedes the airways to the lungs and/or damages the delicate structures deep within the lungs. COPD is the fourth leading cause of premature death among men. It's also a major cause of disability that decreases quality of life, the ability to work and be self-sufficient, and the capacity to enjoy life's simple pleasures.

The five-year life expectancy for people with COPD ranges from 40% to 70%. That means 40 to 70 out of 100 people with COPD will be alive five years after their initial diagnosis. COPD is a chronic, gradually progressing lung disease that is not entirely curable.

Cigarette smoking is the leading cause of COPD and most people who have COPD smoke or smoked in the past. However, most people aren't aware that that there are other factors besides smoking that cause COPD. In fact, less than 40% of people with COPD are smokers at the time of their diagnosis. Further, estimates of *non*-smokers with COPD range from 10% to 30%, so long-term exposure to other lung irritants such as air pollution or workplace toxins apparently also contributes to COPD.

> *In the U.S., more than 32 million people have COPD and 140,000 die each year. Lung cancer is responsible for another 145,000 deaths annually. In addition, pneumonia takes almost 50,000 lives.*

DEFINING COPD

Your lungs are supplied by your airway, the trachea. When you're healthy, your airways are open and elastic, which allows fresh oxygen to come into your lungs, be picked up by your bloodstream, and nourish your entire body. Obstruction or damage in any area of the lung is classified as COPD.

Chronic bronchitis. Your airway branches into two bronchial tubes, one leading to each lung deep within your chest. When these bronchial tubes become inflamed and swollen, that narrows the airways and blocks smaller structures within the lungs. The airways can

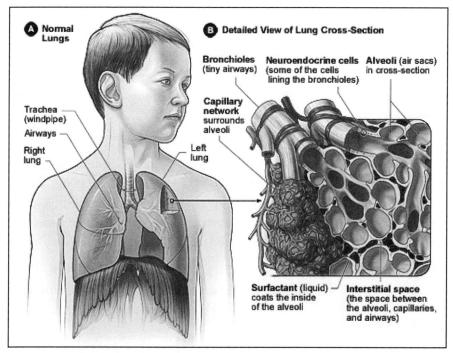

Figure 11.1. The lungs and airways, with a close-up of the alveoli where oxygen is infused into the bloodstream via tiny blood vessels.

become clogged with mucus, causing a chronic cough and discharge. As a result, less air flows into the lungs.

Emphysema. This devastating condition involves damage to the tissue deep within the lobes of the lungs. Seen under a microscope, the lungs are made up of groups of tiny air sacs (called alveoli) that resemble clusters of grapes. Each individual air sac is smaller than 1/100 of an inch (0.2 millimeters).

This intricate tissue absorbs oxygen, which is picked up by fine blood vessels, capillaries that are just 6 microns wide. (Contrast that with human hair, which averages 70 microns wide.) All these delicate lung structures can be damaged by inhaling smoke, particles such as soot or sawdust, or harsh chemicals.

As emphysema progresses, the alveoli can become damaged and distorted, with large irregular pockets or even gaping holes in the walls of each tiny air sac. This damage reduces the amount of oxygen that reaches the bloodstream, draining physical and mental energy.

MAJOR RISK FACTORS

The three most significant risk factors for COPD are smoking, exposure to pollution or toxins, and a family history of respiratory illness (genetics). Other risk factors include:

- Infectious diseases that damage lung tissue, in childhood or adulthood
- Chronic asthma
- Immune deficiency syndromes
- Inflammation of blood vessels
- Connective tissue disorders.

Smoking. Tobacco use is by far the most significant risk factor:

- Between 80% and 90% of people diagnosed with COPD are over 40 years old and either smoke now or used to smoke.
- In addition, 90% of COPD-related *deaths* occur in current or former smokers.
- In general, the more cigarettes smoked and the longer someone smoked, the worse their symptoms.
- While cigarettes cause most lung disorders, pipes, cigars, marijuana overuse, and second-hand smoke are also associated.

Second-hand smoke. Children who are exposed to passive smoke have almost double the risk of developing COPD in adulthood. It usually takes years for lung damage to manifest as chronic respiratory disease, so most people develop it after the age of 60.

Air quality and other environmental factors. Constant exposure to poor quality air laden with particles of soot, dust, or toxic chemicals can irritate your lungs, increasing the risk of COPD. The body of research on these exposures is compelling.

A clever study conducted in London with COPD patients compared their experience walking on a busy city street (Oxford Street) with a walk in Hyde Park. Participants included 40 seniors with COPD, 40 with ischemic heart disease, and 39 healthy age-matched volunteers. Monitoring patient symptoms during a two-hour walk, researchers reported that those with COPD walking on a busy London street experienced twice as much coughing, twice as much shortness of breath, three times the level of mucus, and four times the wheezing. In contrast, after a walk in the park, their lung function was improved for more than 24 hours.

Occupational hazards. Men are subject to a wide range of exposures on the job that put their lung health at risk. These exposures are involved in the production of petroleum, steel,

Environmental and Workplace Exposures	
Smoke and Fumes	**Invasive Particles**
Smoke and industrial emissions, smoke from burning waste or brush, wind-blown dust, pesticides, pollens, smoke from forest fires, bacteria.	Asbestos, coal dust from mining, demolition debris, fiberglass, sandblasting, sawdust from mill work and carpentry.
Chemical emissions from power plants, manufacturing, and cars, including ammonia, carbon monoxide, metals such as lead or mercury, nitrates, nitrogen dioxide, ozone, sulfur dioxide.	PM10 – particulate matter 10 microns or smaller, such as industrial ash and soot (black carbon), dust from construction sites, landfills, and agriculture.
Aerosols, solvents, fumes from welding, numerous other chemicals. In offices, toxins in building materials and furnishings, cleaning products, pesticides.	PM2.5 – fine particles or droplets 2.5 microns or smaller; incomplete combustion of fossil fuels such as coal, diesel fuel, wood, and particulates in auto emissions.

Figure 11.2. Potentially damaging exposures.

chemicals, lumber, and fuels such as coal, as well as the manufacturing of automobiles and in the aerospace, electronics, and consumer goods industries.

Administrative jobs (about one-third of the workforce) are not immune to harmful exposures. Although modern office parks look good, "sick building syndrome" has become another risk in the workplace. Both buildings and furnishings are constructed with artificial materials that off-gas a wide range of chemicals such as formaldehyde. Additionally, a vast array of chemical products are used to clean and maintain these buildings.

COPD from occupational exposures also reflects the interplay between exposures and genetic risk. The frequency, intensity, and duration of the exposure are all factors.

Genetics. Studies of twins in Scandinavia and Holland provided our first real insights into the genetics of COPD:

- The Finnish twins study discovered that people who began smoking before the age of 18 had a 70% risk of retiring from their job early due to disability from COPD.

- The Swedish twins registry reported that about 40% of chronic bronchitis was inherited.

- Dutch researchers found that early antibiotic use increased the risk of asthma by more than 50%. A study of Swedish children found that the risk was doubled.

HOW IT HAPPENS

Chemicals and fumes damage the lungs as irritants. In other cases small particles get deep into the bronchi and into the alveoli. These tiny air sacs, just 1/100 of an inch thick, feed oxygen to the fine blood vessels of the lungs. Large particles cannot lodge there, but extremely fine ones like fiberglass or silica can become embedded, with risk of tremendous damage.

The body creates *granulomas* around foreign particles as a form of protection (just as oysters create a pearl around a grain of sand). That sounds like a good thing, but the presence of granulomas decreases the surface area available for transferring oxygen into the bloodstream. Oxygen is what keeps our cells and tissues alive and functioning.

COPD SYMPTOMS

In the early stages, the symptoms of COPD can be so mild that you may not notice them. Or if you did notice them, you might brush them off as "no big deal" or "it's just part of getting older." Some people even develop workarounds to make the symptoms less of an inconvenience. For example, someone who finds himself breathing hard after going up a flight or two of stairs may start taking the elevator more often. However, the underlying problem is still there. As with any health issue, it's essential to pay attention to your body.

- *Shortness of breath.* Your doctor may describe this as *dyspnea*—the feeling that breathing is hard work or that you can't seem to get enough air. This happens especially when exercising, but it can even happen when even you're doing something as simple as carrying groceries, taking a walk, or going up a flight of stairs.

- *Chronic cough.* A constant cough that produces a lot of mucus (often called "smoker's cough") means that the body is trying to get rid of excess mucus or debris such as dust.

- *Wheezing.* A whistling sound when inhaling or exhaling is usually a sign that the airways are blocked to some degree.

- *Chest pressure or tightness.* Blocked airways create the sense that you can't breathe or can't take a deep breath.

Not everyone who has these symptoms has COPD, and not every person with COPD has these symptoms. If you think you have any of these symptoms, the safe thing to do is to see your healthcare provider and let him or her make a diagnosis.

WHAT YOU CAN DO FOR YOURSELF

Quit smoking. If you're a smoker, quitting is by far the best thing you can do. If you're having trouble quitting on your own, talk to your healthcare provider about prescription options, which may include patches, gum, or prescription medication.

Monitor air quality. When you have COPD, the key is to prevent flare-ups. Minimize your exposure to outdoor air pollution, since the research shows that is a major source of inflammation. Avoid cold dry air, hot humid air, and high altitudes. Higher humidity increases the penetration of particles in the lungs.

Take warnings on air quality seriously. A study at Ohio State University of patients with COPD reported that "exposures even *below* those of air quality standards may still pose significant risks to severe (COPD) subjects."

Preventing flare-ups. Pay close attention to public service announcements about air quality and stay inside when the air outside is especially polluted. If you cannot avoid air pollution, wear an air pollution mask to minimize your exposure.

Signs of Worsening COPD

If you've been diagnosed with COPD, you know how alarming a flare-up can be. Patients usually keep their inhaler and/or oxygen nearby. A pulse oximeter can be an effective tool to measure your actual oxygen level, and they are widely available and affordable. If COPD is a new or emerging condition for you, be on the alert for these symptoms of a potential flare-up.

- Coughing or wheezing more often

- Having to work extremely hard to breathe

- Coughing up more mucus than usual, or mucus that indicates an active infection (darker and thicker mucus)

- Losing weight. For some people with COPD, breathing is so difficult that they burn off more calories inhaling and exhaling than they take in through their food.

- Swelling in the feet, ankles, or legs

- Having a fever.

If you experience any of these symptoms on a regular basis, seek medical attention.

When to call 9-1-1:

- If you're finding it so hard to breathe that you can't walk or talk without gasping

- Sudden mental confusion or inability to think, a sign that your brain is deprived of oxygen

- Visible signs of low oxygen, such as fingernails, lips, or skin that is turning blue

- Coughing up blood

- Having a fever or flu-like symptoms.

People with COPD can die during a flare-up. These are true emergencies that should be handled only by medical experts. Seek emergency care immediately!

- Make sure your employer provides masks, air filters, and other protective equipment. Good ventilation is also vital.

- Avoid dust and places with high levels of dust, cigarette smoke, or other irritants.

- For cleaning, whenever possible use natural products that are less likely to irritate your lungs than bleach and other harsh chemicals. That said, when mold is present, consider spraying it with bleach and then eliminate the bleach residue with soap and water.

Beware of that romantic fireplace or campfire if you have COPD. Avoid backyard barbeques and fire pits, as well as indoor fireplaces and wood-burning stoves. Wood smoke and smoke from burning other natural materials (biomass) is associated with increased risk of COPD, as well as a higher risk of cardiovascular disease, deep respiratory infection, lung cancer, and cataracts.

Filter the air in your home. HEPA filters can be invaluable. Air conditioners can also be effective, although they create extremes of temperature in the home.

Clean house. Keep your home clean and free from excess dust.

- Minimize home accessories that can harbor dust, dust mites, and molds, such as throw pillows, drapery, and rugs. Wash bedding and comforters frequently.

- For dusting throughout the house, spraying surfaces with an aerosol such as CitriSafe or a spray solution (four parts water to one part rubbing alcohol with three drops of essential oil, such as lemongrass or lemon). For bathroom cleaning, you can use this product daily if needed and save the bleach for periodic deep cleaning. Another option if you're sensitive to chemicals but prefer cleaning with bleach is a solution of four parts water to one part bleach.

- Ensure that your cooking vent is working correctly so cooking fumes will be drawn up and out of the house. This is surprisingly important because some burned fats are carcinogenic (meaning that they cause cancer). Good ventilation is also essential when using a gas stove.

- Consider containing your mattress and your pillow in a dust-mite and allergy mattress cover or wrapping your mattresses in heavy plastic to cut down on dust and mold. Allergy covers are also available for pillows.

Dealing with damp areas and mold. Avoid mold and mildew, which occur when there is too much moisture. Install air filters and use a dehumidifier. This matters. Mold can be drawn into the general ventilation system, where it can persist for months or years.

- When mold is severe (in the shower or on the windows), try using a small spray bottle filled with full-strength bleach. (Keep the windows wide open, ventilating the room well.) Within 15 minutes, you can clean the bleach off those surfaces with soap and water to minimize your exposure. Some molds can be removed effectively with a weak solution of one or two parts water to one part bleach. For other types, such as black mold, undiluted bleach appears to be essential.

- Inform yourself about the chemical products you use to clean your home and to maintain your yard or garden. With the exception of killing mold, use chemicals very sparingly.

Talk with your physician about supplements that support lung health. At the top of your short list might be a quality multivitamin, vitamin A, C, and D3.

Identifying food sensitivities. Undiagnosed food allergies and sensitivities can be a major factor in COPD. Dairy products, for example, can trigger respiratory symptoms in someone who is sensitive. According to the National Library of Medicine, about two-thirds of humans can't digest lactose after infancy. (Casein, the protein in milk, can also trigger reactions.)

Tommy and his brothers were all known for their antics. His first asthma attack at the age of 8 was triggered by his big brother's science experiment, with a dramatic release of sulfur that shut down Tommy's bronchi. Later in life, he found that fruit preserved with sulfur made him wheeze and so did wine with sulfur preservative. To keep food additives at a minimum, he shopped in the farmer's markets and the organic section of the grocery store, and was able to avoid further flare-ups.

An elimination diet is something you can explore on your own. This can be surprisingly useful in figuring out whether certain foods or food additives are a factor in your health. The top five foods that tend to cause the most reactions are milk products, wheat, corn, soy, and eggs. Food reactivity is highly individual, and there are wide variations in food tolerance from one person to the next.

When you reintroduce foods into your diet, there is the risk of a flare-up, so talk with your doctor before starting an elimination diet.

COMPLEMENTARY ACTIVITIES

Staying active. Talk to your healthcare provider about how much physical activity and what kinds of activities are best for you. These might include stretching, yoga, or tai chi, mild forms of aerobic exercise such as walking, or adapted weight training.

Walking. If you want to get back in shape, you'll be encouraged to know that the majority of the studies report some degree of benefit from walking. Ideas to consider included the use of a pedometer. A joint study in Chile and the U.K. on COPD found that patients using pedometers averaged 3,000 more steps a day compared with patients who didn't use one.(6)

Yoga. The potential benefit of yoga in the care of COPD patients has been researched at medical schools and hospitals that include the Chicago Medical School, the University of Vermont, and Baylor College of Medicine in Houston. Yoga was found to be beneficial in all the studies: The Chicago study reported better lung function, improved vital capacity, and higher quality of life. A Swedish study on yoga for COPD patients reported: "improved physical symptoms...greater energy, stamina, and body awareness, and a new sense of control over their breathing in different situations." (For more information on yoga practice, see chapter 40, "Yoga for Real Men.")

Among the various types of exercise suggested by your physician, the best are the ones that you *enjoy* and can maintain.

Acupuncture in the treatment of COPD. Of 18 recent studies on acupuncture treatment for COPD, none found harm and 16 reported measurable benefit, including: better exercise tolerance and reduced shortness of breath, superior exercise time, better oxygen saturation, improvement on the 6-Minute Walk Test and in quality of life, reduced acute flares in 80% of participants, and improved blood oxygen levels.

RESOURCES

American Lung Association, available at www.Lung.org.

COPD Foundation, www.copdfoundation.org.

Aly Cohen, MD, Frederich vom Saal, PhD. *Non-Toxic: Guide to Living Healthy in a Chemical World.* Oxford, U.K.: Oxford University Press, 2020.

N. Wise. *The Modern Organic Home: 100+ DIY Cleaning Products, Organization Tips, and Household Hacks.* New York, N.Y.: Good Books, 2018.

For information on the work of Armin Brott, please see:
www.MrDad.com.
For the work of Nancy Faass, please see:
www.HealthWritersGroup.com.

Chapter 12
Environmental Allergies
Matthew Lodewick, MD, Allergist

A new study found that a mother's diet affects her baby's allergies. Which can only mean one thing. My mom ate cats.
— Jimmy Fallon

It is difficult to feel genuinely optimized when you have allergies. You may not die of hay fever, but your quality of life will undoubtedly suffer. Hay fever is like having the common cold, but it lasts for weeks or even months. Who wants to wake up every day with itchy eyes, a runny nose, sneezing. That negatively impacts mood, sleep, energy level, and cognitive function. If this sounds like you, get help!

A third of all men suffer from allergies, and managing the symptoms can improve your mood, sleep, energy and mental processes.

UNDERSTANDING ALLERGIES

What is an allergy? Your immune system has evolved to recognize invaders—to differentiate self and not-self. An allergy occurs when your immune system overreacts to a foreign substance that is not usually dangerous. When you come into contact with that material, your immune system generates inflammation that can range from itching to difficulty breathing that is life-threatening (anaphylaxis).

Your immune system produces substances known as antibodies. If you have allergies, your immune system makes antibodies referred to as IgE (immune globulin E antibodies) that identify specific allergens as harmful, even though they aren't. The allergic response is immune controlled through the IgE antibodies, which recognize specific protein structures. Their response is clear and targeted.

If you come into contact with that particular allergen, your immune system's reaction can inflame your skin, sinuses, airways, or digestive system.

When an allergy-causing molecule triggers an allergic reaction, your immune system unleashes a protective response. First, it sends a chemical signal to *mast cells* that are located

Mechanism of allergy

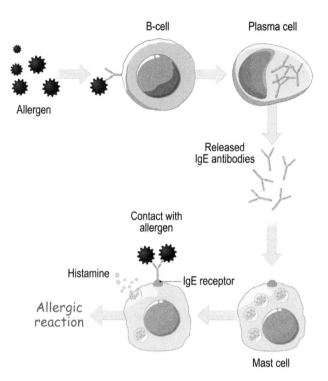

Figure 12.1 Recognition by IgE antibodies drives the release of histamine and the rapid development of symptoms.

in your skin, mouth, nose, lungs, gasrointestinal system, and blood. The chemical signal causes the mast cells to release histamines (stored within the mast cells), causing inflammation and increased blood flow in the area of the allergen. Histamines activate receptors to increase the production of mucous, making you cough and sneeze to dislodge and remove the allergen, inadvertently clogging your nasal passages. Histamine is the chief driving factor involved in allergies, causing a range of responses in different systems. For the eyes, this can mean tearing, itchy, and red eyes. For the nose, it can mean sneezing, nasal congestion, and a runny nose. And for the chest, it can mean chest tightness, wheezing, and shortness of breath.

Common allergens. Men and women are prone to the same types of sensitizations, which include dust mites, pet dander, and pollen. However, as we enter into our later years (70s and 80s), like the rest of our immune function, the allergic response begins to weaken.

ENVIRONMENTAL CONTROL

A cornerstone of allergy management is knowing your triggers and altering the environment to reduce exposures. Some measures like dust mite control are straightforward and hinge on encasing the bedding (pillow, mattress, comforter/duvet), vacuuming and dusting regularly, reducing upholstered furniture, eliminating carpets, having heating and air conditioning ducts cleaned, and reducing humidity below 50%. Other control measures are less feasible.

HEPA filters. People often ask about the value of HEPA (high efficiency particulate air) filters to control allergies. For years, there was hope that they could keep a home allergen free. Unfortunately, they do not. However, they can help some. I would recommend a HEPA filter in a home with a pet as another means to reduce the full extent of pet allergen exposure, as well as in a home where vacuuming and cleaning are not routine. Additionally, HEPA filters are beneficial in reducing indoor particulate matter when air quality indexes move into unhealthy ranges. There are a number of manufacturers of HEPA filters. When making a choice, it is important to look at the volume of the room that the filter will be cleaning. It is also important to look for a unit that operates quietly. Some top brands include Blueair, Rabbit Air, and Honeywell.

Pet ownership. Pets can be a particular challenge, and the only effective means of environmental control is to remove the animal from the indoor living environment. Allergy shots are a particularly useful idea to explore in a situation where removing the pet from your home will make the other members of the family extremely upset. If a member of the household experiences wheezing and poorly controlled asthma from the pet's presence, remove the pet. Two of every three homes has a pet, so allergy shots (allergen immunotherapy) should be considered the cornerstone of management for an individual whose occupation or lifestyle involves recurring exposures to others' homes.

A full discussion of environmental control to the varying air-borne allergens is beyond the scope of this book, but can be found through a local allergist and resources such as the American Academy of Allergy, Asthma and Immunology (AAAAI.org) and the National Institute of Environmental Health Sciences (niehs.nih.gov).

Testing. I do not believe there is an area of medicine that is more suffused with quackery than allergy testing. Skin sensitivity tests and specific IgE serologic (blood) tests are accurate. Avoid laser allergy testing, IgG allergy testing, and muscle strength testing for allergies (these are but a few of the tests to avoid).

Validated allergy tests are very sensitive at identifying substances that cause an individual to make allergic antibodies, but they are not good at evaluating the severity of the allergy.

Severity is best evaluated by seeing the results through the filter of a person's responses to the specific allergen exposure. Keep in mind that year-round chronic exposure is likely to present chronic symptoms like nasal congestion whereas acute, sudden exposures may lead to striking presentation of new symptoms such as sneezing. As a result, for many people it is harder to recognize perennial allergies triggered by frequent exposure because they experience these symptoms daily.

TREATMENT

Once you identify your allergic sensitizations and control your environmental exposures, you can proceed with medication management. Fortunately, the medical options for allergy management are excellent and the majority of these are available over the counter.

ANTIHISTAMINES

Because of the ease of use, antihistamines tend to be the first medication instituted for management. There are first-generation and later-generation antihistamines (minimally sedating).

Increased risk of dementia. I would advise avoidance of first-generation antihistamines, as long-term use may be associated with an increased risk of dementia.

In a study of individuals 65 and older, daily use of Benadryl (and similar agents) for three or more years increased the risk of dementia by more than 50%.

First-generation antihistamines include Benadryl (diphenhydramine), Atarax (hydroxyzine), Chlor-Trimeton (chlorpheniramine), Dimetapp (brompheniramine), and Dramamine II (meclizine). These over-the-counter medications are also associated with drowsiness.

Later-generation antihistamines do not appear to have this problem. Products considered safer include Zyrtec (cetirizine), Claritin (loratadine), Allegra (fexofenadine), Xyzal (levocetirizine), and Clarinex (desloratadine). The later-generation antihistamines tend to be a nice "go-to" medication because they seem to have minimal side-effects (few experience drowsiness) and are long-acting (lasting 24 hours). Since they have a rapid onset of action, they can be used on an as-needed basis. Still, regular use is likely to be more effective than as-needed use in an allergy sufferer experiencing repeated exposures. These medications tend to be most helpful for symptoms of itchy eyes and nose, sneezing, and nasal discharge.

ALLERGY MEDICATIONS

Nasal steroids. The most effective allergy medications are the nasal steroids, which are now available over the counter. Nasal steroids actively reduce the number of inflammatory cells that drive the inflammation, rather than just blocking the release of histamine. The challenge with nasal steroids is that they require consistent use to achieve the benefit, and the onset can be slow, with maximal benefit achieved after 1 to 2 weeks of regular use. The other hitch is that they need to be squirted up the nose. Fortunately, nasal steroids have an excellent safety profile with daily use. However, I recommend that those who have year-round need of nasal steroids consider allergen immunotherapy since safety studies for the use of nasal steroids over many years duration are limited.

However, seasonal use for an individual with spring or fall allergies has an excellent safety profile (chief side effects include headache and bloody nose, which can be reduced by reviewing proper techniques for administering the medication). Furthermore, for the seasonal allergy sufferer, the use of a nasal steroid preceding the onset of pollen season and throughout the season can decrease the exponential rise in allergic antibodies (and associated exponential rise in seasonal sensitization) that commonly occurs in the allergy sufferer with seasonal allergies.

Side effects:

With any over-the-counter medication, I think it best to always consult with the local pharmacist. These professionals are an under-utilized resource.

Risks of oral decongestants in combination with antihistamines. These medications can have an additive effect when taken in combination with oral antihistamines.

Hypertension associated with oral decongestants. Sudafed and other oral decongestants have a number of side effects including hypertension, headache, and insomnia. Oral decongestants have notable stimulant properties that can interfere with mood and cause agitation. As a result, I recommend against using oral decongestants. These should be avoided in those with underlying medical conditions such as heart disease, glaucoma, thyroid disease, and bladder conditions.

Risks of nasal decongestants. Even more troubling are the nasal decongestants which reduce congestion almost instantly, but whose use over just a few days will lead to a congestion more profound and severe than the initial congestion. This is thought to be the result of the downregulation of receptors on the nasal mucosal surface.

Herbal medications. There are a number of other over-the-counter touted allergy medications. Please realize that any medication that is labeled as homeopathic is driven completely by the placebo effect. They tend to be ineffective. Additionally, there are a lot of over-the-counter touted naturopathic/herbal remedies such as stinging nettle, quercetin, and local honey that also likely work as a result of the placebo effect (if they work at all). Butterbur is an herb that has shown some benefit, but it should be recognized that herbal preparations such as butterbur have no meaningful safety monitoring, poor quality control, commonly contain multiple ingredients/chemicals/metals, and are not risk free just because they are herbal products. Butterbur, for example, has been associated with cancer and liver disease, including cirrhosis. I would strongly recommend avoiding these products.

Prescription medication with an FDA warning. If you are experiencing allergies that are not controlled by an oral antihistamine or nasal steroid, then a leukotriene blocker such as Singulair (montelukast) and/or a nasal antihistamine such as Astelin (azelastine) ought to be considered. Despite their prescription status, these medications are rarely game changing for achieving allergy control. The leukotriene blockers don't help everyone, but can be surprisingly useful in the responsive individual. Unfortunately, the FDA recently added a boxed warning note as possible psychiatric side effects have been experienced in some individuals taking leukotriene blockers.

However, the oral antihistamines and the nasal steroids, either alone or in combination, work the best. Nasal antihistamines are much more likely to be helpful than leukotriene blockers, particularly for those experiencing sneezing and runny nose.

The trouble with medications is that they are a temporary fix for a chronic condition. They have no long-term efficacy, and when a man stops his medications, he is symptomatic again.

IMMUNOTHERAPY

Fortunately, allergy desensitization (allergy shots) offers a long-term solution.

Immunotherapy shots. Treatment with immunotherapy reprograms the immune system's response to an exposure to allergens and creates long-term tolerance. This effect can be long-standing, persisting for years and even decades.

The challenge of immunotherapy is that it involves slowly increasing exposures to allergens, and there is a risk for an anaphylactic reaction. (Anaphylaxis is a severe allergic reaction to a specific food, medication, or venom, such as bee sting. The reaction can include a rash, low heartbeat, shock, or difficulty breathing.) As a result, shots are delivered in the physician's office with a 30-minute observation period before you are allowed to leave.

The other challenge is that the dose of immunotherapy has to start at a very low level in order to assure that it is unlikely to cause an allergic reaction. These shots are then increased gradually (up to twice a week) until you reach the goal dosage. This requires approximately

30 to 35 visits. Once at this dose, immunotherapy is traditionally continued once a month for five years. While the commitment to immunotherapy can seem daunting, it allows a man to be free of allergies and allergy medications.

Oral immunotherapy (sublingual). Other developments provide additional options beyond allergy shots. There is another form of immunotherapy called sublingual immunotherapy that involves taking drops of the allergen at very low doses under the tongue or the use of a dissolving tablet. Sublingual immunotherapy is widely available in Europe.

In the United States, sublingual immunotherapy is just becoming available, and FDA approved options are limited to ragweed pollen, grass pollen, and dust mite allergen. Allergy shots are likely to be more effective than sublingual in most patients. Sublingual immunotherapy likely is best when an individual is being desensitized to one or just a few allergens.

One advantage sublingual immunotherapy has over traditional allergy shots is reduced risk of an anaphylactic reaction. After an initial dose in the office with observation, a person traditionally can continue their immunotherapy from home. Sublingual immunotherapy is available through allergists. It is best to find a reputable allergist for sublingual immunotherapy as the benefit can vary by dosing, and there are many who prescribe a dose that is too low to likely yield significant benefit.

Steroid injections. Some clinicians consider a steroid injection to be an "allergy shot." A seasonal dosage of an intramuscular steroid is not an actual allergy shot, but it can give an individual relief that lasts days to weeks. The benefit of steroid injections can be variable, but they have the risk of systemic side-effects associated with steroids such as increased appetite, changes in mood, or lower resistance to infection. In contrast, nasal steroids have minimal systemic side effects.

ADVERSE REACTIONS

Asthma. While the focus of this chapter has been environmental allergies, I did want to take some time to speak briefly about other allergic conditions. Environmental allergies are a common cause of asthma. Asthma treatment is straightforward and effective. Symptoms of asthma include cough, wheeze, chest tightness, and shortness of breath. The key feature of asthma is that it is a reversible state and symptoms wax and wane (particularly in response to triggers). Rescue inhalers like albuterol should temporarily alleviate symptoms. Some common triggers for asthma include viral infections, stress, and exercise. Tobacco smoke is a notable trigger associated with heightened risk for accelerated and persisting loss of lung function and even death. The good news for men is that they tend to be less predisposed to the late onset of asthma we see in women unless there is chronic pet exposure.

Penicillin allergy. There are many other allergic conditions not covered here, but special attention is merited by penicillin allergy because it is of significant medical importance. Those who have penicillin allergy are at much higher risk of drug-resistant infections due to the substitution of more broad-spectrum antibiotics. Additionally, penicillin sensitivity resolves over a ten-year period in approximately 80% of those with a history of this allergy.

There are other forms of life-threatening adverse drug reactions, so it is imperative that a careful history be conducted to clarify the type of reaction that occurred and determine if skin testing and a graded challenge are indicated. Validated drug testing is currently limited to the penicillin/amoxicillin class of medications, but the penicillin skin tests are of high quality. Almost all of the individuals with negative penicillin skin tests tolerate penicillin well, with less than 3% experiencing mild symptoms on re-exposure and virtually no reports of severe symptoms with re-exposure. One last note with respect to penicillin testing is that while the skin test is valuable and accurate, the currently available blood test has no value and can add confusion to care, as it is prone to false positives (inaccurately showing potential reactivity to penicillin when there is none).

Insect stings. Reactions due to honey bees, wasps, yellow jackets, and hornets are also worth a brief discussion as there is highly effective management available, and many patients are unaware of the options. Stings from Hymenoptera provoke anaphylaxis in less than 1% of the population. However, once individuals become sensitive, subsequent stings precipitate anaphylaxis 30% to 60% of the time in them. Allergen immunotherapy (allergy shots) can reduce this risk to 5% or less. Fire ant immunotherapy may have less efficacy, but remains the best option for an individual who has experienced an allergic reaction to fire ant stings.

HOW TO FIND A GOOD ALLERGIST

The value of seeking the care of the best-qualified physicians in your area cannot be overstated. Often there are many competent allergy physicians available. A quality primary physician is an excellent resource for helping you find a good allergist. A good allergist has undergone rigorous training, completing medical school, a residency in either pediatrics or internal medicine, a combined adult and pediatric allergy/immunology fellowship, and received board certification through the American Board of Allergy and Immunology (ABAI.org). They may also be certified by the National Board of Physicians and Surgery (NBPAS.org).

For more information on the work of Dr. Lodewick, please see:
www.BayAreaAllergy.com.

Chapter 13
Circulation: Your Life Depends on It!
Michael Ingegno, MD, Vascular Surgeon,
Judson Brandeis, MD, Urologist,
& Nancy Faass, MSW, MPH, Medical Writer

Perfect health depends on perfect circulation.
— Ellen G. White

Peripheral artery disease (PAD) is a circulatory condition in which narrowed arteries reduce blood flow to the legs and arms. As it progresses, PAD also has the potential to compromise the blood flow to your brain, heart, and genitals.

Deep vein thrombosis (DVT) is a disorder involving plaque or a blood clot in the veins of the leg. A pulmonary embolism (PE) occurs when a large blood clot breaks free and floats up into the lungs.

Acute episodes of peripheral artery disease and deep vein thrombosis are potentially fatal.

Always a golfer, Bill was looking forward to playing more often now that he'd retired. Yet over the last several months, he found himself really dragging by the time he reached the back nine. He needed to stop and rest at every hole. Instead of seeing his doctor, Bill started using the electric golf carts. Gradually the pain got worse until it was constant and sometimes excruciating. At that point, he picked up the phone.

His primary care doctor suggested that he see a vascular surgeon. When the specialist reviewed Bill's health history, it looked like a checklist for diseased arteries—aging, a history of heart disease, smoking, weight gain, and limited physical activity now that he couldn't play golf.

Ultrasound imaging at the doctor's office showed plaque buildup and narrowing of the large arteries in his thighs. When he was resting, his circulation was about 70% of normal, which is why he had no symptoms if he was lounging around the house. The golf course was a different story. His pain occurred whenever he tried to walk any distance.

The diagnosis—peripheral artery disease—didn't seem like that big a deal.

But the doctor cautioned him: Over a six-year period, half of men with peripheral artery disease die from a cardiovascular event.

Bill's surgeon outlined the various options—exercising more and smoking less, managing his blood pressure, managing his weight. He decided to try lifestyle changes before considering surgery. After three months of conservative therapy, it was clear to Bill that the pain was still too much for him to tolerate. He wanted to be able to be active and to play golf again.

Further discussions ensued with his vascular surgeon. The options included angioplasty (balloon expansion of a narrowed artery), possible plaque removal (atherectomy), stenting, or a surgical bypass of the blocked artery in his thigh.

The surgeon pointed out that angioplasty was minimally invasive and seemed like a good option for him. A week later he underwent the procedure at his doctor's office, with mild sedation, local anesthesia, and excellent results. His surgeon confided that ten years ago this technology did not exist, and Bill would have required open surgery in the hospital and a synthetic bypass.

The treatment required follow-up with his surgeon and an occasional ultrasound. Bill takes statins, low-dose aspirin, and tracks his blood pressure. And he's absolutely serious about his lifestyle—tobacco free, back in shape, optimal weight, and best of all, pain-free.

THE SECRET LIFE OF ARTERIES AND VEINS

If you lined up all the arteries in your body, they would encircle the earth. How can a muscle the size of a cantaloupe pump blood 25,000 miles? It has to do with the structure of the arteries.

Although the heart is a pump, maintaining blood pressure requires assistance from the arteries. The wall of an artery is composed of muscle and stretchy connective tissue. When the heart pumps, the artery facilitates the passage of blood by stretching and widening. The artery itself then contracts to push blood forward into progressively smaller and smaller arteries and then into finer and finer capillaries. The inner lining of the arteries (the intima) is covered with specialized smooth muscle tissue, the endothelial cells, which enable easy, unhindered blood flow.

The endothelia prevent clotting, plaque build-up, and resistance to blood flow. The blood vessels continue to branch out like the limbs of a tree as the structures become smaller and smaller in order to nourish every cell in the body. In the fine capillaries, blood provides oxygen and nutrients directly to the cells and tissues in exchange for carbon dioxide and waste.

Here's where it gets interesting. Blood must return to the heart through the *veins*, which lack the thick, muscular wall of the arteries.

The Structure of an Artery Wall

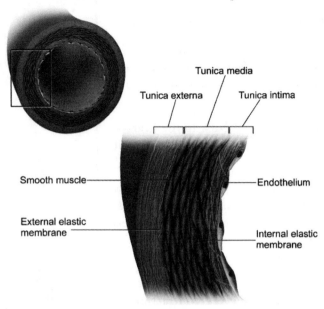

Figure 13.1 The structure of an artery wall, showing the multiple layers of muscle.

PERIPHERAL ARTERY DISEASE (PAD)

As men age, plaque (fatty and fibrous material) accumulates between the layers that line the inside of the artery walls, which causes narrowing of the arteries.

A 50% narrowing of an artery results in a 75% reduction in blood flow.

Deposits of fats gradually become calcified and stiff, especially at branching points of the arteries where there is turbulence in blood flow. These areas include the branching of the arteries that supply the pelvis and legs (and hence the association between poor circulation and erectile dysfunction). In fact, researchers now consider conditions such as atherothrombosis as a single disease, an underlying disorder that can manifest as:

- Impaired circulation (intermittent claudication)
- Erectile dysfunction
- Angina (both stable and unstable)
- Coronary artery disease
- Heart attack
- Stroke due to a blood clot
- Critical limb conditions due to a blood clot (gangrene, necrosis)
- Sudden death.

Why It's Important to Stay Active

Once blood reaches the tips of our toes, given the distance from the heart, how is it possible to get blood back up the legs, working against the force of gravity?

The veins must move blood back to the heart—yet the veins are too far from the heart to benefit from its pumping action.

Instead, blood is moved through the veins by the action of the large muscles in our legs, progressively squeezing the veins. With each step we take, our thigh and calf muscles squeeze the veins as we walk or move.

Within the veins are a series of one-way valves that trap the blood after every contraction of the muscles to keep the blood from draining backwards, due to the pull of gravity. Every step as we walk literally moves the blood forward to the next compartment of the vein, as the contraction of the muscle squeezes the veins.

Our system of veins works only when we are physically active. Before the development of mechanical transportation, most people walked everywhere they needed to go, so getting enough physical activity to keep circulation up was not an issue. Today, however, our sedentary lifestyle is a mismatch for our physiology.

We need to be physically active in order to pump blood back to our lungs for fresh oxygen.

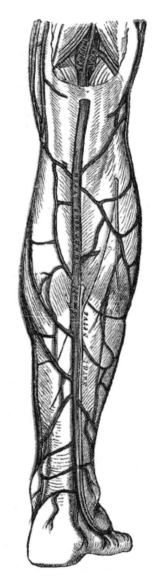

Figure 13.2 Major veins of the leg.

Researchers point out that although antithrombotic therapies (including "clot busters") are safe and efficient, disease and premature deaths are still unacceptably high.

Risk factors. At least 10% of men over 55 have a significant decrease in blood flow to their legs. Risk factors include age, tobacco use, elevated cholesterol, high blood pressure, diabetes, and sedentary lifestyle.

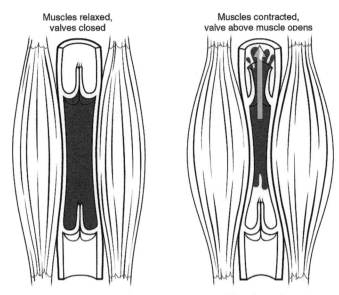

Figure 13.3. How the leg muscles move blood up the veins toward the heart, against gravity.

Progression. Just as one car accident can block traffic on an entire highway, one area of serious atherosclerotic disease can significantly reduce blood flow to an organ or limb. Chronic circulatory insufficiency develops over years, as plaque slowly accumulates and calcifies inside the arteries. Acute insufficiency can occur when a piece of plaque breaks off, usually from a larger vessel, and blocks another blood vessel, reducing or obstructing circulation.

Symptoms. Typical symptoms and presentation of peripheral artery disease include:

- *Pain with exertion (claudication).* Claudication is pain that occurs with increased activity, as the leg arteries become increasingly diseased and narrow. Symptoms in the legs include fatigue and cramping or pain, commonly in the feet, calves, thighs, or buttocks. These symptoms are worse with exercise, because of the increased demand for oxygen, and they improve with rest.

- *Rest pain.* As the blockage worsens, pain progresses to pain without exertion. This condition is referred to as *ischemic* rest pain, describing a condition in which there is a lack of oxygen to the tissues. If circulation is severely compromised, patients may experience ongoing discomfort and pain, even at rest, limiting activities and restorative sleep.

- *Non-healing ulcerations.* Some men present with chronic or slow-healing lower leg wounds. These wounds start as accidental cuts or scrapes and develop slowly as pressure ulcers on the legs or toes due to poor circulation.

■ *Cold hands and feet.* Poor circulation is a classic cause of cold hands and feet, which are the furthest points from the heart.

No symptoms? It is estimated that there are three times as many men with peripheral artery disease who have no symptoms compared with symptomatic patients.

However, be honest with yourself. If you have sores that take forever to heal, leg pain after walking up the stairs, and chronically cold feet and hands, you now know enough to seek medical advice.

Diagnosis and treatment. The initial diagnosis of peripheral artery disease of the legs is made by comparing resting systolic blood pressure at the ankle to the higher systolic blood pressure in the upper arm. If there seems to be a significant difference, an ultrasound of the blood vessels is commonly used to identify the location and severity of the blockage.

Prevention of arterial blockages. Physicians typically recommend a strategy similar to that for reducing the risk of heart disease, including:

■ Smoking cessation

■ Lipid and cholesterol-lowering medication

■ Aggressive treatment of high blood pressure and diabetes

■ Antiplatelet therapy to prevent clots.

Surgical procedures. Reduced blood flow and oxygen to the tissues is termed *chronic ischemia.* Some men have circulatory issues that are either so painful, or so threatening to their health, they require surgery to open the blockage or to create a bypass. Major circulatory issues are addressed with procedures performed inside the artery (endovascular interventions). This is achieved by puncturing the femoral artery at the groin and advancing a balloon, and sometimes a stent (a tube), to the area of narrowing. By dilating the narrowed area and placing a permanent stent, the artery will remain open. For men with difficult anatomy, open surgery with an arterial bypass using a synthetic graft is an option.

DEEP VEIN THROMBOSIS (DVT)

Bruce was flying high. The meeting in Shanghai could not have gone better. The months of preparation and time away from his wife and three children finally seemed to have paid off. Two days of straight meetings and intense negotiations with his Chinese supply chain sealed the deal. Bruce's company would have a huge leg up on their competition. On the flight home, Bruce did a few celebratory whiskey shots with his colleagues and quickly drifted off to sleep. Amazingly, when Bruce woke up, he could see the Golden Gate Bridge in the distance. He made a futile attempt to stretch his legs and then gave it up. Now that the deal was in place, next time Bruce would fly business class. He wanted to get up and use the bathroom, but the seatbelt light was on.

Finally, Bruce was able to get his carry-on and headed off the plane. He realized that he was walking rather gingerly on his right leg. An old soccer injury and cramped plane, he thought. Strange how he could barely put on his right shoe. At the baggage carrousel, he called Elaine to tell her how well the meetings went. His wife was excited to see him, and he could hear his kids jumping up and down in the background. Finally, his baggage came, and Bruce started limping to the curb where his Uber was waiting to pick him up. Again, he noticed how strangely his right leg felt, like a log.

The black Hyundai rolled to the curb, and Bruce stuffed his large frame into the back. The traffic on the 880 was crawling. Bruce was checking his email when he felt a pang of chest pain. And then sudden shortness of breath. His mind started racing. "What is going on? I'm only 38, and no one in my family has heart disease. I eat pretty well and stay in shape as best I can. Maybe it is just anxiety." Sweat began rolling down his forehead, and Bruce frantically rolled down the window to get some air.

"You all right back there?" the Uber driver questioned. Bruce knew something was wrong. "I need to go to the Emergency Room right away!"

Fortunately, there was a hospital at the next exit. Bruce called his wife. He didn't know what to say. He didn't want to scare her, but at the same time, something was dreadfully wrong. Rolling up to the Emergency Room, Bruce was laboring to breathe. The triage nurse took one look a Bruce and his swollen right foot which was no longer able to fit into his shoe. "How long was his flight?"

The rest of the day was a blur. IV fluids, oxygen, CT scan, the ICU, and clot-busting drugs. The triage nurse had seen this many times before. An otherwise healthy businessman is sleeping on a long flight, gets dehydrated, and develops a blood clot in his leg, which travels up to the lungs, causing a pulmonary embolism. In fact, she had one last week who didn't make it. She was determined not to have that happen again. The image of the wife and young family sobbing in the Emergency waiting room was still fresh in her memory.

It took a week in the hospital before Bruce was released. They even had to place an umbrella-shaped filter in his vena cava to prevent the rest of the clot in his right leg from dislodging. As it turned out, Bruce had a common genetic clotting disorder that had gone undetected, but the two days of negotiations and the long flight had created the perfect conditions for forming a blood clot. Fortunately for Bruce, he made it, but a quarter of men with pulmonary emboli die suddenly.

A blood clot in your lung (pulmonary embolus) CAN KILL YOU, even if you are otherwise healthy. This is more common than one would think.

Risk factors for chronic vein disease. Increased risk is associated with advancing age, family history of venous disease, obesity, smoking, prolonged standing, and sedentary lifestyle.

Symptoms of poor vein circulation. Symptoms that your circulation is becoming impaired include changes such as edema; dry, peeling, or shiny skin; changes in skin color on feet or toes; brittle nails; or skin ulcers.

Progression. Damaged or incompetent valves can result in blood pooling or flowing backward. Slow-flowing venous blood can lead to clotting (*thrombosis*) of veins as well as dilated veins.

Triggers of an acute DVT episode. Situations that increase the threat of DVT include a history of immobilization, recent surgery or trauma, obesity, heart disease, or a vascular disorder. DVT is common after long plane flights and after orthopedic hip or knee surgeries.

Symptoms of acute DVT. Deep vein thrombosis should be suspected in men who present with sudden leg swelling, pain, warmth, and redness of the calf or the entire leg.

Surprisingly, DVT can occur in individuals who are otherwise fit and healthy.

On physical exam, there will be dilated superficial veins and swelling, warmth, and pain on one side greater than the other. Some men present with sudden chest pain or shortness of breath.

If you have symptoms of DVT or a pulmonary embolism, and especially if you have recently been on a long, confining airplane flight or had hip or knee surgery, seek medical attention IMMEDIATELY.

Testing. An ultrasound is a simple and non-invasive diagnostic test used to diagnose suspected deep vein thrombosis. Ultrasound with Doppler flow is highly accurate in making a definitive diagnosis. Situations that involve leg pain without deep venous thrombosis are likely the result of muscle strain or tear, lymphatic obstruction, cellulitis, or superficial thrombophlebitis.

Incidence. The precise number of people affected by deep venous thrombosis/pulmonary embolism is unknown, although as many as 900,000 people could be affected (1 or 2 per 1,000) each year in the United States.

- Estimates suggest that 60,000 to 100,000 people in the U.S. die annually of DVT/PE (also termed *venous thromboembolism*).

- It is estimated that 10% to 30% of people with DVT die within one month of diagnosis.

- Among people who have had a DVT episode, one-third to one-half will have long-term complications (post-thrombotic syndrome) such as swelling, pain, discoloration, and dry skin of the affected limb.

- One-third (about 33%) of people with DVT/PE will have a recurrence within ten years.

- Approximately 5% to 8% of the U.S. population has one of several genetic risk factors, also known as *inherited thrombophilias,* in which a genetic defect can be identified that increases the risk for thrombosis.

Sudden death is the first symptom in approximately one-quarter (25%) of people who develop a pulmonary embolism.

VARICOSE VEINS

Chronic vein abnormalities are present in up to 50% of men as they grow older, and the abnormalities manifest as varicose veins in the legs and purple discoloration of the skin. Although varicose veins appear serious, they tend to be superficial. In contrast, deep vein thrombosis occurs in the veins deep within the body and is potentially life threatening.

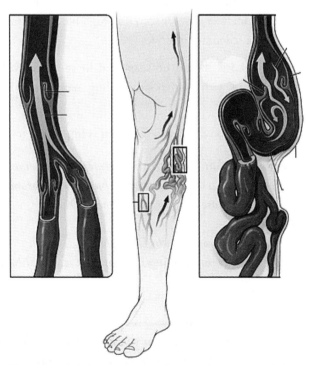

Figure 13.4. An illustration of the one-way valves in the veins and the risks of poor circulation when the valves and the veins become impaired.

Symptoms. Varicose veins are characterized by aching or heaviness, swelling (edema), dry skin, tightness, itching, irritation, muscle cramps, or pain. Visible signs include dilated veins, swollen legs with skin color changes, and/or skin ulcers. At least 20% of older men have varicose veins—swollen, tortuous, dilated veins that can eventually progress to swollen feet and ulceration of the veins.

Treatment. Individuals with dilated veins who have no symptoms and do not find the appearance of the veins concerning do not need intervention. Men who are concerned about the unsightly appearance of these veins should consult with a vascular surgeon. These specialists typically recommend liquid sclerotherapy or surface laser treatment. The results of sclerotherapy are generally thought to be superior to those of laser therapy. Laser therapy is usually reserved for needle-phobic patients or those who are allergic to sclerosing agents.

KEY TAKE AWAYS

- The piece of the puzzle that is often over-looked is the fact that we must be physically active periodically throughout the day in order for our veins to pump our blood back to the heart efficiently.

- At least 10% of men over 55 have a significant decrease in blood flow to their legs. Risk factors include age, tobacco use, high blood pressure, diabetes, elevated cholesterol, and a sedentary lifestyle.

- Deep vein thrombosis should be suspected in someone with any of these risk factors who presents with sudden leg swelling, pain, warmth, and redness of the calf or of the entire leg.

- These conditions can be deadly, so we feel it is important to repeat the warning:

It is estimated that there are three times as many men with peripheral artery disease who have no symptoms as those diagnosed with the disease.

A pulmonary embolus CAN KILL YOU.
This occurs more frequently than one would think.

For more information on vascular disease, please see the website of Dr. Ingegno: www.vasculargroup.com.

Chapter 14

Lowering the Risk of a Stroke
Armin Brott & Nancy Faass, Medical Writers,
& Judson Brandeis, MD, Urologist

The brain is like a muscle. When it is in use, we feel very good.
— Carl Sagan

Michael Johnson is one of the greatest sprinters the world has ever seen. He won four Olympic Gold Medals and held the world record in the 200 and 400 meters. Johnson's nickname was "Superman," and he was named the top athlete of the year in any sport in 1996.

At age 50, Superman had an ischemic stroke caused by a blood clot and suddenly lost the function of his left leg. Fortunately, his wife called a doctor immediately and then drove him to the hospital, and he received medical care right away. However, even with a rapid response and outstanding treatment, it was months before this Olympic superstar could even walk *again and almost a year before he was back to good physical condition.*

Many stroke victims don't receive timely medical care, don't have the determination of a world-class athlete, and lack the financial security that would allow them the time to rehabilitate fully. Strokes have devastating consequences for men, even Olympic heroes.

Strokes are the leading cause of long-term disability in the United States.

A stroke is a sudden interruption in the arterial blood supply to the brain. Since the brain requires oxygen and nutrients, shortly after the blockage occurs, nerve cells in the brain start dying. As they die, the brain and body functions they control stop working.

If the damage occurs in the occipital lobe of the brain, you will become blind. If the damage occurs in the parietal lobe, you may lose your ability to speak or think. If the damage occurs in the right hemisphere, you may lose all function of the muscles on the left side of your body. You may never walk again. You may end up in a wheelchair. Someone will have to help you eat and wipe your butt. Strokes are serious.

This damage is usually irreversible, resulting in permanent disability and loss of quality of life.

SYMPTOMS OF A MAJOR STROKE

Strokes generally don't give you much advance notice. Symptoms come on suddenly and unexpectedly. If you notice any of these symptoms in yourself or anyone around you, call 911 or your local emergency number immediately. Remember, every second counts. Major symptoms of a stroke include:

- Sudden numbness on one side of the body
- Sudden weakness of the face, an arm, or a leg
- Sudden confusion, trouble speaking, or understanding
- Sudden blurred or double vision or temporary loss of vision in one or both eyes
- Sudden trouble walking, dizziness, loss of balance, or poor coordination
- Sudden severe headache with no known cause.

HOW CAN YOU TELL IF IT'S A STROKE?

If you think you or someone you know may be having a stroke, act FAST, and do this simple test:

F — FACE:
Ask the person to smile. Does one side of the face droop?

A — ARMS:
Ask the person to raise both arms. Does one arm drift downward?

S — SPEECH:
Ask the person to repeat a simple phrase. Is his or her speech slurred or confused?

T — TIME:
Call 9-1-1 immediately. Every second without oxygen worsens the damage.

If you suspect a stroke, get to the nearest hospital as fast as you can.

There are clot-busting drugs that could save your brain and your life.

SYMPTOMS OF A MINI-STROKE (TIA)

TIAs are a warning sign. One of every three people who suffers a TIA will experience a major stroke soon after the TIA episode.

TIAs (temporary ischemic attacks—sometimes called mini-strokes) occur when a clot lodges in a blood vessel. These clots cause symptoms, but if they dislodge, the symptoms resolve. As a result, people may experience a brief period of impairment—half of all people experiencing a TIA recover within an hour or so.

Symptoms could include some loss of vision, slurred speech, dizziness, weakness, or unusual clumsiness. Although TIAs are temporary, people who experience them have increased risk of a full-blown stroke. If you've had a TIA, you need timely assessment and support from your healthcare provider or a hospital. Some people may have no symptoms at all, while others may notice one or more of the following:

- Racing, irregular heartbeat
- Chest pain (angina)
- Sudden confusion
- An unusual or intense headache
- Symptoms of going into shock, such as sudden sweating, dizziness, or fainting.

Take this seriously. If you have any symptoms, call an ambulance immediately.

Every year, almost 800,000 Americans have a stroke and an estimated 500,000 have a TIA. Strokes degrade quality of life perhaps more than any other type of injury or disease. Over 70% of those who suffer a stroke are older than 65 and almost 60% are men. Men die younger—and in greater numbers—of heart disease and stroke. Of those who experience a stroke, nearly one-third are so drastically disabled that they can no longer care for themselves.

Patients who arrive at the emergency room within three hours of their first stroke symptoms often have less disability three months after a stroke than those who received delayed care.

HOW STROKES HAPPEN

A stroke can cause blindness, difficulty walking, the inability to talk, physical paralysis, or death. When one of the blood vessels in the brain becomes blocked or bursts, the brain no longer receives the oxygen it needs to function. Although your body replaces dead cells everywhere else in your body, brain cells often are not replaced, which means that much of the damage done by a stroke can be permanent. The CDC reports that 87% of all strokes are caused by a clot or blocked blood flow in the brain (ischemic strokes). About 10% of strokes are caused by bleeding in the brain (hemorrhagic strokes).

Ischemic strokes caused by blood clots:

- Blockage in a blood vessel in the brain

- Destruction of brain tissue due to lack of oxygen-carrying blood

- Half of all strokes are caused by clots that travel from somewhere else in the body.

Hemorrhagic strokes due to internal bleeding:

- Ruptured blood vessel(s) that result in bleeding within the brain

- Bleeding between the brain and the skull

- An aneurism (a weakened area in the wall of an artery)

RISK FACTORS & CAUSES OF STROKE

Primary risk factors:

- **Hypertension.** High blood pressure is the leading cause of stroke, doubling the risk compared with normal blood pressure.

- **Tobacco use.** Smoking more than a pack a day increases stroke risk by 250%. Less than a pack a day still doubles the risk of stroke.

- **Obesity and diabetes.** Two of every three people with diabetes will die of a heart attack or a stroke.

Known risks:

If you have one of these factors, you need to understand that you have an increased risk, and you should take preventive measures seriously. You don't want to become a burden to your family.

- **Age.** Of the risk factors that can't be modified, age is the most significant.

- **Genetics and ethnicity.** Risk is higher for people of Hispanic heritage, and for those from the Mediterranean region and the Middle East or Asia. African-American men are almost twice as likely to suffer a stroke and have the highest death rate from strokes.

- **Family history and lifestyle.** When there is a pattern of stroke or heart disease in the family, that requires a careful assessment in partnership with your doctor. Clearly, genetics is often a factor, but lifestyle can also increase your risk.

Health issues:

- **High blood pressure.** At least a quarter of American men have consistently high blood pressure, the leading cause of both strokes and heart attacks.

- **Diabetes.** High blood sugar is a factor in atherosclerosis, causing the buildup of fatty deposits in the blood vessels. This is another example of the counter-intuitive link between simple sugars in the diet and harmful fats in the body.

  (For additional insight, and for ideas on how to change your daily menu to fresh, whole food, see Part 4. Food.)

- **Plaque and blood clots.** Buildup of plaque on the inside of the arteries can limit blood flow to the brain. (This disorder used to be called *hardening of the arteries*.) The more plaque, the less circulation. The real danger with plaque occurs when it ruptures, releasing clots that can block an artery. As mentioned, this starves brain cells of oxygen, causing major and often permanent damage.

- **Heart arrythmias.** Tachycardia (a pulse over 100 beats a minute), mitral valve prolapse (when a heart valve doesn't close fully), and A-Fib (atrial fibrillation) are considered a possible factor in one-fourth of all strokes. Although A-Fib is primarily associated with aging, tachycardia can affect individuals at any age (even infancy). Mitral valve prolapse can also occur in a younger person, especially in midlife when our hormones start dropping and our stress level increases.

- **Sickle cell anemia.** Symptoms may include headaches, poor circulation, and/or sores on the legs and ankles, as well as stroke.

- **Low testosterone.** Men with low testosterone have been found to have a 10% higher risk of a cardiovascular event, coronary heart disease, heart attack, or stroke and 20% slower recovery. The research also associates low testosterone with obesity, high blood glucose, insulin resistance, metabolic syndrome, high triglycerides, hypertension, and diabetes, as well as erectile dysfunction.

Lifestyle issues:

- **Smoking.** Looking down the road, ten years after you quit, your risk of stroke will be about the same as a non-smoker's.

■ **Nutrition.** The EPIC (European Prospective Investigation into Cancer and Nutrition) study assessed the health of more than 400,000 individuals in ten European countries and shed new light on nutrition. Researchers found *reduced* stroke risk with higher intake of "either fruit, vegetables, fiber, milk, cheese, or yogurt."

If you've ever been confused by the recommendation of 5 to 13 servings of fruit and vegetables a day, this study offered some clarity. Half a pound of fruit and vegetables reduced risk by almost 15%--that translates to a salad and an ample serving of cooked vegetables (think Chinese style stir-fry or grilled veggies or a sautee). Double that by having an apple in the morning and a bigger salad and your risk is reduced by 30%.

■ **Hydration.** Researchers report that men who drank at least five 8 oz. glasses of water a day (2 ½ 16 oz. bottles of spring water, for example) cut their stroke risk by half (53%) compared with those who drank less than three glasses of water a day.

■ **Alcohol use and abuse.** One or two drinks a day used to be considered beneficial. More recent studies report that even one to two drinks daily *increase* stroke risk by as much as 15%. Alcohol overuse raises stroke risk by as much as 35%, because it raises the number of blood platelets and also activates them. Both processes contribute to the formation of blood clots.

■ **Unrelenting stress.** The stress response speeds up your heart rate and spikes your blood sugar (giving you energy so you can escape from danger). But if you're experiencing high levels of stress every day, those same dynamics set you up for heart disease, diabetes, and stroke.

■ **Dental health.** Heart disease has been linked to poor dental health, and both issues are implicated in stroke risk.

■ **Street drugs.** If you become addicted and use drugs for an extended period, your health risks go way up, including the risk of stroke.

■ **Certain prescription drugs:**

Anticholinergic drugs. Commonly taken for allergies, heart disease, and Parkinson's, anticholinergic medications are associated with a 59% percent increased risk of a stroke and an 86% increased risk of dying from stroke (based on a 20 year study of more than 25,000 participants).

Benzodiazepines. Commonly used for sleep and anxiety, benzodiazepines have been linked to strokes caused by blood clots (almost 90% of all strokes). A study monitoring insurance claims for stroke from more than 75,000 people reported that a high intake of benzodiazepines (meaning taking more than four grams annually or using them more than 95 days in a year) increased risk of stroke in all age groups.

Blood-thinning drugs. Although intended to reduce the formation of blood clots, blood thinners have been found to increase the risk of stroke.

NSAIDs (**non-steroidal anti-inflammatory drugs**). Medications such as ibuprofen (Advil), diclofenac, naproxen (Aleve), and diclofenac have been implicated in both cardiovascular disease and stroke.

LAB TESTING FOR RISK

In addition to standard lab tests for cardiovascular risk assessment, such as cholesterol, hemaglobin A1C, and C-reactive protein, additional tests can be helpful in assessing your stroke risk and are available from major laboratories such as LabCorp and Quest. Ask your doctor about them at your next checkup.

- **Testosterone level.** Low testosterone is associated with increased risk of cardiovascular events and stroke. Testosterone levels can be measured in blood, saliva, and urine. Blood measurements are the most commonly used.

- **Homocysteine (imbalanced body chemistry).** Elevated levels of homocysteine are clearly associated with increased cardiovascular risk and stroke. Typically, these levels are addressed with a nutritional supplement designed to reduce homocysteine, often based on B-complex vitamins in the active form.

- **Oxidized LDL.** This aspect of cholesterol is an important recent addition to cardiovascular risk testing. The test measures the most harmful form of cholesterol, which is a reflection of the level of oxidative stress in the body and is currently available through all major laboratories with a lab slip from your doctor.

- **D-dimer.** This recently developed test measures body chemistry involved in the process of clot formation. Elevated levels indicate increased blood clot and stroke risk.

HIDDEN CAUSES OF A STROKE: A-FIB

In the U.S., someone has a stroke related to A-Fib every 12 seconds.

A-Fib (atrial fibrillation) is characterized by an irregular heartbeat, a type of *arrhythmia,* which is a disorder of the heart rate (pulse) or heart rhythm. Other types of arrhythmia include tachycardia (when the heart beats too fast) and bradycardia (when it beats too slowly). A-Fib is the most common type of persistent arrhythmia and affects more than five million people in the United States today.

Increased risk of developing A-Fib is associated with genetics, aging, smoking, excessive alcohol or caffeine use, and high stress. Anyone with heart disease, including valve problems or a history of heart attack or heart surgery has an increased risk of A-Fib. Other conditions that increase risk of A-Fib and stroke include:

- Tachycardia (Some types of tachycardia can double the risk of stroke.)

- Mitral valve prolapse (a heart valve that doesn't close fully) can have similar effects.

- Heart disease present at birth

- Congestive heart failure

- Cardiomyopathy (affecting the heart muscle)

- Pulmonary embolism (blood clot in the lungs)

- Chronic lung disease.

Conditions involving arrythmia are harmless in some cases. However, in other cases, arrythmia can pose an immediate danger to health, increasing the risk of heart failure, stroke, sudden cardiac arrest, or even death. (For additional information on A-Fib, please see chapter 6, "Reducing Your Risk of Heart Disease.")

EMERGING TREATMENTS FROM THE RESEARCH

Recovering from a stroke is a complex process. There is an entire medical specialty, Physical Medicine and Rehabilitation (PM&R) devoted to rehabilitating people with disabilities after suffering a stroke or some other disabling condition. Do not take this journey on your own!

At the same time, treatment and recovery is not a passive process. Since brain injury can really wreak havoc with your quality of life (and that of your caregivers), if you've had a stroke, you or a member of your family needs to become expert at researching the latest science-backed treatments for brain injury. The following are a few promising therapies to complement what a PM&R physician might offer.

Acupuncture. More than 2,000 years old, acupuncture has been shown to be useful in recovery from neurological damage caused by strokes. Over the past ten years, nearly 300 clinical trials have been conducted on every aspect of acupuncture therapy in stroke treatment. Acupuncture has also been found effective in reducing high blood pressure, one of the major risk factors for stroke.

Most major cities have numerous acupuncture centers, and it may be covered by your health insurance (progressive health systems such as Kaiser Permanente provide acupuncture, and in New York City, it's offered at Memorial Sloan-Kettering Cancer Center). You'll want to do your homework to find a provider with in-depth experience at a comfortable price point. (Be sure to work with an accupuncturist who uses disposable needles.)

Hyperbaric oxygen therapy (HBOT). This is an FDA-approved treatment for severe conditions such as wound healing (diabetic foot, diabetic neuropathy, crush injuries, brain abscess, radiation injury, and thermal burns). The Mayo Clinic, for example, uses HBOT to treat gangrene, frostbite injuries, and carbon monoxide poisoning.

Dr. Paul Harch, a professor at the Louisiana State University Medical School, has applied HBOT in the treatment of 18 different types of disorders affecting the brain, including stroke, traumatic brain injury (auto accidents), concussion/blast injuries (military personnel), multiple sclerosis, Parkinson's disease, and mild cognitive impairment. He reports that "Hyperbaric oxygen therapy is the most effective treatment known for brain injury of all types, at all stages of the condition, at all points in time, and all levels of severity."

Although most hospitals have a hyperbaric chamber, treatment is typically provided only for the 14 FDA-approved conditions, due to lack of insurance reimbursement. However, most large cities also have private centers, some managed by medical doctors. Post-stroke, this therapy is worthy of exploration.

rTMS. Repetitive transcranial magnetic stimulation (rTMS) is a sophisticated therapy provided in hospitals and large medical centers. Approved in 1979 for wound healing of tissue and bone, rTMS has been in extensive use for more than 20 years and has been found to be a safe form of treatment for stroke, depression, and other brain disorders. Over the past ten years more than 280 clinical trials have been conducted on rTMS in the treatment of stroke. Currently it's also used for a range of neurological and psychiatric disorders, including Parkinson disease, spinocerebellar degeneration, epilepsy, movement disorders, chronic pain, and migraine, as well as anxiety, depression, OCD, and psychosis. In terms of stroke recovery, a study conducted at a medical facility in Budapest reported that patients who had suffered a stroke ten years earlier and were treated with rTMS experienced improvement. These treatments would be authorized through a neurologist or psychiatrist.

For recent information on treatment using rTMS, see *The Angel and the Assassin* by Donna Jackson Nakazawa (New York: Ballantine, 2021).

What you can do for your recovery once your condition is stabilized, with clearance from your physician:

■ Meditation and breath work. Breath work can have value even when it is difficult to get out of bed. Video or audio coaching can be relaxing and motivating.

■ Walking. Following a stroke, once one has been cleared for physical activity, walking can make an enormous difference and can be surprisingly healing to the brain. To ensure safety, walk sessions need to include supportive care (such as a walker and the assistance of a caregiver) to avoid the risk of a fall.

■ Yoga and qigong are therapeutic interventions. Here too, the goal is to structure your practice so there's no risk of a fall, and to be sure you're exercising at your own comfort level.

For more information on the work of Armin Brott, please see:
www.MrDad.com.
For Nancy Faass, please see:
www.HealthWritersGroup.com.
For additional information:
please see www.Stroke.org.

Chapter 15
The Alzheimer's Tsunami
Judson Brandeis, MD, Urologist
& Michael Abassian, MPH, Researcher

I can still hold my Dad's hand, but I miss him every day.
— Anonymous

- The adult brain weighs about three pounds, which is around 2% of your body weight.

- Your brain uses 20% of the oxygen and nutrients in your body, and in extreme circumstances, your brain may use almost half.

- Brain cells need a constant supply of glucose to stay alive, yet cannot store energy—one of the reasons insulin resistance in the brain is so devastating. As a backup, the liver can break down stored fat to produce ketone bodies that can be used as a substitute fuel when blood glucose is not available.

- More than 60% of your brain is fat, which is why healthy fats, such as omega-3s and omega-6s are vital for brain health. Healthy fat is essential to stabilize the walls of every brain cell and has been found in numerous studies to reduce inflammation.

- In total, the brain contains approximately 100 billion neurons, and this constitutes only about 10% of brain tissue.

- The human brain will triple its size during the first year of life and continue to grow until about the age of 18.

- At 25, the human brain reaches full maturity but keeps developing until the late 40s.

- At about the age of 50, the brain begins to shrink.

- At ages 60 to 74, one person in ten or less has cognitive impairment (3%–10%).

- In those 75 to 84, about one person in six has impairment (17%).

- At age 85 and above, one person in three has some form of dementia (32%).

Optimizing health means maximizing brain health. Our bodies are exposed to harmful environmental effects and lifestyle risks over the course of our lives. Fortunately, there are a number of things we can do to protect our brain and help prevent the onset of dementia.

DEMENTIA DEFINED

Dementia is not a single disease but a broad term that describes impairment in memory, communication, and thinking, declines that are severe enough to interfere with daily life. The impairment is caused by damage to nerve cells of the brain and their connectivity. Alzheimer's disease causes about 60% of progressive dementia in older adults, but there are many other causes of dementia. The second most common type of dementia, termed vascular dementia, is caused by damage to the arteries that supply blood to your brain.

Alzheimer's disease is now the sixth leading cause of death in the United States, and its prevalence is increasing. More than five million Americans currently live with some form of Alzheimer's.

SYMPTOMS

At first, memory loss can begin innocently enough, in an individual who:

- Is often late
- Misses appointments
- Loses things frequently (always looking for their keys, their phone).

MILD COGNITIVE IMPAIRMENT (MCI)—A state between normal brain health and dementia

About 20% of people age 65 or older have mild cognitive impairment:

- Decline that is mainly noticeable to the individual or to close family and friends
- Short-term memory loss and impairment of some mental skills
- Changes in personality and mood such as irritability, anxiety, depression, aggression, or apathy
- Impact on judgment, problem solving, and the ability to conduct complex tasks
- Greater risk of developing Alzheimer's or other dementias.

Unfortunately, there are no FDA-approved medications for treating MCI. Drugs designed to manage symptoms of Alzheimer's have not shown long-term benefits. Later in the chapter, we explore ways to optimize your brain health and reduce your risk for cognitive decline. (In chapter 16, "Reversing Early Dementia," which follows, we will also report on emerging research on reversing mild cognitive impairment.)

DEMENTIA—Memory loss and decline in cognitive function

Dementia involves memory loss and impairment of at least one other mental function, such as language, visual-spatial perception, or reasoning and judgement. The term dementia implies reduced capability that is severe enough to interfere with daily activities. In contrast to mild cognitive impairment, dementia can also result in loss of independence. Many dementia patients are unaware of their memory loss, and often a family member or friend brings the problem to the provider's attention.

Changes in intellect:

- Forgetfulness (the most common chief complaint)
- Difficulty retaining new information
- Getting lost in familiar places (while walking or driving)
- Inability to handle complicated tasks (like balancing a checkbook)
- Loss of executive function, decision making, and problem-solving skills
- Less adaptability, unable to cope with unexpected events
- Becoming less verbal, having difficulty finding words or communicating
- Less acute visual and spatial perception
- Difficulty with balance, coordination, and other motor functions
- As memory loss worsens, confusion and disorientation

Mental/emotional changes:

- Altered personality
- Depression or anxiety
- Anger or moodiness
- Inappropriate behavior
- Paranoia or agitation
- As cognitive losses continue, psychosis (hallucinations)

VASCULAR DEMENTIA—Reduced circulation in the brain

The second most common form of advanced cognitive impairment, vascular dementia is exceeded only by Alzheimer's disease in prevalence. Vascular dementia refers to any type of dementia that is caused by impaired blood flow in the brain due to plaque build-up or blood clots. Imaging with an MRI can evaluate patterns of cerebrovascular disease and atrophy to evaluate the risk of converting from mild cognitive impairment to dementia.

NEURODEGENERATIVE DISEASE

Neurodegenerative disease refers to any condition that involves the death of brain cells. In addition to dementias, neurological conditions include:

- Brain injuries due to physical trauma
- Brain cancer and tumors
- Neurodegenerative diseases like multiple sclerosis and Parkinson's disease
- Seizure disorders
- Mental disorders such as depression, addiction, or schizophrenia
- Clotting or circulatory conditions causing clogged arteries, strokes, or TIAs (transient ischemic attacks).

When any of these conditions is present, the individual is more vulnerable to dementia and Alzheimer's disease.

ALZHEIMER'S—A more severe form of dementia

More than five million Americans currently live with this condition, 80% of them 75 or older. Deaths due to Alzheimer's have increased by almost 150% over the past 20 years. Alzheimer's disease progresses in stages, each more invasive than the prior one. (For additional information on new therapies for Alzheimer's, see chapter 16.)

Mild Alzheimer's disease:

- Losing things or misplacing them in odd places
- Memory loss
- Getting lost, wandering
- Poor judgment leading to bad decisions
- Loss of spontaneity and sense of initiative
- Taking longer to complete normal daily tasks
- Difficulty handling money and paying bills
- Mood and personality changes
- Increased anxiety and/or aggression
- Alzheimer's disease is often diagnosed at this stage.

Moderate Alzheimer's disease:

At this stage, more intensive supervision and care become necessary due to symptoms such as:

- Increased memory loss and confusion
- Shortened attention span
- Inability to learn new things
- Problems coping with new situations
- Difficulty carrying out multistep tasks, such as getting dressed
- Impulsive behavior such as undressing in inappropriate places or using vulgar language
- Outbursts of anger or agitation
- Restlessness, anxiety, tearfulness, wandering (especially late afternoon or evening)
- Repetitive statements or movement, muscle twitches
- Inability to recognize family and friends
- Hallucinations, delusions, or paranoia.

Severe Alzheimer's disease:

People at this stage cannot communicate and are completely dependent on others for their care. They may be in bed most of the time as their body shuts down with symptoms that include:

- Inability to communicate beyond groaning or moaning
- Weight loss
- Seizures
- Skin infections
- Difficulty swallowing
- Loss of bowel and bladder control
- Increased sleeping.

A common cause of death for people with Alzheimer's disease is pneumonia, which develops when a person cannot swallow properly and takes food or liquids into the lungs instead of air. This is a devastating way to end one's life.

EVALUATION

RULING OUT POSSIBLE CAUSES

Now more than ever, it is worth examining the risk factors, what the scientific and medical community knows, and what you can do to minimize your risk of neurodegeneration and cognitive decline. It is essential to rule out the other causes of dementia—especially those that are reversible, such as:

- Low testosterone
- Low thyroid
- Deficiency of vitamin B12 or intrinsic factor
- Sleep disturbances, including sleep apnea
- Drug/alcohol overuse
- Insulin resistance
- Infections such as Lyme disease.

MEDICATIONS THAT CAN WORSEN BRAIN HEALTH

Researchers have identified medications that can lead to cognitive impairment if taken for an extended period of time by an older adult:

- Antianxiety drugs (benzodiazepines such as Valium and Ativan)
- Anticholinergic medications such as Oxybutynin and Ditropan
- Antidepressants (tricyclic antidepressants)
- First-generation antihistamines
- Antinausea medication
- Antipsychotics and mood stabilizers
- Antiseizure drugs
- Chemotherapy
- Cholesterol-lowering drugs (statins)
- Hypertension medications (beta blockers)
- Incontinence drugs (antimuscarinics)
- Opioids such as Norco, Vicodin, Percocet, morphine, and numerous others
- Parkinson's drugs (dopamine agonists)
- Sedatives

- Surgical anesthesia and pain medications associated with "sundowner syndrome" (symptoms getting worse toward the end of the day)
- Sleeping medications such as Elavil, Doxepin, Seroquel and Trimipramine.

RISK FACTORS

Givens:

- APO E4 gene variant and/or a family history of dementia
- History of stroke (three times more likely to have dementia)
- Advanced age

Lifestyle factors. A study of 15,000 adults in midlife (44–66) tracked their health for a period of 25 years, reporting that the top three risk factors associated with dementia were:

- Diabetes (and weight gain—BMI >25)
- Smoking
- Hypertension.

IS DEMENTIA PREVENTABLE OR REVERSIBLE?

Surprisingly, the incidence (new cases) of all-cause dementia has been declining in high-income countries over the past several decades. This reduction is likely due to more education around brain disorders, reduction in vascular risk factors, and lifestyle modifications.

Evidence of recovery from mild cognitive impairment. A study carried out in France (2008) recorded the health of 7,000 people 65 and older over four years. At the beginning of the study, 42% had mild cognitive impairment. Researchers found that about 7% got worse, over half stayed the same (57%), but more than one-third (37%) returned to normal levels of functioning. This study shocked the scientific community because it revealed that mild cognitive impairment isn't necessarily a progressive condition that worsens for everyone. (For additional information on reversing mild cognitive impairment, see chapter 16.)

Research review by the Cleveland Clinic. Research on the effects of lifestyle on dementia compiled by the Cleveland Clinic reported protective effects for:

- **Exercise.** We've known for some time that exercise improves blood flow, memory, the capacity to think, and the ability to learn. What we did not know until recently is that people who exercise regularly have a lower risk of Alzheimer's disease.

- **Nutrition.** Oxidative stress is a chemical process associated with dementias that can result from diets high in sugar and harmful fats, and from obesity. Fresh fruits and salads, which are high in antioxidants, are especially protective against oxidation.

- **Sleep and relaxation.** Researchers have found that sleep reduces the build-up of amyloid plaque, which is typically present once Alzheimer's develops.

- **Mental exercise.** The brain pares away connections between neurons that aren't used—hence the concept of "use it or lose it." Minimize the tendency of the brain to downsize by staying mentally active.

- **Social interaction.** People with an active social life tend to have less memory loss (a finding verified by autopsy in research such as the Nun's Study). This makes it clear that social networks and support systems are important to both quality of life *and* health.

- **Medical management.** It is clear that obesity, hypertension, and diabetes increase the risk of dementia and require ongoing follow-up.

PREVENTION

TREATMENT

At the time of this writing, there is no FDA-approved medication for the treatment of mild cognitive impairment and currently no cure for dementia.

> *Just as cancer is an umbrella term for uncontrolled cell growth, dementia is a general term indicating memory loss and declining cognitive function, so there is not one single cause, and there is not likely to be one cure.*

LIFESTYLE

Physical exercise. Numerous observational studies have found that exercise reduces the risk of dementia. In particular, midlife levels of cardiorespiratory fitness may predict dementia later in life. When you exercise, that pumps your blood throughout your body *and* your brain, reducing the risk of vascular dementia. As an additional benefit, individuals who exercise have more positive emotional states and reduced stress, leading to lower susceptibility to Alzheimer's disease (the stress hypothesis). The American Heart Association recommends that adults get at least 150 minutes of moderate-intensity aerobic activity per week. (See Part 5, "Exercise," for inspiration.)

Sleep disorders. Sleep disturbances, including fragmentation and reduction of sleep, are common in patients with dementia and are also risk factors for cognitive decline. Obstructive sleep apnea in particular is a double whammy, because not only is the patient sleeping poorly, they are also experiencing periodic decreases in brain oxygen that can cause gradual brain impairment.

Mental and social stimulation. Learning and social interaction prevent or reduce cognitive deficits by activating brain plasticity and reducing brain atrophy. A remarkable study published in 2006 compared MRI brain scans of London taxi drivers to those of bus drivers. The taxi drivers who memorized the entire city and drove multiple routes had larger brains (and better brain connectivity) than the bus drivers who drove a predictable route every day.

Memory training. Memory training has shown to improve cognition in healthy older adults. At present, there is no evidence to support the notion that computerized brain training programs marketed commercially have benefits beyond short-term gains in the specific cognitive tasks that are being reinforced. Researchers find benefit from exercises that keep our brains mentally fit, including crossword puzzles, card games, carpentry, art, enthusiastic library use, and online or in-person classes. Keeping our brains fit is much like keeping our bodies fit: we need to stay engaged.

NUTRITION

Inadequate nutrition is common in patients with Alzheimer's disease and is associated with increased morbidity and mortality. The emerging research is taking a systems approach, identifying multiple factors that move the individual toward or away from health:

Mediterranean diet. Studies have shown that those on the Mediterranean diet had a lower incidence of mild cognitive impairment and Alzheimer's disease and slower rates of cognitive decline in population-wide comparisons. Foods found to support brain health include:

- *Fatty fish* due to their omega-3 fatty acids (salmon, herring, tuna, lake trout)
- *Egg yolks,* which provide choline with its anti-inflammatory properties
- *Blueberries and other berries*, low in carbohydrates and high in antioxidants
- *Cruciferous vegetables,* such as broccoli, are high in minerals and cancer-fighting properties
- *Nutrient-dense leafy vegetables* such as spinach and arugula, which provide high levels of vitamin E and vitamin K
- *Walnuts,* which contain DHA (docosahexaenoic acid, a type of omega-3 fatty acid that fights inflammation)
- *Coffee* (neuroprotective when taken in moderation)
- *Dark chocolate* (rich in beneficial antioxidants and flavonoids).

Incorporating these foods into your diet could potentially be health supportive and also displace less healthy foods. When trying any new food, it is vital that you take into account your own individual responses and food sensitivities.

Vitamin supplements. While many aspects of a healthy diet correlate with positive health outcomes, including cognitive health and freedom from dementia, the evidence is insufficient to conclude that any specific nutrition or dietary supplement in isolation reduces the risk of dementia.

- **Antioxidants to counter oxidative stress.** Autopsy studies suggest that oxidative stress may be significant in the development of Alzheimer's disease and other forms of dementia. Studies have found an association between higher dietary intake of antioxidants and lower risk of Alzheimer's disease.

- **B-complex vitamins to normalize homocysteine levels.** There is evidence from the Framingham Study (the longest study of human health in the history of medicine) that high homocysteine (a harmful biproduct of our own body chemistry) and *low* levels of B-complex vitamins are associated with risk of dementia. It is important to take the entire B-complex, but B6 in the active form, folate (B9), and B12 have been shown to be particularly important.

- **Vitamin D deficiency.** Vitamin D deficiency has been associated with cognitive impairment in older adults. The available data suggest that vitamin D (2000 international units/day) confers a modest benefit in delaying functional progression in patients with mild to moderate Alzheimer's disease. It is also recommended to get a blood test for vitamin D levels to detect inadequate levels of this vitamin.

- **Flavonoids.** In the Nurses' Health Study, dietary intake high in flavonoids such as blueberries and strawberries, slightly slowed the rates of cognitive decline. Nutritional scientists theorize that the antioxidant and anti-inflammatory actions of flavonoids may contribute to a protective effect.

Emerging research is likely to reveal the ways in which nutrients support brain health, but ideally supplements should be seen as one aspect of a comprehensive lifestyle program.

SCREENING

There is currently no single, specific lab test for cognitive impairment or dementia.

Basic online screening. The Cleveland Clinic offers a 20-minute, free online brain checkup tool. The results will give you a brain health index score, a brain health guide, a memory score, and recommendations and tips tailored specifically to your responses. Tests that are available as apps on your smartphone can give you quick insight on your cognitive abilities, including attention, memory, and processing speed. These apps include CNS Vital Signs and BrainHQ. These online surveys help gain a general understanding of your mental functioning.

Screening tests used by physicians. Consult your physician or neurologist to see if you could partake in more accurate surveys, such as as the Mini-Mental State Examination or the Montreal Cognitive Assessment. As mentioned, your doctor should also screen you for low testosterone, low thyroid, B12 deficiency, and depression.

Imaging studies and lab testing. Physicians can order a brain MRI for patients with onset of cognitive impairment and neurologic deterioration. The American Academy of Neurology recommend structural neuroimaging with MRI in the routine initial evaluation of all patients with dementia. An MRI provides more detailed information than a non-contrast CAT scan.

The following biomarkers can be detected and monitored in blood and cerebrospinal fluid testing as well as on PET scans and MRI (magnetic resonance imaging):

- Type 3 diabetes—decreased glucose metabolism
- The accumulation of beta-amyloid plaques in the brain
- Brain shrinkage (atrophy).

GENETIC TESTING

With the increasing availability of genomic testing, some healthcare providers are beginning to focus on prevention and holistic medicine guided by their patients' genetic blueprint. Providers can use both genotype (the genetic code) and phenotype (physical and clinical characteristics of the patient) to tailor treatment. Generally, this is good news.

APOE 4: Genetic testing for APOE 4 (pronounced A P O E4) provides an important marker for assessing the risk of Alzheimer's disease. Of the four variants, E4 is associated with major risk of late-onset Alzheimer's disease. This gene is involved in managing inflammation and in clearing amyloid plaque, a protein found in the brain of many Alzheimer's patients on autopsy. The presence of the APOE4 variant in combination with another variant for inflammation (high levels of TNF-alpha) increases Alzheimer's risk seven-fold.

Presence of the APOE4 gene from both your mother and your father can increase risk the risk of Alzheimer's disease by 12 times.
If this applies to you, you need to know that, so you can optimize your lifestyle.

Caveat Emptor (Let the Buyer Beware)

The field of brain health is currently packed with false information and fraudulent marketing. I am constantly seeing TV ads for Prevagen, for example, and wondered if it actually works. In 2015, Quincy Bioscience raked in almost $200 million in sales. In 2019, the makers of Prevagen spent $67 million on TV advertising

According to the company's website, people who use Prevagen *"experience improved memory, a sharper mind, and clearer thinking."* But is that really true? The short answer is a resounding no! In fact, the FDA warned Quincy Bioscience against claiming Prevagen could treat brain disorders and for failing to report adverse reactions. The FDA has also claimed that the main ingredient, apoaequorin, is not acceptable as a dietary supplement. There are no studies showing that oral apoaequorin crosses the blood-brain barrier or reaches the brain.

The two studies that Quincy Bioscience claims to support Prevagen were not blinded or placebo-controlled. The third study, published entirely by employees of Quincy Bioscience, was placebo-controlled and double-blind, but showed no overall benefit for Prevagen. In January 2017 the Federal Trade Commission (FTC) charged Quincy Bioscience with making *false and unsubstantiated claims.*

When you get an infection, the clearly effective treatment is usually anti-biotics, but with conditions like dementia, there is no silver bullet. This void leaves the door open for slick marketers making false claims and products that sound too good to be true. A quick internet search is usually all it takes to get the real answer. Please make sure that you always use reputable sources to research anything that you put inside your body.

Source:
https://www.consumerlab.com/answers/does-prevagen-really-improve-memory/prevagen-memory

Physicians and counselors with expertise in genomic testing can assess your overall risk by evaluating your genetic profile and make dietary and lifestyle recommendations based on your risks. Speak to your physician or neurologist to see if you would benefit from genome sequencing.

Action Steps to Prevent Alzheimer's

Take the major contributors to this terrible affliction seriously:
diabetes (high-carb diet), smoking, and hypertension (lack of exercise).
- Improve your nutrition, and if you need help to do that, get it.
- Stop smoking, if you smoke.
- Exercise like your life depends on it—it does.

KEY TAKE AWAYS

Around the globe, 50 million individuals live with Alzheimer's disease. This number is projected to reach 80 million by 2030 and 150 million by 2050. In the U.S., Alzheimer's disease cost the healthcare system $300 billion in 2020 and is estimated to cost $1 trillion per year by 2050.

In short, this is an enormous problem for humanity.
We don't want you to become another one of the statistics.

- The emerging thinking in this field points out that there are more than 35 known contributors to the development of dementia, so one of the best *preventive* strategies is to optimize lifestyle, using a common-sense approach.

- Mild cognitive impairment is an intermediate state between normal cognition and dementia: it typically does not severely interfere with lifestyle. However, even mild cognitive impairment impacts quality of life with symptoms that include irritability, anxiety, aggression, or apathy.

- There are two points in the development of dementia when you can make a real difference. The first is prevention. The second is reversing mild cognitive impairment, which requires a great deal more effort. These mild conditions are frequently a sign of ongoing memory loss and should be taken seriously. (For more information on therapies for mild cognitive impairment, see the next chapter.)

This is your chance to be a hero and save your own life.

For additional information,
please see the website of the Alzheimer's Association at www.alz.org.

Chapter 16
Reversing Early Dementia
Nancy Faass, MSW, MPH, Medical Writer

There's someone in my head, but it's not me.
— Pink Floyd, Brain Damage

We all know men in their 70s and 80s who are sharp as a tack,
and we also know men who have slowed down or are slipping into
dementia. Why is there such a vast difference?

The short answer is that we do not know. The more accurate answer is that brain health is a complex process that is influenced by a multitude of factors. There will likely never be a single pill or procedure that can restore a man's mental sharpness. The standard solutions are detailed in the previous chapter, which discusses improving general health and circulation. The recommendations in this chapter are more cutting edge and at an early stage of development, but hold great promise.

Men tend to be more vulnerable to conditions that affect the brain
than women. There could be a genetic reason for this.

Of the chromosomes that define gender, females have two X sex chromosomes while males have only one X chromosome (men have an X and a Y). In a female, if one of those sex chromosomes is damaged, it becomes inactive, silent, and the healthy chromosome is activated. In contrast, in a male, that single X chromosome must serve, regardless.

If that X chromosome is damaged by exposure to radiation or chemicals, for example, there is no second X chromosome to replace it.

We don't yet know exactly how that plays out in terms of human growth or brain development. We do know that boys have two to three times higher risk for hyperactivity. Their risk of delayed development is two to three times that of girls. A study by the CDC (2011) on neurological conditions reported: "Boys had twice the prevalence of any developmental disability and excess prevalence for attention deficit hyperactivity disorder, autism, learning disabilities, stuttering or stammering, and other developmental delays." This further highlights the increased vulnerability of the male brain. We know that among men 70 and older, more than 10% have some form of dementia.

THE BREDESEN PROTOCOL—NEW RESEARCH ON DEMENTIA

The work of Dr. Dale Bredesen, MD, reflects more than 30 years of research exploring the underlying causes of cognitive decline. Dr. Bredesen has held faculty positions at UCLA, UCSF, and UC San Diego. He is also president and cofounder of the Buck Research Institute on Aging, in Marin County, California.

In these various roles, he and his team have explored the underlying causes of dementia, predominantly Alzheimer's disease. The understanding of dementia that has emerged sheds new light on cognitive impairment and its treatment. When applied to patients, many experience documented improvement. Working with other physicians, he is currently conducting a clinical trial on the effects of a medical and lifestyle program for the treatment of mild cognitive impairment.

The recent clinical trial of the Bredesen Protocol found that 84% of patients improved, 12% declined, and 4% had no change. This is an exceptionally positive outcome by any standard.

CAUSES OF DEMENTIA

The Bredesen Protocol organizes risk factors for cognitive impairment into six categories, based on the mechanism of action.

Type 1. Inflammatory—Chronic inflammation

These conditions are characteristic of people who carry one or two of the APOE4 genes, which tend to promote inflammation. Although the APOE4 gene represents a major risk factor, the typical American lifestyle includes a number of other major causes of inflammation. We now know that the inflammatory response can increase the production of amyloid, so there is a direct link between inflammation and the development of Alzheimer's.

Type 1.5. Sweet—High insulin and high blood sugar

This form of Alzheimer's is due to glycation, which causes stiffening of the brain cells and possibly chronic inflammation. Levels of insulin and glucose are both high in this pattern, but the insulin is no longer effective. This can result in the destruction of the communication networks in the brain—the synapses.

Type 2. Cold—Low levels of nutrients and hormones

The inability to form new memories can indicate low levels of vitamin D and other nutrients, as well as low levels of hormones, and may include insulin-resistance and high homocysteine. Without sufficient nutrients, the brain's 500 trillion synaptic connections cannot be maintained.

Type 3. Toxic—Exposure to toxins such as metals or molds

In this type of dementia, the brain is breaking down. Both recent short-term memory and earlier memory are being degraded. Toxins can include mercury, lead, arsenic, cadmium, toxins molds, or harmful chemicals. The key steps in treatment involve 1) minimizing exposures, 2) identifying the toxins to which we are exposed, and 3) supporting their detoxification.

Type 4. Vascular—Effects of cardiovascular impairment

These dementia disorders are associated with cardiovascular disease, vascular leakiness, and vascular dementia.

Type 5. Trauma— Brain injury

Injury to the brain from head trauma or accidental injury of any kind increases the risk of dementia later in life. (The brain "insult" could be due to a motor vehicle accident, a fall, a sports-related concussion, or even an injury or illness sustained in childhood.)

A surprising number of lifestyle and environmental factors are harmful to the brain. To date, Dr. Bredesen and his team have identified at least 36 direct causes of memory loss that can be tested for, quantified, and countered with a medical or lifestyle protocol. Some of these "insults" to brain health are environmental (such as pesticides), while others are internal (such as high insulin). Examples include those listed in Figure 16.1.

GENETICS	INFLAMMATION	INFECTION
High body mass index	High homocysteine	Toxic exposure
High fasting insulin	Leaky blood-brain barrier	Gut infection
Prediabetes	Depleted hormones	Shrinking brain volume

Figure 16.1. Aspects of health with the potential to cause memory loss.

By the age of 85, one of every three Americans has dementia. Fortunately, new research is uncovering ways to interrupt the decline caused by cognitive impairment.

TESTING

The initial goal is to identify which one, or more, of these processes is impairing brain function in a given individual. The risk factors can be identified on laboratory tests and then addressed systematically. Once identified, by tackling each factor specifically, physicians have a greater chance to slow memory loss and then gradually reverse it. The protocol includes removing toxic exposures, rebalancing systems that are out of balance, and rebuilding the neural network. The following are brief examples of testing included in the protocol and the treatment applied if the test comes back positive:

- Insulin resistance can be tested very efficiently with a single blood test, the hemoglobin A1C, and improved through guided nutrition and nutritional supplements.

- Hormone levels are evaluated in blood or saliva and can be brought into a comfortable range with hormone-replacement therapy.

- Homocysteine is measured in a simple blood test, available from all of the major labs. If the level of homocysteine is too high (which is potentially harmful), that can be corrected with a B-complex vitamin supplement.

TREATMENT

The greatest potential for success at this time is early intervention. The more accurately the condition is diagnosed, the better the chance of success because treatment can be targeted to the specific problem. This approach involves working with a healthcare professional to get testing, treatment, and guidance on lifestyle. The ReCODE protocol includes many daily activities that people can do at home once they have the input of their physician, to gradually begin reversing cognitive decline.

Assessment:

- Medical history and testing
- MRI of brain volume
- Evaluation of findings

Optimizing metabolism:

- Assess and improve insulin resistance.
- Optimize nutrients, hormones, and growth factor levels.
- Minimize inflammation.

■ The ketogenic diet employed in the Bredesen Protocol is plant-based and rich in nutrients, with adequate protein and healthy fats. It is designed to support optimal brain health and to prevent or reverse cognitive decline. Recognized benefits include normalizing blood sugar and insulin levels, improving insulin sensitivity, reducing inflammation, and promoting detoxification.

Lifestyle as medicine. In this protocol, lifestyle is a major aspect of healing:

■ Ketogenic diet

■ Personalized supplements based on the test results

■ Optimized hormones

■ Exercise 30 to 60 minutes, five to six times a week

■ Sleep at least seven to eight hours or more

■ Stress management

■ Brain training, mental activities, and stimulation

EMERGING THERAPIES FOR COGNITIVE IMPAIRMENT

COMPLEMENTARY THERAPIES

In addition to the therapies we've just discussed there are other emerging therapies that also show benefit. In the past, the consensus was that the brain had no capacity to heal once it was damaged. We now know that a certain amount of healing and growth is possible. The therapies listed below are among the most promising of the treatments that address impaired brain function.

Pulsed electromagnetic fields (PEMF devices and rTMS). Electromagnetic therapies range from hand-held devices that you can purchase and use in your own home (to improve sleep quality, for example) to professional electromagnetic devices that are used in hospitals and large medical practices. The home devices have about 2% of the power of the large devices or less. To date, there have been about 500 studies on PEMF devices, both low-power personal PEMF units and high-powered r-TMS devices. The research is summarized in a book by William Pawluk, MD, MSc., titled *Power Tools for Healing*.

Light therapy—photobiomodulation. More than 200 clinical trials have been held to date on the use of light therapy, ranging from wound repair to performance enhancement. Various spectra of light are applied briefly to stimulate basic functions such as circulation, stem cell production, and energy production to promote healing and growth. Devices that have gotten good reports include Vielight and Bales Photonics. For more information on the use of light, please see Ben Greenfield's book, *Boundless.*

Hyperbaric oxygen therapy (HBOT). More than 600 clinical trials have been conducted on the healing benefits of hyperbaric oxgen therapy. HBOT was first used by the U.S. Navy to treat divers who had suffered decompression sickness. Currently it is approved for 14 different conditions, including diabetic foot ulcers, wound healing, radiation damage following chemotherapy, flesh-eating staph bacteria, and carbon monoxide poisoning. Hyperbaric oxygen has been used in the treatment of 18 different neurological disorders by Dr. Paul Harch, a professor at Louisiana State University School of Medicine and detailed in his book, *The Oxygen Revolution.* You'll also find informative videos on YouTube, including Joe Namath, the New York Jets quarterback, who has used HBOT to heal the after-effects of concussions suffered over the course of his career.

Additional therapies for mild cognitive impairment:

- Walking
- Yoga, qigong, or t'ai chi
- Acupuncture

Additional resources:

Dan Engle, MD. *The Concussion Repair Manual.* Las Vegas, NV: Lifestyle Entrepreneur's Press, 2017.
Datis Kharrazian, PhD, DC. *Why Isn't My Brain Working?* San Diego, CA: Elephant Press; 2013.

IMAGING AND ASSESSMENT

Imaging is an emerging field that now includes a range of technologies capable of assessing the brain in real time through video-like sequencing to define not only brain structure, but how the brain is actually functioning, second to second and minute to minute. A number of imaging techniques are now available which show the brain in action. Each of these tests requires a referral from a physician or a specialist such as a neurologist and follow-up interpretation by a specialist such as a radiologist.

- Functional MRI (fMRI) is comparable to traditional MRI technology, but images the brain continuously in real time.
- LORETA software, used for qEEG evaluations, goes beyond traditional EEG assessment to document subtle patterns of brain function.

- MEG (magneto electroencephalograph) documents electromagnetic brain activity.

- PET scans measure glucose use, recorded in a series of images of the brain in action.

- SPECT scans indicate the regions where the brain is active and which brain cells are "firing."

- Spectroscopy has been used experimentally to assess levels of specific nutrients in the brain.

- Volumetric MRI such as the NeuroQuant can indicate in detail when the brain is losing gray matter and shrinking. Following treatment, imaging can be used to document when repair is occurring, maintaining the size of the brain.

The problems associated with the tremendous rise in dementia is spurring the development of improved assessment and treatment. The emerging approach to therapy is a genuine partnership between the physician and the patient. The cornerstone of success in the Bredesen Protocol, for example, is the major role that the patient plays in implementing lifestyle and nutritional recommendations. The good news is that real improvement in dementia is now possible if we intervene early enough in the process.

RESOURCES

Dale Bredesen, MD. *The End of Alzheimer's*. New York, NY: Avery Publishing; 2017.
Dale Bredesen, MD. *The End of Alzheimer's Program*. New York, NY: Avery Publishing; 2020.
Dale Bredesen, MD. *The First Survivors of Alzheimer's*. New York, NY: Avery Publishing; 2021.

For additional information on the Bredesen Protocol, please see:
www.ApolloHealthCo.com.
For more information on the work of Nancy Faass please see:
www.HealthWritersGroup.com.

Chapter 17
Why You Should Care About Your Weight
Judson Brandeis, MD

The rise of childhood obesity has placed the health
of an entire generation at risk.
— Tom Vilsack

Obesity has surpassed smoking as the #1 cause of preventable disease and disability. For the first time in human history, obesity has become a greater threat than starvation. This is a global epidemic that is increasing in prevalence, affecting over 100 million children and 600 million adults.

People with weight issues are at risk of decades of suffering due to the 230 health conditions known to be associated with obesity. The suffering occurs on a physical level, but also on emotional, psychological, and social levels.

Given the seriousness of the statistics, it would be easy to interpret the intent of the data as fat shaming. Nothing could be further from the truth. It is vitally important to separate these two issues. The tremendous risk associated with obesity is a reality. It is also a reality that people struggling with weight issues experience a great deal of physical discomfort, pain, illness, and loss of wellbeing.

So this information on obesity is not about shaming. It is intended to give readers factual information and encouragement to seek assistance with weight management.

The worldwide prevalence of obesity has almost doubled over the past 40 years. In the United States, the incidence has increased from 20% in the 1980s to nearly 40% in 2020. Among adults in midlife (40–59), the rate of obesity in 2018 was 44.8% and among older adults aged 60 and older, 42.8%. If the current trends continue, by 2030, half of all American adults will be obese, and one quarter will be severely obese.

The treatment of obesity and obesity-related conditions can create financial hardship due to healthcare expenses, lost work productivity, and lower household income. Nationwide, obesity cost the United States an estimated $1.4 trillion in 2017. This is an international trend. In a Swedish obesity study, individuals with obesity were three times more likely to require a disability pension, use twice the number of sick days, and had significantly higher healthcare costs.

Obesity leads to underlying health conditions that include insulin resistance, with impairments in glucose metabolism and the effectiveness of insulin in regulating blood sugar. This condition is also described as prediabetes.

Obesity is associated with a significant increase in morbidity, including diabetes, sleep apnea, high blood pressure, high cholesterol, heart disease, stroke, cancer, and dementia as well as early death. Extreme weight gain strains other systems in the body, increasing the likelihood of back injury or knee replacement, with a trend of worse surgical outcomes when surgery is required. In terms of body chemistry, weight gain reduces testosterone levels and increases the risk of depression, in part due to unstable blood sugar. Weight loss is associated with a reduction in morbidity and mortality.

MEASURING RISK

Waist measurement is straightforward. A waist circumference of greater than 40 inches is considered high risk. Waist measurement also suggests the degree of increased heart disease risk.

Waist-to-hip ratio. Considered by some to be even more clinically useful than body mass index, you may find this measure helpful. Standing, measure your waist at the narrowest point between your hips and your belly button. Now measure your hips and butt at the widest point. Men should have a waist measurement that is not larger than their hips. A waist measurement larger than the hips reflects an abdominal weight that is a predictor of type 2 diabetes later in life.

The body mass index (BMI). Conversion calculators for BMI are abundant on the internet, and much of the medical research still uses that measurement. The body mass index is equal to body weight in kilograms divided by height (height in meters squared). Overweight is considered a BMI of 25 to 29.9 kg/m^2, and obesity is defined as any BMI over 30 kg/m^2.

In general, a higher body mass index increases the rate of death from all causes and especially from cardiovascular disease. Excess body weight contributed to four million deaths globally in 2015 and more than 320,000 deaths in the United States in 2014. In an analysis of almost a million North Americans and European adults followed for eight years, mortality was lowest among men with a body mass index between 22 and 25, with a 30% increase in overall mortality for each 5 kg/m^2 increase in body mass index.

For men with a BMI of 30 to 35, longevity is reduced by two to four years, and for those with a BMI of 40 to 45, lifespan is reduced by eight to ten years.

Years of life lost were highest for people who became obese at a younger age and lived with obesity longer. Medical issues associated with obesity are often accompanied by loss of function, reduced productivity, and poor quality of life.

Type 2 diabetes mellitus. Obesity causes more than 80% of cases of type 2 diabetes, and weight loss can reverse this. Obesity increases blood pressure, especially in men with upper body and abdominal obesity. Coronary artery disease, heart failure, and mortality from heart disease are associated with increased BMI. Obesity is associated with an increased risk of stroke and multiple types of cancers. The effects of excess weight have also been associated with mild cognitive impairment, through a mechanism termed *glycation* in which brain tissue becomes more brittle, with accompanying loss of function. Obesity also affects psychosocial function, including an increase in depression and job discrimination.

Chronic pain. Obesity is a strong independent risk factor for pain. It nearly doubles the risk of chronic pain among the elderly, causing pain in soft tissue such as tendons and ligaments and worsening existing pain in muscles and joints.

Joint damage. Osteoarthritis is a progressive wear-and-tear disease of the joints. Every pound of extra body weight places four to six pounds of pressure on each knee joint, which then wears away the joint. Consequently, the need for knee replacement is estimated to be at least 8.5 times higher among obese men. The likelihood of accidental injury causing musculoskeletal damage also increases significantly with weight.

Orthopedic injuries. Morbidly obese patients need to seek treatment for hip and knee replacement a decade earlier than those with a healthy body mass index. The stress on the joints isn't just from weight gain. The inflammation associated with obesity directly impairs the body's normal joint repair and maintenance, with increased prevalence of self-reported pain, including back pain. Obese individuals have a higher rate of meniscal tears and rotator cuff tendinitis than nonobese patients, often requiring surgical repair. Unfortunately, obese patients also have an increased risk of post-surgical infections, complications, and surgical failure as compared to men with a healthy body mass index.

Obesity is a global epidemic. It significantly decreases health-related quality of life and contributes to millions of deaths annually. In the reduction of orthopedic, cardiovascular, and endocrine problems, every pound matters.

**For more information and resources, please see
www.TheTwentyFirstCenturyMan.com.**

Chapter 18
Avoiding Diabetes
Jerry Stine, Nutritionist,
Armin Brott & Nancy Faass,
Medical Writers

Sugar is responsible for a lot of deaths. Arguably more than crack cocaine.
— Guy Ritchie

Diabetes is easy to diagnose with one simple blood test. And diabetes is the leading cause of heart disease, strokes, blindness, and amputation. So why are men often diagnosed with diabetes 15 years later than women? At that point, there is 15 years of damage that has been done— damage that may be undoable.

It's the stereotype of men and health: we don't go to the doctor, we don't go for follow-up, and we don't finish our medication. It's great to be rugged individualists, except that it's killing us.

So our goal in this particular chapter is to encourage you to build a relationship with a provider you trust. You want a relationship with someone you feel you can talk to— someone who can order tests and medications if you need them, keep an eye on your progress, give you feedback when you get off track, and refer you as needed.

Men are about half as likely as women to go to the doctor. If you haven't been to see a doctor, you don't know your blood sugar level. You don't know whether your blood sugar is too high or too low.

If you haven't seen a doctor, nobody else can tell you how you're doing.

DIABETES MATTERS

- According to the CDC, more than 34 million people in the United States have diabetes, and one in five of them don't know they have it.

- More than 88 million US adults—over a third—have *prediabetes*, and more than 84% of *them* don't know they have it.

- In the last 20 years, the number of adults diagnosed with diabetes has more than doubled as the American population has aged and become more overweight.

- Medical costs for people with diabetes are twice as high as for people who don't have diabetes.

We will offer you some diagnostic self-assessments and a few key lab tests (that you can obtain directly, without seeing a doctor) so you can see whether you are at risk or not.

Our goal here is to provide you with information, so if you are diabetic (and it hasn't been diagnosed), you can catch it as early as possible.

RISK FACTORS AND SYMPTOMS

TYPE 1 DIABETES (no insulin produced by the body)—almost 2 million in the U.S.

Type 1 accounts for only 5% to 10% of cases and most commonly develops in childhood. It appears to be hereditary in about 40% of cases. In this disorder, the body produces little or no insulin, so daily injections of insulin are necessary. Type 1 diabetes tends to make an individual more vulnerable to other serious health issues. Know that type 1 diabetes develops very quickly—usually over a few days or weeks—and the symptoms are often severe, including:

- Sudden feelings of fatigue
- Unexplained major weight loss
- Blurry vision
- Frequent urination and larger-than-normal amounts of urine, especially at night
- Dry mouth and excessive thirst.

(To the reader: If you already have type 1 diabetes, you need to be seeing a doctor for management, not reading this book. However, you will also want to put extra effort into getting your diet right, because it is possible to develop insulin resistance—type 2 diabetes—in addition to type 1 diabetes.)

PREDIABETES (the initial stage of insulin resistance, which precedes type 2 diabetes) —88 million in the U.S.

In prediabetes, the body's cells are becoming less effective at absorbing blood sugar (glucose) and metabolizing it. This process is termed insulin resistance and underlies the whole spectrum of blood sugar issues that people encounter. As a result, blood sugar levels are typically higher than normal, but not quite high enough to be diagnosed as diabetic. A large percentage of people with prediabetes eventually develop diabetes, either type 2 or 3.

These conditions develop slowly, and the symptoms have a gradual onset. At the start, they're barely noticeable. In fact, by the time people are diagnosed with type 2 diabetes, they've had the disease for more than five years without knowing it.

The keys to prevention and treatment are the basics: 1) Eating a healthy, balanced diet that supports normal insulin sensitivity and helps maintains a healthy weight. 2) Getting more exercise. 3) Managing high blood pressure. The benefits of this approach go beyond the prevention of diabetes, by reducing the risks of heart disease.

- *Prediabetes* is not simply a matter of high blood sugar or high insulin. When we test, we are not testing for "prediabetes," which is a broad term, but rather for markers for insulin resistance.

- *Low insulin? Maybe.* Although the general impression is that insulin output is low in diabetes, physicians report that in many cases, the pancreas is pumping out high levels of insulin. Unfortunately, the insulin is not interacting properly with the cells. These conditions do not fit a single cookie cutter pattern.

- *High blood sugar? Maybe.* The common perception is that prediabetes involves a blood sugar level that is higher than normal (hyperglycemia), but not quite high enough to be diagnosed as diabetic. However, in reality you could also have blood sugar in the normal range or have periods of low blood sugar (hypoglycemia).

In cases of prediabetes or diabetes, the condition is not simply low blood sugar. In reality, blood sugar goes too high, then goes too low, and then slowly recovers. This does not fully capture how emotionally and physically stressful these highs and lows are on our mood, our energy, and our health.

The take away? The hemoglobin A1C blood test is an exceptionally useful test to identify an emerging situation of insulin resistance.

TYPE 2 DIABETES (insulin resistance)—34 million in the U.S.

In these conditions, the body produces some insulin, but the cells no longer respond to the insulin. Type 2 accounts for 90% to 95% of all cases and is most common among people over 40 who are overweight. With changes in the American diet and a more sedentary lifestyle, type 2 diabetes has become more common even among children and teens.

Risk factors:

- Having a parent, brother, or sister with type 2 diabetes
- Belonging to a high-risk ethnic group (African American, Latino, Asian American, Pacific Islander, Native American)

- Being 45 or older

- Being overweight, especially abdominal weight around the midsection

- Having high blood pressure and/or high cholesterol

- Sedentary lifestyle, exercising less than two times a week

Advanced symptoms:

- Major thirst

- Huge food cravings and possibly the desire to binge eat

- Being overweight and having difficulty losing weight

- Erectile dysfunction (See Part II, Sexual Healing.)

- Changes in patches of skin color, on the back of the neck, armpit, groin, knuckles, shins, or elsewhere, which could mean too much insulin in the blood, often a sign of prediabetes

- Tingling or numbness in the feet or hands (peripheral neuropathy)

- Urinary tract infections

- Difficulty healing from cuts and sores (When that occurs, the condition is fairly serious, bordering on full-blown diabetes.)

There is no known cure for diabetes; however, it can be managed and treated. Unfortunately, more than five million people have type 2 diabetes and don't know it. Potential complications of untreated diabetes include blindness, kidney disease (often leading to dialysis), and increased risk of heart disease and stroke.

TYPE 3 DIABETES (insulin resistance in the brain) — six million in the U.S.

Type 3 is a recently identified aspect of dementia. It describes insulin resistance *in the brain cells*, a major contributing cause of Alzheimer's disease. One study found that 32% of patients with Alzheimer's disease also had type 3 diabetes.

LOW BLOOD SUGAR (hypoglycemia) — millions of undiagnosed people

If you have hypoglycemia, you will usually feel a lot better after you eat—your energy will go up and your mind will clear because the food is raising your blood sugar to a normal level.

With insulin resistance, you are more likely to feel fatigued after eating because your body is unable to dispose of the sugar by storing it in your cells. Unmanaged hypoglycemia is associated with fatigue and/or depression and/or mood swings.

AUTOIMMUNE DIABETES — an estimated 25% of young American diabetics

In very broad strokes, diabetes takes two forms. Being overweight is one of the markers of diabetes. Then there is a different group of people who are diabetic, but they are thin. This is usually an autoimmune problem, and treatment, diagnosis and care tend to be more complex. If you suspect autoimmune diabetes, you will want to work with a healthcare provider with training and experience in the management of autoimmune disorders.

Autoimmune diabetes has slow onset and is found in 10% of hereditary type 2 diabetic patients. However, among those below the age of 35 with diabetes, the autoimmune form affects 25%. This suggests that younger people are becoming more prone to autoimmune-related disorders.

HOW DO YOU KNOW IF YOU ARE PREDIABETIC?

MEASURING WEIGHT GAIN

Weight gain and/or difficulty in losing weight are key indicators of insulin resistance and prediabetes. One of the common causes of insulin resistance is a diet high in simple carbohydrates and sugars. The obesity that results is clear a sign of insulin resistance. This is not an issue of appearance or fat shaming. Obesity is directly linked to all major serious illnesses, including hypertension, heart disease, cancer, Alzheimer's, kidney failure, and autoimmune conditions.

Keeping track of your weight is a simple method of assessing whether you are in need of lifestyle support.

Waist measurement is straightforward. In most individuals, a waist circumference of greater than 40 inches is considered high risk.

Waist-to-hip ratio. If your waist is as large as your hip/butt measurement, that means you're carrying extra belly fat, always a sign of higher risk and a call to action.

The body mass index (BMI). Conversion calculators for BMI are abundant on the internet and much of the medical research still uses that measurement. Remind yourself that for folks with a BMI of 40 to 45, lifespan is tragically reduced by 8 to 10 years.

SELF-ASSESSMENT CHECKLIST

Each question is scored from zero to three, depending upon frequency and severity. Basically, ignore zeroes and ones. However, if you are scoring many threes in a particular category, get a follow-up with a healthcare provider.

Score: 0 1 2 3 for frequency and severity, three being the most severe or most frequent.

A. Prediabetes Symptoms (Insulin resistance, high blood sugar)					
	0	1	2	3	Total
Craving sweets during the day					
Eating sweets does not relieve cravings for sugar					
Must have sweets after meals					
Fatigue after meals					
Increased thirst and appetite					
Frequent urination					
Waist girth is equal to or larger than hip girth					
Difficulty losing weight					

Figure 18.1 Symptoms of prediabetes.

B. Hypoglycemia Symptoms (Low blood sugar)					
	0	1	2	3	Total
Depends on coffee to get started/keep going					
Light-headed if meals are missed					
Irritable if meals are missed					
With low blood sugar, feeling shaky, jittery, agitated, or easily upset					
If low blood sugar persists, may crash (intense anger or tearfulness)					
Craving sweets during the day					
Eating relieves fatigue					
Sweets are a quick pick-me-up but trigger a plunge in energy 30 minutes later					

Figure 18.2. Symptoms of hypoglycemia.

WORKING WITH A HEALTHCARE PROVIDER

If your waist measurement or your checklist suggests risk, you will want to find a provider who can help you move towards better health. The catch is that first you have to go in.

Diagnosing diabetes. Type 2 diabetes can be difficult to recognize, so often the diagnosis is only made during a routine medical checkup. Prediabetes, which has no visible symptoms at all, is even harder to diagnose.

Sometimes the only clue to potential diabetes is being overweight. Blood tests to measure blood sugar levels and your hemoglobin A1C can clarify your situation.

Who to see for prediabetes. If you are experiencing any of the risk factors or symptoms listed earlier, schedule an exam right now. A primary care doctor, nurse practitioner, osteopathic doctor, or naturopathic physician all have a background in diabetes management and training with an emphasis on nutritional therapy. If you have a healthcare professional who feels that they are not qualified to take you to the next step, they will make a referral.

If you have frank diabetes. In that case, you need to be seeing an internist or an endocrinologist, someone who can deal with your condition in greater detail. You should not attempt to manage diabetes on your own, since poorly managed diabetes can result in a heart attack or blindness at a relatively young age.

DIRECT-TO-CONSUMER LAB TESTING

We are not in any way encouraging you to treat yourself for prediabetes or diabetes—just as we would never suggest do-it-yourself brain surgery. However, we *are* encouraging you to find out your health status, so you know if your body needs essential maintenance.

Direct-to-consumer testing (DTC). If you are someone who hasn't been to the doctor in ten years, know that direct access to lab tests have become more available. Life Extension Foundation, for example, and a number of other organizations provide online portals where people can obtain reliable, legitimate laboratory testing. With these portals, you do not have to see a physician. You simply order the test online and obtain the blood draw from a local blood draw station (phlebotomist). However, it is important to have medical expertise to interpret the tests and to know what to do if the results show a problem.

Hemoglobin A1C. Hemoglobin A1C has been the gold standard for a decade. A test for hemoglobin A1C, along with a panel of markers for prediabetes, costs about $130. These are easy tests to do. A single test for fasting blood sugar can cost as low as $10. The results tend to be fairly straight forward. There are predefined ranges for safety, risk, and frank danger.

If you get diagnosed 15 years after this process has started, you may already be in really big trouble. This is a small investment to make in your health. The A1C test is a reliable picture of blood sugar levels over the last three months, so that one test alone is useful as a first step in determining when someone is at risk.

You can't really do this on your own. If your lab work indicates that you're prediabetic, you are going to need a healthcare professional who can advise you on how to take care of yourself. Even if you get the blood test on your own, you need a healthcare provider who can help keep you on track.

Insulin levels may look normal on the lab tests, despite the presence of prediabetes. In one study, researchers reported that in testing a group of individuals with insulin resistance, 80% were in the *normal range for insulin.* The point of this finding is that type 2 diabetes is not a disease of not enough insulin, but a problem of insulin no longer able to do its job.

The bottom line. These conditions can be fairly complex and require expert care.

WHAT YOU CAN DO FOR YOURSELF

- Get the blood test for hemoglobin A1C.

- If you need to see a provider, make the appointment.

- Make a plan for your exercise. (For ideas on changing out your exercise routine, see Part 5. Exercise.)

- Start transitioning to healthy, fresh food. (For a range of options, please see Part 4. Food.)

- Pick up a bottle of a supplement formula aimed at improving insulin resistance. (See the section "Nutritional supplements for insulin resistance," below, for specific suggestions.)

- Keep a journal/diary to track your weight and your symptoms.

- If you haven't seen any improvement in two months, pick up the phone and make an appointment with a healthcare professional.

The short list. Losing just a few pounds can make a big difference. When someone has prediabetes, the difference between weighing 200 and 250 pounds can be significant.

That is discouraging if you are gaining weight, but it is encouraging if you are losing, because as your weight begins to drop, you will feel the difference, and it will show in your appearance, personal charisma, and sex appeal.

The behavioral piece. If weight is an issue, consider changing your circle of friends. Get support from people with similar goals and challenges. (And stop hanging out with people who don't get it, who are still eating junk food, binge eating, or drinking a great deal of alcohol.) Research has shown that a person's chance of becoming obese increases by 57% if a close friend is obese, 40% if a sibling is obese, and 37% if a spouse is obese, according to the *Thinfluence* authors, Walter Willett, MD, DRPH, and Malissa Wood, MD, of Harvard Medical School.

Find a different group. We already know that when someone has an alcohol issue, if they don't change their circle of friends, they're not going to have much of a shot at sobriety. In sum, limit your exposure to temptation. Avoid people in bars and ice cream shops.

Dairy products can play a role in diabetes. If lab tests are showing a high A1C or blood glucose, avoiding milk products (milk, cheese, yogurt, etc.) can help with recovery. (Research shows that the phosphorous compounds in milk products interfere with the digestion of chromium, a key mineral in insulin response.)

Nutritional supplements for insulin resistance. There are a number of companies that manufacture pharmaceutical-grade nutritional supplements available through physicians, nutritionists, and other healthcare providers, and in health food stores. The best of these products contain minerals, amino acids, and plant extracts that have been demonstrated to have some beneficial impact on insulin sensitivity, and, when you combine them in a good formula, you can get real traction on insulin resistance.

Two good examples of this type of formula are Glucose Support Formula from Pure Encapsulations (available from Amazon.com and Vitacost.com) and Glysen from Apex Energetics (available through physicians and nutritionists).

Health journaling. Journaling is a way of streamlining the medical history process. This is more important than you would think—despite all the technology we have, your medical history is still the biggest diagnostic tool available to your doctors. Your journal could be something as simple as a little pocket notebook that you write things down in on most days.

Even if your symptoms are mild and your A1C is low risk, it's ideal to start keeping a journal, and make note of your worst symptoms and every bit of progress you make. Health journaling can be incredibly powerful. Providers love it when they get a patient who has done the work. Then you can walk into the doctor's office and say, "Here's my weight variation from the last three months" (or blood pressure variation or whatever you are working on at home). That information gives you a running start.

AVOIDING DIABETES **187**

A Doctor's Perspective

As an eye surgeon, I encourage my patients to track their blood sugar because my primary goal is to save their vision.

In this country, we need to be more proactive in fighting diabetes. In medicine, we know that you can't really improve what you don't measure. So let's measure 1) blood sugar control, 2) sugar intake, and 3) exercise.

Know your hemoglobin A1C. Your blood sugar will vary constantly. So a fasting blood sugar check is probably not representative of the true average. However, the test for hemoglobin A1C provides an incredible window into your health. The A1C measures how much sugar is stuck to the outside of your red blood cells. Since they live for a few months, the hemoglobin A1C tells you how thick the syrup is that they swim in. Think of it as the "drug test of sugar." It measures sugar control every minute of every day for the last three months. Patients often tell me their sugar levels are pretty good, but don't actually know their A1C. When we test, it's usually worse than the patient thinks. Patients who know their A1C often have better A1Cs. That's because they know what they are eating, how active they are, and whether that is making the number go up or down.

Discover how much sugar you're eating. Refined sugar is added to many foods in the U.S., and they keep adding more. We need sugar, but just not as much as we are fed. Three hundred years ago, unless you were the King of France, you probably would not have eaten more than 4 pounds of sugar a year. Now, people eat that in a single week. A colleague of mine who struggled to lose weight was shocked when she used an app (like MyFitnessPal or Lose It!) to figure out what she was eating. Her two gummy vitamins and coffee creamer were 37 grams of sugar alone. Measure what you eat and you might be surprised by the opportunities to get rid of unnecessary sugar.

Track your exercise. Although walking is a start, I don't think taking a walk is meaningful exercise. Most of us have been walking since age one. It isn't new, and you aren't going to build muscle by doing the same old, same old. Ever see a 300-pounder walking around the hospital track? Chances are they will never make significant health progress. Its not so much about building muscle but stopping the muscle loss that comes with age. To do that, you need to introduce your muscles to something new and keep the exercise routines fresh.

At the end of the day, the goal is to build diabetes fighting muscle, eat better, and effectively lose weight.

— Ahad Mahootchi, MD, Ophthalmologist and Eye Surgeon

(Please see chapter 24, "Protecting Your Vision," for insight from Dr. Mahootchi on preserving your vision.)

Health apps for prediabetes. Managing your intake of carbs (starches and sweets) is key to managing your weight, so an app that alerts you to the carbs in common foods can be invaluable. The key here is to track carbs and not just calories, since carbs are one of the keys to weight loss, by using an app such as Carb Manager, MyFitnessPal, or Atkins Carb & Meal Tracker.

For additional information, please see the website of the American Diabetes association at www.diabetes.org.

For information on the work of Jerry Stine, please see:
www.LifespanInstitute.com.
For information on the work of Armin Brott, please see:
www.MrDad.com.
For the work of Nancy Faass, please see:
www.HealthWritersGroup.com.

Chapter 19
Infectious Conditions in Men
Josh Perlroth, MD
Infectious Disease Specialist

It's always an uncertainty. We are always
at the infectious disease roulette table.
— Dr. William Schaffner

It is well known that the strength of the immune system declines with age. Everyone eventually experiences the ravages of aging, which includes greater susceptibility to cancer, injury, and cognitive decline. Yet men tend to overlook their vulnerability to the infectious diseases that occur with age.

CHRONIC INFECTIONS

Infections can take a toll not only during their acute phase, but also during the recovery phase, which in many cases, is prolonged and brings its own set of challenges.

Diverticulitis. The instances of this disorder have been increasing along with the prevalence of diverticulosis. This is particularly true in western countries where approximately 50% of the population 60 years of age and older have diverticulosis, attributed primarily to a lack of dietary fiber, particularly that found in fresh fruits and vegetables. Up to 25% of those patients will suffer at least one bout of diverticulitis. By the age of 80, almost everyone has symptoms of diverticulitis.

Sexually transmitted infections. Unfortunately, sexually transmitted infections such as syphilis, gonorrhea, chlamydia, and even HIV continue to circulate, not just among the young. These infections are still on the rise, with nearly 2.5 million combined cases of chlamydia, gonorrhea, and syphilis in 2018. (See chapter 93, which is devoted to this topic.)

Prostatitis. Prostate inflammation has a lifetime risk of occurrence of up to 8.2%, with almost two million physician visits each year. Risk factors include sexually transmitted infections, bacterial bladder infections, and prior instrumentation of the prostate. Prostatitis can increase the potential for prostate cancer, so these conditions are to be taken seriously.

Herpes zoster (shingles). These painful conditions are a generally localized recurrence of chickenpox, which has been a vaccine-preventable disease since 1994. However, men over 40 typically have had chickenpox infections as children, which puts them at risk for shingles later in life, accounting for the one million cases reported annually. The incidence of shingles is approximately four cases per 1,000 in the U.S. annually, but among people 60 years and older, it is about 1% (one in one hundred) annually, according to CDC data. Unfortunately, shingles can be extremely painful, and prolonged pain ("post-herpetic neuralgia") occurs in up to 19% of people. Its incidence is usually age-dependent; the pain can be difficult to manage and decreases the quality of life. The prevalence of herpes zoster is as follows:

- 2% in patients younger than 50 years of age

- Over 20% in those older than 50 years

- More than 35% in those over the age of 80 years.

Skin infections such as abscesses ("boils") and cellulitis. These infections become more common (up to 200 cases per 100,000 patient-years) and have multiple risk factors found in middle-aged men, including skin barrier disruption due to trauma, edema due to impaired lymphatic drainage, or venous insufficiency, obesity, and immunosuppression (such as diabetes or HIV infection).

Dental cavities (caries). I have personally been involved in the care of hundreds of patients with dental infections that did not resolve with standard care. (Also see chapter 53 on optimal dental care to minimize oral infections.)

SEVERE INFECTIONS

Infections that become more common among middle-aged men and beyond include sepsis, pneumonia, and cancers that follow bacterial infections.

Sepsis. When an infection reaches the blood stream, that can result in a systemic or body-wide reaction that causes fever and a dangerous drop in blood pressure. Not only is the acute infection itself taxing on the system, but recovery can be prolonged, particularly if surgical intervention is required. These infections can result in sepsis or septic shock when bacteria enter and multiply in the bloodstream to such an extent that the condition becomes life-threatening. CDC data show that 1.7 million Americans develop sepsis annually, and 270,000 patients die. One-third of hospitalized patients who die have sepsis.

Influenza and pneumonia. These disorders continue to be a leading (among the top 10) cause of mortality. Per CDC data, 250,000 people have to seek care in a hospital due to pneumonia each year. Unfortunately, about 50,000 people die.

RISK FACTORS

Obesity. Weight gain makes the treatment of infections more complicated in terms of antibiotic dosing, recovery times, and surgical outcomes.

Aging. As we age, our ability to fight infections decreases. This phenomenon is correlated with a decrease in T cells, which is not well understood, but seems to correlate with atrophy of the thymus, an important immune organ. Bone marrow production of immune cells also tends to wane as we age. Evidence for waning immune response is well known in the case of decreasing response to vaccines, particularly in those over the age of 65.

Stress. We know from the research literature that stress can be a factor in poor immune health.

Excessive alcohol consumption. Chronic alcohol use over time can damage the liver, which plays an important role in immune function. For example, significant alcoholic liver disease increases the risk of *Vibrio vulnificus*, which can be contracted from eating raw shellfish, particularly oysters. This infection can be life-threatening. Even bacterial infections that may not generally be severe can be worsened by chronic liver disease.

Common viral and bacterial infections. Many men over 40 have families including small children that put them in the crosshairs for common infections that in youth are nearly inconsequential, but in the adult can be much more difficult to negotiate. These include viral infections such as parvovirus and Coxsackievirus (hand, foot, and mouth disease), as well as common viruses such as influenza and chickenpox. In the priorly uninfected adult, these infections and others such as strep throat (*Streptococcal pharyngitis*) can be surprisingly serious.

Travel exposures. The increase in disposable income often allows for more extensive travel experiences. Travel to certain regions of the world presents its own set of potential exposures, including:

- **Malaria.** Exceptionally widespread, malaria is prevalent in Central and South America, Africa, India, and Southeast Asia.

- **Tropical viruses.** Potentially serious viral infections in the tropics include dengue and chikungunya.

- **Norovirus.** Cruise ships are notorious for norovirus outbreaks.

- **Lyme disease and coinfections.** Even camping in North America can put one at risk for Lyme disease, tularemia, and in some cases, plague.

- **Traveler's diarrhea.** This is a risk nearly worldwide. Pre-travel vaccines reduce this risk, particularly vaccines against typhoid fever and yellow fever. Alternatively, antibiotics can be packed and taken as needed should diarrheal illness strike.

Immune-suppressive medications. We are seeing increased prevalence of chronic medical conditions that require immune-suppressing medication regimens, such as rheumatologic disorders, autoimmune conditions, and cancer. As a result, men with these conditions can be at risk for another set of secondary, opportunistic infections not typically seen in the general population.

Antibiotic overuse. Resistant bacterial infections have become increasingly common, so avoidance of unnecessary antibiotics has become a major emphasis of the medical community over the past decade, at least. A large percentage of prescribed antibiotics have been retrospectively deemed unnecessary and are often prescribed for viral illnesses against which antibiotics have no effect.

More than 2.8 million antibiotic-resistant infections occur in the U.S. each year (per CDC data), and more than 35,000 people die as a result. As a practitioner, today I frequently deal with infections that in the past were easy to treat and that now require very broad-spectrum antibiotics or combinations of antibiotics to eradicate.

Antibiotic side effects. Antibiotics also alter the gut microflora and put people at risk for antibiotic-associated diarrhea, and worse, particularly *Clostridium difficile* (*C. diff.*) infection. These bacteria produce a toxin that can cause severe diarrhea, inflammation of the colon, and in extreme circumstances, colon resection surgery or even death. In 2017 there were almost 224,000 cases of this infection, and at least 12,800 people died.

Other potential side effects of unnecessary antibiotics include allergic reactions, fatigue, and even tendonitis or tendon rupture in the case of the fluoroquinolone antibiotic class, which includes Cipro and Levaquin.

Antibiotic-resistant bacteria. Another challenge facing the world is the proliferation of antibiotic-resistant bacteria that are outpacing the development of effective antimicrobial agents. While these bacteria have traditionally been isolated from institutionalized or frequently hospitalized people, it has become more common to find resistant bacteria in people without any history of recent antibiotic use or hospitalization or with limited exposure to prior courses of antibiotics. Resistant bacterial infections are associated with prior exposure to antibiotics, which makes the prospect of facing infections while aging all the more unsettling.

LIFESTYLE FACTORS

Fortunately, there are a number of promising steps we can take to maintain the health of our immune systems, which will be discussed further in chapters 20 and 21.

Lifestyle risk factors tend to be more important than any specific behavior in terms of susceptibility to infectious disease. There is very little strong science behind any supplements or medications to achieve better "immunity." Healthy lifestyle choices are frankly the most significant actions we can take. These include avoidance of smoking, eating a healthy diet high in fruits and vegetables, sleep, and exercise.

Restorative sleep. Many of us also do not get enough restorative sleep, generally thought to be 7 to 8 hours a night, but also likely an individual requirement.

Exercise. The beneficial effects of physical activity on mental health are well established, but less so in regards to immune health.

- Acute exercise increases blood and lymphatic flow, causing more of our infection-fighting white blood cells to circulate in the bloodstream, according to a scientific review in the *Journal of Sport and Health Science* (2019).

- Aerobic exercise at least five days a week can lower the number of upper respiratory infections such as colds over three months by more than 40%, as reported by the *British Journal of Sports Medicine* (2011).

Probiotics. This is a hot topic today, but in fact, probiotics have not been shown to improve infectious disease outcomes. They may help reduce the chances of *C. difficile*–associated diarrhea when we take antibiotics to treat an infection.

Vitamin supplementation. In the healthy individual who gets enough vitamins through his diet, supplementation has not been shown to improve infectious disease incidence or outcomes despite many studies. However, vitamin deficiency is a well-established risk factor for infections linked to increased respiratory infections and increased length of stay in the ICU, according to the *American Journal of Surgery* (2012). As such, the likelihood of benefit from an infection standpoint applies only if the individual has a deficiency. Evidence for other mechanisms of immune modulation with vitamins A, B-complex, and C through data regarding supplementation and immune protection or decreased infection risk are lacking.

Handwashing. Soap and water sanitizing, notably since the COVID pandemic, has again appropriately risen to the forefront of infection prevention. There is no evidence that specifically-branded antibacterial soap has any benefit over regular soap.

MEDICAL INTERVENTIONS

There are many interventions, both in terms of lifestyle and in the medical realm, that have been proven beneficial in preventing infections.

Vaccines. Aside from widespread public sanitation, no intervention in human history has prevented more deaths than vaccines, which have been proven to be safe and effective for decades. Vaccination is the sole reason smallpox was eradicated from the world, and the second infectious disease that has been nearly wiped out is polio. Children now receive vaccines for measles, mumps, rubella, chickenpox, influenza, hepatitis A and B, diphtheria, polio, tetanus, whooping cough, pneumonia, and Haemophilus influenza. As we enter adolescence, vaccines to prevent HPV (human papillomavirus or warts which are precancerous) and meningitis are given. For Americans over 40 years old, the primary vaccines available to decrease infections and their complications are for COVID-19, influenza, pneumonia, and shingles.

The newest shingles vaccine (Shingrix) is more than 90% effective at preventing shingles and post-herpetic neuralgia, and the protection stays at 85% for at least four years per the CDC.

There are two types of pneumonia vaccines that protect against infection by the bacterium *Streptococcus pneumoniae,* which is one of the most common and dangerous causes of pneumonia. The 23 serotypes found in the Pneumovax vaccine are 60% to 70% effective in preventing invasive disease due to these serotypes. Prevnar (13 serotypes) is reported to prevent hospitalization from pneumonia caused by these bacteria in 73% in adults 65 years and older.

Influenza vaccination development must start before the flu season in order to produce enough doses for those who need it. Vaccines are designed to protect against either three or four types of influenza – typically two influenza A strains (such as H1N1 and H3N2) and one or two type B strains. Historically, the effectiveness in preventing flu illness ranges from 40% to 60%.

Health screenings and testing. Just as vaccines are designed to prevent infection, health screening is a crucial component of preserving health as we age, and screening is applicable in some situations to infectious diseases. In particular, colonoscopy, while used primarily as a cancer screening tool, can identify the presence of diverticulosis, which could prompt recommendations for a higher fiber diet or a bowel regimen to prevent constipation.

Good dental health. Dental disease is discussed in more detail elsewhere, but poor dentition and periodontal disease are important primary infectious issues that are thought to contribute to cardiovascular disease.

**For more information on the work of Dr. Perlroth,
please see www.IDDoctors.com.
For additional information on infectious disease, please see www.cdc.gov.**

Chapter 20
How Your Immune System Works
Judson Brandeis, MD, Urologist
& Scott Lu, MD, Clinical Researcher

The most powerful therapeutic system in the world is our own immune system.
— Francis deSouza

Until the early 20th century, infectious disease was the number one killer of humanity. As deaths from infections declined, life expectancy increased from the mid-1930s to the mid-1970s. As a result, we became somewhat complacent about the importance of our own innate immunity, relying heavily on antibiotics and technological medicine.

The recent COVID-19 pandemic has reminded us of the importance of the immune system, and the vulnerability of immunity as we age, especially in those with chronic health issues.

Modern medicine and the public health system have made great strides in reducing illness and premature death from infectious disease.

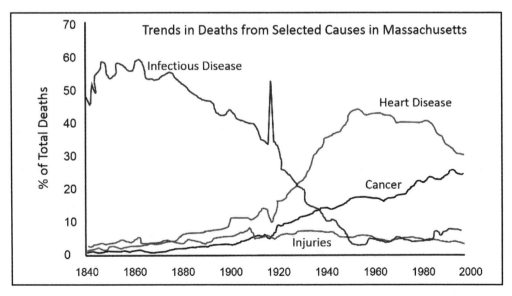

Figure 20.1 Reductions in infectious disease and the rise of chronic, fatal disorders.

- **1890.** Infrastructure was developed in major cities to provide trash and waste removal. (This may sound mundane, but at that time, the average city street was ankle- to knee-deep in garbage, debris, and animal waste.)

- **1900.** With the cleanup of major cities, infectious disease continued to decrease significantly. As germ theory became more widely accepted, the importance of personal hygiene (such as handwashing) was taught in the public schools and was practiced more in the home, further reducing infectious illness.

- **1910.** Chlorine was introduced into the public water supply to reduce bacteria levels, improving water quality in major cities.

- **1932.** The discovery and distribution of sulfa drugs increased defensive measures against infection.

- **1945.** Penicillin vastly expanded pharmaceutical treatment and ushered in a new era in medicine.

- **1955.** Dr. Jonas Salk created the first vaccine to be used population-wide. The concept of vaccination was known since colonial times, but was not an aspect of a coordinated public health effort. Since then, vaccines for a wide variety of illnesses have become more commonplace.

Despite the major extension in lifespan, as Americans became predominately city dwellers, the industrial diet and sedentary lifestyle have increased premature deaths from chronic conditions such as cardiovascular disease and cancer. In spite of the astonishing breakthroughs of science, our most important protection is still the immune system.

THE FIRST LINE OF DEFENSE

THE SKIN

Our protection against infectious disease begins with our built-in defenses. Our skin (and mucous membranes) provide barriers that physically resist the entry of microbes. Skin functions like a massive layer of Saran wrap, covering and protecting the entire body. Close up, it's a complex, multi-layered structure that includes fatty acids, connective tissue, and blood vessels. These different structures and functions protect us from the external environment.

- **Hand washing and showering.** Washing mechanically removes microbes from your skin. Research shows that using soap definitely kills more microbes than just rinsing your hands with water.

- **Mucous.** Humble mucus stands guard in key areas where microbes would be likely to invade the body—the nose, sinuses, mouth, throat, and lungs, as well as the stomach and intestines. Although the structure of each of these areas is different, the function of the mucus is the same throughout. In the nose and throat, for example, mucus traps bacteria and particles such as dust for removal.

- **Mucous membranes.** Lining the respiratory and gastrointestinal (GI) systems, the mucous membranes are home to beneficial bacteria that protect us by providing competition to harmful pathogens. Some of the mucous membranes also feature cilia, microscopic hair-like structures that move germ-laden mucous out of the body in coughs and sneezes. (Note that exposure to tobacco smoke in the lungs can damage the cilia.)

TEMPERATURE AND ACID-ALKALINE BALANCE (PH)

Body temperature. Fever can be an important means of inhibiting the growth of harmful bacteria. Microbes function within a specific temperature range, and the high temperature of a fever essentially cooks them.

Tip. You can recreate a therapeutic fever by doing a sauna. Saunas, sweats, and sweat lodges have been used worldwide since ancient times to recover from acute illness, manage chronic conditions, and support detoxification.

Beneficial stomach acid. The body also destroys bacteria and parasites with hydrochloric acid in the stomach (an important reason to go easy on antacids, since your stomach acid is generally protective rather than harmful). Stomach acid in this way helps to protect against food poisoning.

Tip. Rather than an acid stomach (too much acid), a surprising number of people have low levels of stomach acid. That can be tested, but one can also do a simple trial using a low-strength, over-the-counter supplement containing betaine hydrochloride (HCl) (try 250 mg., for example). If digestion is improved by taking a capsule with a meal, that can be continued. If the supplement causes a little temporary heartburn, that indicates that your stomach acid (HCl levels) are adequate, a good state of affairs.

INFLAMMATION

Inflammation is the body's response when infection or tissue damage occurs, a sign of immune activity. Although we may be bothered by it, the symptoms of immune activity are a clear indication that the body is trying to accomplish something. Familiar examples of inflammation include:

- **An acute, emerging infection.** We think of this type of inflammation as beneficial because it's an aspect of the body's attempts to control an infection such as a cold or the flu. In truth, this applies to any infection.

- **Low-grade, chronic infection.** With an ongoing, chronic situation, the inflammatory process has been triggered, but the normal response isn't enough to resolve the infection. When inflammation becomes constant, more serious conditions can result. In the case of stomach ulcers, people may put up with an upset stomach for years, assuming that the problem is either too much stress or too much stomach acid. We now know that gastritis can be caused by *Helicobacter pylori* bacteria, which can initiate stomach cancer if left untreated. (Dr. Barry Marshall, an Australian researcher, proved that *H. pylori* causes ulcers by drinking a beaker of the bacteria. He developed ulcers in a matter of days and won a Nobel prize for his effort.)

- **Food sensitivity.** Foods that trigger either classic allergy symptoms or some type of food sensitivity can cause chronic inflammation. Gluten sensitivity is a good example.

- **Environmental toxins.** Ongoing exposures can occur at home or at work. Often these exposures are so familiar, they are taken for granted. Environmental contaminants include toxic mold, metals such as lead or mercury, or chemicals (pesticides in the home or garden and household cleaning products).

- **Systemic inflammation.** In a healthy immune system, excessive inflammation is managed by a series of checks and balances. With chronic inflammation, immune activity can make other conditions worse, with an impact on health issues such as arthritis, heart disease, diabetes, cancer, or Alzheimer's disease.

To recap, these four mechanisms serve to prevent harmful microbes from causing an infection:

- The protective barrier provided by our skin and mucous membranes

- Body temperature, including fever

- Acid-alkaline balance, including the stomach acid that protects us against food poisoning

- Inflammation, which is our first response when these mechanisms are breached and pathogenic microbes gain access to the body.

Immune memory is vast. The immune system is able to recognize millions of different types of microbes and particles (antigens). If bacteria or viruses overwhelm our natural barriers, an entire army of immune cells usually provides a targeted response.

IMMUNE CELLS — FOOT SOLDIERS OF THE IMMUNE SYSTEM

Our targeted immune defenses are made up of two systems working together, functioning as foot soldiers (immune cells) and artillery (antibodies). The immune cells (logically described as *cellular* immunity) consist of trillions of microscopic cells that occur in a number of shapes and sizes, with a range of functions. These cells are tasked with identifying and attacking potentially harmful bacteria, viruses, molds, fungi, and parasites as well as cancer cells, allergenic food particles, and cellular debris.

The body's military police. We know that our immune cells can target specific types of bacteria that it "remembers" from past encounters. But our first line defenses will go after anything that looks dangerous.

The white blood cells we learned about as kids go by the fancy name of phagocytes, and the average man has 24 to 33 billion phagocytes in his bloodstream. These ancient foot soldiers of the immune system are comparable to military police, cruising the bloodstream and lymph on the lookout for strange microbes up to no good.

Phagocytes roam the body, engulfing and digesting microbes. Any microbe not recognized will be consumed—literally swallowed whole and digested with enzymes similar to meat tenderizer.

Immune cells, locked and loaded. The armies of immune cells that roam our body are comparable to an elite military force, equipped with spies, troops, demolition experts, and peacekeepers. Their job is to protect us from viruses, bacteria, and molds in the air we breath; bacteria on our skin; bacteria, mold, and parasites in the food we eat: and even the exchange of microbes that occurs during sex.

> *Our greatest exposure is usually from food, which explains why an astounding 70% to 80% of the immune system is located in the gut.*

Peacekeepers. The microbiome refers to beneficial bacteria in the intestinal tract, which protect us by destroying the microbes that cause food poisoning. Antibiotic use can kill the good bacteria, allowing harmful bacteria such as *Clostridium difficile* to flourish. Research has demonstrated that ingesting probiotics and foods rich in probiotics can strengthen our barrier against infection.

Tip. Probiotic-rich foods include live culture yogurt, kefir, and kombucha; uncooked sauerkraut, cultured pickles, olives, and other types of fermented vegetables; and Asian specialty products such as kimchi, miso, and tempeh.

WHITE BLOOD CELLS

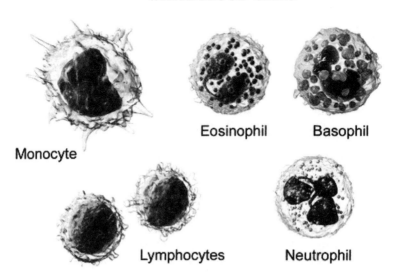

White Blood Cells (WBC)			
Type of WBC	**%**	**Target / Task**	**Lifespan**
Neutrophils	62%	Destroy bacteria and fungi	6 hours to a few days
Lymphocytes	30%	*B cells* release antibodies (artillery) which target antigens *Cytotoxic T cells* and *natural killer cells* target virus-infected cells and any form of tumor or malignancy	Weeks for T cells; Years for memory cells
Monocytes: 2–3 times the size of other WBC	5%	Are transformed into macrophages to target bacteria and phagocytes in the liver to break down red blood cells.	Hours to days
Eosinophils	2%	Larger parasites Modulate allergy-related inflammation	8—12 days
Basophils	0.4%	Release histamine for inflammatory responses	A few hours to a few days

Figure 20.2 Major types of white blood cells and their function. Our protection against bacteria, molds, parasites, fungus, viruses, and malignancies.

The demolition crew. Specialized T cells come equipped for chemical warfare.

- **Natural killer (NK) cells.** Related to T cells, NK cells seek out viruses and emerging cancer cells. Both viruses and malignancies tend to hide *within* our own cells. NK cells destroy viruses, for example, by blowing up not only the virus, but also most of the cell that it's hiding in. Pus is often the remnant of this activity, which helps to explain why infected tissue can be such a mess. Sometimes the immune system causes collateral damage in its efforts to protect us. (Case in point is the cytokine storm associated with acute COVID-19.)

- **Cytotoxic T cells.** These T cells are weaponized with corrosive compounds similar to bleach and peroxide, and like natural killer cells, target hidden viruses and budding cancer cells.

Command central. T cells have activity that ranges from destroying infected cells to various leadership roles, calling up other immune cells to active duty, sending messages, and generally regulating the immune response.

- **Regulatory T cells.** Known informally as T regs, these T cells help manage the immune response by communicating with suppressor and helper cells using messenger chemicals such as cytokines.

- **T helper cells.** These T cells amplify the immune response and help regulate the B cells (which make antibodies) and the T cells. HIV infections destroy T helpers, leaving the body vulnerable to potentially fatal secondary infections.

- **T suppressors.** Functioning as peacekeepers, they turn off the immune system once the threat of infection is over and also prevent autoimmunity.

Insight on the blood tests for your annual physical. If you review the lab slip from your last annual exam, your doctor probably checked to be sure you have enough white blood cells. (Most labs measure neutrophils, lymphocytes, monocytes, eosinophiles, and basophils.) Your physician will be looking for patterns of high or low levels of white blood cells. At times, these patterns suggest an activated immune system. The pattern of white blood cells may also differentiate an acute (immediate) infection from a chronic condition.

ANTIBODIES—IMMUNE ARTILLERY

The antibodies are microscopic fragments of protein comparable to artillery or shrapnel. An antibody can neutralize a microbe directly or simply *tag* the microbe (or the cell where it is hiding) for attack by other immune agents.

Antigens. Anything that can trigger an immune response is considered an antigen, including microbes, large undigested food particles, allergenic foods, or debris from cells.

Targeted immune cells respond to these threats through a lock-and-key process, reading the detailed structure of the antigen's cell membrane and marking them for destruction.

Immunoglobulins—the antibodies. Antibodies *bind* to antigens, coating them with microscopic fragments of protein, creating a sticky surface somewhat like Velcro. When the antibodies become snagged in mucus, the microbe is trapped and can be ejected from the body in a sneeze, a cough, or in stool.

Types of Antibodies

Both immune cells and antibodies have a general (*non-specific*) system that destroy any life form suspected of being dangerous. There is also the *targeted system* that identifies specific invaders and primes the immune cell for a search-and-destroy mission. Each of the five classes of antibodies has a different function:

- **Secretory IgA (SIgA) antibodies.** Broad-spectrum IgA are found in tears, saliva, sweat, and colostrum, and in the GI tract, the lungs, and the prostate. SIgA provide peacekeeping functions and are found in great numbers in the digestive tract. The friendly bacteria in the gut (the microbiome) consists of *trillions* of bacteria tasked with digesting our food, so these bacteria are essential to our survival. However, spoiled food laden with bacteria or mold is one of the greatest threats to our health.

  SIgA are able to differentiate the good guys from the bad guys. (For example, SIgA tolerate bacteria such as acidophilus that digest milk for us, while targeting harmful E. coli bacteria, a common cause of food poisoning that can be fatal in the very young and those of advanced age.)

- **IgA antibodies.** These immunoglobulins play a crucial role in the function of our protective mucous membranes.

- **IgG antibodies.** IgG are often involved in delayed responses. They are considered evidence of food sensitivity in contrast to rapid response antibodies (IgE) that can trigger life-threatening allergic responses. When testing for infection, IgG are considered evidence that a particular infection occurred in the past.

- **IgE antibodies.** IgE are generated in "crisis" situations involving full-blown allergies, which are life-threatening in some cases. IgE antibodies can mount inflammation so rapidly that the airway swells closed, causing difficulty breathing. Classic IgE allergies include intense reactions to peanuts and shellfish, as well as bee stings. Note that these responses are always individual. (For more on IgE, see chapter 12 on environmental allergies.)

- **IgM antibodies.** IgM are produced in response to an active infection only; they do not reflect past infections. (For example, if you've had COVID-19, recovered, and now have immunity to COVID, your IgG levels for COVID antibodies will be higher, but you will have no IgM antibodies for COVID.)

As one way of thinking about IgM antibodies, imagine a library that has one copy of every book, but if a particular book becomes popular, the publisher must begin producing thousands of copies. When a bacteria or virus enters the bloodstream, the IgM antibodies bind to the microbe, and white blood cells (foot soldiers) mount an attack.

However, if there are more microbes than IgM, then the B cells must produce IgG antibodies (another type of artillery) to mark the dangerous microbes. Unfortunately, this takes time. However, after the infection is defeated, IgG antibodies hang around so it is less likely that the same microbes will cause future infections. (This also serves to develop an immunologic memory that can quickly eliminate the same infection if it occurs again.)

Although antibodies can recognize an antigen and lock onto it, they can't destroy it without help. That's the job of the T cells, which signal other cells like phagocytes to fight infection.

Tip. If you find that you're getting sick a lot, as a first step, it's useful to be tested for "total immune globulins." If the level of antibodies your body produces is too low, that could suggest depressed immune function. Low levels also indicate that the results of *all* antibody testing will be less accurate.

At the time of this writing, major labs use antibody testing to check for ten different types of infections including Epstein-Barr (mononucleosis); herpes 1, 2, and 6; mycoplasma (a potential cause of pneumonia); and Rocky Mountain spotted fever (tick-borne infection), as well as allergens to more than 10 different types of mold.

For more information on immunity and health please see
www.TheTwentyFirstCenturyMan.com.
For more information on immunology, see the site of the American Academy of
Allergy, Asthma & Immunology at www.aaaai.org.

Chapter 21
Boosting Your Immunity
Jerry Stine, Nutritionist
& Nancy Faass, Health Coach

The four components that keep our immune system healthy are good nutrition, exercise, breathing, and meditation.
— Ann Boroch

The immune system goes about its business most of the time without our awareness—until it doesn't. What can you do to maintain good immune function, and what can you do when there's a problem?

THE BASICS

Multivitamin. There is a great deal of research showing that a quality multivitamin helps to maintain immune function day to day. Look for a multivitamin formula that contains a broad-spectrum of vitamins, including vitamin A, B-complex, and vitamin C as well as trace minerals (particularly copper, manganese, selenium, and zinc) to support your immune function.

Omega 3. This is a supplement that benefits every cell and tissue in the body, since fatty acids are key constituents of cell walls. You'll want a quality brand to ensure higher potency, better absorption, and low mercury content (harvested from fish in clean deep ocean waters).

Vitamin C. Many of us benefit from additional vitamin C. We now know that vitamin C levels can be depleted by stress, whether our body is fighting an infection or coping with some other type of stressor.

Vitamin D. Most multivitamins contain vitamin D and for many people that is sufficient. However, vitamin D deficiencies are not at all unusual, so we recommend getting vitamin D levels tested on a regular basis.

Magnesium. There's strong evidence that the stresses of modern lifestyle can deplete magnesium with potential impact on cardiovascular health, the immune system, energy production, and digestive function. Lack of regular bowel movements is one symptom. Fatigue is another common symptom of low magnesium.

Food choices. A quality diet and good food choices are an essential aspect of maintaining strong immune function. Since reactive foods can wreak havoc with your immune system, check out the sections in this chapter on Food Reactions and on "The Immune System on Sugar." Also see chapter 31 ("What Is Food?"), especially the section "Fast Carbs, Slow Carbs" and chapter 35. Food Allergies.

Does Your Immune System Need Extra Support?

If you're having trouble shaking a cold or experiencing chronic inflammation reflected in arthritis, digestive issues, or psoriasis, ask your doctor to check your nutrient levels with simple blood tests.

Nutrient testing. Typically, lab work to check nutrient levels includes vitamins A, D, folate (B9), and B12; these tests are available from any large medical lab, such as LabCorp or Quest. If your condition is not severe, you may decide to see a health coach or nutritionist for guidance on how to maintain your health and immune function within the context of your lifestyle.

Levels of immune cells. Important immune system markers are frequently part of a standard chemistry (chem) panel, which may include basophils, eosinophils, lymphocytes, monocytes, and neutrophils (see the preceding Chapter 20. How Your Immune System Works) for more on the importance of these immune cells. Patterns of high or low levels of these immune cells can indicate acute or chronic bacterial or viral infection or a generally suppressed immune function. If you get sick frequently or if you have chronic illness, your physician will want to test and track these levels over time.

With any supplement that is new to you, only make one change at a time to be sure it agrees with your system.

CONDITIONS RELATED TO IMMUNE FUNCTION

AUTOIMMUNITY

Common autoimmune diseases include rheumatoid arthritis and lupus erythematosus. Autoimmune activity is also present in certain types of thyroid disorders, celiac disease, diabetes mellitus type 1, Graves' disease, inflammatory bowel disease, multiple sclerosis, and psoriasis.

Autoimmune activity refers to disturbances that result in attacks by the immune system on our own body, as if our cells or tissue were foreign. There are at least five common underlying causes of this type of autoimmune activity that tend to be underappreciated:

- Food-related issues caused by excessive carbohydrate and sugar intake

- Consumption of reactive foods

- Low-grade or silent infections

- Mold exposure

- Toxic substances in the environment, such as metals or toxic chemicals.

In the last decade there have been great advances in our understanding of autoimmune activity and in the development of interventions to help regulate the immune system. Physicians and health coaches trained in functional medicine often have expertise and experience in the management of autoimmune disorders.

Resource. *The Autoimmune Paleo Cookbook*, by Mickey Trescott. (2003)

BRAIN-ASSOCIATED SYMPTOMS—Brain fog, lack of focus, declining memory, depression, or anxiety—and surprising links to the immune system

The fact that the brain has a separate, independent immune system was just discovered in the last ten years.

One of the major players in this unique system are the glial cells—the microglia (micro-glee-uh). If you happen to have an autoimmune disorder, a head injury, or a neurological condition such as Parkinson's disease, these little cells can make your life hell. With a neurological crisis such as infection or injury, the brain's immune system may become primed, moving into a constant state of "red alert" that is easily triggered.

Immune reactivity anywhere in the body can also trigger inflammation in the brain. The brain's immune system lacks the mechanisms to counter this inflammation, to downregulate excessive activity. The result is delayed or incomplete management of brain inflammation.

Anti-inflammatories to calm the brain's immune defenses. The microglia protect you against bacteria or toxins that happen to cross the blood-brain barrier. Like any defender, they can become overly enthusiastic about their job and cause collateral damage. Here are some nutrients that can reduce brain inflammation when these little immune cells become overly active:

- **Glutathione.** The most important antioxidant in the body

- **Resveratrol.** Extract of grape (skins)

- **Curcumin.** An extract of turmeric (related to ginger), a mainstay of Indian cuisine

- **Green tea extract.** Consumed as a beverage in China for 4,000 years

Coping with brain fatigue. If mental activity tires you quickly, you may be experiencing brain fatigue. This type of fatigue can also reflect depletion of nutrients vital for brain function. These include free amino acids derived from dietary protein, which our body uses for ongoing operation and repair. Amino acids are utilized at a rapid rate under stress and can become depleted. A number of amino acids provide the building blocks for neurotransmitters, and if our levels are low, mental energy and moods can suffer. There are a variety of amino acid blends aimed at various types of stress that can be helpful.

Resources. If you struggle with brain fog or depression, a recent book of interest explains the immune-brain connection and disorders such as depression and brain fog with new approaches to treatment: *The Angel and the Assassin: The Tiny Brain Cell that Changed the Course of Medicine* by Donna Jackson Nakazawa.

Supplements. Two useful amino acid products are NOW Sports Amino Complete (available from Amazon.com and Vitacost.com) and Montiff amino acid formulas (available from Amazon.com and Pure Formulas.com).

CANCER PREVENTION—Your body's every-day efforts to deter cancer

How your body protects you. Our bodies randomly produce cancerous or malfunctioning cells on an ongoing basis. One of the major jobs of the immune system is to identify and destroy these dangerous cells as a form of daily housekeeping. Cancer can gain a foothold if the immune system can no longer rid us of these abnormal cells.

Natural killer cells (aka cytotoxic T cells) are the immune agent tasked with roaming the body searching for cancerous cells. When they find a cell with malignancy inside, they punch holes in the cell's outer membrane and inject enzymes similar to meat tenderizer, dissolving the cancer cell. This strategy is also used to destroy viruses harbored within our own cells.

Cancer cells can be caused by:

- Ongoing or massive chemical exposures (including cigarette smoke)
- Smoldering viral infection, (such as cytomegalovirus, Epstein-Barr, hepatitis B or C, human herpesvirus 8, or human papilloma virus)
- Chronic infections of any type
- Repeated injury
- Genetic sensitivities
- Poor diet choices (The data associate a high-carb diet with cancer, and we know that cancer cells thrive on glucose.)

- Oxidative stress, which can be compared to a form of rust that degrades cells and tissue.

Oxidative stress and cancer. The caustic chemicals the immune system uses in our defense are similar to the bleach and peroxide we all use to clean our homes. These chemicals, produced by our bodies, result in oxidative stress. Excessive levels of oxidative stress is a confirmed precursor to cancer, so it is vital to help your body clear this stressful chemistry with a healthy daily intake of *anti*-oxidants. These nutrients, found in fresh fruits and vegetables, provide the antidote to oxidative stress.

Resource. An astonishing book on the underappreciated role of lifestyle in preventing cancer is by David Servan-Schreiber, MD: *Anticancer: A New Way of Life* (New York: Penguin Books, 2017).

COLDS AND FLU—What you need to know to fight cold and flu viruses

Nutrients that help to prevent viral infections:

- The Basics, listed on the first page in this chapter.

- Medicinal mushrooms. During cold and flu season, these can provide a form of tonic. There are a number of effective formulas, which typically include beta-glucans. Try different variations to determine the product that is most effective for you.

If you suspect that you are actively fighting a virus. The following is a list of potentially useful supplements. To support your immune system, you will want to be sure to take the basics and then choose two or three key supplements from the following:

- Vitamin D

- Monolaurin and echinacae, taken in combination

- Colloidal or nano silver

- Elderberry syrup

- Zinc lozenges (not to exceed 150 mg per day)

DIGESTIVE ISSUES—How the body protects us from food poisoning

As much as 80% of the immune system is apparently located in the gut, tasked with ongoing surveillance every time we eat. We come equipped with a series of protective systems:

- **The stomach destroys bacteria in food with beneficial stomach acid.** Ever wonder why we don't get food poisoning every day? We are protected by the miracle of our stomach acid, which kills invading microbes, literally dissolving them. (So only take antacids if you really need them. Your stomach acid is there for a *very* good reason.)

- **In the gut, the immune system monitors incoming food to verify whether it is safe or harmful.** The purpose of the immune system in the gut is to recognize friend from foe. This means differentiating trillions of friendly, beneficial bacteria (probiotics) from mold and bacteria in food and water and destroying any suspicious microbe that has made it through the stomach acid.

- **If the invader is potentially harmful, it is bombarded with artillery, the antibodies.** Antibodies can be compared to a form of shrapnel, coating invading microbes with projectiles. This creates a surface like Velcro, so the pathogen gets caught in the conveyor belt of mucous that continually moves through the gut and is disposed of.

- **When any of these systems go out of balance, the result is dysbiosis.** This is an unhealthy balance in the microorganisms of the gut—for example, an overgrowth of *Clostridium difficile*, which is known to proliferate after antibiotic overuse, or bacterial biofilm that flourishes with a high sugar diet, at your expense.

A broad-spectrum probiotic. Research continues to show the benefits of taking probiotic supplements. However, it is important to understand that probiotics alone will not usually overcome poor diet choices. There are many different formulas with different strains of probiotic bacteria. It may take a certain amount trial-and-error to find a product that works well for you. Another complementary approach is to be sure to include a range of fermented foods in your diet:

- **Dairy.** Yogurt, kefir, acidophilus milk, fermented cheeses (cheddar, Gouda, mozzarella, cottage cheese)

- **Staples.** Miso for broth, tempeh, natto

- **Vegetables.** Home-style pickles, brine-cured olives, pickled vegetables, sauerkraut, kimchi

- **Carbs.** Sourdough bread

Food sensitivities. As a personal experiment, for two weeks cut out grains and milk products (just those two types of foods), and see if there is an improvement in your health.

Strategies from functional medicine. The impact of poor digestive function on overall health has spurred the development of a wide range of new laboratory tests to explore underlying causes of disturbed gut function. If you have persistent GI problems, consider consulting a functional medicine physician or health coach.

Resource: *Optimal Digestive Health,* by Trent Nichols, MD and Nancy Faass (Rochester, VT: Healing Arts, 2005).

FATIGUE

Often, we feel profoundly exhausted when we are coming down with a cold or the flu. That reflects the huge drain on our energy from fighting a virus. Immune system activities also interfere with energy production. While fatigue from a viral infection is to be expected, chronic fatigue that persists for more than two weeks is not normal and indicates that it is time to check in with your doctor or health coach.

FOOD REACTIONS

You may be wondering why information on food reactivity is included in a chapter on immune function. The research shows that food reactions can disrupt the immune system, reflected in conditions ranging from mood swings to brain fog. Here's how that manifests:

- Reactions to food can trigger leaky gut syndrome (aka intestinal permeability).
- When that occurs, particles of undigested food or bacteria are released into the blood stream.
- This places a burden on the liver, which attempts to detoxify the debris.
- If the liver is unable to remove and detoxify the food particles or bacteria, they begin circulating in the blood stream, triggering inflammation.
- This can activate the entire immune system, manifesting as inflammation.

Possible symptoms. The response to food reactivity and leaky gut is totally individual, involving different systems throughout the body. Prime examples include:

- Fatigue that is not improved with sleep
- Brain fog, spaciness, lack of focus, or memory problems
- Mood swings, anxiety, depression, or irritability
- Skin disorders and conditions, including acne, eczema, psoriasis, or rosacea
- Joint pain and stiffness
- Worsening problems with digestion and gut function.

THE IMMUNE SYSTEM ON SUGAR

Sugar and other simple carbohydrates are composed of empty calories. This means that sugary foods provide calories, but none of the nutrients the body requires to function. This depletion of vitamins and minerals can reduce the effectiveness of white blood cells.

Sugar drops your white blood cell count. When you eat sugar, the number of your white cells drops to such an extent, it can be measured with a lab test.

Sugar can also make your white blood cells less effective. Researchers have coined the term "lazy leukocytes" to describe white blood cells that are unable to combat microbes. A diet high in sugar can cause this condition. Unfortunately, this compromise in immune function does not always show up on in a blood test. Blood test results may look normal, but immune function may be subpar.

What you can do. If you have a sweet tooth, find other foods that you can eat and enjoy in place of sugary foods. Take a look at the content on fast carbs, slow carbs in chapter 31, "What Is Food?" Start by substituting foods low on the glycemic index, like berries or luscious salads, for foods that are too sweet or starchy. Make good food a habit and an absolute priority.

William seemed to develop a cold every two weeks, like clockwork. No sooner did he shake one cold when a new one would start. He was able to get feedback from a buddy of his who was an amazing nutritionist. Once he lowered his carb intake, the colds just stopped. (He also lost 30 pounds in the bargain.)

INFECTION, LOW GRADE

One heart attack in four occurs with no sign of warning. We know that heart disease can be increased by an infection such as *Chlamydia pneumoniae* (a type of chlamydia that is *not* sexually transmitted). Infectious illness is now recognized in the medical literature as a contributor to heart disease, cancer, and autoimmune activity, as well as risk of dementia.

A stressful lifestyle and normal aging can contribute to reduced immune system function, increasing our vulnerability to stealth infections. Low-grade infections range from viruses to bacteria—like the ones that cause Lyme disease, cat scratch fever (bartonella), or yeast overgrowth. Chronic low-grade infections can be harbored in the gums, the sinus, the gut, bladder, or the joints.

INFLAMMATION

Chronic inflammation means that the immune system is frequently triggered. What makes this condition so tricky is that it can be invisible—utterly silent. Chronic undetected inflammation is dangerous because it can contribute to almost all of the major disabling illnesses, including:

- Heart disease

- Cancer

- Dementia and memory loss

- Joint disease

- COPD.

Major causes of ongoing immune activation include:

- Consuming foods to which you are sensitive

- Simple carbs that spike blood sugar

- Low-grade infections

- Repeated chemical exposures, which could involve smoking, excess alcohol use, or toxins in the worksite, even at low levels

- Obesity (see the following for more on this subject).

INFLAMMATION DUE TO OBESITY

Fat cells are a source of inflammation and the result of several different types of inflammatory activity:

- Insulin resistance occurs when the body cannot properly manage blood sugar. A diet high in simple carbs contributes to frequent spikes in blood sugar, which is a form of metabolic stress.

- Once prediabetes develops (insulin resistance), the body shifts into a chronic state of inflammation.

- In the case of obesity, the fat cells produce additional inflammatory compounds.

Fat cells produce estrogens, driving down testosterone levels. For men in andropause, it is important to know that estrogen is four times more powerful than testosterone in influencing the brain signaling that controls testosterone levels. The estrogen drops testosterone and then creates a negative feedback loop that drops it further.

The solution to this type of inflammation is to reduce insulin resistance by:

- Reducing simple carbs
- Lowering consumption of reactive foods
- Managing leaky gut
- Supporting detox pathways.

Resource. Mark Hyman, MD, *The Blood Sugar Solution 10-Day Detox Diet: Activate Your Body's Natural Ability to Burn Fat and Lose Weight Fast* (New York, NY: Little, Brown, Spark, 2014).

SKIN

For minor skin problems such as bites, cuts, scrapes, and burns:

- **Nutrients vital for skin healing.** Vitamin B complex with the active form of B6, vitamins A and D, and the minerals silica and zinc

- **Topicals.** Aloe vera, calendula ointment, Chinese burn ointment (Ching Wan Hung, an external analgesic)

Slow healing. If a minor wound is not healing, increase your level of vitamins A and D and zinc.

Serious skin conditions such as acne vulgaris, psoriasis, eczema. When there is a serious skin disorder, it is vitally important to detect any underlying issues in your body that may be contributing to the problem. Step 1 is to cut out sugar, grains, and dairy for two weeks and see how you are doing. If that brings only minor benefit, the next step is comprehensive lab testing. Major chronic skin issues require medical support.

STRESS—How stress depletes your immune system

High stress comes from many different sources: examples include psychological stress due to work-related demands or family issues; physical stress caused by too much work, or not enough sleep or exercise; and bio-chemical stress due to substance abuse or workplace exposures to toxins.

When stress takes the form of an immediate emergency, like running from an angry dog, adrenaline goes up, sounding the alarm throughout your body to mobilize you for action.

Cortisol goes up, releasing stored energy (glucose) from your liver to power your legs for running and your arms for fighting or protecting yourself. However, when stress is

Rebuilding Immunity

Whenever there is an infection, the first priority is to identify and treat the infection. The doctor may initially prescribe an antibiotic or other medication to clear the infection.

- **Restore good nutrition.** When people become ill and lose their appetite, they may become protein deficient. To support good nutrition, a number of predigested protein powders can be helpful as supplements, including fortified rice protein or whey.

- **Provide basic nutrients.** Sometimes all that is needed is zinc and a good multivitamin (one that includes vitamin A and B6) to restore immunity, since these are key nutrients. However, zinc intake should not exceed 150 mg a day, since excessive levels have been found to depress immunity.

- **Replenish nutritional deficiencies.** Lab tests can be used to measure the level of specific nutrients so deficiencies can be addressed. The levels are later remeasured to be sure they have been restored.

- **Check immune function.** Tests are available to measure macrophage levels, T cell count, and antibodies. You can ask to have "total antibody levels" checked for IgA, IgE, IgG, and IgM to be sure your body is producing enough antibodies.

- **Enhance depressed immunity.** Herbal and vitamin supplements to improve immune function can be prescribed based on the findings in the lab work. Supplements are targeted to the specific needs of the individual, whether the goal is to stimulate T cells, macrophages, or antibodies.

- **Check hormone levels.** Most men, as they age, experience drops in testosterone, adrenal hormones such as DHEA, and growth hormone. Immune function suffers as a result. These hormones can be measured through simple blood tests and then replenished to appropriate levels and monitored periodically through retesting.

frequent, intense, or relentless, the continual demand shifts from adrenaline to cortisol in an effort to keep you going.

Cortisol is a normal and appropriate response to stress. However, chronic stress can cause hormone imbalance. Cortisol begins to drop and hormones such as DHEA can become depleted, lowering testosterone and progesterone levels.

Resources. There are so many interesting books on stress, we are going to leave this to your discretion.

VACCINES

Vaccines trigger "active immunization" in the body. This involves injecting antigens from identified pathogens (for example, the influenza virus) to trigger the immune system and activate B cells. The vaccine primes the body to produce these antibodies, creating a permanent memory in your immune system of that specific infection. The general goal of the vaccine is to simulate disease without the detriment of a full infection. Active immunization includes a vaccine-response, but also the body's natural production of antibodies. In some cases, one vaccine injection is enough to develop life-long immunity. However, some viruses, such as the seasonal flu, undergo rapid changes to their surface proteins. Every year new flu viruses emerge, and a new flu vaccine must be developed in response, containing the viral strains most likely to cause an infection that year.

**For more information on nutrition and the services of Jerry Stine, please see: wwwLifespanInstitute.com.
For more on nutrition and coaching with Nancy Faass, please see:
www.TheNeverDietDiet.com**

Chapter 22
Reducing the Risk of Disability
Max Lippman, DC, Chiropractor

The pain is still there. It goes from my lower back into my right leg.
It started in my back because of my hamstring....
I can't swing a bat, and I can't even bend over for a ground ball.
— *Cesar Izturis, Ex-Professional Baseball Player*

As a chiropractor, my primary role in healthcare is to manage back pain using a conservative approach. I oversee a clinic in the San Francisco Bay Area that has treated more than 7,000 patients, including pro athletes, tech CEOs, gym franchise owners, and everyday men just looking to live a pain-free life. My primary goals are to identify the causes of dysfunction, reduce pain, and improve functionality.

I see people with back pain every day, so I understand the concern that a random injury may worsen and become disabling. Yet in the majority of cases, the risk of disability doesn't come from The Big Incident.

Accidents are something you can't necessarily avoid. You may be involved in a car crash for which you bear no responsibility. Clearly such things happen, and we provide rehabilitation in our office for people dealing with those types of injuries. That experience has proven a useful frame of reference for understanding the major causes of disability.

MAJOR CAUSES OF DISABILITY

Surprisingly, the most common disabling conditions over which you have some control are those that start small, due to:

- Fatigue, deconditioning, and atrophy from working at a desk job
- Repetitive motion injuries, especially in the workplace
- Weekend warrior syndrome
- Unconscious dysfunctional movement patterns.

SITTING IS THE NEW SMOKING

It's not just the technology we use that puts us at risk, but also the amount of time that we spend sitting that becomes problematic. The longer you sit, the fewer years you live and the less vitality you have. A sedentary lifestyle more than increases the risk of heart attack and stroke (by 147%), it almost doubles the increased risk of death from cardiovascular events.

Avoiding sitting disease. The biggest concerns with inactivity are weight gain and inflammation. If you're lethargic and you're not moving, that's a recipe for disaster.

- **Weight gain.** One of the major issues with weight gain is that it puts tremendous pressure on the joints. Consider your knees. All the weight you are carrying falls directly on your knees, so if you were 160 pounds and you put on another 40 pounds, that's a 20% increase bearing down on your knees.

- **Impaired circulation.** Without good circulation the fine network of small blood vessels (capillaries) can no longer do the work of delivering oxygen and nutrients to the cells.

- **Inflammation.** Another major concern is low-level inflammation throughout the body, due to lack of activity and poor circulation.

In our society, we SIT far too long, staring at screens for eight hours a day at work, then SIT and drive home in our cars, where we SIT and have dinner, and then SIT for a few more hours and watch TV or read. This pattern starts when we are young, when we are forced to sit in school, crammed into small desks with little room, stuck in poor posture.

WEEKEND WARRIOR SYNDROME

The majority of injuries involve some type of disc event, which can be avoided by doing the following:

- Prevent deconditioning with regular exercise.

- If you are not exercising regularly, think twice about taking on high-impact activity.

- Recognize when something is too heavy to lift as you usually would, and figure out how to move it safely.

- Be proactive. If you need to move a refrigerator, do you need a dolly or a buddy?

The majority of back injuries involve disc herniation.

Most of the severe injuries I see are from somebody trying to move something like a 500-pound fire pit by themselves—situations in which people think that they can handle it, but common sense would make it clear that they can't.

The situations that are the most avoidable are the ones in which you say, "I'm just going to quickly unload this truck full of dirt," and then do it in an idiotic way rather than an informed, intentional way. Usually, that happens to someone who's become deconditioned. If you spend 50 hours a week sitting in a chair and then go work in the yard for five hours or go to the gym and lift big weights, it's not surprising that you could blow out a disc.

OSTEOARTHRITIS

Arthritis tends to be an umbrella term. To manage arthritis effectively, it's important to differentiate between osteoarthritis and any of the autoimmune disorders such as psoriatic arthritis, rheumatoid arthritis, and a plethora of other arthritic conditions that are beyond the scope of this chapter. (Rheumatoid arthritis, for example, is an autoimmune disorder that requires a completely different approach, because it's an actual disease.)

Among these various conditions, osteoarthritis is the most prevalent type of arthritic disorder. Fortunately, it's also the one that you can do something about. In contrast to rheumatoid arthritis, osteoarthritis is not a disease, but the aftereffects of wear and tear and old injuries.

Genetic risk of inflammation. Some people are at greater risk of bone spurs and joint inflammation. They may take all kinds of supplements to reduce the inflammation, but they are simply more prone to arthritis than the average person. When we look at their spine on X-rays or MRIs to assess the condition of the discs, we can see additional evidence of osteoarthritis as well.

Genetic aspects of bone health. Some people have stronger, more resilient discs, and some don't. Typically, arthritis comes from some sort of abnormal biomechanical stress on the body. With chiropractic care, if we are providing periodic adjustments and keeping the biomechanics in good condition, then hopefully that will minimize arthritis.

If you have a family history of osteoarthritis, especially at an earlier age, it is important to build protective and supportive activities into your lifestyle, including adjustments to keep your biomechanics functioning smoothly, as well as regular exercise, a high quality diet, and minimal alcohol and sugar.

MANAGING OLD INJURIES

Folks who played football in high school and college are probably going to have more arthritis than someone who didn't. So if you're one of those guys who beat his spine up at the age of 20, how do you prevent a big disaster at 40?

- The best approach is to think in terms of how you move. How can you keep your spine moving fluidly, comfortably, segmentally?

- Get evaluated by a chiropractor, physical therapist, or movement specialist, because if some area of your spine is "stuck," they can help you get it moving again.

- Relearn how to move your body to minimize joint stress. If you have an arthritic joint and you load it correctly, that will slow the level of degeneration.

- Globally, focus on how much you're sitting every day (and *how* you are sitting).

- Include some type of stretching and strengthening exercise, such as yoga or Pilates.

Silent inflammation. A low level of inflammation present throughout the body can interfere with the normal repair and maintenance of joints and connective tissue. This is sometimes called silent inflammation, which can persist for years before obvious symptoms of pain become apparent.

Inflammation is the wakeup call. Although the initial stages of arthritis are also silent (before structural deterioration occurs), inflammation can occur early on as tendonitis, discitis, or some sort of inflammation. The pain is not in the bone, but in the joint, tendons, and connective tissue around it. The inflammation, although painful and inconvenient, will alert you to the developing arthritis, which offers the opportunity to intervene earlier.

Reducing inflammation is key to managing pain. Once you reduce the inflammation, even if you still have the same compromised discs, there's a good chance the pain will be gone. There will be less inflammation in the surrounding tendons. Additionally, if you improve the biomechanics of your chair, desk, car seat, and couch, you've removed some of the triggers. (You're not making it worse every time you sit on the couch to watch a movie.)

The structure does not always correlate with pain. It's important to know that arthritis does not necessarily correlate with pain. Obviously, the more arthritis you have, the more likely you are to have pain, but it is not a one-to-one correlation. I see people with terrible looking MRIs who have no pain, and I have patients who have beautiful MRIs, who are in a great deal of pain.

Referred pain. I had a patient last week who had failed physical therapy. I realized that the pain "in his hip" was not coming from his hip. It was referred from the L4 disc in his spine. Once we freed up that disc, he was able to start walking again for exercise.

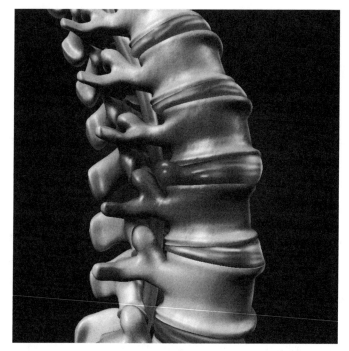

Figure 22.1. The majority of back injuries involve some type of disc event.

PREVENTIVE CARE

At times, selfcare, stretching, sitting less, and squatting more are not enough. That could be a good time to see a chiropractor or physical therapist. Chiropractors are the premiere low-back specialists for mild to moderate symptoms and early intervention. Our goal is to help manage spinal conditions without drugs or surgery, utilizing manipulation, massage, therapeutic equipment, and exercise to retrain the biomechanics of the back and bring integrity back to the nervous system of the spine.

Early intervention. The sooner a patient can be evaluated, the easier it is to manage the case, and the less likely that they will develop chronic pain and need ongoing pain medication, surgery, or both. If you are managing a spinal condition, here is a helpful decision tree you can use to sort out the next step in early intervention, starting with the most conservative options:

- Ergonomics and posture

- Stretching, exercise, supplements

- Personal training/athletic training

- Over-the-counter pain killers

- Chiropractor/physical therapy/acupuncture

- Prescribed medications

- Imaging: X-rays/MRIs

- Injections

- Surgery.

Applying an ounce of prevention. In our office, we have healthcare providers who see people with acute conditions and others who see patients with chronic issues. We also have therapists whose specific expertise is in the management of mild, moderate, or severe disorders. If you have an immediate, acute injury that is mild, you may see us once or twice. We will give you some exercises, and you're on your way. If you have a condition that's chronic and severe, it's a six-month program.

Finding the right provider. This can be a challenge, because there are some chiropractors who overstep their scope of practice or use predatory sales tactics. Some chiropractors will try to scare you into care and have you sign a long-term contract. If you feel like you are buying a used car, instead of receiving personalized healthcare, that is a good sign that you are in the wrong office. To find a great chiropractor, I would start by:

- Reading reviews

- Calling the office to ask about a typical visit

- Inquiring about a typical care plan for someone with your condition

- Requesting a ballpark estimate of the cost of care. If they cannot give you an estimate, they are probably going to try to sign you up for a long-term plan.

Imaging. I do imaging in my office primarily to rule out possible reasons a patient is not getting better. If I've adjusted someone for four weeks and they still don't seem to be improving, I take an X-ray. I might find, for instance, that they have severe spinal stenosis (narrowing of the space within the spine, which puts pressure on the spinal nerves). The imaging can provide evidence of why they are not healing as fast as expected, and that informs my clinical strategy.

Taking a science-based approach. A chiropractor grounded in the research literature will give you specific exercises to complement manipulations and offer you the option of being released from care when an acute injury has been corrected.

WHAT TO DO IF YOU GET INJURED

It's helpful to understand the role that a chiropractor can play in helping a patient heal from an injury. We see a great many worker's comp patients in my office, and our approach is to move the patient toward healing using manual therapy and exercise. Quarterbacking the case, there are a number of decisions involved:

- Does the patient simply need to be adjusted?
- Is the main concern that they're stiff and have abnormal biomechanics?
- Do we need to get them in to see the physical therapist?
- Do they need to see an ergonomic specialist or an occupational therapist?
- Is the next step a referral to a pain management specialist?
- Do they need a referral to be assessed for spinal surgery?

Who to see first? If you begin with an orthopedist or a spinal surgeon, there is a 50% chance of eventually getting spinal surgery. If you go to a chiropractor, physical therapist, or a pain management specialist, there is less than a 10% chance of surgery. Clearly, this is a skewed number, because if you have horrific back pain, you're going to go to the orthopedist first. That said, the vast majority of people who start with a chiropractor are going to be able to avoid surgery for lower back pain.

Why earlier is better. It's much easier to fix things when they're early and fresh, rather than having to work through scar tissue, poor patterning, and inflammation. Yet out of force of habit, 90% of the population will just go to their primary care provider and ask for pain meds. That works fine if you have a mild problem, and you know that it's probably going to heal.

However, if the injury is more complex or severe, you may simply be masking the pain and deferring treatment of the injury. It's good to be seen by some type of manual therapist or movement specialist who has expertise in the type of injury you've suffered, someone who can provide therapy and coach you on making deliberate, intentional changes in your movement patterns to maximize healing and avoid reinjury.

Integrative medicine. There are always times when surgery is the right intervention and medications are the right intervention. That's why they make the drugs, so you can get out of pain and back to work and being yourself. But as a society, we tend to lean too heavily toward medications, imaging, and surgeries. We lean away from physical interventions, even when study after study makes it clear that for lower back pain, many patients are able to heal effectively with a combination of manipulation and exercise.

Direct access to treatment. You can now see a chiropractor or a physical therapist without a referral. Working with these providers, you are using a physical solution for a physical problem. (The emphasis wouldn't be on pharmaceuticals, since neither of these providers are legally empowered to prescribe.) However, you may get a better solution in contrast to masking the pain with pharmaceuticals and allowing the injury to get worse. That can lead to injections and surgeries, which can be problematic and should be reserved for more extreme cases.

Depth of training. Graduates of chiropractic college have the same number of hours of education as medical doctors. However, they usually do not train in a hospital as medical doctors do. Both chiropractic college and physical therapy (PT) specialization are typically three-year doctorate programs after undergraduate school. Like PTs, chiropractors guide patients in therapeutic exercise, and perform manipulation and other therapeutic modalities. Chiropractors also tend to take a holistic approach, by providing interventions such as nutrition counseling. Both chiropractors and physical therapists are empowered to diagnose patients within their scope of practice, which reduces the cost of care and means that people are seen sooner after an injury.

Periodic checkups. To me, getting a checkup by a chiropractor or a PT when there are no symptoms present is similar to going to the dentist when you're not in pain. It makes sense to periodically be evaluated. However, this is not the norm in our society. With that said, the most common time to see a PT or chiropractor is when a condition does not seem to be getting better.

The continuum of care. If you're already seeing a chiropractor or would like to see one and may be wondering about communication with your primary care provider, know that the overall climate is changing for the better. In my own office, I take care of patients for 30 different medical doctors. Today, many more physicians are open to chiropractic care and are comfortable referring patients. For the vast majority of insurance plans, chiropractors and physical therapists provide entry-level care.

Educate yourself. We don't come into this world with an instruction manual. The most challenging aspect of health and the human condition is that there is no single solution for everyone. There is no perfect diet for everyone and no perfect exercise for everyone. If you have back pain or joint pain, you will want to learn about your body. Learn how to use it as if it were a beautiful instrument.

For more on the work of Dr. Max Lippman and on chiropractic care, please see www.BlackHawkChiropractor.com.

Chapter 23
Spine Care
Max Lippman, DC, Chiropractor

If your spine is inflexibly stiff at 30, you are old.
If it is completely flexible at 60, you are young.
— *Joseph Pilates*

Train for your job as if it was an athletic event...

If you were a football player, how would you become more dynamic, more explosive? Would you do interval training or intense muscle development? If you work in an office ten hours a day, how do you train so you don't become deconditioned? What do you need to do to preserve your body and your spine, given the stress of inactivity?

Develop awareness. To conserve the health of your spine, you will want to notice what you're doing day after day, in terms of your posture and how you move. You want to create the conditions for success. This is not a matter of set-it-and-forget-it. That's not going to happen with just a five-minute stretch in the morning. Rather, it means increasing your awareness, by becoming mindful of your body throughout the day:

- How do you sit in your car?

- How do you sit at work?

- Do you have a sit-stand desk?

- How do you hold your ribcage?

- Are you breathing deeply or shallowly?

- How are you training your body for the job that you do every day?

Do a self-assessment. One of the most effective things you can do is an audit—record your sleep habits, do an audit of your work environment, and document your daily movement and exercise. (Suggestions for a sleep audit are included in chapter 29 on sleep.)

Practice intentional awareness. Your increased awareness is a tool you can use to stay in touch with your physical reality.

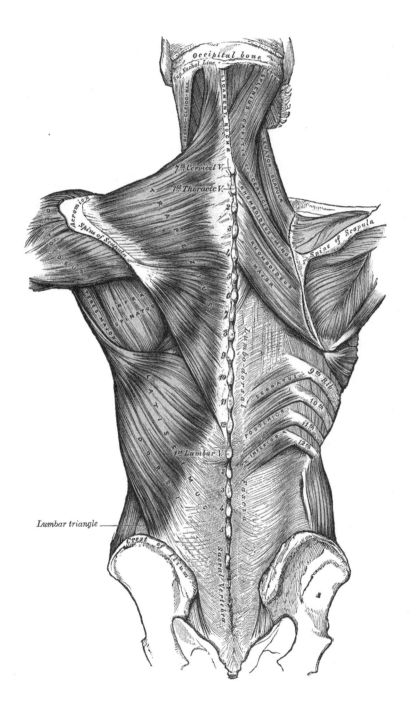

Figure 23.1. The magnificent spine. (Henry Vandyke Carter. Gray's Anatomy.)

The Magnificent Spine

The spine is an incredible structure that offers strength, flexibility, and protection for our nervous system. The strength stems not just from the 26 bones in the spine or the muscles surrounding those bones, but from the very architecture of the spine and its shape. Every step we take, every lift, and all the pressure from day-to-day activities are distributed through the natural S curve of the spine. If the structure of the spine was absolutely straight, that would cause rigidity throughout the back. However, the curves of the human spine (neck/cervical, midback/thoracic, and low back/lumbar) are designed to take on tremendous loads of stress and absorb them, while maintaining the ability to be flexible and dynamic. Most of us can move our spine in all sorts of directions while bearing weight, yet rarely does that cause injury. As we age, if we lose those curves, we start to see diminished function.

The flexible portions and curves of our spine transition into the pelvis, which acts as a foundation for the torso. The torso has very little dynamic motion, but a massive amount of strength. It is built as a foundation, a bowl to anchor and distribute forces from our upright bodies, without tearing, ripping, or breaking. Thus, many of the bones of the pelvis are fused together, including the five bones of the sacrum, the two bones of the coccyx (the lowest area of the spine), and the ilium, ischium, and pubis (the pelvic bowl).

When working perfectly, the spine and skull house all of the central nervous system, protecting it from damage. The pelvis acts as an anchor point for our strongest muscles to keep us moving and erect.

Between each vertebra, the spine is composed of discs that act as cushions that distribute forces exerted on the spine by daily activity. Each disc is made up of two parts, an extremely fibrous material (annulus fibrosis) on the outside and a jelly-like inside (nucleus propulsus). The outside is woven together and is incredibly durable, while the inside acts as a shock absorption mechanism comparable to what you would see in the inner sole of a shoe. The discs allow the spine to flex, extend, rotate, and be compressed without compromising power.

Although the spine is an incredible structure in our body that allows movement, protection, and strength, it can be injured in any number of ways. Car accidents, athletic injuries, or heavy lifting without training can all result in traumatic injury to the spine. There are several types of arthritis that can attack the spinal joints, the most common being osteoarthritis, which can destroy the spine in the process of aging.

If you're not intentional about the way that you're sitting and moving, you're probably not going to be as intentional about the way that you're eating and exercising. Rather, you want to be checking in with yourself: "How am I taking care of my body? How's my back doing? How's my gut? Is there a better way to exercise? To rest? To eat?"

Build good daily habits. If you start thinking along those lines, you'll start moving away from the idea that there's one single intervention that you need to be doing. It's more a matter of asking, "What are the daily habits that I need to develop?" Once you see things from that perspective, your intention, the way you move, and your posture will start to shift, and that will change everything for the better.

For example, if you're a restaurant server, you're walking (or running) and moving your body all day, and you probably don't need to go home and take a 30-minute walk. You've already gotten your stretching and movement. But if you're a tech worker, maybe you need to incorporate a walk after dinner because you haven't moved all day.

Balance sitting with activity. What can you do to counter the effects of a sedentary workstyle?

- Stretch before and after you sit.

- Make sure your hamstrings are loose.

- Loosen your hip flexors (the muscles that run from your hip joints to your knee joints).

- Make sure you're sitting in the correct way.

- Consider using a sit-stand desk or a sit-stand riser on your existing desk.

- Stand up and stretch several times an hour so you don't get locked in.

- Go walking or running daily.

Improving Your Circulation and Muscle Tone With a Sit-Stand Desk

This is a basic fitness strategy you can build into your day, by alternately sitting and standing while you work. In addition to improving your circulation, you'll probably find that you have better muscle definition in your calves and improved tone in your thighs within a matter of weeks. Many people also report a noticeable increase in energy.

Whether you work in an office or at home, this work style can be achieved through the use of an affordable sit-stand riser that you place on your desktop or with an automated sit-stand desk. For your home office, you can create an excellent sit-stand work surface with a credenza (such as those available from Ikea) or by using a dresser appropriate to your height and proportions. The work surface should be elbow height, so your arms hang comfortably at your sides and your forearms can rest on the desktop (your arms should form the letter "L").

As with squatting, be sure to ease into this work style, perhaps starting with 30 minutes standing, alternated with 30 minutes sitting, and gradually increase the time you spend standing.

The large muscles in your thighs (your glutes) are the secret to good circulation. Your heart pumps blood throughout your body via the arteries, but getting blood back to your heart from your toes, your veins must move the blood against gravity.

Your toes are a long way from the mechanical pumping action of your heartbeat. Instead, the veins move your blood through the action of your leg muscles, up a series of one-way valves. Whenever you walk, the tightening of your leg muscles squeezes the veins, moving the blood up toward your heart inch by inch, up the veins through the one-way valves.

If you sit at a desk all day, and only get up for lunch, as about one-third of Americans have for the past 70 years, your circulation will be seriously impaired. As a result, you may feel sluggish and fatigued much of the day. This sedentary work style also puts you at risk of health issues that include type 2 diabetes and heart disease. What's more, your lymph system operates in a somewhat similar manner to the veins, relying on the action of your muscles as you walk to circulate the lymph. Clearing the lymphatic system is essential to the daily housekeeping that moves debris and toxins out of the cells and tissue. (Before the industrial revolution, almost everyone walked everywhere all the time, so this was not an issue.)

You can also become more active by varying tasks (moving the printer across the room, making phone calls standing), taking a stretch break every 20 minutes, getting up and walking around once an hour, and getting outside for a 20-minute walk on your lunch hour. The basic idea is to build more movement and activity into your day using a number of different strategies. This trend toward a more active work style was first innovated in the Netherlands, and is now also practiced in Scandinavia and the U.K.

BASICS

Be sure to stretch:

- When you stretch, stretch fully.

- Make sure you're stretching both sides of your spine.

- Don't just stretch your hamstrings and your back.

- Be sure to include stretches for your quads, your hip flexors, and your abs.

- Consciously minimize the face-forward position that most of us assume much of the time, given cell phones, computers, TVs, and classrooms. People come in to see me with neck pain, back pain, and shifts in posture so pronounced they show up on X-rays.

Hinge at the hips. The easiest way to avoid blowing out a disc is by relearning how to lift. First off, learn to hinge at the hip to reduce stress on the discs. If you've been doing it wrong, you're not alone. Lots of people at the gym are doing squats and doing them incorrectly. (You'll find a number of useful videos on Youtube.com that explain how to do this.)

Relearn how to squat. Our bodies are not built to sit, and we have learned this unnatural position through years of training. Looking at modern day hunter-gathering societies, like the Hadza in Tanzania, their lifestyle involves the same amount of sedentary time as that in our industrial society, but it is spent in a squatting position. As a result, they have much less chronic disease and back pain. According to a 2020 USC study, the simple transition from a sitting position to a squatting position can have massive health benefits, including increased fat metabolism and improved muscle tone.

You don't need to squat 400 pounds; you just need to squat your own body weight. Of course, you can't always be squatting. If you are forced to sit for long periods of time, develop a game plan to unwind the confinement of a sedentary workstyle. That means learning how to activate your psoas muscles, while also lengthening the front of your hips.

How sitting deactivates the lumbar spine. Strong muscles protect the discs and joints in the spine. As the back muscles weaken after years of chronic sitting, fat infiltrates these muscles, which renders muscle tissue not only weak, but stiff and less able to contract. Thus, the integrity of the muscles is deteriorated, and when we challenge the spine, injury is more likely to occur, potentially resulting in chronic back pain.

Engage the glutes. We also need to learn how to engage the glutes (the three large muscles on each side of your butt). The goal is to engage those muscles in tandem with the lumbar spine, pulling as a unit, to keep the body erect. A great resource for this is Foundation Training (see www.foundationtraining.com). There has been a huge amount of focus on the posterior chain by physical therapists, athletic trainers, and chiropractors over the last ten years. Learning how to master this powerful (and underappreciated) part of your body can be the key to relieving stress on joints and discs in the spine.

Use a hip hook to strengthen your pelvic floor. Another unfortunate result of sitting too much is that we have lost control of our pelvic muscles, which can cause anything from back pain to tight legs to a lackluster sex life. It is high time to regain control of those muscles. Learning how to pelvic thrust, how to take decompressive breaths, and how to stretch the hip flexors and open the rib cage is the best way to avoid low-back pain. This type of exercise will protect your spine from degenerative disc disease, sciatica, muscle spasms, and arthritis. You will probably find it exceedingly beneficial to learn how to stretch the pelvic muscles and the deep hip flexors like the iliacus using tools such as a hip hook or a Pso-Rite.

To learn, to teach, and to love are basic to the meaning of life. How can you learn more about yourself? How can you learn more about other people's perspectives? How can you teach what you've learned and be able to convey that to build a foundation of love? All the best in your quest to sit less, stretch more, and live a healthy, pain-free, and vital life.

For more on the work of Dr. Max Lippman and on chiropractic care, please see www.BlackHawkChiropractor.com.

PART 3
ADVICE FROM SPECIALISTS
Introduction
Judson Brandeis, MD

The more you learn about the human body, the more you appreciate the amazing complexity of how each system works, what happens when it breaks down, and the intricacies of how to fix it. This section will cover some of the specialties that help men function at their best.

- Human vision is astoundingly complicated. Our eyes see 24 million different images over an average life with a resolution of 576 megapixels and the ability to see 500 shades of gray. At least 80% of our memories are based on what we see, and so about half of the human brain is dedicated to our vision. The eye muscles are the most active and fastest in the body.

- Our ears turn soundwaves into mechanical energy, which is then converted into chemical energy and finally into an electrical signal. Hearing allows us to enjoy the subtleties of a Mozart symphony, the sound of our children, or localize danger. On top of that, our hardworking ears never turn off. Even when we are asleep, our ears protect us by hearing all of the sounds around us.

- The foot is one of the most overworked, under-appreciated parts of the human body. Your feet are the foundation that supports your entire body weight and three to four times body weight when you are running. My Fitbit tells me that I take 10,000 steps a day, and the average person walks about 100,000 miles in a lifetime. That's a lot of stress on the 52 bones of the feet.

- Our hands are magnificent tools that can play Chopin, perform microsurgery, and climb Half Dome. Over a lifetime, our durable fingers are bent and stretched about 25 million times. Curiously, the right and left hand are each controlled by the opposite side of the brain.

- Humans have only been walking on two feet for four million years, and evolution has not perfected the design. Your spine is a work in progress, which is why back pain is the leading cause of disability in the U.S. The spine supports your body, allows flexible movement, and protects your spinal cord. I injured my back lifting rocks in the garden and suffered the consequences of a spine out of alignment. Once you experience pure nerve pain, you come to truly appreciate your spine when it is functioning well again.

■ Sleep is vital, and sleep deprivation will kill you more quickly than food deprivation. The most extended period of sleep deprivation recorded was 18 days versus 74 days for food deprivation. Sleep provides downtime for our brains, a time when our body temperature and metabolism drop. During the two hours a night of REM sleep, we dream and get erections, which is one of the reasons that men with sleep apnea are more likely to suffer from erectile dysfunction.

I hope these chapters will lead to a greater appreciation of the miracle of your physical being.

Chapter 24
Keeping Your Vision Sharp
Ahad Mahootchi, MD,
Eye Surgeon

Just because a man lacks the use of his eyes
doesn't mean he lacks vision.
— Stevie Wonder

There's no Saturday 5K run for people who develop presbyopia ("old vision"). Some of the vision problems that come with age are annoying, but easily solved. Others are devastating and can lead to vision loss that is not correctable with glasses. Does it have to be this way?

Almost all vision loss in the U.S. is preventable, yet the 2010 U.S. Census found that about 90 million of the 142 million adults over 40 had vision problems.

The truth is that many of the things you need to do for your eyes should be done long *before* you are older. As an ophthalmologist, I have spent the last 25 years treating and preventing vision loss. In my experience, age 35 seems to be prime time for an intervention.

Let's skip interventions that require maximal effort for minimal gain. After all, who wants to do 1,000 push-ups a day if it only makes you .01% stronger? We are going to cover important things you should do and those you should not. Mainstream medicine is paid primarily to treat disease, not prevent it, so these simple and inexpensive interventions are frequently overlooked. The most common causes of blindness have years of repeated research that shows how to avoid them, yet they are still all too common. Fortunately, simple prevention can have major benefits.

BASICS

The eye can be compared to a very elaborate video camera. We have two "lenses," the cornea on the outside and the natural lens on the inside which focuses light onto the "retina" in the back. Comparable to the film in a camera, the cornea is of fixed power, while the lens within the eye varies as it focuses, adjusting to the light.

- **The iris** is the colored portion of the eye, which has an invisible opening in the center that varies in size to adjust how much light comes through, like the lens on a camera.

- **The retina** is a thin layer of tissue that lines the back of the inside of the eye, behind the iris. The *retina* receives the light that the lens has focused and converts the light into neural signals that are sent to the brain for visual recognition.

- **Rods and cones** line the retina. *Rods* are responsible for vision at low light levels with no color and low spatial acuity. *Cones* are active at higher light levels and are capable of color vision and high spatial acuity. The fovea, the middle of the retina, is the primary focus of your vision and is populated exclusively by cones.

- **The optic nerve** transfers visual information from the retina to the vision centers of the brain via electrical impulses.

Within the brain, neurons devoted to visual processing make up about 30% of the cerebral cortex, compared with 8% for touch and just 3% for hearing.

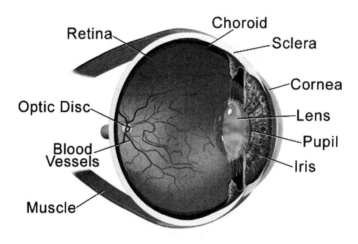

Figure 24.1. Anatomy of the eye.

PREVENTING VISION PROBLEMS

Vision loss occurs along a spectrum, ranging from visual impairment correctable with glasses, to visual disability, legal blindness, or blindness with no perception of light. Most of us would recognize a vision loss at the 20/50 level. That means that what a normally sighted person can see at 50 feet, a partially-sighted person must be only 20 feet away (30 feet closer) in order to see. This is not the technical meaning of the term 20/20 or 20/50, but is a good practical translation. Legal blindness means that, even with glasses, one's best vision is 20/200 in the better-seeing eye. Most visually disabled patients can see some light. However, problems start with vision loss that is much less dramatic.

Causes of Low Vision

The most common causes of low vision and vision loss in Western countries are:

#1 Cataracts – impact 25 million people age 40 or older (by age 75, half of the population)

#2 Age-related macular degeneration – 11 million Americans, more prevalent in men

#3 Glaucoma – impacting almost 3 million Americans, but the second leading cause of blindness

#4 Diabetic retinopathy – affects 2.6 million over the age of 40 and blinds 400,000

#5 Eye injuries – 2.4 million eye injuries occur annually, and 65% involve people over 45. Fully 90% of these injuries can be prevented simply with protective eyeware.

DIABETIC RETINOPATHY

Diabetes is the leading cause of visual disability in the Western world. It's completely preventable, yet still common. Think about how crazy that is.

Diabetes causes the blood vessels in the back of the eye to leak and then bleed. This debilitating condition is termed diabetic retinopathy. Diabetics with good long-term control do not develop serious retinopathy. There are laser surgeries and eye injections that can help, but it's best never to get to that point in the first place.

In this country, we are too lax about taking action early. We often give medication for prediabetes, but we need to provide meaningful resources for better nutrition, weight loss, and exercise to build diabetes fighting muscle.

CATARACTS

Cataracts are common. Almost everyone will develop cataracts if they live past 55. The surgery to fix cataracts is the most common in the U.S. and almost four million operations are performed on cataracts each year. Fortunately, the complication rate is very low. Often, a skilled surgeon can also reduce the need for glasses.

These conditions involve a clouding of the natural lens that occurs with age. When we are born, our lenses are clear and flexible. As our body chemistry changes with aging, lenses stiffen so that focusing between far and near becomes more difficult. Later these changes in body chemistry make the lens less clear, like looking through smoky glass.

Clear Lens Exchange is an outpatient procedure designed to reduce (or eliminate) dependence on glasses, as an alternative to laser procedures or other types of procedures. Clear Lens Exchange can be very effective for some with impaired vision due to aging. However, although cataract surgery can be helpful, macular issues afterward can reverse the benefits of surgery.

As a physician and a biochemist, I see problems with flexibility (presbyopia) and with clarity (cataract) as part of a continuum. Taking a lutein supplement will help your lenses in both regards.

MACULAR DEGENERATION

The macula is the most important area of the retina, a focal area about the size of the letter "e" on this page. We employ this area of the eye for our best central vision, for reading, and to distinguish color. Macular degeneration develops when the central portion of the retina, the *macula*, becomes impaired. Macular degeneration involves vision loss in the center of the eye, often with some vision intact in the periphery of the eye. In dry macular degeneration, the center of the retina deteriorates. With wet macular degeneration, leaky blood vessels grow under the retina, and blurred vision is a key symptom.

Macular degeneration is the most common cause of vision loss for older people in Western countries. However, changes are seen in the eye decades before we lose vision. At first, our vision may be 20/20 by the chart, but it may take more effort to get reading done. If it took you three minutes to read the front page of a newspaper, it may take you five the following year, and then seven, at which point the print has to be a larger font. Glasses don't help. Think of it as having a cheap film in the back of your expensive camera. Buying the latest lens technology won't help you to take a better photo because the film is terrible and slowly getting worse.

GLAUCOMA

This is a disease of the optic nerve that connects the eye to the brain. Early changes are often seen decades before serious vision loss occurs. Early detection is key. What you lose, you don't get back.

Marijuana. There is no legitimate reason to smoke pot for glaucoma. You would need to be stoned out of your mind 24/7 for it to begin to work. Even in that unworkable stupor, it isn't a fraction as effective as other forms of treatment. No legitimate ophthalmologist would recommend pot for glaucoma.

Sleep apnea can mimic glaucoma. Unrecognized or untreated sleep apnea can damage the optic nerve in a way that can be confused with glaucoma. In the U.S., up to 70% of glaucoma cases may be due to sleep apnea, particularly in patients whose eye pressure is not high. This is another good reason to keep your weight down and stay trim, since that reduces your risk of sleep apnea.

UNEXPECTED RISKS TO VISION

The Devastating Effects of Smoking

Now let's cover what you shouldn't do. Cigarette smoking is disastrous for the eyes. It takes 15 years after quitting to reduce the risk of vision impairment due to smoking. Many of these patients feel caught between a smoking addiction and the risk to their eyesight. They didn't get to that point quickly. It happened slowly.

Smoking increases the risk of macular degeneration by 400%.

If you already have macular degeneration, smoking increases your risk of blindness by 400%.

Smoking hastens the necessity for cataract surgery.

On average, smokers need surgery ten years before non-smokers. To make matters worse, they are more likely to have a rocky road postoperatively due to a number of possible complications.

A number of additional eye diseases are associated with smoking.

There are so many harmful effects on vision that, frankly, it makes no sense to smoke. Visual disorders worsened by smoking also include vein occlusion and artery occlusion.

Sex Meds and Vision

Cardiovascular disease is bad for your libido, as the other chapters in this book will attest. But the treatments can cause visual side effects and even blindness if you have trashed the blood supply to the optic nerves. Viagra, Levitra, and Cialis work great for some, but the risk of losing vision just when the fun starts is real, and that vision isn't coming back. All those drugs lower blood pressure in the eye, and if the blood supply is compromised, that can cause a "stroke" of the optic nerve—anterior ischemic optic neuropathy (AION). My advice is, don't smoke if you use those drugs. Be open with your ophthalmologist when considering their use, and ask if you have a "disc at risk." People with this condition are more likely to have AION.

Nutritional Supplements to Prevent Macular Degeneration and Cataracts

Lutein. A biochemical cousin of vitamin A, lutein is found in large amounts in dark green, leafy vegetables. Lutein is essential for macular function, and studies show it decreases the chances of developing age-related macular degeneration by 30%. (Westerners have diets notoriously short on dark greens and also have more age-related macular degeneration.)

It takes five servings a week of dark-green, lutein-rich foods, like spinach, collards, or kale to achieve proper lutein levels. (Greens like spinach, for example, contain four times the amount of lutein compared with the amount in lettuces and cabbage.) While a diet rich in green leafy vegetables is excellent for reducing colon cancer risk (and as part of a plant-based diet with cardiovascular benefit), it's hard to do. You are also playing catch up. Your colon probably can't learn to absorb that much, that quickly. There is also some evidence that your stomach chemically destroys the first 6 mg of lutein you consume. Typically, 20 mg capsules of lutein are widely available, effective, and affordable.

Vitamin A. In third-world countries, vitamin A deficiency leads to the deterioration of eyesight. Vitamin A is a fat-soluble vitamin, and if you don't have fat in your diet, you don't get vitamin A. However, vitamin A simply isn't a concern for most of our readers.

Omega-3 oils. Although the last word is not in on omega-3 oils for heart health, it is a settled matter for the eyes. Omega-3s reduce the risk of age-related macular degeneration by 40%. Case closed. AMD is an eye disease that can worsen over time. It's the leading cause of severe, permanent vision loss in people over the age of 60. In short, you can achieve a 40% risk reduction in age-related macular degeneration just by taking lutein and omega-3 oil supplements.

SOLUTIONS FOR VISUAL IMPAIRMENT

Previously, we only worried about distance vision (more than 20 feet away) and up-close vision for reading. The computer has changed that. Now we frequently spend hours in front of a computer. The focal distance to the computer screen is considered intermediate vision. It is a challenge for eyeglass technology because trifocals or bifocals may require you to tilt your head while you look at the screen. This can cause a serious neck issue if not corrected. The choice of how to fix things depends on your occupation, your lifestyle, and how much time you spend on a computer and outdoors. There isn't one fix for all.

Monovision. This is an approach in which the doctor, either with surgery or contact lenses, tries to focus the dominant eye for distance and the non-dominant eye for near vision. This may be effective, but it has some pitfalls:

- The amount of correction you need for near vision changes throughout life.

- Some doctors are not precise about how they check for dominance. The difference between the two eyes may be okay for a cocktail hour, but not so good for sustained reading.

Note: The contacts used as a trial of monovision can be irritating to the eye, particularly if you have dry eye disease. Contacts are worth a try, but they are not the only solution.

Multifocal contact lenses and natural lens replacements. These lenses are getting better, but they work by splitting light between distance and near targets. As a result, visual images can appear slightly dimmer and not as sharp in some cases.

- A contact lens trial is always a good idea. If you don't like it, then you probably should not proceed with the surgical options using this technology. The near vision can be excellent, but the night vision tends to be bothersome for 6% to 20% of patients. Your ability to read without glasses can give way later to annoyance with side effects in night-time vision.

- There is also some concern that, if you develop eye problems later, you may be worse off. There is no free lunch here.

- There are also surgeries to make the pupil effectively smaller in the non-dominant eye. This pin-hole effect helps the near vision, but may cause some issues at night. There is a contact lens version of this that may be worth your time to evaluate.

Note: Don't sleep with your contacts in. This raises the risk of problems later if you decide to get laser vision correction.

Accommodating lens implants. These lenses seem to be the holy grail of ophthalmic surgery. This is a replacement lens that gives you distance, intermediate, and near vision without splitting light—just like your eyes do at their best. One type of lens implant, available in the U.S. since 2004, is Crystalens. Generally, there are no night-time issues with these implants, and the distance and intermediate vision are excellent.

- The near vision is 20/40, so not 20/20. For the far-sighted who are 55 or older, I don't think this is a controversial choice.

- To those who are younger or are near-sighted, there are barriers. There are other versions of this type of lens available internationally that seem to work quite well for healthy eyes.

Laser vision correction. This is one of the most successful surgeries available, with a low incidence of problems. It is great at fixing distance vision. However, it will not give you both distance and near vision if you are 45 or older.

Using common sense when choosing the provider of laser vision corrective procedure (or any other surgery) is a good idea. Be alert to red flags. Go someplace else if the procedure is bargain basement priced (such as $500 per eye), if you have limited knowledge of the surgeon and have not met him/her beforehand, if you have to pay before the screening exam, or if everyone on the staff seems to be in sales and marketing.

Dry eyes afterward can be an issue. Pre-treating with Thera-Tears Extra three times a day or more (starting a month before surgery) seems to eliminate the problem, in my experience. You want a surgeon who recognizes dry eye as a potential problem and alerts you to that fact before the surgery. (This is another reason to be cautious about your choice of an eye surgeon.)

Be forewarned that there are many instances in which the referral involves money going between the referring doctor and the surgeon. That can influence who you are referred to and what you are sold, so do your research.

UV protection and polarization. For quality vision in bright sun or near the glare of water, nothing beats polarized sunglasses. They can be filled by prescription almost any-where. I see imposter polarized glasses for sale commonly in stores and flea markets. The lenses sold at your doctor's office are usually noticeably more clear and scratch-resistant than the type you get at the mall. It's easy to test for yourself whether polarized glasses are real or bogus.

UV protection isn't polarization. There is a great deal of marketing these days around UV protection. UV does have a small impact on cataract formation. However, its benefit is almost 100 times less than the negative impact of smoking or poor diet. Stay focused on the big impact items.

Protective eye wear. Bottle rockets, racquetball, and weed eating are words that make my heart sink when I'm at work. It is not only the guy setting off the fireworks at risk, but also the people around him. It's the 11-year-old kid standing 100 feet away from the guys lighting the fireworks who gets the bottle rocket to the eye. No joke.

Before OSHA, industrial accidents were the most common cause of vision loss among workers. Once safety glasses were required, we fixed that.

Many of us now wear eye protection at work, but at home we are often lax. We need to be smarter about where and when to wear eye protection. Whenever you are around high-risk activities, impact resistant glasses should be the first thing that comes to mind. Find a pair of safety glasses with a stylish frame for your workshop and get an extra pair for the glove compartment, so it becomes second nature to put them on.

For additional information on vision care and the work of Dr. Mahootchi, please visit: www.SeeBetterFlorida.com.

Chapter 25
Preventing Hearing Loss
Michael Murphy, MD, MPH,
Ear, Nose, & Throat Surgeon
& Toby Hill, BC-HIS, ACA,
Hearing Instrument Specialist

It's not the hearing that improves life, but the listening.
— Mihaly Csikszentmihalyi

Our sense of hearing is fundamental to both our safety and our quality of life. With respect to safety, our hearing warns us of potential threats: a fire alarm, a car horn, or a siren. Our quality of life is significantly improved with good hearing and compromised when hearing is lost.

A good sense of hearing allows us to fully enjoy nature around us, pleasures such as music, and our relationships with family and friends. When hearing is lost, these very things become sources of frustration. Family relationships may become strained by miscommunication and misunderstandings. Most concerning is the fact that when one loses hearing, often the instinct is to retreat socially and withdraw. Someone with a fun-loving or social personality may withdraw due to concerns about saying the wrong thing or sounding stupid. Ultimately, this can lead to reduced mental acuity and cognitive function.

The good news is that the vast majority of hearing disorders can be effectively diagnosed and treated. In this chapter we will discuss the anatomy and physiology of the ear, the classification of hearing disorders, and the diagnosis and treatment of common causes of hearing loss.

The effective diagnosis and treatment of hearing loss will likely require a medical evaluation. Often the initial assessment can be made by a primary care provider, using screening tests for hearing that are performed during the visit. A visit to a specialist, usually an otolaryngologist (an ENT, an ear, nose, and throat doctor), will allow for a definitive evaluation. In addition, a formal evaluation of hearing by an audiologist is required.

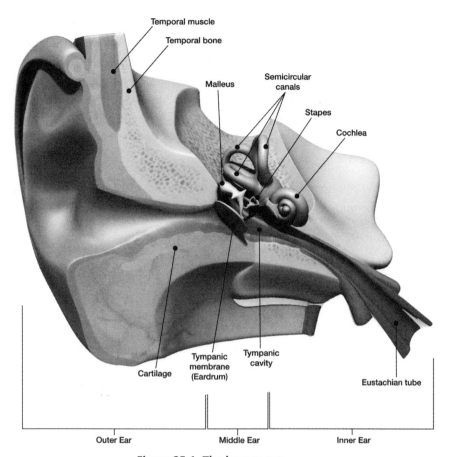

Figure 25.1. The human ear.

THE ANATOMY OF THE EAR

The basic anatomy of the ear is composed of three areas: the outer, middle, and inner ear (see Figure 24.1).

THE OUTER EAR

The outer ear is composed of the *auricle* and the *external auditory canal*.

■ **The *auricle*** is the visible part of the ear on the side of the head, and is also called the pinna (Latin for wing/fin). The main function of the auricle is to collect sound and direct it to the external auditory canal.

- The *external auditory canal* runs from where the auricle attaches to the side of the head to the eardrum (the tympanic membrane). This canal is essentially a cylinder measuring 1 inch long and 1/3 of an inch wide. The outer third of the canal is composed of cartilage and subcutaneous tissue and is lined with skin. Wax glands (the cerumen) and hair follicles are located in this portion of the canal. The inner two-thirds of the canal is composed of skin, which is directly on top of underlying bone. This portion of the canal is extremely sensitive.

THE MIDDLE EAR

The middle ear is composed of 1) the ear drum, 2) three tiny hearing bones that amplify sound, and 3) the middle ear space.

- The *ear drum* **(the *tympanic membrane)*** is an important structure within the ear. It separates the outer ear from the middle ear. The tympanic membrane is essential for hearing, collecting sound waves and then transforming these waves into vibrations that are transferred to the hearing bones.

- The *hearing bones* **(the *ossicles)*** are three small, connected bones that transmit the movement of the ear drum to the inner ear. The malleus (Latin for hammer) is the first of the three bones and is attached to the ear drum. The incus (Latin for anvil) is the middle bone. The stapes (Latin for stirrup) attaches to the oval window of the inner ear and acts like a piston, creating waves of energy that are essential to the process of hearing.

- The *middle ear space* is the air-filled space behind the ear drum. It has a close relationship with the eustachian tube, which runs from the back of your nose to the middle ear space. The function of the eustachian tube is to ensure that the pressure behind your ear drum is the same as the pressure around you. (You become aware of these changes in pressure when you travel to a higher elevation in the mountains or on a plane, and feel the need to clear your ears.) When this tube is not open and functioning properly, medical problems, including hearing loss, can occur.

THE INNER EAR

The inner ear is composed of a series of tube-like structures: 1) the cochlea, 2) the semicircular canals, and 3) the internal auditory canal.

- The *cochlea* (Greek for snail) is the hearing side of the inner ear. It is essentially a fluid-filled sac rolled up on itself, making almost three complete turns. The cochlea converts the vibrations created by the stapes bone within the middle ear into an electrical signal to be sent to the brain.

- **The *semicircular canals*** within the inner ear are vitally important to our sense of balance. They are three fluid-filled tubes connected to the cochlea: the horizontal, superior, and posterior canals. These canals provide our sense of balance. Vertigo, the sensation of dizziness, originates when there is dysfunction or injury to the semicircular canals of the inner ear. Often disorders of hearing loss within the inner ear are associated with vertigo and/or balance symptoms.

- **The *internal auditory canal*** is a bony canal that connects the inner ear to the area of the cranial cavity that contains the brainstem, arteries, and nerves (the posterior cranial fossa), including the vagus nerve. The auditory canal is about 3 ½ inches long and 1 ½ inches wide (8.5 mm by 4 mm), on average. The main structure in the canal is the vestibulocochlear nerve, which transmits information on balance from the semicircular canals and supports hearing through the cochlear nerve from the cochlea. The facial nerve also travels through the canal, transmitting information that creates facial movement.

The Physiology of Hearing

The outer, middle, and inner ear structures work together to convert sound waves into electrical impulses, to be transmitted by the cochlear nerve to the brain, in the following sequence.

1. Sound waves are gathered by our external ear and transmitted to the ear drum by the external auditory canal.

2. The sound waves create vibrations of the ear drum, which are transmitted through the three ossicle bones in the middle ear to the cochlea in the inner ear.

3. The piston-like action of the stapes creates waves in the fluid of the snail-shaped cochlea.

4. These waves ultimately cause movement of hair-like nerve cells (the cilia) within the cochlea. There are about 30,000 cilia within the cochlea, and the movement of these hair-like cells creates electrical signals that are sent to the brain via the cochlear nerve. The cochlea determines the frequency pattern of sound based on the waves created.

ASSESSMENT OF HEARING LOSS

TYPES OF HEARING LOSS

Given the complexity and delicacy of these structures, it is easy to see how hearing can become impaired. Hearing loss is classified in three types: conditions of the external or middle ear (conductive), conditions affecting the inner ear (sensorineural), or mixed, involving both types of impairment.

Conductive hearing loss. This type of hearing loss is caused by conditions involving the external and/or middle ear including the ear drum. These forms of hearing loss can often be treated medically or surgically.

Sensorineural hearing loss. This form of hearing loss is caused by conditions involving structures of the inner ear: the cochlea, semicircular canals, and/or the auditory nerve.

Mixed hearing loss. As the name implies, this form of hearing loss involves both conductive and sensorineural hearing loss.

THE EVALUATION

The assessment of hearing loss should start with a *physical exam* by a medical provider, which is essential because many causes of hearing loss involving the external and middle ear can by diagnosed and treated based on a physical exam.

Tuning forks can be used to assess hearing status. Typically, tuning forks that vibrate at a frequency of 256 Hertz (Hz) and 512 Hz are used. This type of evaluation can be helpful in determining if hearing loss is present and, if so, the type of hearing loss and basic degree of severity. In the absence of a formal audiologic assessment, the tuning fork evaluation can be used in making a diagnosis and in initiating treatment. (As an ear, nose, and throat doctor, I rely on the tuning fork evaluation in the initial assessment of every patient who reports having hearing loss.)

Audiologic Assessment

The only way to accurately know your hearing thresholds is to have a hearing test. At a minimum, a hearing test should be administered by age 50, performed by a qualified hearing professional, ENT, audiologist, or hearing instrument specialist. A sound booth should be used to ensure accurate results. The hearing professional will first perform otoscopy, visualizing the outer ear and the external auditory canal to ensure there is no blockage. Your ear drums should be visualized and any abnormalities or fluid in the middle ear noted.

The audiometric assessment consists of a series of tests referred to as pure tone air, bone, speech, speech in noise (SIN), and, in some cases, further evaluation of the ear drum (tympanometry). The hearing professional determines the patient's ability to hear a tone at frequency patterns of 250, 500, 1,000, 2,000, 3,000, 4,000, 6,000, and 8,000 Hz. The threshold for each frequency is determined by a correct response 50% of the time.

Air conduction testing is performed using headphones, either over the ear or in the ear. Pure tones are presented and travel through the ear canal to the ear drum (TM), then through the middle ear system to the cochlea. Bone conduction testing uses an oscillator placed on the mastoid process (the bone behind your external ear). The oscillator vibrates at each specific frequency and bypasses the outer and middle ear. Bone conduction testing determines whether there is an air/bone gap, which would be consistent with a conductive or mixed hearing loss.

Speech Audiometry

This type of testing consists of three parts: speech reception threshold (SRT), word recognition scores (WRS), and speech in noise (SIN) (which provides the speech to noise ratio—SNR).

Speech reception threshold (SRT). This is the softest level at which a patient correctly repeats a word 50% of the time. Spondee words are two-syllable words in which each syllable is stressed. These are words like baseball, hot dog, staircase, etc. This threshold is used to verify accurate results from the pure tone audiometry and is used to approximate the most comfortable volume level for normal hearing. It is also instrumental in determining candidacy for amplification.

The word recognition score (WRS). This score is calculated by using a list of 25 or 50 phonetically balanced words. These words are then presented to the patient at their most comfortable listening level (MCL). Each word can either be spoken directly to the patient or through recorded speech. Recorded speech is the standard of care because it eliminates the variability of accents and pitch of the presenter. The purpose of the word recognition score is to determine candidacy for amplification and to determine if there is a possible tumor on the auditory nerve.

Speech in noise (SIN). This test determines the level at which a patient begins to have difficulty hearing in a noisy environment. This evaluation is instrumental in establishing the level of technology needed for the patient's lifestyle, as well as reasonable expectations of how the patient will perform in a noisy environment. Speech in noise testing involves a series of sentences spoken by either a male or a female voice at 70 dB or higher. Noise is introduced to the signal in the form of multi-talker babble at 25 dB lower. With each consecutive sentence, the noise will increase 5 dB until the speech to noise ratio (SNR) equals zero—i.e., the point at which the noise is as loud as the volume of the spoken word. When the patient can no longer hear the speaker, and the noise overwhelms the speech, the speech to noise ratio is determined.

The testing information is recorded on an audiogram. The audiogram is a visual and numerical representation of the patient's hearing, including recommendations for treatment. Not all patients who are struggling to hear in quiet and noisy environments are candidates for hearing instruments. This determination is made by the professional and the patient when discussing the patient's complaints. The cost-to-benefit ratio is one of the criteria your professional will use to determine treatment. For patients who are audiometrically normal, or who have a very mild hearing loss, there are options other than hearing instruments if that is what is most appropriate.

TREATMENT OF DISORDERS OF THE EXTERNAL EAR CANAL

IMPACTED EARWAX

Overview. Earwax (cerumen) is a mixture of sebum and sloughed skin cells. Sebum is an oily, waxy product of the sebaceous glands that lubricates our skin and hair. Cerumen acts to lubricate, clean, and protect the ear canal, migrating from the inside of the ear canal outward. The movement of the jaw assists in the migration of the cerumen out of the ear canal. In the process, cerumen can combine with hair and debris to form a blockage. A cerumen impaction occurs when the accumulated cerumen causes symptoms, which can include the following: ear fullness, itching, ear pain, vertigo (dizziness), a reflex cough, and/or hearing loss. Cerumen impaction is a frequent (and reversible condition) that can cause a significant degree of hearing loss. The hearing loss can reduce the ability to hear by as much as 5 to 40 dB depending on the degree of blockage. Cerumen impaction can also cause hearing aids to malfunction.

Indications for treatment. Treatment for cerumen impaction is indicated when symptoms develop, most commonly ear fullness or blockage and/or hearing loss. Patients who seem to be having difficulty hearing, but are unable to express symptoms should receive a hearing evaluation that includes checking for impaction. This is especially important for elderly patients, patients with cognitive impairment, and young children, since the hearing loss associated with cerumen impaction can impair cognitive function in these patients and is usually treatable.

Methods of treatment. General earwax removal can be performed by a primary care physician, nurse, audiologist, or in some cases, hearing aid dispenser. If the ear is impacted, see an ear, nose, and throat specialist (otolaryngologist). It is important that cerumen removal be performed with proper tools and techniques. If not, complications can occur. Complications can include laceration of the ear canal with bleeding, secondary infection of the ear canal, dizziness, or perforation of the ear drum. The method of removal often depends on the experience and training of the provider, available equipment, and the time needed for removal. If necessary, treatment by an ENT can definitively address the situation.

TREATMENT OF DISORDERS IN THE MIDDLE EAR

THE EUSTACHIAN TUBE

This structure (pronounced "u-station") is a surprisingly important aspect of the ear and of hearing. The eustachian tubes are canals on each side of the face that run from the back of the nose and upper throat to the middle ear. The most important function of the eustachian tube is to assure that the pressure behind the ear drum is the same as the pressure around us. When we are able to "clear" our ear during a plane flight or when changing elevations, the eustachian tube is functioning properly. In contrast, most of us have experienced the feeling of a "blocked" or "plugged" ear when the pressure in our middle ear does not equalize properly. The same lining that coats the back of the nose also lines the opening of the eustachian tubes. Common causes of eustachian tube dysfunction include:

- Nasal and sinus infections

- Allergic rhinitis

- Acid reflux (laryngopharyngeal acid reflux—reflux into the throat)

- Barotrauma due to inability to equalize pressure (plane flights, trips to higher elevations, SCUBA diving)

- Irritants such as smoke and/or air pollution

- Tissue growth in the back of the nose or nasopharynx such as polyps or enlarged adenoids.

OTITIS MEDIA

Otitis media (inflammatory conditions of the middle ear) can take several forms.

Acute otitis media (AOM) involves acute inflammation with the classical signs of heat, redness, swelling, pain, and loss of function. These conditions most often occur in children five years old or younger.

Otitis media with effusion (OME) often occurs after treatment for AOM when the infection has resolved and antibiotics have converted the signs of infection (purulent secretions) to clear, sterile fluid. Other causes of OME include dairy allergy or sensitivity, viral infections, and barotrauma. Patients with OME report ear fullness/pressure and hearing loss. Pain is typically not present in the ear. When the ear is examined, the fluid in the middle ear is often clear or light yellow in appearance. A bubble (air-fluid level) may be seen. Patient may also experience "popping" or "crackling" in the ear due to swelling at the opening of the eustachian tube. An audiologic evaluation will reveal a flat ear drum and a mild to moderate conductive hearing loss in the involved ear.

Therapy for OME depends on the underlying cause. Typically, I tell my patients that we treat their ear by treating their nose. I have patients use a nasal steroid spray once a day. (Nasacort and Flonase are now available over the counter. The recommendation is two sprays in the nostril on the side of the bad ear once a day for 10 to 14 days.) If the spray fails to resolve their symptoms, then I offer patients a short course of oral steroids (prednisone).

If you have OME and the fluid in your middle ear persists, referral to an ENT doctor is necessary for a procedure in which an incision is made in the drum (myringotomy) and the fluid is removed with suction. At that point, an ear tube (tympanostomy tube) may be placed in the ear drum through an incision referred to as the myringotomy site.

INJURY TO THE BONES OF THE MIDDLE EAR

Otosclerosis is a condition in which there is abnormal breakdown and reformation of bone that can eventually result in complete conductive hearing loss and severe overall hearing loss. The hearing loss can occur at any time, but usually begins in young adults (in their twenties to thirties). About 60% of cases are genetic, so this condition runs in families, but not everyone with the gene will develop otosclerosis. These changes involve the stapes bone (the third of the three ossicles in the middle ear). Normally, the stapes bone acts like a piston to create a fluid wave in the cochlea of the inner ear. This movement of fluid within the ear is ultimately converted to an electrical signal, which is sent to the hearing area of the brain. When abnormal bone forms around the stapes bone, a gradually worsening conductive hearing loss occurs in the affected ear. Ultimately, a maximal hearing loss can occur. At this point, the stapes bone becomes fixed and cannot move, so the individual becomes unable to perceive any sound.

Treatment. Early in the course of the condition, patients are typically administered periodic serial audiograms to follow the progression of hearing loss. Hearing aids are initially an effective intervention when the hearing loss begins to negatively affect the patient's quality of life. At that point, a surgical procedure (either a stapedectomy or stapedotomy) can be performed. The surgery is performed in an operating room using a microscope to monitor the procedure.

Either the entire stapes bone is removed and replaced with an implant, or a portion of the bone is replaced (stapedotomy). The success rate for treating the conductive hearing loss with this procedure is over 90%. There is approximately a 1% chance of a complete loss of hearing in the ear during the procedure.

EAR DRUM PERFORATION

Trauma to the ear drum (tympanic membrane) can cause significant hearing loss. The degree of hearing loss depends on the size and location of the perforation. Ear drum perforations can be caused by ear infections, barotrauma (due to increased water or air pressure, for example, during SCUBA diving or an airplane flight), a foreign body in the ear canal, Q-Tip injury, or trauma to the ear. If there is any question of an ear drum injury, the patient should be seen by a provider as soon as possible. If the perforation does not heal, a more formal surgical procedure called a tympanoplasty can be performed to "patch" the defect in the tympanic membrane.

TREATMENT OF INNER EAR AND NEUROLOGICAL HEARING LOSS

Sensorineural hearing loss (SNHL) is caused by conditions affecting the cochlea, cochlear nerve (8th cranial nerve), internal auditory canal (for example, acoustic neuroma tumors), or involving the brain. Most often the hair cells in the cochlea are damaged. These cells are vital to hearing because they convert the mechanical energy of the fluid wave within the ear to an electrical signal to the brain.

AGE-RELATED HEARING LOSS

Aging can result in a progressive hearing loss (termed presbycusis) in the higher frequencies (higher-pitched sounds), the most common cause of hearing loss. Patients most often report difficulty hearing in settings with background or competing noise. In addition, patients report having difficulty understanding speech, even when the sounds are sufficiently loud. This is confirmed by a decreased word recognition score on the audiologic evaluation. Tinnitus is often present as well and varies in severity. The tinnitus is typically more bothersome in quiet settings.

NOISE-INDUCED HEARING LOSS

Damage to the cochlea due to loud noise is another common cause of sensorineural hearing loss. Data from the 2011 and 2012 NHANES surveys (the National Health and Nutrition Examination Survey) found that 24% of adults aged 20 to 69 had evidence of noise-induced SNHL. Loud noises can cause direct mechanical damage to cochlear structures. Over time, with age-related hearing loss, frequencies above 4,000 Hz decline as well.

Recreational exposures. Even a brief exposure to very loud noises can result in severe hearing loss. This usually involves exposure to noise greater than 120 to 155 decibels (dB). This can occur when patients experience elevated sound levels with:

- Firearm-related noise close to the ear
- Recreational activities such as concerts
- Sporting events.

People at sporting events may be exposed to average sound levels of 81 to 96 dB, with peak sound levels of 105 to 124 dB. In these settings, protecting hearing with ear plugs or muffs is recommended.

Occupational exposures. OSHA (the United States Occupational Safety and Health Administration) has set guidelines to protect workers from noise exposure. All employees exposed to noise levels greater than 85 dB must be provided with hearing protection and be enrolled in a hearing protection program. Exposure to noise needs to be limited, based on how loud the noise is on a time-weighted average: workers with an exposure to 90 dB (the noise level of a power lawn mower) may be exposed for eight hours; limited to four hours at 95 dB; and not to exceed two hours at 100 dB.

DAMAGE DUE TO MEDICATION

A number of drugs are toxic to the inner ear (ototoxic) and can cause hearing loss. The most common of these are antibiotics and chemotherapy agents. The hearing loss usually starts in the higher frequencies and worsens with continued exposure. If you have any question about the potential of a medication to cause hearing loss, inquire about the possibility with your pharmacist or the prescribing provider.

OTHER DISORDERS

Tumors. Most tumors involving the inner ear are benign. The most common tumor causing hearing loss is a benign tumor of the vestibular (balance) portion of the vestibulocochlear nerve (8th cranial). These are termed vestibular schwannoma (or acoustic neuroma). This typically presents as an asymmetric hearing loss in just one ear. Other symptoms can include tinnitus, dizziness, or balance symptoms. Any patient with hearing loss that is worse in one ear should be evaluated by an otolaryngologist to rule out an acoustic neuroma.

Meniere's disease. This is a condition in which too much fluid builds up in the inner ear. Patients will have a sudden "attack" with typical symptoms of hearing loss, tinnitus, or ear fullness involving the cochlea side of the inner ear and/or spinning vertigo involving the vestibular side of the inner ear. Attacks typically cause severe symptoms that can last for hours. The inner ear is injured or compromised in some way and milder symptoms persist after the initial episode. Any patient with the sudden onset of significant hearing loss (with or without vertigo) should be evaluated as soon as possible, and Meniere's disease should be considered.

SUDDEN HEARING LOSS

Sudden hearing loss can occur with the rapid onset of significant hearing loss in one or both ears. The hearing loss may be conductive, sensorineural, or mixed in nature. The evaluation should include a physical exam and tuning fork test if possible.

> *Any patient with a sudden hearing loss*
> *should be evaluated by a provider as soon as possible.*

A sudden hearing loss requires prompt diagnosis and treatment to optimize the chance of partial or complete recovery of hearing. Any patient with a significant hearing loss should be seen by an otolaryngologist for confirmation of the diagnosis.

Timely evaluation. Ideally an audiologic evaluation should be obtained at the soonest possible opportunity, either immediately or within a matter of days—no later than two weeks after the onset of the hearing loss, but hopefully much sooner.

Patients with sudden hearing loss should be evaluated for other possible conditions, including autoimmune inner ear disease, Meniere's disease, stroke, multiple sclerosis, or a vestibular schwannoma (a type of tumor of the inner ear).

A magnetic resonance imaging (MRI) scan of the brain and internal auditory canals is the gold standard test for the imaging diagnosis of vestibular schwannomas and is also indicated in patients with sudden sensorineural hearing loss. Often CT (computed tomography) scans are obtained when patients initially present for evaluation. Patients experiencing sudden hearing loss frequently go to the emergency room with concerns about a possible stroke. The CT scans obtained in this setting are not sufficiently detailed to rule out a vestibular schwannoma. Thus, patients are exposed to the radiation of a CT scan without getting a definitive diagnosis.

Treatment. Typically, patients with a suspected (or confirmed) sudden hearing loss are treated with high-dose oral steroids (prednisone 60 mg daily for seven days until reassessment). Ideally, patients return in seven days, and an audiogram is obtained. The clinician diagnosing the patient with SNHL will utilize serial audiograms to manage patient care effectively. At the appropriate time, the steroid medication is tapered off. Hyperbaric oxygen treatments may be offered as well. To reiterate, these treatments should be started within two weeks of the onset of hearing loss. The injection of steroid medication into the middle ear space can be offered as an additional treatment after two weeks if oral steroids (and hyperbaric oxygen treatments, if ordered) are not effective.

Ongoing observation. If, after a thorough evaluation, no underlying medical issues are identified, hearing loss becomes a quality of life issue. If patients are functioning adequately, I typically arrange for a follow-up audiogram in one year. Timing of future audiograms is based on the presence and degree of subsequent hearing loss progression.

HEARING ASSISTANCE DEVICES AND HEARING AIDS

If the patient is a candidate for amplification, the next step is to determine the most appropriate treatment plan. The hearing professional will make a recommendation based on a number of factors: the patient's hearing loss, lifestyle, work environment, physical limitations, and cosmetic considerations. Hearing aids have advanced significantly in the last ten years.

With the inclusion of low-emission Bluetooth, hearing aids have evolved far beyond the earlier technology. These are no longer your grandparent's hearing aids. Even behind-the-ear styles (known as a *receiver in the ear* or RIE) are now very small, and the cosmetic aspects are appealing. These devices are so small and cleverly disguised, most people have no idea that the patient is wearing hearing aids. The advantage of Bluetooth in the hearing device is the capacity to stream audio directly from a cell phone or tablet into the hearing device. The Bluetooth also enables the user to take part in private conversations on a cell phone or listening to audio hands-free.

These hearing aids can be adjusted in very challenging listening environments. For example, when going to a noisy restaurant, the patient can use an application on their phone to change the settings in their hearing aid for a restaurant environment, whereby reducing noise occurring behind them. Using this new technology, some hearing aid wearers hear better in noisy environments than individuals with normal hearing.

How hearing aids work. There is a great deal of technology packed into these tiny, sophisticated instruments. All hearing aids share certain features: a microphone, a classifier (which analyzes incoming sounds and classifies them according to different listening environments), an amplifier, and a receiver. Some manufacturers include other components that add levels of complexity; however, all contain at least the following basics: When sound reaches the wearer, the microphone picks up the sound and the classifier then determines the nature of the sound (whether the sound is speech, noise, speech-in-noise, and where the speech or noise is coming from). The hearing aid performs a spectral analysis to determine:

- Whether to alter the sound by reducing background noise.

- Whether to turn on additional microphones, shaping the sound field to maximize hearing in noise, music, or wind, for example.

The amplifier then amplifies each frequency based on the patient's audiogram. The signal is sent to the receiver, and the sound generated in the ear canal travels to the tympanic membrane in seven millionths of a second (seven milliseconds) and, in most cases, slightly over three milliseconds.

Types of hearing aids. The size and style of hearing device is dependent on the patient's hearing loss, the size and shape of the ear canal, and of the outer ear, as well as lifestyle and cosmetic preferences. The hearing professional will consider all this when making a recommendation. Hearing aids now come in many sizes and types:

- Behind the ear (BTE)
- Receiver in the ear (RIE)
- In the ear (ITE)
- In the canal (ITC)
- Completely in the canal (CIC)
- Invisible in the ear (IIC)
- Extended-wear deep insertion.

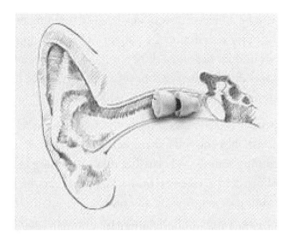

Figure 25.2. Completely in the canal hearing aid (CIC).

Insertions are devices that are placed very deep in the ear canal by the hearing professional, and are kept there for up to three months, allowing the user to live their life and even shower. It is also possible to swim while wearing an insertion if one's head is not submerged.

Personal sound amplification devices. Amplification products are available for people who have normal hearing but struggle in meetings or moderately noisy environments. These devices are designed for people who are not candidates for a hearing aid or who have not accepted the need for hearing aids. A personal sound amplification product (PSAP) can be an app used with headphones, earbuds, a handheld microphone, or an over-the-counter (OTC) amplifier.

- **Bone anchored hearing aid (BAHA).** These surgically implanted devices work by creating vibrations in the bone around the ear. The vibrations stimulate the cochlea of the inner ear, bypassing the conduction of sound through the ear canal and middle ear. Because the BAHA device bypasses the conductive components of hearing in the ear canal and middle ear, these devices are typically used for patients with significant conductive hearing loss. The BAHA devices require adequate sensorineural hearing for good results.

- **Cochlear implant.** Surgically implanted devices are available that bypass the damaged cochlea and directly stimulate the auditory (cochlear) nerve, sending the information to the brain. However, the implant does not provide normal hearing. Hearing through the implant has a different quality than normal hearing, but with effort and training, people are able to recognize speech and sounds in the environment, which enables them to communicate and function effectively.

Having a basic understanding of the anatomy of your ear and the mechanisms of hearing make you a more informed patient. As we have discussed, the majority of medical causes of hearing loss can be effectively treated. While sensorineural hearing loss cannot be cured, hearing aids provided under the direction of an expert can minimize the negative effects of the hearing loss on your quality of life. If you have concerns about your hearing, see a provider and effectively address the situation.

KEY TAKE AWAYS

- Any significant hearing loss should be immediately evaluated by a competent provider. Many causes of hearing loss are treatable, especially if addressed early on.

- Protect your hearing by using hearing protection in loud settings.

- Surgical options exist for patients with hearing loss who are not functioning well with hearing aids.

For information on the work of Dr. Michael Murphy, please see: https://stanfordhealthcare.org/medical-clinics/diablo-valley-ent.html. For more information on corrective hearing devices and the work of Toby Hill, please see: www.ContraCostaHearing.com.

Chapter 26
Stronger Bones
Judson Brandeis, MD, Urologist

Many a man has failed because he had a wishbone where his backbone should have been.
— *Ronald Reagan*

Although more common in women, osteoporosis is an important cause of morbidity and mortality in men. After the age of 65 or 70, men and women lose bone mass at about the same rate. Approximately 2 million men over the age of 65 in the United States have osteoporosis. In 50% of men with osteoporosis, a cause cannot be identified, and there may be a genetic factor for these patients.

Another 3.5 million men have osteopenia. Osteopenia refers to bone loss that is not as severe as osteoporosis. An individual with osteopenia is more likely to fracture a bone than someone with a normal bone density, but less likely to fracture a bone than someone with osteoporosis.

In men, bone mineral density increases markedly during the testosterone surge of puberty until it peaks at age 20. After attainment of peak bone mass, men lose approximately 20%–30% of their bone mass during their lifetime. Most of the adult skeleton is replaced about every 10 years. Decreased bone mass can occur due to low peak bone mass at age 20 or as the result of bone loss later in life. A 60-year-old man has a 25% chance of having an osteoporotic fracture during his life. By the age of 90, one of every six men will have a hip fracture.

PRIMARY RISK FACTORS

Increased risk of bone loss in men is associated with:

- A family history of osteoporosis
- Poor bone growth in childhood and adolescence
- Low hormone levels.

Hormonal effects:

Low testosterone. Levels of testosterone are the best-characterized risk factor for osteoporosis in men. Researchers report that bone loss increases in men with a serum testosterone level that is below 200 and bone density decreases.

Researchers conducting a large study of older men with low testosterone reported that after supplementing testosterone for a year, significant improvements were noted in the volume of bone density and estimated bone strength, particularly in the spine. Generally speaking, testosterone supplementation:

- Improves bone mineral density

- Slows the rate of bone loss

- Reduces the incidence of fragility fractures.

Blood testing for total testosterone is recommended after the age of 50.

Low estrogen. Estrogen regulates bone metabolism in both men and women and preserves bone density in both genders, so a certain amount of estrogen is protective. Researchers reported that a decline in blood levels of estradiol (a form of estrogen) below 15 was linked to declines in bone health.

SECONDARY CAUSES OF BONE LOSS

Loss of bone mass can be caused by nutrient deficiencies, lifestyle/behavior, diseases, or medications.

Low levels of essential nutrients:

- Vitamin D deficiency, which is associated with osteoporosis, reduced physical performance, and increased risk of fractures

- Low calcium levels due to an inadequate diet

- Low levels of healthy stomach acid, with less ability to break down mineral content in food

- Gastrointestinal disease, which results in lower levels of mineral absorption

- Celiac disease, impairing the ability to absorb minerals

- Higher levels of inflammation

Lifestyle factors:

- Both cigarette smoking and excess alcohol intake are associated with increased rates of bone loss and fracture.

- Low levels of physical activity are associated with bone loss and a higher risk of fracture in older men. A sedentary lifestyle doubles the risk of hip fracture. Immobilization due to illness or injury also increases risk.

Diseases and medications that can accelerate bone loss:

- Chronic conditions that affect the kidneys, lungs, stomach, and intestines or alter hormone levels

- Taking steroid hormones like prednisone for conditions such as asthma or rheumatoid arthritis

- Other immune-suppressive drugs

- Seizure medication, which is associated with bone loss and abnormalities in bone and mineral metabolism

- Androgen deprivation therapy for the treatment of prostate cancer, which can result in rapid bone loss.

Note: Finasteride does not cause bone loss. This medication, which blocks the conversion of testosterone to DHT, is used by many men for prostate shrinkage and hair growth.

TESTING AND TREATMENT

Routine bone mineral density testing in men is not currently recommended. However, bone measurement density is prescribed in men with clinical manifestations of low bone mass such as osteopenia evident on X-rays, a history of low-trauma fractures, or a loss of more than 1.5 inches in height. Risk factors for fractures such as long-term steroid therapy, androgen deprivation therapy for prostate cancer, low testosterone, primary hyperparathyroidism, or intestinal disorders also suggest the importance of bone density scans.

In men who are candidates for bone mineral density testing, dual-energy X-ray absorption symmetry, or DXA measurement of the spine and hip, is also recommended. Fractures at these sites have the most significant impact on a patient's health.

Lifestyle measures:

- Weightbearing exercise such as walking, jogging, or dancing

- Jogging on a treadmill or using a Stairmaster

- Playing non-contact ball sports such as tennis, softball, soccer

- Weight training and use of resistance machines.

Specific therapies:

- Testosterone replacement is beneficial, especially for men with a testosterone level below 200.

- Total calcium intake from diet and supplements should be 1000 mg/day for men up to the age of 70 and 1200 mg/day after 70. When blood levels of calcium are low, calcium supplements have been found clearly beneficial.

- For vitamin D, the recommended daily allowance is 600 international units for men up to 70 and 800 international units for men 71 and older.

- Regular checks of vitamin D levels in blood tests are essential to monitor levels of this vital nutrient. Risk factors include lack of sunlight during the daytime and/ or consistent sunscreen use. Your doctor can obtain reliable testing of vitamin D through any medical laboratory such as LabCorp or Quest.

- Vitamin K is another essential nutrient that aids vitamin D in maintaining healthy bones.

- Magnesium is also supportive of bone health and is available in many nutritional supplements. (Magnesium citrate is the best-absorbed form.)

- Steroid-induced bone loss should be treated aggressively, especially in older individuals.

- Men being treated for prostate cancer with androgen deprivation therapy should also be treated aggressively for osteoporosis.

- Men with celiac disease, Crohn's disease, ulcerative colitis, or low production of protective stomach acid (hydrochloric acid—HCl) are at risk of poor digestion, poor absorption of the mineral content in their food, and low vitamin D levels.

- It is also important to avoid smoking and excessive alcohol.

For men who fail conservative measures, oral bisphosphonates like alendronate or risedronate are good initial therapy because they have been found to be effective and are inexpensive. There are even intravenous formulations for individuals who cannot tolerate oral bisphosphonates. However, these medications should be used under a physician's direct supervision.

**For additional information on bone health,
please see: AmericanBoneHealth.org.**

Chapter 27
Foot Health
Jonathan Steinberg, DPM, Podiatrist

The human foot is a masterpiece of engineering and a work of art.
— Leonardo da Vinci

The feet are the foundation of the musculoskeletal system. As with a house, if the foundation is not level, the structure above will not function well. We each inherit a foot type that is stable or unstable. Depending on the stability, it is possible to predict future orthopedic issues of the foot and ankle, as well as the knees, hips, and lower back. Instability usually presents as excessive motion.

An unstable foot has excessive motion in one of three planes; front/back, side to side, and up and down (frontal, transverse, and sagittal). This motion affects the delicate balance of muscles and tendons that connect all 26 joints of the foot. Out-of-balance muscles and tendons can cause a variety of pathologies, including bunions, hammer toes, neuromas, plantar fasciitis, or painful skin lesions, as well as arthritis within the joints themselves.

Fortunately, many biomechanical imbalances can be controlled with orthotics, which can range from over-the-counter inserts for minor issues to custom orthotics for more control of unstable foot types.

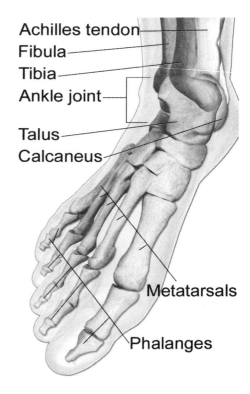

Figure 27.1. Anatomy of the foot.

The bottom line is that you should be aware of any instability and correct it before you get injured. As you get older, it is harder to heal these problems.

Consulting a board-certified podiatric physician can prevent complications resulting from instability, slowing progression of bunions, decreasing arthritis, and preventing knee and lower back issues. Podiatry should also be considered preventative medicine for athletes who use their feet.

COMMON SYMPTOMS THAT MERIT CARE

PAIN CONDITIONS

Heel pain. Plantar fasciitis is heel pain that can develop quickly without trauma in both athletes and in men carrying out normal activities. Excessive motion (the foot flattening in the sagittal plane) puts undue strain on the plantar fascial ligament, which runs from the heel to the forefoot. Chronic excessive pressure creates painful inflammation in the area of attachment in the heel. X-rays show a small heel spur at the attachment of the ligament on the heel bone called the calcaneus. This spur is a symptom of long-standing irritation to that bone by excessive pulling of the fascia forward. It tells us you need orthotics to decrease the flattening and to reduce the fascial strain and inflammation that causes pain.

Pain on the inside of the knee joint. Pain can also result in a biomechanical imbalance. Pain caused by excessive pronation (leaning in) can create deviation in the joint. The poor alignment affects balance and creates abnormal pressure and dysfunctional glide. Overcompensation for this can damage the cartilage of the knee joint, hip, and lower back.

Gout. Gout presents as a painful great toe, foot, or an ankle that is inflamed and swollen. It is caused by excess uric acid that forms crystals in and around the joints. The body's reaction to these crystals causes inflammation, swelling, redness, and pain. With repetitive episodes, uric acid deposits, called tophi, can develop, which can further damage the joints.

Men are more likely to have gout than women. Health issues such as obesity and increased cholesterol increase the risk of these painful episodes. Dehydration, alcohol, sugary soft drinks, and diuretics can also precipitate an episode of gout. If you have genetically increased uric acid production, a medication such as allopurinol as well as adequate hydration can help block the uric acid pathway and reduce your risk of gout.

FUNGAL INFECTIONS

Fungal infections are seen most commonly as athlete's foot (tinea pedis) and nail infections. These are caused most often by a fungus (mold) called a dermatophyte, which causes dry, itchy areas between the toes and yellow-brown thickened nails. Often moist areas between toes can have fungus as well as yeast and sometimes bacteria. Fungus thrives on hot, moist, dark spaces, explaining its preference for our sweaty feet enclosed in athletic shoe gear.

Genetic susceptibility. There is also significant evidence that there is a genetic susceptibility to developing these infections. The skin's immunologic system simply does not recognize the fungal elements as dangerous and allows them to thrive. Fungal nails, once established, can be more challenging to treat due to the fungal elements not only in the nail, but in the nailbed and the nail root.

Athlete's foot can also present with small vesicles when infected with inflammatory fungal elements. Because it is also in the dermatophyte group, standard antifungal cream can treat this variant.

A podiatrist will diagnose athlete's foot and fungal nails with microscopy and culture. Treatment of athlete's foot will range from antifungal powder, creams, and sprays to oral antifungal medication such as Lamisil.

Topical creams such as Lotrimin Ultra or Clotrimazole AF are generally effective. Keto-conazole 2% cream is also effective and has a broader spectrum of activity, eradicating yeast such as candida. Ultraviolet shoe trees are also available ("Steri Shoe"), which will keep your shoes free of fungal elements as well as bacteria. The creams should be applied two times daily for seven days, after having washed and dried the area between the toes. If clearing is not seen, or if redness or swelling is noted, see your doctor immediately. Secondary bacterial infections can occur on occasion. Remember, after the infection has cleared be sure to exercise anti-fungal hygiene:

- Dry off feet thoroughly after showers or swimming
- Alternate shoes, allowing each pair to dry out for a day
- Dry between toes
- Spray shoes with Lotrimin powder
- Apply antifungal cream to feet once weekly
- Change socks not only daily, but also after workouts
- Avoid public showers without wearing flip-flops.

Fungal nails. Treatment of fungal nails is more complicated. In my experience there are only two treatments that cure onychomycosis—oral medication such as Lamisil (terbin-afine) or pinpoint laser treatment. Topical medications cannot reach the fungal elements beneath the nail or in the posterior nail fold. The oral medication is taken for 90 days and has a significant side effect profile. The laser treatment in my experience has no complications and is pain-free. Generally, laser debridement of the nail or oral medication in conjunction with topical medication is most successful in eradicating the infection.

ARTHRITIS

Arthritis is inflammation within and around the joint, but there are different types of arthritis. Osteoarthritis or degenerative arthritis is the result of wear and tear over the years. Systemic diseases, such as rheumatoid or psoriasis of the joints, can also produce arthritis.

Degenerative arthritis is the most common condition in which cartilage becomes worn or damaged, causing stiffness and aching. As the cartilage degenerates further, bone-to-bone contact creates pain and swelling. Bone spurs can develop around the joint, inhibiting motion and creating a stiff joint. This type of arthritis can be treated with medication to decrease inflammation, like a nonsteroidal anti-inflammatory such as ibuprofen or a steroid injection, depending on the specific area of inflammation and its severity.

Surgical intervention can include removing bone spurs with a joint "cleanup" or may involve a fusion to prevent bone-to-bone movement and pain. A recent development is joint implants. These have been utilized in the forefoot successfully for many years, especially for the great toe joint. These joint implants are also available for the ankle.

Systemic manifestations of autoimmune arthritis, such as rheumatoid arthritis and psoriatic arthritis, will need to be managed by your physician. Good management will help decrease inflammatory changes from the disease and decrease damage to the joints.

Alternative medical techniques like cannabis-based oils, acupuncture, and reflexology have been used to decrease discomfort. Lack of extensive scientific research makes it challenging to evaluate their true efficacy. Examples of supplements thought to decrease inflammation and pain include: curcumin (from turmeric root), Omega-3 fatty acids, glucosamine, and chondroitin sulfate.

PLANTAR WARTS

Viral warts or *Verruca pedis* (plantar warts) are skin conditions arising in both children and adults. The human papillomavirus (HPV) is responsible for plantar warts. Both skin abrasions and a transiently impaired immune system are necessary to infect the skin. The virus can exist on nonorganic material such as concrete walkways, grass, dirt, and swimming pools with abrasive nonslip surfaces, which are a high risk for harboring the virus and causing skin abrasions.

Warts may clear spontaneously in about 30% of patients, but those that do not are often painful, irritating, and cosmetically distressing to the patient. Generally, it may take up to six months for a wart to spontaneously resolve on its own. These warts are usually well-circumscribed lesions with thick skin overlying the growth. When the lesions are debrided, pinpoint bleeding is noted. If the wart is adjacent to a nail, the nail itself may have a distorted shape. These lesions are painful with compression but also can be discomforting with direct pressure when walking. No single treatment technique and/or specific antiviral therapy is successful in all cases. Treatment depends on the patient, lesion, and location. It's best to address these lesions when they are small, with less viral load.

- Salicylic acid is a first-line conservative treatment when combined with regular debridement by your doctor. In about 70% of patients 40%–60% salicylic acid is effective, but takes weeks of treatment. Over-the-counter medications such as Occlusal HP, Duofilm, and Compound W all contain 40% salicylic acid and work well.

- Cryotherapy with liquid nitrogen is available from your podiatrist. It is generally painful and works by destroying the viral cell membrane and stimulating local inflammation—a cell-mediated response.

- Surgical excision of the lesion with destruction at the base is effective but will take several weeks to heal and can be painful. Laser destruction and surgical excision can leave scars.

- Other treatments available at the podiatrist include topical retinoids, topical 5-fluorouracil, and cantharidin (a blistering agent).

BUNION

A bunion is a bony bump that forms on the joint at the base of the big toe. The big toe pushes against the next toe forming the bunion. Tight shoes, foot stress, and arthritis are causes.

The main symptoms are bone deformity, pain, and stiffness. There are two types of bunions: One is a misalignment caused by

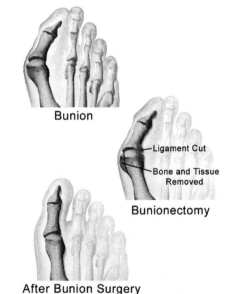

Bunion

Ligament Cut
Bone and Tissue Removed

Bunionectomy

After Bunion Surgery

Figure 27.2. Surgical correction of a bunion.

improper biomechanics, and the other is a juvenile bunion that is genetic and noted in younger patients. A positional bunion develops when there is bone growth on the side of the metatarsal head, forcing the joint capsule and tendons into malalignment.

A structural bunion involves the widening of the first metatarsal and second metatarsal space. The increasing angle between them in turn pushes the great toe toward the second toe. This can result in pain and swelling as well as skin irritation, including pressure ulcerations. Treatment will depend not only on the severity of the deformity, but also on the clinical symptoms, such as pain, stiffness, swelling, and painful calluses that affect a person's lifestyle.

■   The most conservative treatment consists of shoe gear adjustment and nonsteroidal anti-inflammatory medication.

■   A podiatrist can inject cortisone and platelet-rich plasma.

■   Surgical intervention depends on the severity of the deformity and will involve soft tissue rebalancing around the joint as well as removing excessive bone. An osteotomy with screw fixation will be carried out in more structural deformities to correct the widened metatarsal angle.

Biomechanical stability and appropriate shoe gear will play an important role in preventing the initial problem and decreasing progression.

HAMMER TOES

These are contracted lesser toes caused by inherited muscle imbalance or abnormal bone length. When the toes buckle (flex) abnormally, tissue contracts. Use of orthotics for an unstable foot can decrease the progression of the contracture. The foot will function more normally, creating less compensation. Early evaluation is preferable while the condition of the toes is still flexible.

Treatment depends on the rigidity of the contracture. If the fifth toe is flexible (can be easily straightened) then a simple procedure involves cutting the tendon and releasing the contracture. There is a two-week recovery period as the soft tissue heals, during which you can be fully functional. If the deformity is rigid, then an arthroplasty needs to be done, removing bone to decompress the joint and straighten the toe. This does take more time to heal, about four weeks in a surgical shoe. The timing of surgical intervention is based on severity, failure of orthotic stabilization, and the effect the hammertoe is having on your activities of daily living.

NEUROMA

A neuroma causes a sharp pain under the ball of the foot, which occurs when one of the toe nerves becomes inflamed. This usually occurs between the third and fourth metatarsal heads (Morton's neuroma). The neuroma is caused primarily by irritation as it sweeps through the intermetatarsal ligament. The bone and ligament create chronic irritation, with the resultant perineural fibrosis–thickened nerve.

- Self treatment consists of wearing wider shoes, taking nonsteroidal anti-inflammatories like Alleve, and wearing a metatarsal pad under the point of discomfort. However, early evaluation should be done to rule out other problems such as a stress fracture.

- Cortisone injections and use of a nonsteroidal anti-inflammatory are the standard of care. A metatarsal pad will be utilized to decrease inflammation and separate the metatarsal heads, relieving pressure on that nerve. If this is successful, no further treatment will be necessary.

- Surgery is performed if the thickened, inflamed nerve is not responding to conservative treatment. A neurectomy involves surgically excising the thickened portion of the nerve with residual minor numbness noted to the adjacent toes.

ANKLE SPRAINS

Ankle sprains are a common injury that occur due to the overstretching of a muscle or muscle groups. An ankle sprain can also involve injury to the tendons, ligaments, and soft tissues surrounding the joint.

The most common ankle sprain is an inversion sprain, in which the ankle turns in, stretching, or tearing the three most prominent ligaments that stabilize the lateral ankle. Generally, when there are black-and-blue tissues, severe swelling, and pain, then there is at least some damage to one or more of these ligaments. The initial injury should be treated with the classic RICE–rest, ice, compression, and elevation. If a fracture is suspected, splinting will be necessary and further immediate evaluation recommended.

In moderate to severe sprains in which tendons and ligaments have been stretched, ankle bracing should be carried out as soon as possible to partially immobilize the joint, allowing soft tissue to heal in a configuration that is not stretched or contorted. An air-cast ankle support will allow the tissue to heal in a more normal position.

PREVENTING INJURIES

■ Warmup before exercise—cool down and stretch after activities.

■ Increase intensity and duration of activities gradually—as fitness improves, it will be possible to do increasingly more strenuous activity without injury.

■ Use proper sports techniques and equipment.

■ Alternate hard workouts with easy ones to let your body rest.

■ Cross train—alternate types of activity regularly.

■ Do not ignore aches and pains. A few days rest may help you avoid more serious injury.

DIABETES

Having diabetes can directly affect the feet, due to issues relating to diminished circulation, peripheral nerve dysfunction, and decreased effectiveness of the immune system to combat infections.

Signs of changes in skin temperature, skin color, and/or breaks in skin integrity can all be precursors to more serious problems and need to be evaluated by a physician.

■ Redness, swelling, and drainage can indicate an infection that needs to be aggressively treated.

■ Cool temperatures can indicate diminished peripheral circulation.

■ Decreased sensation can indicate peripheral neuropathy.

Diabetics need to pay special attention to their feet with daily inspections, meticulous hygiene, and proper shoe gear. Exercise and proper nutrition are equally important. Careful control of glucose and regular lower foot examinations are the best preventive care.

For more information on foot health and podiatry, please see the website of the American Podiatric Medical Association at www.apma.org. For more on the work of Dr. Steinberg, please see: www.muirfootandanklecenter.com.

Chapter 28
Hand Health
Greg Horner, MD, Orthopedic Surgeon

*Often the hands will solve a mystery that the intellect
has struggled with in vain.*
— Carl Jung

*My interest in medicine developed from the uncommon experience of being a Big Ten wide
receiver while studying mechanical engineering. It wasn't just that I was far better at physics
than football. My growing awareness of the myriad of injuries incurred by my Northwestern
teammates, paired with a clear connection to the engineering principles underlying their treatment, caused me to fall in love with orthopedic surgery.*

*I changed my major to biomedical engineering and subsequently gained early admission to the
top medical school in the country to become a team physician. As fate would have it, my men-
torship would include Dr. A. Lee Dellon, one of the world's top hand surgeons and the authority
on peripheral nerves. That experience led to a 21-year career in microvascular hand surgery
packed with more than 100,000 patient visits. Here I offer the insight I wish my patients would
have had before the episodes that led them to me.*

The way a man considers his hands is quite different from the perspective of a woman. This
chapter has a focus that is broadly applicable, but written with men in mind. The basis
for the content is the types of questions I have received from men over the years regarding
their hands. While it is not meant to be exhaustive, I have sought to focus on the patients
I have seen and what I might have told them if I had had the chance, long before I became
their doctor. In other words, this is a discussion of prevention. I will focus on the most
common injuries that I see, and how to avoid ever coming to my office.

MAJOR FACTORS IN HAND HEALTH

NERVES OF THE HAND

When you think of your hand nerves, you probably think of lacerations that could get you
in trouble. It turns out that you should be more aware of a much more insidious threat.
Peripheral nerve compression, such as carpal tunnel syndrome, affects more than 10% of

American adults. Untreated, peripheral nerve entrapment can lead to permanent loss of muscle function and to decreased sensation, and it may contribute to degeneration of the joints with significant loss of function as well. This is terrible stuff.

Carpal tunnel syndrome, cubital tunnel syndrome, neural entrapment at Guyon's canal, thoracic outlet syndrome, and neural foraminal stenosis . . . these are all fancy words for the various sites where you are most likely to get a pinched nerve at some point in your life. These locations include the neck (foraminal stenosis), elbow (cubital tunnel), and the wrist (carpal tunnel syndrome and Guyon's canal). Technically these conditions are straightforward to describe. A nerve must pass through various points of potential constriction as it moves from your spinal cord to your hand or your brain.

The carpal tunnel is the most common site of nerve compression, a tunnel-like space comprised of the wrist bones, forming an arch bound at the top by a ligament. Your tendons may swell or increase in size, the joints between the bones may widen, or lesions, such as ganglia, may form in the tunnel. However, whatever the problem affecting that space, the space has only so much room. The nerve at any site of compression is the most fragile structure. It is highly sensitive to pressure and swiftly begins to lose function.

When a nerve fails to perform its function, the first thing you notice is tingling (such as that you experience when you wake up after sleeping awkwardly on your arm). Left untreated, the muscles controlled by that nerve begin to shrink or *atrophy*. Atrophy is a late sign, and it tells the clinician that the problem has become irreversible. Loss of muscle strength causes imbalances of forces across the joints of the hand. This can result in arthritic degeneration, which is always irreversible. Therefore, prevention is critical.

The cause is multifactorial and includes metabolic dysfunction, such as diabetes mellitus. Although prevention is beyond the scope of this discussion, it is worth stating here that general health is inextricably linked to hand health. Our everyday body mechanics and activities provide the best pathway for direct prevention of nerve compression affecting the hand. The hand tends to be a barometer of the general health of an individual.

POSTURE

You may be reading this manuscript on a handheld device rather than a book. Americans spend more than four hours per day on mobile devices and computers. The typical posture associated with digital device use is abysmal. Your neck is usually in a flexed position (bent forward) that causes a dramatic increase in pressure in the cervical spine. This stress is compounded by fatigue due to the efforts of the stabilizing muscles of the neck to support your head while it is cantilevered out in a face-forward position. This combination can lead to degeneration of the cervical spine and neural foraminal stenosis (pinching of the nerves in your neck). Slumped posture also reduces space in the thoracic outlet, the place where your nerves enter your arm. Thoracic outlet pressure and pinched nerves in the neck are not just problematic on their own. They can profoundly worsen nerve compression elsewhere, causing what we refer to as a *double crush phenomenon*.

Elbow flexion beyond 90 degrees increases pressure in the important ulnar nerve within the elbow, aka the funny bone. This nerve is essential for the function of most of the small muscles in your hands and transmits sensation at the ring and small fingers. Wrist extension or flexion (bending up and down) beyond eight degrees increases pressure within the carpal tunnel and on the median nerve therein. This nerve is vital for the rest of the small muscles in your hands and most of your fingers.

You don't need to commit any of that to memory. These disorders are surprisingly simple to prevent, with just two rules to follow:

- **When using computers and digital devices, sit up as straight as possible.** You want to hold your head erect, facing forward, even if that means holding your phone at eye level manually or using a support device like a stand or a riser. (Stands are available for use with laptops, tablets, and even phones.) This erect posture is crucial on trains and planes. I always wear a soft neck brace when I fly or take trains. The brace prevents neck flexion and profoundly decreases pressure in cervical disks, even when sleeping in flight.

- **When typing, keep your elbows at 90 degrees (like the letter L).** Hold your wrists and forearms flat on the desktop or table surface, or slightly extended. Adjust your chair to keep your elbows at or slightly above table height. Fold the legs on the keyboard so it lies flat on the table, to avoid excessive wrist extension or flexion. Be especially wary of your posture when using laptops and tablets.

Hand numbness, tingling, or weakness that is severe or has lasted more than four weeks necessitates consultation with a physician. Generally, a brief telemedicine discussion is adequate to determine the next steps.

JOINTS OF THE HAND

The natural question that comes to mind is, "What is a joint, and what is hand arthritis?" Simply put, a joint comprises the soft ends of the bone known as *cartilage* (such as the end of a chicken bone), which is always concave on one side and convex on the other. This configuration allows one bone to pivot on the other like a ball in a socket. The joint is enclosed in a *capsule* that keeps it lubricated with a slippery glucose and protein mix. In fact, the slippery nature of cartilage on cartilage in this fluid bath is 100 times as slick as ice on ice.

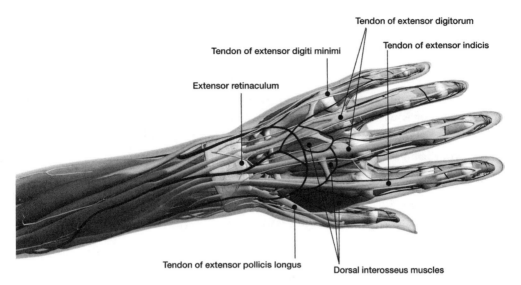

Tendon of extensor digitorum

Tendon of extensor digiti minimi

Tendon of extensor indicis

Extensor retinaculum

Tendon of extensor pollicis longus

Dorsal interosseus muscles

Figure 28.1. Structure of the hand.

So how does cartilage wear out if there is no friction? It doesn't. Cartilage damage only occurs from compression, the result of too much pressure on the fragile cells in the cartilage matrix. Overload obviously can occur due to impact force, but it is more likely that the bone will fracture than that the cartilage will become damaged. The cartilage is generally a precise fit, so any pressure is evenly distributed across its full surface regardless of the joint angle. However, mechanical misuse of the hand can lead to cartilage overload. Your joints are heavily dependent on your nerve and muscle function.

THE OPPOSABLE THUMB AND FINGERS

Our opposable thumb describes the ability to turn our thumb to face or *"oppose"* our fingers. In contrast, the finger joints primarily bend and straighten. Given their structure, pinching causes the finger joints to deal with forces in the wrong direction, or "orthogonal" to the normal motion of the joint. This counter pressure generates a high compression force on the far side of the finger joints, referred to as eccentric force. It may come as no surprise that the far side of the finger joints, or the "ulnar" side, is where arthritis usually develops. Once the cartilage is damaged, the degeneration will spread progressively across the joint.

There are a surprising number of other situations in which one might unevenly load their finger and threaten the cartilage. Think about pinching keys or holding flat, heavy objects. A rule of thumb (pardon the pun) that captures the concept of eccentric force and protects your fingers from your opposable thumb is:

- When lifting any objects, try to position your fingers to face upward and oppose gravity rather than using your thumb.

- When dealing with small objects, routinely seek to use a light grip, or seek adaptations to increase the size of the object. The best situation that illustrates this concept is writing devices. Always use a wide grip pen or pencil to maximize width. Increasing the surface area and width of the pen increases the contact with your hand and decreases eccentric forces on your finger joints.

- If a power pinch is necessary, pinch to the side of the finger rather than index to thumb tip. This way, all of the fingers bear the brunt of the force, and no force is eccentrically applied to the finger joints.

SKIN

It is true that the best way to estimate a person's age is to look at their hands. Your hands encounter the sun more than any other part of the body. In addition to sun damage, your hands experience extreme environments that no other part of your body must face, by way of chemicals, abrasion, wind, desiccation, water or excessive moisture, and more. Over the years, the skin on your hands accumulate damage from the sun that includes a variety of physiological changes beyond the scope of this chapter. The result is thinning of the dermis, deep wrinkles, laxity, and roughness.

Further, the hand is one of the most likely locations for the development of skin cancer (carcinoma). Part of the skin includes the nail and nail fold of your fingers, the *paryonychium*. These structures are equally susceptible to carcinoma and are particularly vulnerable to excessive moisture and minor trauma. Acute nail bed infections are very common and often caused by minor trauma to the nail or nail bed. Chronic nail bed infections (lasting more than six weeks) are usually fungal and related to occupation or activities involving excessive moisture (think dishwashing). The *cuticle* is a filmy tissue that seals the nail fold and is critical for preventing impregnation of bacteria or fungi in the area and causing infection. Do not remove your cuticle!

- **Sun protection.** Lotions are available that serve the dual purpose of SPF protection from harmful UVB and moisturizing. Apply daily, even in the winter months.

- **Gloves.** There are gloves for nearly all activities. Buy them, wear them, and protect your hands, not just from the sun and elements, but also from potential trauma. Whether cycling, playing water sports, or doing chores such as washing the car, always strive to wear gloves.

- **Nail care.** If you must have a manicure, never cut or push back the cuticle.

THE WRISTS

You have probably heard and likely followed the age-old adage that *if you can move your hand, then it's not broken.* Dear reader, please believe me that this is *not* true, and it is the cause of considerable permanent damage to men arriving too late at the hand surgery office. Although a comprehensive discussion of fractures is beyond the scope of this chapter, please allow me to indicate three sprain/fracture varieties that, although frequently subtle, can ruin your hand.

SNAC wrist. Scaphoid fractures can occur from minor trauma. They are very common and often subtle. The scaphoid is a tiny wrist bone that is precarious because most of its blood flow is cut off if a fracture crosses two-thirds of the bone at any point. Slight tenderness on the thumb side of the wrist may be the only sign or symptom. It is routine for hand surgeons to order an MRI to make the diagnosis because of the subtlety of findings. If not treated in a cast, there's a very high likelihood of the scaphoid not healing. If it doesn't heal, the wrist degenerates into terrible arthritis called *Scaphoid Non-union Advanced Collapse* (SNAC wrist), a very debilitating condition.

SLAC wrist. A scapholunate ligament rupture is a tear of a very small and filmy ligament at the center of your wrist. The symptoms can be as mild as slight tenderness or pain following an injury, often with minimal swelling. You may think it's just a sprain. But once torn, the ligament cannot heal itself. Rupture of this ligament can destabilize the entire wrist and results, inevitably, in wrist degeneration similar to that of the SNAC wrist. Termed *Scapholunate Advanced Collapse* (SLAC Wrist), this condition is also very debilitating.

Articular fractures. Minor trauma anywhere in your hand or wrist can cause fractures that involve the joints. Symptoms can be minimal and even go away after some time. However, in a similar manner to SLAC or SNAC wrist, a fracture through a joint can lead to destruction of that joint and irreversible *post-traumatic osteoarthritis*, a condition that is, once again, debilitating.

These injuries and many others can be surprisingly subtle. You cannot expect urgent care or E.R. docs to catch them. It is best to see a specialist if you have any injury resulting in pain or swelling at any joint in your hand or wrist. Time is generally of the essence, as many upper extremity injuries must be treated within two to four weeks, depending on the injury. Delay can result in irreversible damage and often severe loss of function.

YOUR BRAIN

Yes, your brain is the most important organ involved in protecting your hands. Every year I have the horrifying experience of managing patients who are very intelligent, and even sober, who make extraordinarily poor decisions that will change their lives forever. The type of decision that probably illustrates this point the most clearly occurs each summer when a man (I have never seen a woman make this mistake) decides that, for some reason or other, he should clear grass from the underbelly of a *running lawnmower* with his bare hand. The second most illustrative example is much more common to the degree that there's a name for it, "Thanksgiving finger." Without going into further detail, please observe these easy hand-protective measures:

- **Always cut away from your hand.** I once treated an extraordinary pianist who had the misfortune of using a sushi knife to cut an orange toward her hand. Sushi knives are often cut at an 11-degree angle, and they are far sharper than typical knives. After I repaired her nerves and tendons, the pianist later invited me to a sensational orchestral concert where she brought the house down with her post-recovery performance. There are many others today who will not be nearly as fortunate.

- **Instead of your hand, use tools whenever you can.** Machinery, wild animals, and other sharp things can ruin your hands, as can electricity. As the late-night commercial suggests, the hand cannot be used as a knife. It should never be used as a hammer either. In fact, there is a particularly pernicious problem called *Hypothenar Hammer Syndrome* that results from using the heel of the hand to hammer objects, like a stake or an ill-fitted part into place. The result is occlusion of an artery in the palm and can threaten loss of your hand. The treatment is often microvascular reconstruction.

- **Use common sense.**

WHEN TO SEE A DOCTOR

Your hands and fingers are structures that you really do not fully appreciate until they are at risk. You need to be proactive in seeking a physician's opinion if you have:

- Joint pain or swelling that persists beyond a few days following trauma
- Any infection or signs of infection (redness, swelling, or drainage)
- Any weakness
- Numbness or tingling that persists beyond a few days
- Any apparent deformity
- Unusual skin lesions of any sort.

It is always best to seek a specialist. While a general orthopedic surgeon is usually more than qualified for most bone and joint injuries, always seek a hand specialist when dealing with wrist or hand concerns. I hope that these preventive measures will guide you for years to come. Thank you in advance for taking good care of your hands.

KEY TAKE AWAYS

I get these questions frequently at cocktail parties and holiday gatherings. Since people wonder about these things, they are probably worth clearing up once and for all.

- **What is "knuckle cracking," and does it cause arthritis?** The snapping sound of knuckle cracking is thought to be *cavitation* in the joint fluid. While it doesn't appear to cause arthritis, knuckle cracking is probably not good for your joints.

- **What are some hand exercises you can do to keep your hands strong? Are the squeezing devices good?** To reiterate, general health is inextricably linked to hand health. For example, your childhood experience and current testosterone levels are more important than any exercises in determining grip strength. In fact, getting good sleep is probably as good as any strengthening exercise. I generally do not recommend hand-strengthening exercises except in recovery from disease or injury of the hand.

- **How should you "throw a punch" so that you do not injure your hand or wrist?** *I would recommend not punching anything or anyone.* However, if a punch is absolutely necessary, then here are three recommendations from hand surgeons and boxers alike:

    1. Keep your wrist straight and punch at the end of your reach to avoid wrist "buckling" and injury.

    2. Lead with the knuckle of the middle and/or index finger. The knuckles of the ring finger and the small finger are far weaker. In fact, a term associated with fractures of the ring and small finger is "boxer's fractures."

    3. If you choose to take up boxing, learn from the pros.

- **How can you find a good hand specialist?** The American Society for Surgery of the Hand has a search tool for finding hand surgeons. That is the best way to get started.

For more information on the work of Dr. Horner, please see:
www.trivalleyorthopedics.com/gregory-horner-m-d/.

Chapter 29
Optimizing Sleep
Michael Murphy, MD, MPH
Ear, Nose, & Throat Surgeon
Sleep Specialist

A good laugh and a long sleep are the best cures in the doctor's book.
— Irish proverb

Sleep is the engine that drives our lives. With good quality sleep we wake up feeling ready to conquer the world. We feel sharp, ready, and capable to handle whatever the day throws our way. On the other hand, with poor sleep, life is harder and less enjoyable.

This chapter will focus on simple, practical things you can do to improve the quality of your sleep. We will also briefly discuss the most common sleep disorders affecting men at our stage of life.

THE PHYSIOLOGY OF SLEEP

While I will not go into great detail about the physiology of sleep (it can get complicated), having a basic understanding will provide a sound foundation for the topics we cover in this chapter.

We have a circadian timekeeper in the hypothalamus of our brain. The circadian system helps control our core body temperature, appetite, and sleep. Our circadian system keeps aligned with the 24-hour day by zeitgebers ("time givers" in German). The primary zeitgeber is the light-dark cycle in our environment.

The Two-Process Model of Sleep. The Circadian Process (Process C) drives alertness or wakefulness over the 24-hour period. During the day our alertness gradually increases, peaks, and then declines in the evening as bedtime approaches. The circadian drive is lowest during our biological night. The pineal gland in our brain makes the hormone melatonin, which makes us sleepy, and production of melatonin peaks during our biological night.

The Homeostatic Sleep Process (Process S) indicates our drive to sleep. Our drive to sleep rises steadily until it peaks at night when our circadian drive is reaching a low point. Sleep ensues. As we sleep, our sleep drive declines until it reaches a low point and the circadian drive is increasing. We wake up. The cycle repeats.

Understanding this basic model of sleep is important. Sleep problems ensue when these two processes get out of sync (more on this later). This model also helps form the basis for basic sleep hygiene.

How much sleep do we need? Getting a sufficient amount of good quality sleep is essential for our physical and mental health.

The American Academy of Sleep Medicine and Sleep Research Society state that adults age 18 to 60 need to sleep at least seven hours a night on a regular basis. This is consistent with recommendations of the National Sleep Foundation, specifying that adults ages 18 to 64 need seven to nine hours of sleep a night on a regular basis. Unfortunately, many Americans fail to meet the above recommendations. Nearly 30% of adults in the United States report sleeping six or fewer hours per day. Not getting adequate sleep can have serious consequences in both the short term and the long term. Studies have clearly shown that not getting enough quality sleep can lead to automobile accidents, work-related accidents, poor work performance, health problems (cardiovascular disease, obesity, and poor immune function with the resulting effects), and strained personal relationships.

ANALYZING YOUR SLEEP

Keeping a Sleep Diary

A great way to understand the amount and quality of your sleep is to keep a sleep diary. These diaries are readily available and easy to use. The diary should be kept for seven to fourteen consecutive days. A simple 24-hour log or a more detailed Consensus Sleep Diary can be used. The diary should reflect your typical sleep patterns for both weekdays and weekends. It is best to complete each entry immediately after waking up in the morning. There are also a number of electronic sleep diaries available as apps. Ideally, the sleep diary should include the following elements:

- The time you get into bed
- The time you fall asleep
- The number of times you wake up during the night
- The amount of time it took you to fall back to sleep

- The time you wake up in the morning

- The time you get out of bed to start the day

- The number and length of naps you take during the day

- Caffeine, alcohol, and medication use (very helpful to include).

The following information can be determined from your sleep diary:

- Average sleep time on weekdays

- Average sleep time on weekends

- Sleep latency (the time it takes to fall asleep once the lights are off; 15 to 20 minutes is the goal)

- Sleep efficiency (the percentage of time you are asleep when in bed). The calculation is (time asleep)/(time in bed) x 100; ≥85% is normal.

Consumer Devices for Tracking Sleep

Companies are now recognizing the value of products that help customers analyze their sleep patterns and improve the quality of their sleep. New products are coming to the market all the time, and the technology is continually advancing. It is important to note that the majority of these sleep technologies are not approved as medical devices by the Food and Drug Administration. In addition, there are few published scientific studies validating the accuracy of these devices. Consumer sleep technologies are typically divided into wearables (devices you wear) and nearables (devices that monitor your sleep from a nightstand, mattress, or nearby location).

Wearable devices frequently use an accelerometer to sense motion. They are based on actigraphy, a medical-grade accelerometer that has long been the standard tool for objectively estimating sleep patterns and duration. Wearable devices measure the amount of sleep overnight, but are not as good at tracking the depth of sleep. Examples include:

- FitBit (www.fitbit.com)

- Apple watch with sleep applications such as AutoSleep (by Tantsissa)

- Withings watches (www.withings.com).

Nearable devices include bedside smartphone applications, bedside devices, and devices placed on or under the mattress. Using differing technologies, these devices analyze your sleep.

Examples of nearable devices include:

- Withings Sleep Tracking Mat (www.withings.com)
- Smartphone apps such as Sleep Cycle (by Sleep Cycle) and Sleep Time (by Azumio).

While many of these technologies have not been validated by medical studies, the biggest benefit of these devices is to help you better understand your sleep.

IMPROVING YOUR SLEEP

The most important efforts you can make to improve the quality and amount of your sleep are simple lifestyle choices. We refer to these practices as sleep hygiene. These are easy to understand but sometimes hard to do! Good sleep hygiene includes the following:

Keep the same sleep schedule by going to bed and getting up at the same time, including weekends. Your body will get used to the schedule, making it easier to go to sleep and wake up.

Prepare for sleep by relaxing and winding down.

- Avoid the use of electronics for at least 30 minutes prior to bedtime. The blue light from computer screens and hand-held devices can suppress natural melatonin production, making it difficult to fall asleep. Blue light from a screen also stimulates the rise of cortisol. (Our brain interprets blue light as blue sky. Thinking that it is morning, our body releases glycogen to give us energy, just when we're trying to go to sleep.)
- Minimize stress such as work-related activities or to-do lists prior to bedtime.
- Reading with dim light can make it easier to go to sleep.
- Having a consistent bedtime routine makes it easier to go to sleep.

The proper sleep environment is important.

- A comfortable mattress and pillow(s)
- The bedroom should be comfortably cool.
- The environment should be dark and quiet. Studies have shown that environmental light and noise significantly impact sleep quality and quantity. Use ear plugs, curtains, or opaque shades to create a dark, quiet environment that is conducive to good sleep. If your sleeping environment is uncontrollably noisy, try a sound machine or some type of white noise.

Daily exercise will improve your sleep. Multiple studies have shown that exercise improves the ability to fall asleep faster, extends total sleep duration, and enhances sleep quality. Avoid exercise just prior to bedtime because your body is likely to take a while to wind down after exercise.

If you have trouble sleeping at night:

- Avoid naps, especially in the late afternoon. If you need a nap, try to avoid sleeping longer than 30 minutes. Short naps can help alleviate daytime fatigue, sleepiness, and improve mental function. Naps are often needed for shift workers (more on this later).

- If you wake up and have trouble going back to sleep, do not stay in bed. Get up, go to another room, and do something relaxing (have a cup of decaffeinated tea, and read in dim light for example). When you feel drowsy, return to bed to go back to sleep.

Caffeine, nicotine, and alcohol:

- Caffeine makes it hard to go to sleep. Avoid caffeine for eight to ten hours before you plan to go to sleep.

- Avoid smoking in the evening. Evening nicotine results in more awake time during the night.

- Avoid excessive alcohol in the evening. Although alcohol may make it easier to *go to sleep*, it has several negative effects on your sleep. Alcohol causes us to spend more time in the lighter stages of sleep (making it easier to wake up), especially early in the morning.

SLEEP DISORDERS: THE BIG PICTURE

Understanding the big picture with respect to sleep disorders is helpful because it puts into context problems you may have with your sleep.

The most common system for denoting sleep disorders is the International Classification of Sleep Disorders (ICSD). We are currently on the third edition (ICSD-3). Major categories of sleep disorders include:

Insomnia — Persons who have difficulty going to sleep or staying asleep with daytime consequences (fatigue, difficulty with concentration/performance, mood symptoms).

Sleep-related breathing disorders — Persons with abnormal breathing during sleep. This category includes obstructive sleep apnea.

Circadian rhythm sleep-wake disorders — Persons who have a misalignment between their environment and sleep-wake cycle (an alteration of the circadian system), this category includes jet-lag and shift-work disorders.

Sleep-related movement disorders — Persons who have simple, stereotyped movements that disturb sleep with daytime symptoms (fatigue, daytime sleepiness, insomnia), may experience restless legs syndrome or sleep-related bruxism (teeth grinding).

Parasomnias — Persons who have undesirable physical events (complex movements or behaviors) or experiences (emotions, perceptions, dreams) that occur with sleep are described as having parasomnias. Unlike the stereotyped activity seen with movement disorders, the behaviors with parasomnias are more complex and purposeful. This category includes sleep walking, sleep terrors, sleep- related eating disorder, and nightmare disorder.

Central disorders of hypersomnolence — Persons with a primary complaint of daytime sleepiness (an irrepressible need to sleep or daytime lapse into sleep) not due to another sleep disorder experience conditions that include narcolepsy.

The ICSD-3 includes 60 specific diagnoses within the seven major categories. I would like to briefly touch on several diagnoses that are most relevant to men at our stage of life. A board-certified sleep physician has the training to diagnose and treat the sleep disorders included in the ICSD-3. You can search for local sleep centers (and physicians) at www.sleepeducation.org.

OBSTRUCTIVE SLEEP APNEA

Sleep-related breathing disorders are characterized by abnormal breathing during sleep. Obstructive sleep apnea (OSA) is by far the most common condition in this category. Fundamentally, snoring and obstructive sleep apnea occur when there is a reduction or cessation of airflow due to a narrowing or closure of the upper airway during sleep *while respiratory effort continues;* i.e., the airway narrows while the sleeper is attempting to breathe.

> *Although snoring is a quality-of-life issue for bed partners, obstructive sleep apnea is a health issue. Untreated over time, OSA can lead to serious health problems, because levels of oxygen in the body are reduced, and the individual becomes sleep deprived.*

Obstructive sleep apnea is diagnosed by a test called a polysomnogram. The presence or absence of OSA and its severity are measured by the Apnea-Hypopnea Index (AHI). An AHI greater than five denotes the presence of OSA. Paul Peppard from the University of Wisconsin and colleagues published a paper entitled, "Increased Prevalence of

Sleep-Disordered Breathing in Adults" in 2013, and this study forms the basis of estimates for OSA prevalence in U.S. adults. In the study, adults are grouped from ages 30 to 70. At least 17% of U.S. females (14,682,306) have obstructive sleep apnea.

Based on current population estimates, the data show that up to 34% of U.S. males — more than 27 million men — have obstructive sleep apnea.

While OSA is ultimately diagnosed by a polysomnogram test, there are several practical ways to determine whether you simply snore or actually have sleep apnea.

The first indicator is apnea (altered breathing patterns) witnessed by a bed partner. While this does not prove you have OSA, it is highly suggestive. In this situation, the bed partner is not just annoyed by their partner's snoring, but is worried about their breathing.

The STOP-Bang Questionnaire (SBQ)—included in this chapter—is a useful tool for assessing possible obstructive sleep apnea.

If you suspect that you may have obstructive sleep apnea, you will need to have an office visit with an appropriate provider. Your primary care doctor is a good place to start. The expert in evaluating potential sleep apnea is a head and neck surgeon (an otolaryngologist, commonly known as an ear, nose, and throat or ENT doctor). These surgeons specialize in treating patients with upper airway obstruction (both medically and surgically). You can search for a local ENT doctor at www.entnet.org (www.entnet.org/content/find-ent). Ultimately, you will likely need a sleep study (a polysomnogram test). While traditionally these tests were done in a lab setting, increasingly the tests are done with you at home in your own bed.

Identifying and treating obstructive sleep apnea, if you have it, is one of the most import-ant things you can do for your overall health and quality of life. Your partner will also benefit, sleeping in the same bed and happily in a quiet room!

SHIFT-WORK DISORDER

Individuals who work night shifts commonly have difficulties with alertness at work and trouble getting good quality sleep at home. Shift work is recognized as a risk factor for seri-ous health problems such as weight gain or obesity, cardiovascular diseases, and even cancer.

It is estimated that one-third or more of shift workers have sufficient symptoms to meet the criteria for a diagnosis of shift-work disorder.

The STOP-Bang Questionnaire (SBQ) (www.stopbang.ca)

This questionnaire uses observations about your snoring and basic information about you and your health to determine your risk for obstructive sleep apnea. The test has been scientifically validated and found effective in clinical settings. You can take the questionnaire online at www.stopbang.com or use the version below. To score the questionnaire, "Yes" answers are 1 point each and "No" answers are scored as 0 points.

Question 1. Snoring? Anyone who snores loudly is at risk of obstructive sleep apnea.

Question 2. Tired? Daytime fatigue is one of the primary symptoms of OSA.

Question 3. Observed? I have found in my practice that when a partner observes that the patient stopped breathing or experienced choking or gasping for air during sleep, this is a highly predictive sign of OSA.

Question 4. Pressure? Hypertension (high blood pressure) is one of the most common cardiovascular conditions seen in patients with OSA.

Question 5. Body Mass Index (BMI) more than 35 kg/m²? There is a very clear association between body weight and the severity of snoring and OSA. There are online charts and tools to help you determine your BMI.

Question 6. Age – older than 50 years?

Question 7. Neck size large? (Measured around the Adam's Apple.)

The size measurement is different for males and females, but it still represents a measure of obstruction at the level of the neck in our equation.

Question 8. Gender = Male?

Obstructive sleep apnea has been linked to serious conditions, including stroke, abnormal heart rhythms, and heart attack risk (myocardial infarction).

Interpreting the score on the STOP-Bang Questionnaire

Low risk of OSA: Yes to 0–2 questions

Intermediate risk of OSA: Yes to 3–4 questions

High risk of OSA: Yes to 5–8 questions, or

Yes to 2 of 4 STOP questions + individual's gender is male

Yes to 2 of 4 STOP questions + BMI >35 (kg/m²)

The underlying problem with shift work disorder is the loss of balance between the circadian and homeostatic sleep processes. Under normal circumstances when a person works during the day, they go to bed at night when their sleep drive is high and the circadian signal for alertness is low. When a person works a night shift, these two drives become misaligned. This misalignment between the person's biology and the sleep-wake schedule imposed by their job often leads to severely impaired sleep with associated consequences.

A person with suspected shift work disorder should have a consultation with a sleep specialist. In today's setting of increasing telemedicine visits, this should be relatively easy to accomplish. A local sleep provider can be identified at the website www.sleepeducation.org or by searching for a local sleep medicine specialist.

While many tools can be used to help make the diagnosis, a sleep diary is the key tool for documenting and analyzing the sleep-wake disturbances related to shift work (see discussion above).

Improving wakefulness during the night shift. This is essential. Sleepiness can impair cognition, coordination, and motor control required to drive and operate machinery effectively. Altered moods and emotions can occur. These health risks can occur even if the individual is trying to optimize sleep quality. The following treatments can be effective:

- **Naps.** Naps before the night shift, or late during the night shift if possible, can improve performance. The naps should be short (less than 60 minutes) to avoid entering into the deep stages of sleep.

- **Caffeine.** Small doses of caffeine (approximately 75 to 100 mg – the amount in a small cup of coffee) administered during the shift may help sustain alertness.

- **Wake-promoting agents.** Prescription medications modafinil and armodafinil are options for persons who are still sleepy at work despite the above measures. These medications should be prescribed by an experienced provider.

- **Light treatment.** This is beyond the scope of our discussion, but can be administered by a sleep physician.

Improving daytime sleep. This starts with good sleep hygiene (see above). For persons who still have difficulty sleeping, the following treatment options are available:

- **Hypnotic medications.** A short-acting hypnotic prescription medication may be helpful. These medications need to be prescribed and have potentially significant side effects. They should be prescribed by a provider with sufficient experience. The biggest potential practical problems with these medications is the carry-over sedation effect into the night shift.

- **Melatonin.** Taking melatonin (1 to 3 milligrams) improves total sleep time for shift workers. It should be taken 30 minutes prior to the desired onset of sleep. (Additional information is provided on melatonin later in this chapter.)

INSOMNIA

Insomnia is a common medical complaint. The diagnosis of insomnia requires three things:

- Difficulty sleeping (going to sleep and/or staying asleep)

- Difficulty sleeping despite an adequate opportunity to sleep (as opposed to people who do not get a sufficient amount of sleep but will fall asleep and stay asleep if given the opportunity)

- Impaired function during the day as a result.

Patients with insomnia often enter a vicious cycle. They worry that the lack of adequate sleep will negatively affect their ability to successfully function during the day. This worry about the negative effects of their lack of sleep makes it more difficult to go to sleep and stay asleep.

The compromise in daily function as a result of insomnia can include, but not be limited to, the following: fatigue or malaise, poor attention or concentration, daytime sleepiness, reduced performance at work, and negative behaviors (irritability, hyperactivity, or aggression). Insomnia is categorized as short-term or as chronic, based on the duration of symptoms (three months is the dividing point).

- **Short-term insomnia.** This is typically due to a significant life stressor (relationship difficulties, job stressors or loss, personal or family health problems, death of a friend or loved one). The symptoms typically resolve when the stressor is no longer present.

- **Chronic insomnia.** To meet the criteria for a chronic disorder, symptoms must occur at least three times a week for at least three months. Most patients with chronic insomnia have had symptoms for many years.

Successful evaluation and treatment of insomnia, especially if chronic, requires the expertise of an experienced provider. You can start by seeing your primary care doctor who can make an appropriate referral if necessary. Alternatively, you can seek out a board-certified sleep physician (www.sleepeducation.org). This website contains excellent overviews of common sleep problems, including insomnia.

RESOURCES

Mattresses. The top portion of a mattress may affect the quality of our sleep. Sleeping on a firmer, more supportive mattress topper may improve both sleep quality and performance. Mattress toppers are divided into high- and low-rebound types. High-rebound toppers have a supportive feel and high breathability. Low-rebound toppers are pressure-absorbing and include "memory foam" toppers. Research has shown that sleeping on a high-rebound mattress induces a continuous and more rapid decline in core body temperature during the initial phase of sleep and results in improved athletic performance measures in young, healthy volunteers.

Pillows. Your pillow can also have a significant effect on the quality of your sleep. Ideally, your pillow should maintain the proper alignment of your head, neck, shoulders and spine as you sleep. Improper alignment can cause neck stiffness, neck pain, shoulder pain, or headaches.

Many pillow-related factors come into play: support, comfort, fatigue, height, and the shape of the pillow. Pillow types can be divided into standard and functional pillows. A functional type pillow, in general, has a height difference between the side and center of the pillow. The goal of the functional pillow is to keep the head supported in the proper position. Cervical pillows are functional pillows specifically designed to address cervical spine (neck) symptoms.

A 2017 Korean study showed that "Participants who used a regular-type pillow had poorer satisfaction on multiple comfort and support factors (support, comfort, height suitability, shape suitability) compared with those who used a functional-type pillow. To reduce neck fatigue and shoulder pain, designers should consider the height for neck support in the lateral position. To reduce neck fatigue, it is desirable to use materials like latex or memory foam that provide neck support."

Essential oils. Multiple studies using sleep questionnaires (Pittsburgh Sleep Quality Index, State-Trait Anxiety Inventory, Beck Anxiety Inventory) have demonstrated improved sleep quality and reduced anxiety in patients using inhaled essential oils at bedtime. Lavender oil consistently showed benefit. Lavender essential oil can be placed on a cotton ball at the bedside.

The distraction of artificial light. Artificial light, at the wrong time, negatively affects our 24-hour circadian timing system and our sleep quality. Bright light at night can delay the reduction in our circadian alertness level, making it harder to go to sleep. Bright light too early in the morning can accelerate the increase in our circadian alertness level, causing us to wake up earlier than desired. The effect of bright light on our circadian system can also be used to help treat circadian rhythm disorders (such as jet-lag disorder).

The blue light emitted from electronic devices (such as mobile phones and computers) reduces the body's production of melatonin, which is essential for the onset of sleep. A recent study of college students in Saudi Arabia found that "using a mobile screen >8 hours/24 hours, using the mobile for at least 30 minutes before sleeping after the lights have been turned off, and keeping the mobile [device] near the pillow are positively associated with poor sleep quality."

Melatonin. Melatonin is a natural hormone produced by a small gland within the brain, the pineal gland, which becomes active as darkness occurs. The rising melatonin levels make you feel sleepier and less alert. Melatonin production usually occurs around 9 pm and the levels stay elevated for about twelve hours, falling back to the low daytime levels around 9 am. Being exposed to bright light at night and the blue light of electronic devices directly inhibits the production of melatonin.

In the United States, melatonin is available in tablet form, marketed as a dietary supplement. As a result, it is regulated less strictly by the Food and Drug Administration (FDA) than prescription drugs. Synthetic melatonin is made in factories not regulated by the FDA, and some melatonin supplements may not contain what is listed on the label. Most commercial melatonin products have dosages that cause melatonin levels in the blood to be much higher than natural levels in the body.

Melatonin has shown effectiveness for treating patients with *jet-lag disorder*, *shift-work disorder*, and *delayed sleep-wake phase disorder*. Melatonin is currently not recommended for treating patients with insomnia due to a lack of studies providing strong evidence for its benefit in these patients.

Short-term use of melatonin supplements appears to be safe in most patients. There is not enough information to confirm the safety of long-term use of melatonin. Good, quality medical studies are needed to establish the safety and efficacy of supplemental melatonin in a variety of sleep disorders.

Tryptophan and 5-HTP. The compound 5-Hydroxytryptophan (5-HTP) is made in our bodies from the amino acid L-tryptophan. We get this essential amino acid L-tryptophan from certain protein foods, such as turkey, for example. We can also obtain 5-HTP as a dietary supplement.

- 5-HTP is the intermediate step in the conversion of the amino acid L-tryptophan to the neurotransmitter serotonin in our bodies.

- Serotonin has wide-ranging effects in our body and is a chemical precursor to melatonin.

- While clear scientific studies on the effects of 5-HTP on sleep quality are lacking, experience suggests that 5-HTP may help shorten the time it takes to fall asleep and increase the amount of sleep time.

As a dietary supplement, 5-HTP is not regulated by the FDA. There is no specific dosage for addressing sleep symptoms. The long-term safety of taking 5-HTP is not clear. Doing so may aggravate some medical conditions such as anxiety, depression, or obesity.

RESEARCH ON SLEEPING PILLS — Side effects and cautions

Researchers report that a number of familiar medications can increase dementia risk.

First-generation antihistamines, such as Benadryl (diphenhydramine), are typically taken for allergy symptoms. Drowsiness is a common side effect. As a result, Benadryl has been used as a sleep aid for many years. Many medications, including Benadryl and other first-generation antihistamines, block the action of the chemical acetylcholine, which transmits messages in the nervous system throughout our body. In the brain, acetylcholine is involved in learning and memory and is necessary for cognitive function in general. Medications blocking the action of acetylcholine are termed anticholinergic.

These anticholinergic medications result in cognitive impairment.

While the cognitive impairment typically resolves when people stop taking the medication, several studies have identified a possible link between these medications and dementia. First-generation antihistamines, like Benadryl, were included in one of the original studies, published by the *Journal of the American Medical Association* in 2015. On the basis of evolving medical data, one should avoid the frequent or long-term use of sleep aids containing first-generation antihistamines.

Second- and third-generation antihistamines. Of note, there is no association between second- and third-generation antihistamines (such as Zyrtec, Allegra, Claritin, and Xyzal) with cognitive impairment and dementia.

Sedative medications—benzodiazepines. These sedatives have been prescribed for sleep problems for many years. This class of medication includes the drugs Xanax, Librium, Klonopin, Valium, Ativan, and others. These medications, while effective, have been linked to dementia.

These drugs can impair cognitive function and can be habit forming.

Z-drugs. Another class of medications used to treat sleep problems cause sedation due to effects on GABA receptors in the brain. These medications have been called Z-drugs because they all have the letter Z in their name. The drugs include zolpidem (Ambien), zaleplon (Sonata), and eszopiclone (Lunesta).

The Z-drugs have negative effects on cognition and behavior, as well as on performance, including driving and operating machinery.

Z-drugs can also cause complex sleep behaviors that can result in serious injuries or death. Fatal cases have included the following events: carbon monoxide poisoning, drowning, falls, hypothermia, and motor vehicle collisions, as reported in the journal *Pharmacoepidemiology and Drug Safety* in 2020. Put simply, these drugs are not safe and should be avoided.

Caution: Taking first-generation antihistamines, benzodiazepines, or Z-drugs for sleep problems is not good for your health. These drugs should be avoided if at all possible.

I would recommend that anyone who has sleep symptoms severe enough to require one of these medications see a board-certified sleep specialist for evaluation and future treatment.

For additional information on Dr. Murphy's services as a sleep specialist, please see stanfordhealthcare.org/doctors/m/michael-murphy.html.

Chapter 30
Coping With Jet Lag
Jay A. Olson, PhD, Researcher
Mariève Cyr, MSc, MD Candidate

I think a major element of jetlag is psychological.
No one ever tells me what time it is at home.
— David Attenborough

Jet lag is one of the main downsides of business trips and vacations abroad. Although various remedies, supplements, and gadgets claim to reduce jet lag, many of them do not work. Fortunately, the most reliable way to minimize jet lag is easily accessible and free: light exposure. In this chapter, we outline the practical methods to reduce jet lag, in order to make the most of your trip.

JET LAG DEFINED

Jet lag is caused by disruptions in circadian rhythms, which are approximately 24-hour cycles that influence body processes such as sleep, alertness, hormone production, and temperature. Circadian rhythms are present in bacteria, plants, and animals, as well as almost every cell in our bodies. These rhythms are controlled by internal body clocks that have evolved over millennia to help our bodies synchronize with the day and night cycle.

Normally these rhythms align with the environment, so we feel more alert during daylight hours and more tired during the night. However, when we travel across time zones in a short period of time, the light-dark cycle changes faster than our body clock. When traveling from the United States to Russia, for example, you cross 12 time zones. Upon arrival, your body clock is 12 hours off: it is now telling you to fall asleep during the day and remain alert in the middle of the night. This misalignment is called jet lag.

Jet lag is why we may make worse decisions during overseas business meetings or have trouble sleeping on vacation. It causes excessive daytime sleepiness, reduces cognitive performance, creates gastrointestinal issues, and influences mood.

HOW TO REDUCE JET LAG

The primary way that the body stays aligned with the environment is by monitoring light exposure. Opening the blinds earlier than usual on a sunny morning tells your body clock to shift earlier, so you will be more likely to wake up earlier the next morning. Getting light exposure at night tells your body clock to shift later, so you fall asleep later that night. (Spending time on your phone or computer right before you go to bed could keep you awake when you want to go to sleep.) When traveling, your body will naturally adjust by roughly one time zone per day, but there is a great deal of individual variation. Some people experience minimal jet lag symptoms, while others remain fatigued for weeks. By controlling light exposure, you can help your body clock shift to the new time zone as quickly as possible and minimize the effects of jet lag.

> *When crossing only a few time zones (such as within North America), follow this simple rule: get light exposure in the morning before flying east and light at night before flying west.*

Ideally, this light exposure comes from sunlight, for example, by opening the blinds or going on a short walk outside. Artificial light sources can also be effective, such as turning on as many lights as you can or using a portable lightbox. Lightboxes mimic natural sunlight and are sold in many pharmacies and online to treat seasonal affective disorder (the "winter blues"), misaligned circadian rhythms, and jet lag. When buying a lightbox, look for "10,000 lux" on the label to ensure that the light is bright enough to shift your body clock rapidly. Around 15 to 30 minutes of light should be sufficient; however, the brighter and longer the exposure, the quicker your body will adjust.

Flying up to three time zones east. Suppose you are crossing three time zones from Los Angeles to New York. Two days before your flight, start shifting your sleep schedule by half an hour per day. If you usually wake up at 8:00 am, wake up half an hour earlier (7:30 am) and get light exposure in the morning. That night, go to bed half an hour earlier than usual. The following day, shift your sleep schedule by an additional half hour: wake up at 7:00 am, get morning light exposure, and go to bed half an hour earlier. On the day of the flight, wake up another half-hour earlier (6:30 am) and get morning light exposure. By the time you arrive, you will have adjusted to the new time zone and will experience minimal or no jet lag. Alternatively, by simply by shifting your schedule and getting light exposure on the morning of your flight, you can partially reduce jet lag.

These small schedule adjustments before your trip can help prevent jet lag upon arrival. However, you can also align your body clock after arriving, which tends to be less effective but sometimes more convenient. The process is similar, but it does not require adjusting your sleep times: simply get light exposure for half an hour each morning until you are no longer jet-lagged.

Flying up to three time zones west. For short westward flights, such as from New York to Los Angeles, you will want to shift your body clock in the opposite direction. The night before your flight, get light exposure as late as you can and go to bed one hour later than usual. It is easier for most people to shift their body clock later, rather than earlier, meaning that you typically adjust faster to westward travel than eastward travel. One day of shifting before a short westward flight should thus suffice to prevent jet lag.

Crossing more time zones. When crossing four or more time zones, estimating when to get bright light exposure becomes more complicated. For this reason, researchers have created various apps to help with these calculations. We have created Jet Lag Rooster (JetLagRooster.com), a free website where you enter your flight and sleep details to receive a personalized jet lag reduction plan. Another research group has created an app called Entrain that uses similar principles (entrain.math.lsa.umich.edu). Depending on your trip, the apps may also suggest times to avoid light, in which case using dark sunglasses and a sleep mask may be helpful.

If you are crossing many time zones on a very short trip—such as a three-day business trip from Los Angeles to London—only considerable preparation can prevent jet lag. In these cases, focus on other techniques such as caffeine consumption to boost your alertness when needed.

Melatonin. Melatonin is a hormone produced by the body and is primarily secreted during the night. Taking melatonin supplements can promote sleep, but it can also help shift your body clock. Melatonin is most effective at reducing jet lag when traveling east and when combined with the light exposure strategies described above. Melatonin is typically taken between 10:00pm and midnight at the destination. Small doses (0.5 mg) seem to reduce jet lag as effectively as larger ones (3 to 5 mg) but have fewer side effects. Although melatonin is generally safe, it may interact with conditions such as epilepsy. Consult your doctor or pharmacist before taking any new medication or supplement.

TRAVEL FATIGUE

Travel fatigue is the accumulated fatigue caused by the logistics of flying: waiting around at the airport, sitting for a long time, and being woken up by announcements on the plane. Reducing travel fatigue is relatively easy; avoid alcohol and drink a lot of water either during the flight or after landing. Once you arrive, take a shower or a short nap (ideally under 25 minutes). Even if your body clock remains misaligned, these simple steps will improve your alertness.

Caffeine. Caffeine can similarly improve alertness and reduce fatigue, and it is the only stimulant recommended for general use. Caffeine is best consumed 20 to 45 minutes before its desired alerting effect. To reduce its adverse impacts on sleep, avoid caffeine for at least three hours before bed or more if you are sensitive to caffeine.

Medication. Some of the most common drugs used to promote sleep include Valium (diazepam), Ativan (lorazepam), and Ambien (zolpidem). These medications may offer symptom relief, but they do not help your body clock adjust to the new time zone. Further, many of these drugs have addictive properties and serious side effects. We recommend favoring strategies such as light exposure, the gradual shifting of your sleep schedule, or taking melatonin before resorting to these medications. (For additional information on the side effects of sleep medication, please see chapter 29 on sleep.)

Conclusion. Jet lag results from a misalignment between your body clock and the environment. Timed light exposure is the most reliable and well-researched method to reduce it. Although preventing jet lag requires some preparation, it can keep you at peak performance during business trips and help you make the most of your vacations.

KEY TAKE AWAYS

- To minimize jet lag, make it a point to get additional light exposure in the morning before traveling east, and light at night before traveling west.

- When crossing more than three time zones, use an app (such as JetLagRooster.com) to generate a personalized plan that will suggest the ideal times for light exposure and sleep.

- Strategies for reducing travel fatigue include staying hydrated, minimizing alcohol, and taking a shower or a short nap upon arrival.

Melatonin supplements can help reduce jet lag, and caffeine can improve alertness.

**Information on preventing jet lag can be found at
www.JetLagRooster.com.
For more on the work of Jay Olson, please see:
www.JayOlson.com**

PART 4
FOOD
Introduction
Judson Brandeis, MD

The Power of Food is really Spiritual. It not only brings the whole family together at the same table, it brings the whole world together.
— Vikas Khanna

Food provides the building blocks of life. Proteins make up our muscles and organs. Calcium creates the structure of our bones. Fats and carbohydrates are our fuel. Vitamins facilitate chemical reactions. In this section, we will discuss the foundation of good nutrition and a healthy diet. However, food is so much more than nutrition. Food is connection, memory, adventure, cultural identity, joy, and love.

Animals eat food to survive. We have all seen nature videos in which a pack of lions attacks an animal carcass with a ring of hyenas and vultures salivating and waiting their turn. Contrast this with a dinner of family and friends laughing, relaxing, and enjoying.

For humans, food begins with preparation. A family comes together to shop for the ingredients for grandma's special recipes, inspecting every single celery stalk and each chicken breast in the process. Or a pack of men returns to their women and children with venison, bursting with pride at the accomplishment.

The process of cooking brings a group together through an intricate dance in the kitchen. The smells of the food bring anticipation of the meal. For many families, cooking together is a way to work together and create a family connection essential for bonding and emotional health. Thanksgiving was a way for the Pilgrims to thank their new friends, the Wampanoag Indians, for helping them survive.

Food creates memories. The sight, smell, sound, and taste of food bring us back to some of the most meaningful times in our lives. It also connects us to our ancestors or our culture. Americans from similar cultures have a way to connect over food, and people from different countries have a meaningful way to experience each other's culture through the cuisine. I have never been to Japan, but I sure do love sushi! Eating good food is something that everyone can agree on and enjoy together. Families can resolve problems over meals, and business deals get made over a power lunch. For humans, food goes far beyond protein, fat, and carbohydrates. Food is connection, joy, and love.

Chapter 31
What Is Food?
Judson Brandeis, MD, Urologist
Nancy Faass, MSW, MPH, Health Coach
& Jerry Stine, Nutritionist

Food. 1a: material consisting essentially of protein, carbohydrate, and fat used in the body of an organism to sustain growth, repair, and vital processes and to furnish energy.
— Encyclopedia Britannica

We're all still figuring out what to eat. . . Every year it seems like there's a new fad diet, and the experts are saying that what they told you last year is no longer true. We've all seen rave reviews of low-fat diets, low-carb diets, and everything in between. How can all these diets be correct? In this chapter, we're not going to recommend any one approach to food. Instead, we will provide you with the basic facts so you can assess nutritional information for yourself.

Ever since scientists cracked the code on the human genome in 2003, we have had the proof that we are all genetically unique.

When it comes to food, over the past 60,000 years humans have adapted to the entire span of climates and local foods in every region, which has given us an amazing array of inherited traits. Perhaps you are descended from people of the north, adapted to eat a high-fat diet, or maybe your parents are both from the tropics, so everyone in your family eats vegetables and fish.

But what if your dad was from the north and your mom was from the tropics? In that case, the best food for you is anybody's guess.

To make things even more complicated, a number of different genes affect food metabolism, and we don't know yet exactly which genes matter most or how they interact.

No easy answers. There is no fast and easy way to "read" your genes and determine your optimal diet. In ten years, there may be an app on your phone for that, but today we are still limited to trial and error.

FAST CARBS, SLOW CARBS

This section of the book is intended to help you understand the drawbacks and benefits of different types of food. Our food consists of carbohydrates, proteins, fats, and fiber, but the requirement for each of these ingredients is individual.

What are carbohydrates? The sun is the source of all energy on earth. Every second the sun produces the same *energy* as about a trillion one-megaton bombs and about one billionth of the energy produced by the sun is absorbed by the earth. Each photon emitted by the sun contains a tiny amount of energy.

Plants evolved to trap that light energy with chlorophyl in their leaves and convert it into natural sugars like glucose, fructose, and sucrose, using carbon dioxide from the air and water. These natural sugars are used by plants to grow and flower. Plants store the energy by combining these glucose molecules into long chains called starches. Animals store energy as glycogen, which consists of more highly branched chains of glucose.

Collectively, sugars, starch, and glycogen are known as carbohydrates, and they are an important source of cellular energy. When animals eat plants or each other, they capture this energy.

Slow carbs are rich in fiber. In the Paleolithic, 40,000 years ago, people lived on nuts, seeds, roots, greens, and other edibles. Think fiber. A lot of fiber. These are the original comfort foods—slow foods (a hearty stew simmered over a fire or roasted sweet potatoes). Lots of munchy food, lots of chewing, and long, slow, relaxed digestion.

Ancient grains are slow carbs too and also rich in fiber. Ancient grains first appeared as wild grasses 10,000 years ago. These are all comfort foods—whole grains that fill you up and "stick to your ribs." (Think wild rice with grilled steak.) That means lots of chewing, lots of fiber, and slow digestion, with the gradual release of natural sugars.

Slow carbs take an hour or two to digest. As the digestive tract does its magic, high-fiber vegetables and complex carbs, like whole grains, are gradually broken down in the stomach and passed along to the small intestine for further digestion. As the fiber breaks down, the nutrients in the food are released, little by little, and absorbed into the blood steam.

TIP #1—Managing carbs is one of the keys to managing weight.

What's the story on fast carbs? Let's consider my occasional indulgence in chocolate chip cookies. If I eat a plate of cookies, the sugar (sucrose) that they contain will zip through my stomach and be rapidly absorbed into my blood steam from the gut.

The sucrose in the cookies will quickly be converted to glucose, flooding my bloodstream and spiking my blood sugar.

As soon as my blood sugar starts to rise, my body will respond by secreting insulin, a normal, healthy response. The job of insulin is to move blood sugar into the cells where it can be burned to make energy.

But the sugar and white flour in the cookies will cause a rapid spike in blood sugar, which forces a huge release of insulin to keep my blood sugar at a safe level.

If I binge on sugary foods very often, the repeated strain on the system that controls my blood sugar will start to wear it out.

The cookies, while fun to eat, are a severe stress on my liver, my pancreas, and my body's chemistry. If I develop insulin resistance, I will be plagued by:

- An uneven supply of energy
- Increased inflammation
- Greater tendency to gain weight
- Difficulty losing weight.

In contrast, slow carbs, which are digested and released slowly, cause very little stress on the system. Cells are able to maintain even levels of energy, and there is less likelihood of weight gain.

How sugar packs on the pounds . . .

If these mechanisms are routinely stressed, my body will not be able to manage blood sugar and insulin levels. One result of this is that sugar is converted to fat and stored.

And where does it go? On my gut, my hips, thighs, love handles, and other places where I don't want to gain weight.

Why is it so hard to lose weight? Fat storage began as a survival thing. For hunters in the Paleo, obtaining food was a challenge, and we know that they periodically went for days or weeks between meals, totally without food. The ability to store calories as fat was essential to their survival. They could not call up GrubHub and have a 2,000-calorie burrito delivered in 15 minutes or put the leftovers from dinner into the fridge for the next day.

An extreme (and astonishing) example of this in nature is humpback whales who feed for 23 hours a day for 5 months while they are in Alaska, then swim to Hawaii, have a baby, feed the baby, and then the mother and baby swim back to Alaska, all without eating for seven months. These whales rely on stored fats for seven months while making this perilous 6,000-mile journey. That lifestyle pattern is hardwired into many different species from penguins to people. Looking deep into our history, the ability to store fat was key to our survival . . . until now.

Now we are drowning in a tsunami of sugar.

If I eat a lot of sugar, over time that puts a strain on my body's ability to produce insulin and on my cells' ability to absorb all that excess glucose. (This is insulin resistance— prediabetes.)

And if I indulge in sweet junk food every night, I'll habitually have high blood sugar and high insulin, but my body won't be able to burn the sugar because of the damage to my system.

When I start gaining weight, that will cause wear and tear on my heart, my blood vessels, and my gut, among other things.

THE CARB INDEX: A MEASURE OF FAST AND SLOW CARBS

The Carb Index is a tool you can use to tell the fast carbs from the slow carbs. The Index is a measurement of how quickly any given food is metabolized, and whether it triggers the release of a great deal of insulin or not. Foods rated 55 or below are slow carbs that don't trigger much insulin. (Note: many versions of the Index included on the web are inaccurate.)

To support steady blood sugar or to lose weight, minimize food choices above 55 on the Index. (There are some surprises here. I thought rice cakes were healthy and maybe sweet potatoes weren't.)

First, go through the list included here and check the entries 55 and below that *you like*. Base your menus and your grocery list on these lower Index foods. If your goal is to lose weight, that will take the weight off gradually, and keep it off, without reducing your food intake, so no dieting needed and no skipping meals.

> **The end of dieting:** *For those of you who enjoy food, and don't like dieting, give this system a try. You need never go hungry again.*

WHAT ABOUT PROTEIN?

Proteins are essential to life. Protein foods provide the building blocks for muscles, antibodies, hormones, digestive enzymes, blood, and connective tissue. In order to repair our bodies and maintain our health, cells and tissue are being replaced in an ongoing process, which requires a continuous supply of protein.

THE CARB INDEX
(*The Glycemic Index*)

Foods That Trigger Insulin

Grains, Breads, Cereals, Vegetables		*Sweeteners, Fruits, Dairy*	
White bread, baked potatoes	95	Maltose	105-150
Instant rice	90	Glucose	100
Cooked carrots	85	Raisins	95
French fries, pretzels, rice cakes	80	Honey	75
Corns flakes, corn on the cob, frozen or canned corn	75	Watermelon, dried apricots	70
Plain bagels, crackers, graham crackers, puffed wheat, sweetened cereals	75	Pineapple	65
White rice, taco shells, beets	70	Ice cream, ripe bananas	60
Spaghetti	60		
Foods That Trigger Less Insulin			
Brown rice, wild rice, oatmeal, sweet potatoes	55	Mango, kiwi	50
Yams	50	Peaches, plums	40
Green beans, green peas	45	Apples, oranges	40
Pinto and lima beans	40	Yogurt with fruit	35+
Kidney beans, black beans, butter beans; nuts (30 or below)	30	Milk, whole and skimmed	30+
Asparagus	20	Cherries, grapefruit	25
Green leafy vegetables, tomatoes	20	Yogurt plain, unsweetened	15

Figure 31.1 The Glycemic Index, a measure of how fast specific foods raise blood sugar. (Source: (c) 2021 Nancy Faass, MSW, MPH)

TIP #2. PROTEIN—Protein results in only half the weight gain caused by carbs. Although protein can be converted into energy, its primary job is to provide the raw materials for the structure of the body.

Unlike glycogen and body fat, which are stored as sources of energy in case food is not available, protein isn't stored for future needs. The positive aspect of this is that lean protein foods are not a major source of weight gain.

You can obtain protein from two sources:

- **Animal-derived proteins** include fish, poultry, red meats, dairy products (cheese, milk, yogurt), and eggs.

- **Plant-based proteins** include beans, soybeans, peas, chickpeas, peanuts, lentils, and mushrooms, as well as nuts and seeds.

What kind of protein? Proteins are composed of twenty different essential amino acids, half of which our bodies can make. But nine of these our bodies cannot make, and we must obtain them from our food. Today, we also have the option of taking high-quality amino acid supplements in capsule or powder form, as well as protein foods.

(Amino acids combine to make peptides, which are short chains of two to fifty amino acids. Peptides combine to make proteins.)

How much protein? In terms of *how much* protein we need, there is little consensus. People who advocate for a Paleo or ketogenic diet point to the diet of wild game eaten by our ancestors. On the other hand, advocates of plant-based diets point to compelling research indicating the benefits of lower protein intake. (See chapter 34 for insight on plant-based nutrition, written by a board-certified cardiologist.)

General recommendations suggest approximately 3 to 7 ounces (about ¼ to ½ a cup) of protein for a man who weighs 160 pounds. (Doing the math, that's 0.8 to 1.7 grams of protein per kilogram of body weight.)

Who needs more? Athletes, body builders, individuals with a highly active lifestyle, and pregnant women tend to have higher protein requirements. Some vegetarians may find that supplementing with free amino acids is beneficial. In an interesting study of weight training in older adults (average age, 75), those who supplemented with additional protein gained about 20% additional muscle mass. Factor into the equation:

- Your response to different amounts of protein

- Your response to different types of protein (plant-based, animal-protein, red meat, poultry, seafood, eggs, deep fried tofu, mushrooms, nuts), amino acid supplements

■   If you want to take off a few pounds, remind yourself that *high* protein consumption can contribute to weight gain.

Not enough protein? In the industrialized world, protein deficiency occurs most often among people with chronic illness, older adults, and the poor. Dieters may be tempted to drop their protein intake to a very low level in order to cut out fat. Primary symptoms of protein deficiency include:

■   Thinning of skin, hair, and nails

■   Loss of muscle mass

■   Bigger appetite and increased calorie intake

■   Risk of infections

■   Increased risk of bone fractures

■   Fatty liver.

Too much protein?

■   Short-term symptoms can include indigestion, constipation, diarrhea, dehydration, fatigue, irritability, or headaches.

■   Bone loss can result from a high protein diet, causing osteopenia or osteoporosis.

■   Increased risk of heart disease and cancers from both red meat and prepared meats such as hot dogs are reported in studies involving thousands of individuals.

Optimizing digestion. Protein is broken down by digestive acid in the stomach and then protein-digesting enzymes (protease) made in the pancreas. Absorption occurs in the small intestine. If you frequently have an uncomfortable sense of heaviness or bloating after meals, you may be low on stomach acid or enzymes. Stomach acid (hydrochloric acid — HCl) and/or enzymes can be supplemented with over-the-counter dietary supplements.

Getting complete protein from plants. In North America, about 70% of protein foods are derived from animals. However, globally, about 60% of the protein that people eat comes from plants. Meat contains all 20 amino acids (complete protein), whereas plants are primarily carbohydrate and contain only some of the aminos. To provide complete protein, grains and beans are used in combination. In Central American cultures, for example, cuisine that includes corn, beans, and rice provides a complete array of amino acids.

Amino acid supplements. Today, the quality of both protein supplements and free amino acids have improved so significantly, supplements are worth considering if you:

- Are a vegetarian

- Burn protein at a high rate

- Suspect that you are not fully digesting or absorbing the protein you eat

- Suffer from swings in your mood or mental energy.

Amino acids can now be purchased in powder and capsule form and various blends are available that have been formulated as a buffer against different types of stress.

GOOD FATS, BAD FATS

TIP #3 FATS—Healthy fats support good energy and provide raw materials for hormones and brain function.

Why we need fat. Fats are the most efficient form of energy and are essential to health and life. Fats are the raw materials utilized to make our hormones, comprise more than half of the brain, form the coating on our nerves, and support the health of our skin. However, consuming the wrong fats and oils can be damaging.

Imbalances in fatty acids can be a factor in many health issues, particularly conditions involving myelin destruction (demyelination) such as multiple sclerosis, Parkinson's, and some types of neuropathy.

An efficient source of energy. Essential fatty acids are utilized for energy. Fats and oils are a major source of calories that our bodies burn for energy.

Raw materials for hormones. Although fat has gotten a bad rap in recent years, you actually need it. Your hormones, for example, are made from cholesterol, which is manufactured by the liver from fatty acids.

Vital to brain health. The human brain is 60% fat, confirmed in recent research posted on the website of the National Institutes of Health. If someone calls you a "fat head," this is literally true. (Smile and take it as a compliment.) The point is, you need quality fats to replenish the chemistry of your brain in order to think clearly and to function.

Protection for your nerves. The nervous system can be compared to the electrical wiring in our homes. Like standard electrical wiring, every nerve in our bodies is wrapped in protective coating—myelin—which is made from essential fats. It is vital to replenish that coating with quality fat intake. When myelin is inflamed or destroyed, that results in devastating conditions such as multiple sclerosis, Parkinson's disease, inflammatory neuropathy, or Guillain-Barre syndrome.

Cell function. The human body is composed of 15 trillion cells. Every one of those cells is enveloped in a cell wall, a selective system that controls the full function of the cell. The cell walls (also referred to as cell membranes) require healthy fats in order to function. Without fats, these membranes become brittle and less able to absorb nutrients.

HEALTHY OILS

Extra virgin olive oil. Olive oil, prized by the Greeks and the Romans, has been a staple of human nutrition for thousands of years. Recent research has also found that it is very heart healthy. Nutritious and flavorful, it has better shelf life than most other vegetable oils. The low smoke point makes it appropriate for salads and light sautéing, but less suitable for high heat or deep frying. Olive oils have a strong, distinctive taste, depending on the specific type of olive and the region where it is grown. For those that want a milder flavor, more refined olive oil is available, but has less nutritional value.

Coconut oil has become popular in recent years and can offer a new flavor dimension to sauteed dishes. This oil has a good shelf life and a higher smoke point than olive oil, so it is good for stir-frying vegetables, making omelets, and other stove-top cooking. Coconut oil contains fat in a form that is very efficiently utilized by the body — medium-chain triglycerides. This efficient use can speed up metabolism in a healthy manner, so it has been considered a weight-loss product for a decade. Virgin coconut oil also has a marvelous fragrance and flavor. Recent research has raised the question of whether it is as healthful as olive oil, so the last word is not in on this product. Stay tuned.

Extract of coconut oil (MCT oil). This oil is an extract of the medium-chain triglycerides found in coconut oil. MCT oil is liquid at room temperature, clear, and has no flavor, so it mixes well with both salad dressings and with olive oil and is frequently included in a ketogenic diet (for example, MCT oil can be used in coffee for morning energy, sometimes referred to as bullet-proof coffee, also inspiring a brand by that name).

Clarified butter/ghee. Ghee is a staple of Indian and Ayurvedic cuisine, made from clarified butter. The milk protein (casein) and other solids have been removed, so ghee tends to cause fewer reactions for those who are sensitive to the protein in dairy products. Since clarified butter is more stable at higher temperatures than most oils, it is excellent for cooking over direct heat.

BAD FATS

We know from fifty years of research that some fats *are* bad for you. At this point, there's no question. In other cases, there are big problems that get very little attention. Here's the short list of concerns:

- **Increased cardio risk**, due to higher levels of LDL (the harmful form of cholesterol) and lower levels of HDL cholesterol (the good kind)

- **Increased cancer risk**

- **Disrupted cell function,** replacing healthy fats with harmful fats.

Trans fats are found in French fries, doughnuts, and all other commercially deep-fried foods. Deep frying degrades the quality of fats and oils due to overheating for an extended period of time. In addition, often the fats used by restaurants for deep frying have been hydrogenated.

Hydrogenated fats are found in crackers, chips (yeah, bummer), cookies, cakes, pastries, microwave popcorn, and most snack foods. Hydrogenated fats are manufactured from vegetable oils using an industrial process to make them more shelf-stable and less subject to rancidity. Margarine and Crisco are hydrogenated. Originally intended as inexpensive, healthier replacements for butter and lard, their solidified form is a tip-off that they have been altered.

Saturated fats are found in fatty meats like marbled steaks, poultry skin, high-fat dairy products, and lard. However, although saturated fats from plant sources were associated with cardiovascular risk in the past, recent research is changing our perspective on tropical oils such as coconut oil and palm oil.

Rancid fats. A major problem with vegetable oils is rancidity and oxidation. If these oils are exposed to air and light they can change chemically in a very undesirable way. When these vegetable oils are degraded, they lose their nutritional value and can become harmful to consume. So freshness is one of the keys to healthy fats.

Unstable vegetable oils. Many of the most popular vegetable oils are surprisingly unstable and spoil easily. The bad news is that until they are *really bad*, you can't tell that they've gone rancid. This is one of the reasons that more stable oils, such as olive oil and coconut oil, are replacing former staples of American cooking such as canola, safflower, corn, soy, and sunflower seed oil, which are all less stable than olive oil.

Low smoke point. This is the temperature at which an oil or fat begins to oxidize and burn. You want to cook with oils that are stable in heat. Save more delicate oils for salads and recipes where they won't be directly subjected to high heat.

Dr. Leo Galland, MD, a physician who practices nutritional medicine, recommends discarding any and all oils older than six weeks to minimize risk of rancidity.

FIBER

The award for the most underrated food group goes to fiber, also known as roughage. In reality, fiber is not really food because it is the part of plants (in grains, fruits, vegetables, nuts, and beans) that the body can't break down. Instead, it passes through the body undigested, keeping your digestive system clean and healthy, easing bowel movements, and flushing cholesterol and harmful carcinogens out of the body. If you don't think that is important, ask the thousands of otherwise healthy men who end up with colostomies every year.

A low-fiber diet causes constipation that turns into diverticulosis that can evolve into severe diverticulitis (an infection of the diverticulum similar to appendicitis, but worse), which requires surgical removal of the sigmoid colon and a temporary colostomy. These unfortunate outcomes are more common than you think. A third of men under 60 have diverticulosis, and about two-thirds of men older than age 60 have diverticulosis. In addition, a quarter of a million Americans are hospitalized for diverticulitis each year. These hospitalizations are easily preventable with a diet rich in fiber.

TIP #4. FIBER—Fiber-rich foods support healthy gut function and fill us up without causing weight gain.

My internist recommends eating a bowl of salad as big as my head every day. Fiber keeps food moving and supports the friendly flora (the microbiome) within the gut. The fiber is essential for digestion and regularity, blood sugar control, weight management, and optimal cholesterol levels. In addition, fiber confers protective effects against esophageal reflux disease, duodenal ulcer, diverticulitis, hemorrhoids, and gastrointestinal diseases such as colon cancer. These benefits help to explain why fiber-rich food is a factor in reduced rates of obesity, hypertension, diabetes, cardiovascular disease, and stroke.

Some fiber is soluble, able to dissolve in water, and some is insoluble. Soluble fiber can help lower blood cholesterol and glucose levels, and is found in oats, peas, beans, apples, citrus fruits, carrots, barley, and psyllium. Insoluble fiber promotes the movement of material through your digestive system and increases stool bulk, so it can benefit those who struggle with constipation or irregular stools. Whole-wheat flour, wheat bran, nuts, beans and vegetables such as cauliflower and green beans are good sources of insoluble fiber.

Recommended allowance. The Institute of Medicine has set a recommended daily amount (RDA) for fiber intake. Men ages 50 and younger should consume a minimum of 3 tablespoons (38 grams) of fiber per day, and men 51 and older should consume 2 tablespoons (30 grams).

Ultimately, as long as you tolerate fiber well, you want it to be part of the food you eat, rather than an afterthought. That means beginning the shift to slow food, which is fiber-rich.

When fiber is to be avoided. If you have any gastrointestinal disorder, you will want to avoid fiber until you can consult with your physician. Conditions in which fiber is contraindicated include active diverticulitis, inflammatory bowel disorders such as Crohn's disease and ulcerative colitis, or narrowing or obstruction of the bowel.

Fiber and gluten sensitivity. The initial attention on fiber was chiefly focused on fibers from grains such as wheat, barley, rye, and rice. These grains are a problem for people with gluten sensitivity—people who have a genetic sensitivity to a specific protein in grains, gluten. The degree of gluten sensitivity ranges from mild reactions to total inability to digest grain in any form. For people with true gluetn sensitivity, grains, and the fiber they provide, are not practical. Fortunately, vegetables can provide all the fiber we require if a wide variety of vegetables are consumed.

Fiber and the microbiome. Fiber is critical to maintaining the healthy range of bacteria that make up the huge population of intestinal bacteria in the gut. The microbiome aids in digestion, protects against food allergies, and supports the immune system. The most effective way to support the biome is to eat the widest variety of natural foods that are available, especially vegetables. The bacteria in the gut consume and ferment fiber to produce special metabolites and substances that keep our gut healthy.

KEY TAKE AWAYS

Tip #1. Carbs — Managing carbs is one of the keys to managing weight.

Tip #2. Protein — Protein results in only half the weight gain caused by carbs.

Tip #3. Fats — Healthy fats provide raw material for hormones, brain function, and energy.

Tip #4. Fiber — Fiber-rich foods support healthy gut function, filling us up without causing weight gain.

Resources

Mark Hyman, MD. *Eat Fat, Get Thin: Why the Fat We Eat Is the Key to Sustained Weight Loss and Vibrant Health.* New York, NY: Little, Brown Spark, 2016.

Mark Hyman, MD. *The Blood Sugar Solution: The Ultrahealthy Program for Losing Weight, Preventing Disease, and Feeling Great.* New York, NY: Little, Brown Spark, 2014.

Michael Pollen. *The Omnivore's Dilemma: A Natural History of Four Meals.* New York, NY: Penguin, 2017.

For more information on health coaching with Nancy Faass:
www.TheNeverDietDiet.com.
For more on nutritional consulting with Jerry Stine, see:
www.LifespanInstitute.com,
and the website of the American Academy Nutrition and Dietetics
www.eatright.org.

Chapter 32
Kicking Sugar
Angela Stanford, MBA, RDN, NBC-HWC
Registered Dietician Nutritionist

Sugar is the sociopath of foods. It acts sweet, but it's really poison.
— Karen Salmansohn

Chances are you already know that eating too much sugar isn't good for you, yet you are still overdoing it. On average, American adults consume about 17 teaspoons (270 calories) a day compared to The American Heart Association's recommendation that men consume no more than 9 teaspoons (1/4 cup—36 grams of sugars or 150 calories) of added sugar per day.

> *Two hundred years ago, the average American ate only 2 pounds of sugar a year. By 1970, consumption had increased to 123 pounds per year. Today, the average American consumes a whopping 152 pounds of sugar per year. This equals three pounds (6 cups) of sugar a week!*

Sugar in its natural form, found in vegetables and whole grains (complex carbohydrates), is not the enemy here.

Most people don't overeat fruits or vegetables. They do, however, overeat and drink added sugars in everything from coffee to sodas, breakfast cereal to desserts, and a broad range of packaged, processed foods from vegetables to entrees. Added sugars provide you with calories that have little or no nutritional value (known as empty calories). This is deceptive—after having a sugary snack, you probably feel satisfied, but in reality, your body is starved for nutrients.

The Standard American Diet (SAD) also contains too many refined carbohydrates from "fast carbs"—foods like pasta, white bread, white rice, and potatoes that are easily broken down into sugars. These foods are digested and metabolized rapidly, dumping the excess glucose into your bloodstream. The result is an immediate energy high (and a crash about 30 minutes later). Unfortunately, the extra blood sugar (glucose) is stored as fat.

It is not always easy to detect foods containing added sugars. Obvious items include candy, cookies, desserts, and soft drinks, all loaded with refined sugar. Other seemingly innocent foods like crackers, yogurt, milk, and fruit juice are also culprits. Even savory items like spaghetti sauce, peanut butter, salad dressings, and ketchup can also contain surprising amounts of added sugar.

Sugar is disguised on food labels in many forms including:

- Agave
- Brown rice syrup
- Brown sugar
- Coconut sugar
- Corn sweetener
- Dextrose
- Fructose
- Fruit juice concentrate
- Glucose
- High fructose corn syrup
- Honey
- Invert sugar
- Lactose
- Maltose
- Maple syrup
- Molasses
- Sorbitol
- Sorghum syrup
- Sucrose

When we consume all this additional sugar, it gets stored as fat.

This deception by food manufacturers has prompted the requirement that, by mid 2021, they will be required to list the amount of added sugars in addition to naturally occurring sugars on the Nutrition Facts Label. A recent analysis found that this labeling could potentially prevent nearly one million cases of cardiovascular disease and type 2 diabetes over the next two decades.

Interestingly enough, our bodies main fuel source is glucose—sugar in its simplest form. Glucose is made by breaking down the foods we consume as proteins, carbohydrates, and fats. But most of us are genetically wired by Mother Nature to run on a whole-food / plant-based diet and can get all this premium fuel without ever consuming added sugars.

The primary difference between fast food and slow food is that foods high in fiber are broken down slowly in the digestive track, so the nutrients and glucose are released gradually:

- **Protein** can take four hours to digest.

- **Whole grains** like brown rice or wild rice take about two hours to be digested.

- **Salads and raw veggies** are also "slow food" because of the high fiber content.

(Sound boring? Think Greek salad, for example, with sweet red peppers, olives, cucumber, and tomatoes, topped with lemon juice and olive oil or a tasty dressing.)

SIDE EFFECTS OF SUGAR

The more sugar you eat, the higher your blood-glucose level will be, which triggers the release of the hormone insulin making your body store fat. Eating a high quantity of sugar in one sitting causes your body to remain in the fat accumulation mode for longer periods.

Sugar can drive down your hormones. Increased sugar consumption leads to insulin resistance, which lowers testosterone levels. Low testosterone can lead to erectile dysfunction and decreased sex drive.

Effects of low testosterone. There is also an impact on your general health and well-being, since testosterone supports heart health, lean muscle and corresponding strength, stronger bones, better memory and focus, stronger libido, and positive moods. As testosterone drops, you lose all these health benefits.

Leptin resistance. Leptin is a hormone that helps regulate appetite. It tells your brain when you are full and when to stop eating. If you eat too much sugar, leptin stops working. Your fat cells continue to produce leptin, but your brain's ability to "hear" its message shuts off. This condition of "leptin resistance" also leads to a reduction of testosterone production, with the compounded lowering of sex drive.

Lower growth hormone. Overconsumption of sugar also reduces production of human growth hormone (HGH). Secreted by the pituitary gland, HGH has widely-recognized anti-aging properties. In the presence of increased insulin from excess sugar, HGH drops, which can lead to sexual dysfunction.

Fatigue. Sugar may give you a temporary spike of energy, but too much sugar leads to frequent bouts of fatigue, and you can't perform at work (or in bed) when you are too tired.

Weight gain and difficulty losing weight. High sugar consumption contributes to excess calories and inflammation in the body. These excess calories are stored as fat. Sugar can interfere with hormone messaging, causing us to hold onto unwanted weight.

Inflammation can affect everything from your joints to your heart. Sugar is highly inflammatory, so a diet high in sugar can trigger arthritis symptoms, raise blood pressure, and increase the risk of cardiovascular disease.

Higher levels of stress and anxiety. Elevated blood sugar and insulin lead to chronically higher levels of cortisol, one of the so-called stress hormones that triggers the fight or flight response. Elevated cortisol leads to increased stress and anxiety, both of which can cause decreased libido.

Kidney stones. Sugar, particularly in the form of fructose in sodas, increases risk of kidney stones by more than 23% in people who drink more than one regular soda a day. (That means about one of every four people who are fond of sodas is at higher risk.)

Tooth decay. Excess sugar feeds the bacteria in your plaque to create acids that wear down your tooth enamel, forming cavities over time.

Liver disease. Alcohol isn't the only food that can wreck your liver. Eating too much sugar increases risk for non-alcohol fatty liver disease (NAFLD) or the buildup of extra fat in your liver cells. Effects of NAFLD increase as we get older. In fact, 25% of men over 40 have it, and according to Baylor College of Medicine, 80% of people with NAFLD aren't diagnosed. This is serious because it can lead to cirrhosis, a scarring of the liver that could lead to cancer over time (according to the American Liver Foundation).

Brain fog and attention deficit. Sugar alters the balance between excitatory and inhibitory neurotransmitters resulting in reduced attention, alteration in memory, mood changes, and drowsiness.

Prostate cancer. Inflammation of prostate tissues due to high blood sugar levels in men who are obese has been found to increase the risk of an enlarged prostate and potential cancer. Sugar also encourages the wrong mix of digestive flora (encouraging "bad bugs" in the gastrointestinal tract). Since the prostate is located right next-door to the colon, it is theorized that this encourages low-grade infection in the gut. While this is still a theory to some extent, there is currently consensus in the medical literature that a high-sugar diet is associated with increased cancer incidence.

Joint pain and inflammation. Excess sugar leads to systemic inflammation in the body, which often shows up as pain in the joints. This can create a domino effect, deterring exercise and contributing to weight gain.

Sugar addiction. Sugar stimulates the same areas of the brain as drugs of abuse and alcohol. For this reason, sugar can cause people to lose control over their consumption levels. *Scientific American* reports: "Rats given a choice between highly sweetened water and intravenous *cocaine* overwhelmingly favored the tasty beverage."

> *If you have a history of binge eating, failure at setting rules about your eating (like cheat meals), and repeated failures with "eating everything in moderation," perhaps you are addicted and should avoid sugar completely—just as a smoker serious about quitting must avoid cigarettes or someone with an alcohol addiction must totally avoid alcohol.*

THE BACK STORY ON ARTIFICIAL SWEETENERS

When trying to decrease sugar, some turn to artificial sweeteners like saccharin, acesulfame, aspartame, neotame, or sucralose. These zero-calorie sweeteners are found in packets for your coffee/tea and commonly used to sweeten diet sodas and sport drinks. Although they reduce the calories in diet foods, research over the past seven decades has found that artificial sweeteners are linked to negative health outcomes.

Artificial sweeteners also pack a more potent sweet taste than table sugar. Regular consumption leads to a constant pining for more intense sweets, so naturally sweet food like fruit and unsweetened foods like vegetables are no longer palatable.

Artificial sweeteners may play another trick, too. Research suggests that they can prevent us from associating sweetness with caloric intake. As a result, we may crave more sweets and tend to choose sweet food over nutritious food, resulting in weight gain. Participants in the San Antonio Heart Study who drank more than 21 *diet drinks* per week (3 per day) were twice as likely to become overweight or obese as people who didn't drink diet soda. Research has also concluded that artificial sweeteners contribute to heart disease, diabetes, and cancer.

*A study on daily consumption of diet drinks found a
36% greater risk for metabolic syndrome (prediabetes) and a
67% increased risk for type 2 diabetes.*

HOW TO GET OFF SUGAR

Eat real, single-ingredient foods that grow from the earth, roam the earth, or swim in the sea. Avoid processed foods high in sugar and refined carbohydrates including soft drinks, candy, baked goods, fruit juices, fruits canned in syrup, low-fat/diet foods, and refined white flours.

- **The place to begin is the grocery store.** If we buy sweets, of course we're going to eat sweets.
- **Replace soda and juice** with sparkling or spring water, lemon water, herb tea (great over ice), vitamin water, coffee, or low-carb lattes. Don't add sugar to tea or coffee.
- **Replace sugar** as a flavoring with lemon, lime, ginger, cinnamon, vanilla, or nutmeg.
- **Enjoy fruit** such as berries, an apple, or stone fruit (peaches, plums, cherries) when craving something sweet.

- **Choose recipes that replace sugar** with fruit as a sweetener.

- **Experiment** with natural, zero calorie sweeteners like stevia or monk fruit (lo han guo) when you want a touch of sweet in beverages like coffee or tea.

- **Read nutritional labels** to avoid added sugar disguised in many forms.

- **Get support.** If you find that you are not making the progress you want, explore working with a nutritionist or joining a support group.

When men decrease sugar in their diet, they not only avoid health issues like heart disease and diabetes, they also lower body fat, reduce joint pain, look better (naked), increase their energy, feel more confident and attractive, and enjoy more physical intimacy.

For more about Vital Nutrition & Wellness and the work of Angela Stanford, please see www.vitalandwell.com.

Chapter 33
Weight-Loss Strategies
Peter Vash, MD, MPH, FACE
Endocrinologist & Obesity Expert

My doctor told me to stop having intimate dinners for four.
Unless there are going to be three other people there.
— *Orson Welles*

Losing weight is a hard, frustrating experience, and keeping it off is even more difficult. Overweight individuals who want to lose weight often end up wasting their time and money on fad diets, unproven nutritional products, and unscrupulous, even harmful, weight loss programs. While weight loss is rarely quick and easy, it can be steady, progressive, ongoing, and achievable. Once you know what to do and how to reduce your calorie intake and are committed to doing that over time, you can achieve safe, significant, and sustainable weight loss.

Weight gain with excess fat deposited in the abdominal area (belly fat) puts an increased strain on the body's organs, back, and joints. Excess body fat is strongly associated with increased rates of type 2 diabetes, hypertension, cardiovascular disorders, stroke, elevated levels of cholesterol and triglycerides, gall bladder disease, fatty liver disease, cirrhosis, sleep apnea, degenerative joint disease, psychological and emotional disorders, and dementia. Unfortunately, overweight individuals live shorter lives and have more discomfort, pain, and disability.

Weight gain and obesity are the result of excess calorie intake over an extended period of time, resulting in an imbalance between energy (calorie) consumption and energy (calorie) expenditure. These excess calories are stored in the form of triglycerides that make up most of the fat cells and serve as an energy reserve. There are other factors that often affect weight gain, such as activity level, as well as genetic, environmental, medical, economic, and psycho-social issues that influence the consumption of extra calories. However, it is only the excess calorie intake that causes the storage of these extra calories in the form of fat. While this concept appears simple, and most individuals know it is true, knowing what to do, and how to do it, is more complicated and burdensome.

Weight gain can also be influenced by:

- Medical conditions, such as hypothyroidism (low metabolic rate), excess cortisol levels from Cushing's syndrome, and excess insulin production.

- The use of certain medications, such as corticosteroids, anti-depressants, anti-psychotics, and anti-anxiety and anti-convulsant medications.

These potential factors should be ruled out first by an experienced physician. Once these medical and prescription drug causes have been ruled out, there are several ways to achieve safe, significant, and sustainable weight loss.

Medically Recognized and Accepted Treatments for Weight-Loss:

1) Dietary and Behavioral Life Style Changes

2) Increased Physical Activity

3) Behavioral Modification and Cognitive Intervention

4) Medication and Supplements

5) Bariatric Surgery

The method, or more likely combination of methods, that is best, depends on the individual's decision. It is essential to understand that weight loss will help not only one's physical appearance, but also overall physical, psychological, and emotional health and wellbeing along with a reduced risk for chronic diseases.

SUSTAINABLE WEIGHT LOSS

1. DIETARY AND BEHAVIORAL LIFESTYLE CHANGES

The body burns or metabolizes the calories in food as fuel to provide for the energy, heat, and movement. The body's metabolic rate (total energy expenditure) is comprised of three factors: 1) the resting metabolic rate (the body at rest – 70%); 2) the cost of food metabolism, which is the thermic effect of food being digested to release energy (10%); and 3) physical activity energy expenditure, or movement (20%). Different food groups have varying amounts of energy (calories), and the more energy-dense the food is, the higher number of calories it contains. The calorie content for each gram (weight) of a food group is the following: carbohydrates contain four calories per gram, protein contains four calories per gram, fat contains nine calories per gram, and alcohol contains seven calories per gram. This is why men who eat fatty foods (nine calories per gram) while drinking alcohol (seven calories per gram) quickly put on weight.

All diets, be they keto, Paleo, low carb, low fat, high protein, intermittent fasting, etc., depend on the same energy format to cause weight loss. The fewer calories you eat, the more calories are taken from your fat storage (energy reserve) to keep your metabolic rate stable, and the more weight you lose. Many clinical studies have examined specific diets to determine if there's a single diet that's the best one for weight loss.

However, the research suggests that there is no one best diet for weight loss. While some diets may work for some individuals in the short term, in the long term, all diets of the same calorie content produce very similar weight loss results. For example, a low carbohydrate diet can produce an early increased weight loss, most of which comes from water loss, but after an extended time, the weight loss results are similar to other diets. Different individuals may react differently to the same diet, while other individuals may have the same weight loss from using different diets. All diets work when you stay on them, and all diets fail when you go off them.

There are no best diets for weight loss as all diets will work to some degree for most individuals. But the most critical factor is to adhere to a nutritionally balanced calorie-reduced diet over an extended period.

Clinical studies show that all diets result in about the same amount of weight loss after one to two years if you adhere to them.

The less you eat, the more you lose is an obvious and commonly accepted mandate, but one that is uncommonly followed.

Here is a general and approximate concept to help one lose excess fat. Multiply your current weight by a factor of 10, and this is about (plus or minus 10%) how many calories you need to maintain your current weight. Then by reducing your daily calorie intake by 500, 1,000, or more calories each day, this will result in a steady progressive weight loss. For example, a 250-pound man needs about, plus or minus, 250-pounds x 10 = 2,500 calories each day, on average, to stay at this current weight.

Since it takes, in theory, a deficit of about 3,500 calories to lose a single pound of fat, a daily reduction of 500 calories per day will produce a weekly deficit of 3,500 calories (500 x 7 days) amounting to about 1 pound of fat loss per week.

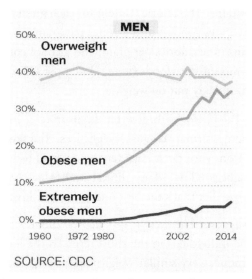

Figure 33.1. Percentage of American men who are overweight.

A deficit of 1,000 calories a day will result in a weekly deficit of 7,000 calories (1,000 x 7 days), which should, in theory, cause a loss of 2 pounds per week (7,000/3,500 calories per pound of fat = 2 pounds). Since the excess weight may not have occurred quickly, it will probably take some time for it to leave. A diet with reduced refined sugars and starches, high in fruit, vegetable, and fiber, moderate amounts of lean protein (eggs, fish, fowl, seafood, lean meats, tofu, legumes), and lower amounts of oils, mayonnaise, dressings, and alcohol has the best long-term weight loss results.

It is important to understand that a large part of any initial weight loss in the first two weeks is water, excreted as urine. Then after this brisk fluid loss, the slow but steady process of fat loss continues. A loss of 1% of your present weekly weight is considered a good goal and a reasonable rate of weekly weight loss. Avoiding foods that contain large amounts of sugars, fat, and salt (such as ice cream, chips, fries, fried foods, pastries, cookies, sugar-sweetened drinks) as well as other snack and junk foods will make a considerable difference with the speed and amount of your weight loss. Eating your meals at specific times and not eating between those times, or after dinner will avoid random emotional eating. It also doesn't matter when you eat, but it does matter what you eat, how much you eat, and how fast you eat – slower is better.

Recommendations for a Healthy Weight-Loss Diet

For a general, well accepted, nutritionally balanced weight-loss diet, a reduced-calorie, reduced refined sugar "Mediterranean" type diet should be considered. It recommends

EXERCISE-CALORIE CHART

Calories burned per hour on average for a 160-pound person

Very Little (50-150 calories/hour)		Significant (300-500 calories/hour)	
Sleeping	60	Hiking	360
Sitting, eating, handwork	90	Aerobics, general	420
Standing	100	Bicycling, light-moderate	420-560
Driving	110	Tennis	470
Housework, office work	140	Weight lifting	520
Moderate (150-300 calories/hour)		**Extreme (500+ calories/hour)**	
Walking, slow pace	180	Basketball	600
Light dancing	220	Moderate dancing	600
Golfing	250	Swimming	620
Yoga	280	Jogging, 6 MPH	700
Walking, moderate-fast	250-320	Running, >10 MPH	900+

Figure 33.2. The number of calories burned during popular types of exercise.

foods such as olive oil, fresh fruits and vegetables, legumes (beans, peas), nuts, seeds, and a limited amount of eggs, cheese, dairy, fish, and lean red meats. A suggested ratio is:

- 30%-45% from unsaturated and monosaturated fats

- 30%-40% from unrefined carbohydrates/organic whole grains

- No sugar-sweetened beverages and reduced amounts of pasta, pastries, cookies, chips, etc.

- 20%-25% from lean meats, seafood, and fish

- Reduced alcohol intake, smaller portion sizes, and no snacking between meals will also help to produce a significant weight loss.

2. INCREASED PHYSICAL ACTIVITY

The general activity time recommendation for weight loss is about 300 minutes of physical activity per week. Aerobic activity (running, walking, cycling, swimming, etc.) is best for fat burning, while anaerobic exercise (resistance training, weight lifting) is best for building lean body (muscle) tissue. Since muscle burns more calories at rest than does fat, an increase in muscle mass means a higher metabolic rate throughout the day. It is challenging to achieve any significant amount of weight loss through exercise alone, simply because it takes a significant amount of exercise to burn fat off, but very little time to put fat on.

3. BEHAVIORAL MODIFICATION AND INTERVENTION

If you have strong food cravings, there are several behavioral strategies that can help change compulsive eating behaviors into healthier weight-losing behaviors. They include:

- Support
- Self-monitoring
- Stress management
- Contingency management (substitution)
- Problem solving
- Stimulus control (planning ahead).

Keeping a food and behavior journal is one of the most effective interventions, especially to help avoid emotional and stress-induced eating.

By becoming aware and mindful of what you eat, when you do eat or snack, and under what circumstances you are triggered to eat, you are then better able to control your eating.

Support. Connecting with friends, support groups, and health professionals can improve adherence to the needed lifestyle changes that result in weight loss. Supportive and positive comments for your weight loss are to be appreciated, but fat shaming is to be avoided and firmly rebuffed.

Self-monitoring. This approach includes:

- Keeping a food journal

- Logging in daily calorie intake

- Regular weight checks

- Documenting time, location, and emotional feelings when eating

- Situations in which you engage in stress-induced and emotional eating.

Stress management. This means being mindful of eating when you are upset, bored, frustrated or angry, etc. The next step is to replace an eating behavior with a non-caloric alternative action/activity such as:

- Meditation

- Talking about your feelings with a friend

- Getting some physical activity

- Resolving upsetting problems quickly and moving forward

- Not holding grudges.

Contingency management (substitution). When presented with an unplanned eating challenge, replace the unhealthy eating situation with another non-caloric reward, substitution, or action. For example, when taken unexpectedly to an Italian restaurant, be prepared to order chicken, fish, or a seafood salad and forgo the pasta.

Problem solving. For a problematic food, snacking, or eating event, replace it:

- With another food choice, time, or place for eating

- By substituting reduced caloric alternatives for higher calorie choices, such as drinking sparkling water instead of alcohol

- Substituting fruits, vegetables, and reduced calorie foods instead of high-caloric, refined sugar and fat-loaded snack foods, junk food, or comfort foods.

Stimulus control. Plan ahead for your meals and avoid eating situations:

- Decide before going into the restaurant or to the meeting what you will eat

- Eat in a structured manner (specific time for the meal) to give you better control over emotional eating situations

- If watching specific television shows usually makes you hungry for snack foods, become aware of what makes you stimulated to eat, and avoid the temptation.

4. MEDICATION AND SUPPLEMENTS

There are six major commonly prescribed weight loss medications the FDA has approved to be safe and effective: 1) orlistat (Xenical), 2) phentermine, 3) phentermine combined with topiramate (Qsymia), 4) lorcaserin (Belviq), which at this time has been withdrawn from the market, 5) naltrexone and bupropion (Contrave), and 6) liraglutide (Saxenda).

Each of these medications has weight-loss benefits, but also some potential side effects. None are addictive, and their use is best explained and prescribed by a knowledgeable and experienced physician.

There are few weight loss-supplements that are documented to be effective and safe, despite the advertising hype. My team of board-certified physicians has developed two herbal products that are scientifically validated and clinically proven to help produce weight loss in a steady and safe manner. *Attenuate* helps to reduce appetite, lower hunger sensation, and control sugar and carbohydrate cravings. It contains an enhanced dose of *Garcinia cambogia* (4,500 mg per day), scientifically recommended and clinically proven to produce significant weight loss.

Attenuslim helps to mobilize and metabolize the stored fat in the abdominal, hip, and waist areas, and it also helps to control appetite and sugar cravings. It contains a unique formulation of two proven herbal ingredients, meratrim and lowat, to reduce the stomach's production of the hunger hormone ghrelin. This helps to control snacking and promotes weight loss.

5. BARIATRIC SURGERY

This is the most effective treatment for extreme obesity (Body Mass Index over 40) or significant obesity (Body Mass Index over 35) with severe chronic co-morbidities (diabetes, hypertension, cardiovascular heart disease, obstructive sleep apnea, etc.). The two most highly recommended procedures for both weight-loss effectiveness and safety are the Roux-en-Y gastric bypass procedure and the Sleeve Gastrectomy. These procedures are not intended for overweight individuals, but rather for those with obesity, and must be performed by well-trained and experienced bariatric surgeons. Many clinical studies report these surgeries can help very obese patients achieve and maintain a healthier weight, free of many of the associated co-morbidities.

However, these procedures are not permanent cures, and follow-up behavioral lifestyle and dietary changes must be implemented to prevent weight regain. Contact the American Society for Metabolic and Bariatric Surgery (ASMBS) at asmbs.org/patients or call 352-331-4900 for answers to your questions and to find an appropriate surgeon.

Five easy strategies for weight loss:

1. Eat in a structured manner at certain times that fit your schedule, two or three meals a day without snacking, eating between meals, or eating after dinner.

2. To lose weight, you must eat fewer calories than you need for your daily physical activity and sustain that effort over time.

3. Stay on your chosen, recommended, or prescribed diet because adherence is the most crucial part of any weight-loss program.

4. Eat only when you are physically hungry (when your stomach indicates hunger), but not when you are psychologically (emotionally) hungry.

5. Losing weight is something that you can achieve. Have a positive attitude and realistic expectations, and remember that reducing calorie intake causes weight loss, while increasing the calories you burn, maintains weight loss.

**More information about the weight-loss strategies described in this chapter
and the products themselves can be found at
www.attenuatepro.com
and in Dr. Peter Vash's book, *Lose It and Keep It Off.*
www.petervashmd.com**

Chapter 34
Plant-Based Nutrition
Joel Kahn, MD, FACC, Cardiologist

Our excessive intake of meat is killing us. We fatten our cows and pigs,
kill them, eat them, and then they kill us.
— William C Roberts, MD

You might imagine that the question of what men should eat for optimal health is a topic with broad agreement worldwide. If you think so, I am sorry to disappoint you. Food wars, sometimes ugly, have dominated the last few decades of nutritional discussion. This started with the Atkin's low-carb movement and then moved on to the Paleo and ketogenic diet groups, the carnivore (all-meat) craze, the Mediterranean and DASH (Diet Approach to Stop Hypertension) data, and the ever-present vegetarian and vegan followers. Any night of the week you can tune in to different national TV specials and hear widely conflicting nutrition information by seemingly credible MDs and PhDs. What are you to do?

On a personal note, I adopted a completely plant (vegan) diet at age 18 when I entered my pre-medical/medical school program at the University of Michigan. I have not touched a beef burger, chicken breast, salmon fillet, or a bowl of ice cream since then. I have been practicing cardiology for over 30 years and every patient has learned of the "diet-heart" connection. The vast majority of science now favors plant-based nutrition.

I literally see health conditions reverse—atherosclerosis and disorders like type 2 diabetes, hypertension, cholesterol disorders, obesity, and psoriasis, all reverse. The requirement for medication also lessens or disappears with plant-based diets.

BENEFITS OF A PLANT-BASED DIET

Plant-based nutrition has been shown to prevent and reverse heart disease, type 2 diabetes, certain cancers such as those of the prostate, autoimmune diseases such as rheumatoid arthritis, hypertension, high cholesterol, and even erectile dysfunction. There are new data that further reinforce the argument that eating primarily or only fruits, vegetables, whole grains, and legumes is optimal for your health. Here are eight reasons to choose plant foods, such as a bean chili over a meat chili.

Type 2 Diabetes. A long-term study from Finland that followed more than 2,000 men over a period of 19 years showed that replacing even 1% of calories from animal proteins with plant proteins lowered the risk of developing diabetes by 18%.

Liver disease. A growing health concern is non-alcoholic fatty liver disease or NAFLD. An analysis of over 3,000 subjects in the Netherlands found that increased levels of dietary protein from animal sources (meat) were associated with a greater risk (reaching 50% higher) of developing non-alcoholic fatty liver disease.

Asthma. A study on the effect of processed red meat consumption on asthma symptoms reported that eating cured red meat more than four times a week increased the odds of having worsened asthma by 76%.

Colon cancer. The world was caught off guard in October 2015 when the World Health Organization announced their results of a comprehensive analysis demonstrating that processed red meats like bacon, salami, and hot dogs cause colorectal cancer. In a more recent analysis, 400 studies were examined. They found that the risk of colorectal cancer increased by 12% for each quarter-pound of meat eaten per day (1/2 cup or 100 gm of red and processed meats). Whole grains and vegetables decreased the risk.

Stomach cancer. Researchers analyzed the results of 42 studies relating diet to stomach cancer. They found that higher intake of red meat increased the risk by 70% while processed red meat (such as luncheon meat and hot dogs) increased risk by 80%.

Head and neck cancer. In a study from the Netherlands of over 120,000 subjects followed for more than 20 years, consumption of processed red meat was associated with developing cancers of the head and neck. The risk was increased by as much as 50% compared to the low or non-meat eaters studied.

Depression. In an analysis of 21 studies examining diet and depression, eating red and processed meats increased the risk of depression by over 25%, while fruits and vegetables had the opposite effect.

Sexual health. Clearly, I am committed to the science of "plant-forward" or plant-only diets, but can it benefit male sexual health too? Eating red meat can increase exposure to TMAO, (a newly identified metabolite that appears to cause clogged arteries), and to neu5Gc, (believed to damage arteries via an antibody pathway), as well as pesticides, hormones, and antibiotics that can all disrupt the health and gland function of men.

Avoiding meat is one of the most important health decisions you can make. Whether meat comes from cows raised on grass or corn or whether you know the farmer or not, meat can be an inflammatory food. Red meat inherently has a chemical structure that drives reactions in the body that promote inflammation, diabetes, heart disease, and cancer growth. The data indicate that the more servings of fruit and vegetables you eat, the more likely you are to avoid chronic diseases and to delay death. Eating meat has the opposite result, leading to disease and early death. Men should limit or eliminate the number of meals and portion sizes that contain red meat, poultry, pork, and even fish.

IDENTIFYING THE OPTIMAL DIET

One basic problem in any discussion of food is that nutrition research is difficult. It is difficult to get large groups of volunteers to eat different diets for long periods of time to evaluate whether they stay healthy or develop diseases such as heart attacks, strokes, cancer, diabetes, or erectile dysfunction. So, what are we to do? Fortunately, two leading nutrition scientists have offered surprisingly similar norms for evaluating nutrition science in terms of longevity and metabolism.

Valter Longo, PhD, is director of the Institute of Aging Research at the University of Southern California, author of *The Longevity Diet*, creator of the Prolon fasting mimicking diet, and internationally known academic researcher. In his book, he teaches the Pillars of Longevity as a practical format that can be used to evaluate optimal human nutrition. These pillars are:

- Biochemical studies that a diet is likely to be favorable

- Randomized studies supporting a diet

- Epidemiology research studies tracking a particular diet in a large population, with indications that it is beneficial

- Studies of people living over age 100 that reflect the food pattern.

If we take the ketogenic diet (an ultra low-carb and high-fat plan) as an example, the analysis would indicate that biochemical studies do not favor it, randomized trials overall do not favor it long term, epidemiology studies indicate a risk of early death, and centenarians do not eat a ketogenic diet. In fact, in his book, Dr. Longo dismissed the entire ketogenic diet craze in one short paragraph as a trend without support.

The other leading scientist who shares his views on how to analyze science is Nobel Prize laureate Michael Brown, MD. He was awarded the Nobel Prize in Medicine in 1985 for his research on cholesterol metabolism. Dr. Brown delivered a lecture entitled "A Century of Cholesterol and Coronaries" in which he described a method of evaluating the literature he called the "Four Lines of Evidence." These four lines are remarkably similar to the Pillars introduced by Dr. Longo. Together they provide a framework for considering new information in a meaningful way, from a big-picture perspective. If you hear about a new diet trend, or if your trainer recommends some new approach to nutrition, remembering the four pillars or the four lines of evidence may give you a platform you can use to evaluate whether there is enough evidence to alter your menu long term. Usually, the solution comes down to fresh vegetables, fruits, legumes, and whole grains.

CONSENSUS FROM THE MEDICAL COMMUNITY

A series of prominent recommendations proposed as models for healthy food choices have been introduced by several major scientific groups. These are generally large and credible organizations that spent many hours developing a consensus on what we should eat. It is worthwhile to study a few of these examples.

Harvard Healthy Eating Plate 2011

The *Healthy Eating Plate*, created in 2011 by nutrition experts at the Harvard School of Public Health and editors at Harvard Health Publications, was designed to address deficiencies in earlier nutritional recommendations such as those of the U.S. Department of Agriculture, in the USDA's MyPlate. The Healthy Eating Plate provides detailed guidance, in a simple format, to help people make the best food choices. The main intent of the Healthy Eating Plate is to focus on diet quality.

The *type of carbohydrate* in a diet is considered more important than the *amount of carbohydrate*, because some sources of carbohydrate — such as vegetables, fruits, whole grains, and beans — are healthier than others. These guidelines also advise consumers to avoid *sugary beverages*, a major source of calories—usually with little nutritional value—that are found everywhere in the American diet. The Healthy Eating Plate encourages consumers to use *healthy oils* (such as olive oil) in place of butter or lard, and it does not set a maximum on the percentage of calories people should get each day from healthy sources of fat. In this way, the recommendations from Harvard are the opposite of the *low-fat message* promoted for decades by the USDA. Specifically, this plate includes 50% fruits and vegetables, 25% whole grains, and 25% healthy proteins such as beans or lean meats. It replaced the glass of milk with a glass of water. The Harvard diet is a great example to consider as a pattern for healthy food choices.

EAT—*The Lancet* Planetary Diet 2019

Food systems have the potential to nurture human health while supporting environmental sustainability. The EAT–*Lancet* Commission addresses the need to feed a growing global population a healthy diet, while also defining sustainable food systems that will minimize damage to our planet. The Commission describes a universal healthy reference diet, based on an increase in consumption of healthy foods (such as vegetables, fruits, whole grains, legumes, and nuts), and a decrease in consumption of unhealthy foods (such as red meat, sugar, and refined grains) to support major health benefits, and also increase the likelihood of attaining Sustainable Development Goals. This is set against the backdrop of defined scientific boundaries that will ensure a safe operating space within six Earth systems in order to maintain a healthy planet. Men should have some concern about the health of the planet and the environment they live in. This food plate is a great reminder that quality matters and that plant foods are less harmful to the Earth than animal food agriculture.

Australian Government Food Plate 2019

Crafted to promote a healthy lifestyle and cut the risk of chronic diseases (which are often fueled by diet choices), the *Australian Dietary Guidelines* were written by a panel of independent experts overseen by the National Health and Medicine Research Council, and based on the most robust nutritional science we have—citing *more than 1,100* scientific papers. They boil the research down to five guidelines:

Guideline 1. To achieve and maintain a healthy weight, be physically active and choose the correct amounts of nutritious food and drinks to meet your energy needs.

Guideline 2. Enjoy a wide variety of nutritious foods from the five food groups every day, and drink plenty of water.

Those five food groups are what nutritionists call *core foods*, because eating them provides the nutrients we require to live well. They are:

- **Vegetables and legumes/beans.** Adults are advised to eat five to six servings of these a day, where a serving is equal to about 2/3 of a cup (75g, 100–350kj/25–85 calories), which essentially equals three cups total of cooked vegetables, salad, and legumes over the course of a day. Examples include half a cup of cooked green or orange vegetables, beans, peas, or lentils; a cup of green leafy vegetables; half a medium potato; or a medium tomato.

- **Fruit.** Two servings a day, where one serving is about one cup (150g, 350kj/85 calories) — but note *one serving of fruit* isn't always equal to *one piece of fruit*. Think of a medium banana, apple, orange, or pear; or two small apricots, kiwis, or plums; or a cup of diced fruit. (Fruit juice and dried fruit are allowed, but only *occasionally*. Fresh whole fruit is preferred.)

■ **Grain-based foods, preferably whole grain or high-fiber sources.** Four to six servings a day, where one serving is equal to 500kj (120 calories). That's about one slice of bread; half a cup of cooked rice, pasta, or similar food; or a quarter-cup of muesli, among others.

■ **Lean meat and poultry, fish, eggs, tofu, nuts and seeds, and legumes/beans.** Eat two to three servings a day, where one serving is 500–600kj (120–145 calories). That's anything from 1/3 to 1/2 cup (65–100g) of meat, fish, or chicken; two eggs; 1/2 cup (170g) tofu; or 30g nuts, which is about a handful.

■ **Milk, yogurt, cheese, and/or plant alternatives such as oats, soy, and hemp, mostly from reduced-fat sources.** Two and a half to four servings a day, where one serving is 500–600kj (120–145 calories). This governmental recommendation is very similar to the 2011 plate from Harvard.

Canada's Healthy Eating Pattern 2019

Canada's Healthy Eating Pattern was developed as a resource for its citizens. The guidelines emphasize three primary issues—1) foundations for healthy eating, 2) foods and beverages that undermine healthy eating, and 3) the importance of food skills. When it comes to nutritional advice, the guide simply says to consume produce, whole grains, and protein foods regularly, with most of the protein friendly for vegetarians and vegans. It also recommends avoiding saturated fat by consuming *unsaturated sources*, which are mostly plant-based foods or fish. It does not endorse dairy consumption. The objective of the healthy eating pattern is to provide more specific guidance on the recommended amounts and types of foods as well as life-stage guidance (such as recommendations for young children and seniors).

■ The intended audience is also health professionals and policy makers.

■ The healthy eating pattern can be used as an additional resource for developing procurement policies in institutions, such as long-term care facilities and hospital settings.

Overall, all the plates have in common an emphasis on predominantly plant food choices, varied and whole, with water being the main beverage. With that, the health of the populace and the planet would flourish. Men should eat a big salad every day, grab an apple, drink a glass of water, tea, or coffee in place of a milk latte, and try the enormous variety of beans, peas, and lentils as sources of plant protein.

EATING FOR YOUR ARTERIES (AND SEXUAL HEALTH)

Men have 50,000 miles of arteries that course through their bodies from head to toe. The layer of cells that lines all the arteries—the endothelium—is just one cell layer thick, yet so extensive, it collectively weighs as much as your liver. Eat to maintain a healthy endothelium.

We all want a healthy endothelium because it boosts sexual health, wellness, longevity, and optimal fitness, preventing heart attack and stroke. Maintaining a healthy weight, avoiding smoking, and practicing healthy lifestyle habits are goals to follow. Certain foods can also boost the production of nitric oxide and reverse endothelial dysfunction to power our health. These foods, rich with concentrations of natural dietary nitrates that support increased nitric oxide production, include: spinach, kale, bok choy, arugula; beets and the beet greens; watermelon, including the rind, and rhubarb; nuts, particularly pine nuts; whole grains such as oats and wheat germ; garlic and onions.

Another approach is to use polyphenol-rich foods or functional foods to boost the enzyme that makes nitric oxide to enhance its production. Apples and grapes have high concentrations of these molecules and have been shown to boost exercise duration. Other foods rich in polyphenols include berries of all kinds; stone fruit such as peaches, plums, apricots, and cherries; and pomegranates, which all have profound benefits when included in our diet.

WHAT SHOULD MEN EAT?

The foods that maintain the healthiest arteries, blood pressure, blood sugar, and cholesterol levels also support good sexual function and vitality. The myth that men need meat has been promoted by the meat lobbyists and does not match the actual data. Learning to love the foods that love you back is key. At least once a day, eat a salad (without meat and cheese) that is colorful and is at least as big as your head! Eat an apple in place of a donut. Make a bean chili in place of a beef chili. Try a plant-based milk, like oat or soy, for a coffee whitener, for cereal, for your oatmeal, for an ice cream treat, and even for a cheese (there are now nut-free products made of oats and sunflower seeds if a nut allergy is an issue). Your buddies may pressure you to join them for a burger, fries, and a malt, but let them know that you care about your endothelium and sexual function and are simply following Harvard Medical School recommendations.

For more information on heart-friendly food, cardiovascular health, and the work of Dr. Kahn, please see www.DrJoelKahn.com.

Chapter 35
Food Allergies
Matthew Lodewick, MD
Allergist

Having food allergies doesn't mean your body is broken.
In fact, it means your body is highly intelligent.
— Gabriela

Although the hot new focus of health concerns is currently on food allergies, the majority of bad reactions people experience with food are rarely classic allergies. When reactions are associated with an allergy (and they may be an important reason for poor health), they can be alarming but the allergen can be quite straightforward to identify, as is the case with a peanut or shellfish allergy.

> *True food allergies are commonly severe, occur within minutes, and are specific to particular foods.*

IDENTIFYING FOOD ALLERGIES

Virtually all my patients with food allergies are already aware of their sensitization when they first become my patient.

It is possible to develop a food allergy at any age. If you suspect a food allergy, see an allergist. If you have a true food allergy, practice vigilant avoidance and have auto-injectable epinephrine readily available.

> *If you have experienced hives, throat tightness, chest tightness, and/or gastrointestinal symptoms with a specific food or food group, see an allergy specialist.*

One common misconception is that there are severe food allergies and mild food allergies. In terms of classic IgE allergies, it is chiefly a matter of the dose of allergen to which one has been exposed. Small doses result in milder symptoms while larger doses are associated with more explosive symptoms. Exposure to the food in the setting of exercise or alcohol may heighten the reaction.

Oral immunotherapy. Studies are ongoing with food oral immunotherapy (OIT) and food sublingual immunotherapy (SLIT). These treatments have demonstrated the capacity to reduce reactivity by increasing the threshold for a systemic reaction, but no study to date has shown prolonged sustained desensitization (lasting more than months) or cure. The thought leaders in the field have become more proactive about treatment, and the next decade or two may prove transformative in how we look at and treat food allergies.

Allergy testing. One of the greatest challenges today is that interpreting food allergy tests is not straightforward (although the allergy can have a clear history and a very selected panel of food suspects). Broad food panels tend to create more questions than answers and often require extended office-based oral challenges to clarify sensitizations. Unfortunately, food allergies commonly are falsely ascribed to patients when the assessment has been in the hands of a provider without the nuanced understanding of food testing and interpretation or who relies on unvalidated food tests.

Digestive symptoms. A common presentation to the allergy office is the patient with ongoing abdominal complaints and concerns about a possible food allergy. These visits are often accompanied by great anticipation that a final understanding of the cause and the relief of symptoms will result from food skin (or serologic IgE) tests. Unfortunately, this is rarely the case. To be clear, isolated abdominal cramping, nausea, vomiting, and/or diarrhea are not uncommon presentations of a food allergy. But in these cases, the cause is often due to ingestion of a specific food, and that food is likely included in the individual's diet. For a food allergy sufferer, the foods to which they are sensitive are of a limited set. For most who present with stomach complaints and hope for a solution, there is no consistent food to which they can attribute symptoms. These patients are better served by considering a low FODMAPS diet and, if that is not effective, by seeing a gastroenterologist.

Oral allergy syndrome. While I have emphasized that true food allergies are severe and pose a life-threatening risk, there is a mild reaction to food called oral allergy syndrome that does not tend to provoke severe symptoms. It is a case of mistaken identity. Certain nuts, fresh fruit, and vegetables have proteins that are structurally similar to pollen. Ingestion of these foods is confused by the immune system with ingestion of the pollen to which the individual is sensitive and leads to mild complaints of itchy mouth and throat. Diagrams that nicely tie the pollen with the associated food are easily found with a simple online search.

A caveat, especially with nuts, is that oral complaints with trace exposures can be misconstrued as oral allergy syndrome when a more serious nut allergy could be present. If uncertain, it is best to assess the question through an allergist.

The complex question of food sensitivities. If you have digestive symptoms and are wondering why there seem to be no easy answers, consider that more than 60% of your immune system resides in your gut. This creates the potential for major reactions from time to time—cramping, diarrhea, pain, or symptoms of full-blown food poisoning.

Today we have a massive supply of relatively safe foods. Yet it has only been a hundred years since humans gained access to refrigeration. For the millennia before the present, there was no easy way to preserve fresh food and guard against food poisoning. Humans were in a constant battle with mold, hostile bacteria, and viruses in our food supply. To cope, the priority of the immune system has always been safeguarding against contaminated food. In response, immunity within the gastrointestinal tract evolved into an incredibly complex system that includes more protective friendly flora than the number of stars in the known universe. It is not surprising that at times we are unable to second-guess the reactions of this vast system.

GLUTEN SENSITIVITY AND CELIAC DISEASE

Gluten sensitivity. This is currently a hot topic that is ripe with misinformation. While there may be a temptation to check for a gluten allergy to account for nasal congestion and fatigue, this is one of the most common food allergy tests reported as a positive when it is in fact negative (referred to as a false positive), particularly in individuals with pollen allergies. Gluten sensitivity describes a mix of different pathophysiologic responses. There are some who are truly gluten allergic, but these individuals know they are food allergic because of the intensity and speed of symptom onset with gluten ingestion.

Celiac disease. The other well recognized form of gluten sensitivity is celiac disease. This can be more indolent and can take years to be diagnosed. The most common symptoms of celiac disease are bloating and diarrhea and, sometimes, weight loss. It has a genetic component, so testing in close relatives should be considered, especially if they have symptoms consistent with celiac disease. Celiac disease can look very similar to irritable bowel syndrome, so ruling out celiac disease in this circumstance is very important. Celiac disease can be associated with other autoimmune conditions, including autoimmune thyroid disease or diabetes. Testing is very good in the right hands and the right situation.

In an individual with celiac disease, the first part of the small intestine (the duodenum) can show damage and flattening of the absorptive surface, which impairs nutrient absorption. Microscopic imaging of the area shows an overabundance of active inflammation. To achieve accurate testing, it is important that an individual who has symptoms suggestive of celiac disease be seen and evaluated by a capable physician (either a primary physician

The key reason that the celiac disease diagnosis is important is because celiac disease is associated with lymphoma and other gastrointestinal cancers. We believe long-term adherence to a strict gluten-free diet can markedly reduce this risk.

comfortable with diagnosing this disorder and/or a gastroenterologist) prior to eliminating gluten from their diet. Prolonged avoidance eliminates the measurable diagnostic markers of this condition. The gold standard test is endoscopy with biopsy, but a blood test (in the right hands) can also be outstanding at confirming a diagnosis.

For those who have non-celiac gluten sensitivity, there is not this risk, and it probably is not a major problem to have occasional gluten. Given the cancer risk, it is vital to know who needs to avoid gluten 100% of the time and who does not. As for non-celiac gluten sensitivity/intolerance, there remains work to do to better understand and define this set of disorders.

Gluten-free lifestyle. There are testimonials from many patients on the benefits of a gluten-free lifestyle, but the science behind non-celiac gluten sensitivity is currently limited. These individuals likely do not have the same need for a tightly controlled gluten-free diet. Elimination diets that improve symptoms should be followed by reintroduction of gluten. These elimination/reintroductions should be repeated periodically to better test if gluten is in fact an issue. The benefits of a gluten-free lifestyle are likely from reduced intake of processed foods, a healthier lifestyle overall, and consumption of more natural, whole foods.

For more information on the work of Dr. Lodewick, please see:
www.BayAreaAllergy.com.

Chapter 36
Finding the Right Diet
Nancy Faass, MSW, MPH,
Health Coach

You don't need a silver fork to eat good food.
— Paul Prudhomme

Dr. Mark Moyad, MD, MPH on Diet & Lifestyle

It is important to empower yourself when it comes to diet and lifestyle. In sorting out the question of diet, most of us want to believe that ultimately there is a perfect diet, one diet that is right for everyone. However, as a public health educator/doctor/clinical researcher working in an academic urology department for almost 30 years, I would consider it myopic if someone tried to convince me that there is only one type of treatment for prostate cancer. Why do we think that diet is any different?

Let's be rational about this. We need to tie diet to objective and subjective outcomes. If we obsess on diet, life becomes an analytical nightmare, and we are tempted to fixate on everything we put in our mouth.

I don't really care what diet you are on, as long as your health is improving, and you are moving objectively in a positive direction. If you are doing the ketogenic diet, good for you. If you're doing the Mediterranean diet, great. If you like intermittent fasting and you only eat one meal a day, that's fabulous. In the near future, we may find that all these diets are healthy and that they all work fine if you adhere to them.

That said, you should also track your lab values working with the medical team you entrust with your health. Currently, we use some of the criteria developed in some of the most comprehensive studies available: for example, a notable review conducted in 52 countries, which identified key laboratory tests and lifestyle factors in defining health. Here is a comprehensive list of some of the priorities everyone should focus on:

- Blood cholesterol (LDL) and inflammation (C-reactive protein)
- Blood pressure
- Blood sugar
- Whether you smoke or not
- Healthy BMI with a healthy waist size
- Healthy mental health/low stress
- Fruits and veggies daily
- Moderate alcohol intake
- Exercise for an average of 30 minutes a day
- Miscellaneous—dietary fiber, supplement and medication awareness and compliance
- Your subjective sense of wellbeing

We want to make sure the basic numbers on your lab work are moving in the right direction with the diet of your choice. If they are moving in a positive direction, and you are working with a doctor you trust, that is the diet that works for you.

Why? Because the biggest problem with diet is adherence, which raises the question of what constitutes happiness. You want to be on a diet that is accomplishing your goals and that you find satisfying. Perhaps it's Paleo or intermittent fasting. It could be keto, vegetarian, or vegan. (Note: some people get upset at me when I say vegetarian/vegan is a "diet," because it is considered a "lifestyle" by many nutritionally dedicated folks, but isn't it really both of those things?) You can find a dietary program, in moderation, that moves your lab values in the right direction.

What diet is best? It's the diet you can stick to. It's the diet that moves your numbers in the direction you want. It is the diet that makes you happy and essentially it is the "diet"/"lifestyle" that increase your chances of living better and longer.

Mark Moyad, MD, MPH, Co-Chair, 2019 Prostate Cancer Conference,
Prostate Cancer Research Institute (PCRI) and
University of Michigan Jenkins/Pokempner Director of Preventive & Alternative
Medicine Education in the Dept. of Urology

For more information on the work of Dr. Moyad, please see
https://medicine.umich.edu/dept/urology/mark-moyad-md-mph.
Dr. Moyad's books on nutritional supplements are available
on Amazon.com and from Barnes & Noble.

THE RIGHT DIET FOR YOU

Good nutrition is one of the most effective tools we have for reducing the risk of heart disease, stroke, cancer, and Alzheimer's. If you have experienced weight gain and your waist is 38 inches or greater, you probably have insulin resistance (or metabolic syndrome, a more severe form of prediabetes). This means that your body is having a hard time getting blood sugar into the cells to nourish you. In the majority of cases, the solution is to manage your intake of carbs, especially sugar(s).

Choose an approach to nutrition that you like and adapt it to the food of your region and your culture. The following are examples of the healthiest weight-loss diets offered over the past 30 years.

DETOX AND RESET

This diet, developed by Dr. Mark Hyman of the Cleveland Clinic, is designed to give your body a breather. There is a 10-day period with limited carb intake and then a plan for progressively phasing in carbs. That breather helps to reset your microbiome (the beneficial bacteria that essentially digest your food) by reducing levels of yeast and bacteria in the gut that drive food cravings. In short, the detox reduces cravings, which is a major key to successfully losing weight.

Mark Hyman, MD. *The 10-Day Detox Diet: Activate Your Body's Natural Ability to Burn Fat and Lose Weight Fast.* New York, NY: Little, Brown Spark, 2014.

Another classic nutrition plan with great recipes that provides a two-week reset: Arthur Agatston, MD. *The South Beach Diet: The Delicious, Doctor-Designed, Foolproof Plan for Fast and Healthy Weight Loss.* New York, NY: St. Martin's, 2003.

ALLERGY AND AUTOIMMUNE DIET

An important framework for thinking about food is that *all* diets are somewhat abstract and do not take into consideration individual variations in food tolerance. Many nutritionists consider food allergies and sensitivities to be among the most underappreciated issues in health. A good autoimmune cookbook will help you avoid the most common trigger foods, yet still keep you well nourished.

You can use lab testing to determine your specific food tolerances to customize your diet program. Recently developed food allergy testing is superior to that available in the past. This will enable you and your physician to determine the foods that are acceptable or tolerated by your individual body chemistry. If for some reason you cannot get tested, you might consider what is termed an elimination diet, considered the gold standard by many physicians.

Mickey Trescott. *The Autoimmune Paleo Cookbook*. Austin, TX: Greenleaf Book Group, 2016. If you suspect you have food allergies, an autoimmune disorder, or some other form of chronic illness, the recipes here brilliantly sidestep almost every major allergen known to man.

CyrexLabs.com – A source of advanced laboratory testing focused on autoimmunity and food reactivity.

ANCIENT GRAINS / WHOLE GRAINS

First, the good news and the bad news about a diet of whole grains. The bad news is that you will probably only lose 2 to 3 pounds a month. The good news is that you need never diet again and never go hungry again. This is a sustainable diet that will just keep shedding the pounds—month in, month out, year in, year out—until you achieve your optimal weight, without cutting back on your food intake.

From the long view, your weight loss could be about 20 pounds a year. By way of comparison, using a medication such as metformin, the research shows that the average weight loss is about 10 pounds a year. (Metformin has been the best-selling drug for prediabetes over the past 30 years.)

You will want to purchase organic, non-GMO grains, since modern forms of grain have a different molecular structure than the ancient grains and are associated with allergies and autoimmune reactions. You'll also need to give up modern wheat products, because today's hybrid wheat contains 500 times the amount of protein (gluten) of that in ancient grains. Many people find that their body simply does not know how to handle the novel protein in modern wheat.

The trick is to find whole grains that you *do* like—are you a rice and beans guy? Serve up your favorite rice (long grain, short grain, basmati, forbidden/black, or wild rice) with your favorite beans (kidney beans, black beans, pintos, refried beans). If you'd like, pair that with roast chicken, fish, or steak. Love lentil soup and tasty dahl? Any traditional cuisine can be adapted to an ancient grain diet, which is the original slow comfort food.

However, if you have a chronic illness, consider a keto or Paleo diet after talking with your healthcare provider. Genetically we are hardwired for a diet of veggies, small roots, and protein foods.

Ann Taylor Pittman and Hugh Acheson. *Everyday Whole Grains: 175 New Recipes from Amaranth to Wild Rice, Includes Every Ancient Grain*. TI Inc., 2016.

Amy Chaplin. *Whole Food Cooking Every Day*. New York, NY: Artisan Books, 2019.

DASH DIET AND THE DASH DIET 2

This diet is especially relevant if there is active cardiovascular illness. There has been a great deal of research involving patients with cardiovascular conditions and/or hypertension applying the DASH diet and its variations. Frequently people are on medication, and the DASH diet is often utilized in conjunction with medical management of cardiovascular illness. The research results suggest that people with stage 1 hypertension using this diet experienced improvement in blood pressure equal to or better than any blood pressure control medication. Reduction in salt intake through substitution is a primary aspect of these diet plans.

The DASH diet focuses on what people should eat, rather than what not to eat. The plan utilizes common foods available in your grocery store. Rich in fruits, vegetables, complex carbohydrates, and low-fat dairy products, the DASH diet is lower in fat, saturated fat, cholesterol, and sodium.

For more on variations of the DASH diet, see the website of the Hypertension Institute of Vanderbilt University: https://hypertensioninstitute.com/nutritional-services/.

GLYCEMIC INDEX DIET

See chapter 31 What Is Food? for an overview of the glycemic (carb) index and how to use it to select tasty, fresh foods that promote stable blood sugar and minimize weight gain.

INTERMITTENT FASTING

This approach involves alternating between periods of *clean fasting*, and periods of healthy nutrition. During the clean fast, the emphasis is on hydration and one consumes water, sparkling water, black coffee, and/or black or green tea (not fruity herbal teas, which mimic food). Clean fasting alternates with windows of time when it is appropriate to eat. Initially, that might mean, for example, not eating after 7 p.m. in the evening and having breakfast at 7 a.m. This particular eating pattern is referred to with a ratio—12:12 (hours).

For someone who wants to lose weight, it could mean a pattern of 16:8, which would mean lunch and dinner, but only coffee or tea for breakfast. The advantages to this particular plan are reported to be a gradual end to food cravings, as well as sustainable weight loss, and the ability to eat higher glycemic foods (starchy comfort foods), in moderation.

Genetically, a certain amount of fasting makes sense because for hunter-gatherers, food stores periodically ran out, requiring people to fast whether they wanted to or not.

This diet is not for everyone and is not considered appropriate for anyone with higher nutritional requirements—kids, teens, pregnant women, and those nursing a baby. It is also not appropriate for people with an eating disorder or for those who want to do extended fasting, given the risk of reactive binging.

Gin Stephens. *Fast. Feast. Repeat.* New York, NY: St. Martin's Griffin, 2020.

KETOGENIC DIET

If you have a chronic health issue, this is a brilliant, science-based approach to nutrition, but like all the other diets, more appropriate for some people than others. Dr. Terry Wahls is a physician, researcher, and university professor of medicine (U. Iowa), who effectively reversed her own multiple sclerosis (MS) using good nutrition. Dr. Wahls' condition was so severe she no longer had the strength to sit up in a conventional wheelchair. She improved this condition by eating a nutrient-rich diet, and since then has led a series of research studies to determine if this approach is helpful to others with MS or Parkinson's disease. A typical menu consists of stir-fried veggies, fresh salad, berries, and meat, poultry, or fish. Suggestions for vegetarians are also provided in the guidelines. The diet has three phases, enabling you to go from where you are now to where you want to be.

Terry Wahls, MD. *The Wahls Protocol: Cooking for Life.* New York, NY: Avery, 2017.

MEDITERRANEAN DIET

Research has found that the traditional Mediterranean diet reduces the risk of heart disease. In fact, the Mayo Clinic has reported that "a recent analysis of more than 1.5 million healthy adults demonstrated that following a Mediterranean diet was associated with a reduced risk of cardiovascular mortality, a reduced incidence of cancer and cancer mortality, and a reduced incidence of Parkinson's and Alzheimer's diseases." This is a very flavorful diet, with a wealth of traditional recipes.

Like most healthy diets, this one includes fresh fruits, vegetables, and whole grains, with fish as an option. The diet limits unhealthy fats. The majority of scientific organizations now encourage healthy adults to adapt a style of eating similar to that of the Mediterranean diet for the prevention of major chronic diseases.

PALEO (PALEOLITHIC DIET)

The rationale for the Paleo diet is explained by the Hypertension Institute of Vanderbilt University: "For millions of years, humans and their relatives have eaten meat, fish, fowl, and the leaves, roots, and fruits of many plants. One big obstacle to getting more calories from the environment is the fact that many plants are inedible. Grains, beans and potatoes are full of energy, but all are inedible in the raw state as they contain many toxins... [The Paleo diet] is the only diet that is coded for in our genes—it contains only those foods that were consumed 'on the table' during our long evolution, and discards those which were not."

This diet focuses on the types of whole foods available in the early stages of human development and avoids modern, commercially manufactured foods. The emphasis in this diet is on the widest variety of vegetables available. However, potatoes, sweet potatoes, corn, and other highly starchy vegetables are omitted, because in part they are the genetic creation of modern agriculture with no equivalent in the natural world. (The ancient form of these vegetables, like Peruvian potatoes and the Indian corn grown in the southwest are one-tenth the size of modern versions of potatoes and corn. The originals are higher in mineral content and much lower in carbs. High carbohydrate vegetables like potatoes and corn cause undesirable, rapid spikes in blood sugar.)

Hypertension Institute, Vanderbilt University. Paleo Diet. https://hypertensioninstitute. com/paleo-diet/. Accessed March 7, 2010.

The primary difference between this style of eating and that of the ketogenic diet is that keto diet has no starchy root vegetables, or high carb fruits (like grapes or bananas). The Paleo diet excludes common foods that induce inflammation and foods that have naturally occurring toxins, such as grains, beans, and potatoes, as well as nightshades. If this topic is of high interest, you may enjoy a review of the insightful research by Dr. Weston Price from the 1930s documenting the health and nutrition of indigenous people across the globe.

Weston A. Price, DDS. *Nutrition and Physical Degeneration, 8th edition.* Lemon Grove, CA: Price-Pottenger Foundation, 2009.

For more nutritional strategies, please see the website of Nancy Faass: www.TheNeverDietDiet.com.

PART 5
EXERCISE
Introduction
Judson Brandeis, MD

Press Release

German Pharmaceutical Company Ubung disclosed today the release of its new, experimental drug XC-100. This new wonder drug has many beneficial effects including:

- Weight loss
- Reduced risk of heart disease
- Reduced risk of type 2 diabetes
- Decreased depression
- Increased mental acuity
- Strengthened bones and muscles
- Reduced risk of colon, breast, uterine, and lung cancer
- Improved sleep
- Improved sexual health
- Reduced blood pressure
- Reduced cholesterol
- Improved longevity
- Improved digestion
- Boosted pain tolerance
- Increased self-esteem and confidence
- Decreased inflammation
- Reduced anxiety

Because of the tremendous benefits of XC-100, Ubung is going to make this available to all Americans for free. They are thinking about calling this new drug EXERCISE.

Chapter 37
Getting Back in Shape
Jerry Stine, Antiaging Coach

If you wait, all that happens is you get older.
— *Larry McMurtry*

As a nutritionist and trainer, I find that frequently my clients are overwhelmed by the idea of getting back in shape. Here's Jon's story:

I feel like a classic example of someone who's deconditioned. I used to run and lift weights. I was pretty strong and had lots of energy.

But as a programmer, I work insane hours, so I'm at the computer for long stretches. How am I ever going to get back in shape? I don't have a lot of time, and I'm frankly at a loss about where to start, given the weight I've gained and the muscle I've lost.

GETTING STARTED

Where to start? Begin with what has worked in the past. Weight training? Jogging? Brisk walking? Yoga? Swimming? The good news is that it's your choice.

- If you were a runner, start with brisk walking; then work up to alternating brisk walking with jogging, and then move on to jogging.

- If weight training appeals to you, start with a lower weight and more reps. Then over the course of the next few weeks, increase the number of reps every few days, using repetition to gain strength rather than moving on to heavier weights.

- Tennis player? If you haven't played in a while, it is important to warm up carefully to avoid high-impact injuries. Start with doubles.

STRENGTHEN CONNECTIVE TISSUE FIRST

Give yourself time to adapt. We can take a cue from the world of bodybuilders. They break down fitness into three different levels of adaptation, of which the first level is the most important. This early stage of training focuses on strengthening connective tissue.

Your connective tissue rebuilds at only 25% the rate of muscle. This means that in the first few weeks of exercise, you need to keep the intensity of your workouts very low.

Your improved muscle tone could mistakenly give the impression that you are ready to step up your game. In reality, you are still in an earlier phase, laying the foundation for joint stability.

Remember that the connective tissue in the joints is lagging *75%* behind in terms of development. You can clearly see the potential for injury here.

The connective tissue is functioning at a lower capacity, slowly building toward a stable base. This process underlies every form of exercise imaginable, including very low-impact activities like brisk walking, swimming, and yoga. The way to achieve strong connective tissue without injuring yourself is to begin with activity levels that don't feel like exercise at all, focusing on the basics, including range of motion.

Emerging from a serious health issue? If you are injured or feeling depleted, begin at a level so moderate, it almost feels like you're not doing anything. There should be absolutely no sense of strain. Your new program probably won't fit your old idea of exercise and fitness, yet a low-impact program can actually do a great deal. Any activity, at any level, can start the process, helping to move the body forward. As your body adapts, you can gradually increase the frequency, intensity, and duration.

To protect your joints, in the beginning use repetition to build your strength, rather than high-intensity workouts.

Be patient. When people are out of shape, often they want to get back in shape as quickly as possible. They become nostalgic, attempting to return to their glory days. In rushing things, they risk becoming extremely sore, or injured if they're unlucky. Have patience and compassion for yourself. Acknowledge where you are and start there.

WARM UP AND CHECK IN

If you're working out or exercising on your own (without a trainer), and you're out of shape, there are some basic strategies that will help you to avoid injury. In terms of the benefits of getting in shape, we could parade out all the facts and figures, but there's another perspective that will enable you to focus your approach and become more grounded.

Tune in to your body. In essence, you want to become more aware of how your body feels. The goal is to exercise in a way that brings that awareness and sensitivity forward, so you are in touch with your body. That is an important step in establishing your routine.

Among folks who are out of shape or overweight, many report that they have little awareness beyond their hands. They simply didn't feel their bodies. This can also be true of people who do mental or creative work, in a job that involves a sedentary workstyle or demands intense concentration. Picasso is quoted as saying, "When I enter the studio, I leave my body at the door . . . ."

Do a quick check-in each time you exercise. One way to increase your awareness of your body is to begin each exercise session with a brief self-assessment. This check-in and warm-up are crucial first steps.

- Each time you exercise or work out, start by doing slow, relaxed stretches: a forward bend, deep knee bend, slow arm circles, and gently twisting your body from side to side.

- As you go through your favorite stretches, your goal is to feel what's working and what's not, what's stiff and what's not, and what's comfortable and what's not.

- This check-in also functions as a warm-up.

- Tune in to your current situation in terms of exercise and progress. Are you seeing improvement in areas that were bothersome? Or are those areas getting worse?

Apply mindfulness. Self-awareness and mindfulness can also be applied to any form of exercise. Every time you work out or exercise, you are tuning in, asking yourself, "How is this feeling? Is this too much?" Then you can quickly regroup when necessary and think it through, "What else could I do that's a little easier?" As a bonus, mindful practice can provide an extra dimension that deepens the quality of your experience. There is extensive research showing that exercising mindfully produces better results.

MANAGING AN INJURY

If you already have an injury, then it's preferable to develop your exercise program by working with a professional such as a physical therapist, a personal trainer, or a chiropractor. And if you've been injured, the warm-up and check-in phase becomes even more important.

It's worthwhile to consider that age can affect recovery from injury. Younger men are less prone to injury and tend to recover more quickly. In older men, age-related changes to tendons and ligaments can increase the risk of injury and recovery may take longer. Respect where you are. Move forward step by step, knowing that if you stick it out, you will get where you want to go. Prevent the frustration of re-injury. Take pain seriously as a warning sign to slow the pace a bit so you can prevail.

Don't ignore feedback from your body. Do not try to push through the pain. Focus on exercises or movements that do not challenge the injured area.

Keep the intensity of your workouts low to reduce the risk of injury (or re-injury). As you exercise, the structures around those vulnerable areas will develop better circulation, inducing real healing and improvement. Again, if there is pain, note your limitations, and don't go beyond them.

Pain is a warning. Pain from an injury is a warning, a sign of damage or substantial loss of function. The purpose of pain is to indicate damage and to motivate us to avoid additional damaging activities and situations. This protects the body and provides an opportunity for healing. Our main focus here is on coping with pain from an injury, but you can also apply the same strategy to deal with pain caused by a disease such as osteoarthritis.

Anti-inflammatories are optimal after your workout (but not before). It is also very important not to use over-the-counter (OTC) anti-inflammatory drugs to help you work through injury or soreness. Anti-inflammatories can mask pain, and you won't know whether you're overdoing it or not. However, anti-inflammatories are good *after* a workout. There are numerous kinds of OTC and nutritional support products that can be helpful with recovery. (For more information, see the Resources section at the end of the chapter.)

PAYOFFS OF EXERCISE

Easing into exercise will enable you to focus your approach and become more grounded.

Building energy and endurance. You may feel that you don't have the energy to begin. People who are deconditioned tend to have low energy due to fewer mitochondria. The thousands of mitochondria within each cell are the sources of your energy production. Know that exercise stimulates the growth of more mitochondria, increasing the capacity of your body to make energy. But that doesn't happen overnight. Premier athletes have tons of mitochondria, which they got by exercising, but it can take years to achieve this level of peak performance.

Supporting longevity. The importance of exercise to health has been very powerfully demonstrated in an ongoing research study at Stanford University with serious runners who have been tracked by a research team for at least 15 years. This is the only human experiment showing an activity that is confirmed to increase longevity.

Using media to stay engaged. If you find low-impact exercise boring, do something that will keep your interest while you exercise. Listen to an audiobook. Listen to music, especially upbeat music. Exercise outside. Watch television or a video. Do whatever suits your preference and keeps you involved. Many men are motivated by videos that are physically inspiring: martial arts movies, Olympic reruns, footage on triathlons, or documentaries about top athletes. Let the exercise engage your body at your level, whatever that level is, trusting that the ongoing process of activity on a regular basis will bring about the result you want without force, strain, inflammation, or injury.

Mixing it up. Cross-training is an important concept, especially for older men. Overuse injuries are prevalent. It's good to include different types of exercise over the course of a week. Jogging or brisk walking (not strolling) pairs well with yoga or resistance training. Or you could use a set schedule, such as swimming during the week and biking on the weekends. Or it can be whatever you want to do that day or time of day. (You might look for opportunities to exercise outside like jogging on the beach, hiking, or doing yoga outdoors.) Switching it up (cross-training) helps prevent overuse injuries.

Most people do better if they schedule time to exercise in their calendar.

Letting go of criticism. Be forgiving of yourself. No criticism. If you miss a day (or a week, whatever it is), let go of self-judgement. Just let it go. Simply come back to your practice and begin again. It's like doing meditation, but you're doing it physically, with physical movement. (For more on coping with self-criticism and negative self-talk, see the invaluable classic by David Burns, MD, *Feeling Good*.)

Drawing inspiration from videos, apps, and online resources. There are a huge number of online resources to instruct, encourage, and track your exercise. Search for the specific video or app for the type of exercise of interest. You will find a wealth of information under search terms such as "weight training videos," or "yoga for men," or "cross-training for runners." You can even focus the search by the level of experience you have, ranging from beginner to advanced. There are video instructions for yoga, tai chi, and qigong. These can be fun even if you have never done these activities before. Try a number of them; you may find that you enjoy all of them. This can be a great source of new ideas for your program and less expensive than a trainer if you are on a budget.

Keeping an exercise journal. It is useful to have a little exercise notebook for jotting quick notes: "Soreness in left elbow has healed / Did 5 more pushups today, total 20! / Still stiff in the morning." Whatever your response or progress, make a note of it. There are also a large number of apps for tracking your exercise. Search for "exercise tracking apps." Some of the fitness trackers styled like a watch monitor your pulse and other data to give a more detailed picture of what your body is experiencing while exercising. This is not just for your own use. It can be very helpful if you need some kind of coaching, adjustment, or treatment from a trainer, a chiropractor, or a physician. The act of keeping track of your exercise in a journal or with an app is also a powerful tool for self-accountability. Maintaining the journal becomes a reward in itself.

KEY TAKE AWAYS

Most of us have a preconceived idea of fitness. When we're out of shape, we're obviously a long way from that ideal. It seems like an impossible gap. And, in fact, it *is* impossible. You can't go from unfit to fit in any kind of short timeframe. No one can.

Rather, begin with a mindset of compassion and acceptance of your current condition, understanding that you're not going to push things, you're not going to try to move huge weights, run long distances, or do any of the exercises that you used to do. The risk of injury or severe soreness has to be respected, so you don't wind up taking one step forward and two steps back. Accept the fact that the pace needs to be slow at the start. This may require you to adjust your expectations in order to set more realistic goals. Simply stay current with your immediate situation and bring the presence of mindfulness to everything you do. Maintain a thoughtful, accepting view of yourself as you move through the process to become more fit.

RESOURCES

Anti-inflammatory products. In addition to over-the-counter anti-inflammatories, there are a variety of well-researched, herbal anti-inflammatory products. They can be helpful in quenching inflammation and can be used on an ongoing basis for pain. Again, we recommend not using any anti-inflammatory *before* you exercise to avoid inadvertently masking pain. You want to be able to feel what's happening in your body while you're exercising so you don't overdo it. For this reason, anti-inflammatories are best taken *after* exercise. They can also be taken with the connective tissue support products discussed below. Many different supplement companies make their own version of these natural supplements.

Connective tissue/joint support. These formulas contain nutrients the body requires to restore, strengthen, and maintain connective tissue. This type of product is particularly useful as you step up the intensity of your exercise program or if you're rehabilitating from an injury. The apparent reduction in pain and inflammation comes about not because of an analgesic effect, but because the connective tissue itself is actually healing and getting stronger.

Nutrient support for performance. There is a wide range of products aimed at maximizing strength, endurance, and muscle growth from exercise, including amino acid blends, protein powders, adaptogenic herbs, and hormone support. These products help you get the most benefit from the time you invest in exercise and can be especially useful for older men. Working with a nutritionist, personal trainer, or health coach can also be helpful in setting up a program.

Amino acids for recovery. There are amino acid supplements that effectively improve the recovery from exercise by providing several benefits. They not only minimize the breakdown of muscle tissue, they also turn exercise into a positive experience by supplying the specialized amino acids that are required for growing muscle and connective tissue.

Quality food and quality sleep. Support your fitness efforts with good food and sleep. The exercise will help improve your sleep. Sleep is the time when the body performs major repair and restoration, so not getting enough sleep handicaps recovery. (For instance, it is during sleep that the body generates new mitochondria.) You don't want to be burning the candle at both ends trying to recover energy and endurance. The combination of more exercise, good food, sleep, and rest is essential to rebuild a strong, pain-free body and develop more energy and stamina.

Bodywork. There are many different types of massage and restorative bodywork. Some of these disciplines have become highly evolved in the assessment of individual structural needs. An in-depth assessment is followed by focused, individualized manual therapy, which can produce remarkable results. This type of comprehensive approach helps return the body to a more normal, supple ease of function. Although there are other schools of bodywork, the best-known of these systems is Rolfing (www.Rolf.org).

PEMF for sleep and recovery. Pulsed electromagnetic frequency (PEMF) devices can provide effective support for quality sleep and for recovery. This type of device first gained FDA approval in 1979 for bone and tissue healing. Dr. William Pawluk, MD, the North American expert on PEMF (with a background in internal medicine and teaching in major medical schools), has 25 years of experience in the research and applications of these devices. For more information, see www.FlexPulse.com, www.DrPawluk.com, or his book, *Power Tools for Healing*.

Foam rollers for stretching and self-massage. Foam rollers are very useful in an exercise or recovery program. For example, you can use a roller at bedtime to help you sleep, to recover from the day's physical stresses, and for relaxation. As always, take it easy when you begin. The rollers are made from a dense foam, are about 5 to 6 inches in diameter, and come in different lengths from 12 to 36 inches. If you are only getting one size, get the 36-incher. They are very popular and available anywhere exercise products are sold. There are many different ways to use a foam roller, with numerous videos online. Just search for "foam roller videos." Some of the best are those by physical therapists and trainers performing entry-level stretches. Check out a few videos to see which exercises with the roller appeal to you.

BOOKS

B.K.S. Iyengar, *Iyengar Yoga: The Path to Holistic Health,* revised edition. New York, NY: DK, 2013.

Mark Stephens and Sally Kempton, *Yoga for Sleep*. Berkeley, CA: North Atlantic Books, 2020.

Jon Kabat-Zinn, PhD, *Full-Catastrophe Living*. New York, NY: Bantam, 2013.

Aaron Alexander, *The Align Method*. New York, NY: Grand Central Publishing, 2019.

Ben Greenfield, *Boundless*. Las Vegas, NV: Victory Belt Publishing, 2020.

David Burns, MD, *Feeling Good: The New Mood Therapy*. New York, NY: Harper, 2012.

**For more information on the work of Jerry Stine,
please see www.LifespanInstitute.com.**

Chapter 38
Joint Health Is the Key to Staying Active
Will Workman, MD, Orthopedist

Everyone pities the weak. Jealousy you have to earn.
— *Arnold Schwartzenneger*

Using our bodies for sports and recreation is a gift that most of us took for granted in our younger years. Those of us who continue to pursue an active life realize that the body doesn't so easily submit to the intense impact and gyrations that we once breezed through. The aches and pains of sore and sometimes injured muscles, tendons, ligaments, or joints were not so common and pronounced in our recollection of the glory years. For some, the response is to increase the intake of anti-inflammatory supplements, brace up, and forge ahead—ignoring signs of strain and the body's cry for recovery. Others will take a more mature, thoughtful approach and commit to conditioning the body so that it remains supple, powerful, and minimally damaged. At some point, this perspective becomes essential if we want sports and recreation to remain an integral part of our life. I want you to be one of those guys.

HOW MOVEMENT MAXIMIZES FUNCTION

Continued participation in sports and activity not only represents a recreational outlet for psychological well-being, but also helps the body run optimally. When it comes to joint health, keeping the joints moving is essential to maximize function. Studies show that passive motion at the knee joint (that is, moving the knee without significant impact) can actually stimulate cartilage growth.

Think preventively. However, being active and in motion with the addition of impact—such as that involved with jogging, full-court basketball, or singles tennis—can hasten the destruction of already vulnerable middle-aged cartilage. This is particularly true if there has been prior trauma. So, often, the little signals by way of aches and pains that we feel in the joint—sharp pain, lingering pain, periodic locking, or clicking—are all signs of a joint at risk. We must heed these signals in order to maintain effective usefulness through middle age and beyond.

Sitting is the new smoking. One of the bigger mistakes one can make when the joints start to demand our attention is to switch to a sedentary lifestyle. Immediately, the lack of activity may lead to weight gain, which is hard on joints, and the lack of movement means that there is no stimulation to keep cartilage healthy. Numerous studies have found that a knee with cartilage damage will have accelerated wear, meaning quicker time to cartilage loss, to bone-on-bone friction, and pain. Heavier patients tend to wear out more quickly.

Solution—low-impact sports and exercise. Clearly, it is important to be active and play sports, but some sports can make your joints hurt. Stopping sports and activity won't help, so the answer is to make better choices of activity. Choose sports and exercise that involve motion without impact, that are kinder to joints:

- Swimming
- Biking
- Canoeing and kayaking
- Surfing
- Tai chi and qigong
- Yoga
- Doubles' tennis
- Golf, walking
- Weight training
- Walking and hiking.

CARE AND MAINTENANCE FOR STRONG JOINTS

There isn't one set way in which the joints wear out. They can wear out from disuse, overuse (alternating disuse/overuse), and, for some, from choosing the wrong parents. Overuse is defined as narrowly constrained activity patterns, a form of repetitive motion, at high volume. (There is risk of these overuse patterns not only in our choice of exercise, but also in the workplace, both in office work and jobs involving physical labor.) Any of these types of unintended abuse can lead to painful joints with limited mobility. So the key to keeping your joints feeling good and functioning well is to:

- Keep your weight down
- Choose lower-impact type sports and activities
- Perform sports, exercise, and activity in moderation
- Maintain a variety of activities and dynamic movement patterns.

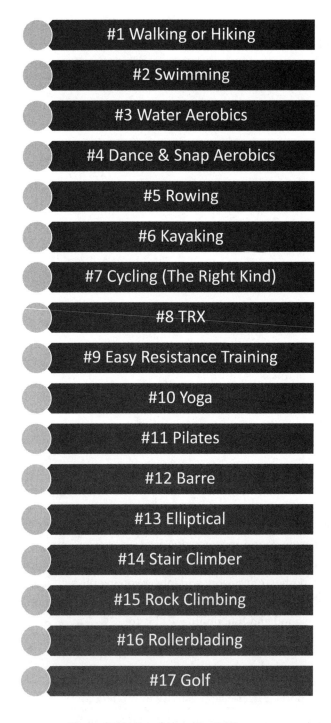

Figure 36.1. Low-impact activities.

Building tendons to support joint function. Finding a way to reliably restore articular joint cartilage remains the holy grail of orthopedic surgery, but there are other ways to positively affect joint function and health. While nothing can be done to bring cartilage back, strengthening the muscles and tendons around the joint effectively unloads the strain on the joint. Studies have shown that tendons become much stronger when they are stimulated by activity.

The stimulus of a strength workout actually results in thickening of the fibers (stronger fibers!) and increased cross-links between fibers (stronger fiber bundles!) resulting in a stronger overall tendon. Think of your tendons as springs (or shock absorbers) attached to your joints. The stronger the spring, the more energy it can absorb. Instead of force being absorbed in the joint surface, your tendons—or springs—will absorb the shock. Think of an old car with worn out springs bouncing down the road versus a well-tuned, race-ready sports car flying down the road. I know which one I want to drive.

Minimizing weight gain and its impact. Getting rid of excess body weight is helpful in reducing the load on the joints and decreasing the breakdown of cartilage. In one study, investigators measured blood levels of a protein from cartilage breakdown after walking exercise. They compared groups differing by 40% in weight. The heavier subjects showed significant increases in cartilage breakdown immediately after walking.

Strength and flexibility training serve many purposes in the quest to maintain an optimally functioning body. We have mentioned its effects on tendons, but it also is associated with weight loss. The more muscle a person has, the higher the metabolism. A stronger and more flexible body makes sports and physical activity all that much better and more enjoyable. Similar to the age-related loss of bone known as osteoporosis, there is also an age-related decline in muscle mass. Building and maintaining that muscle now will make things better in the future.

Strength training. There are many ways to do strength training. As a rule of thumb for middle-aged men, the goal should be to get toned and strong in preparation for activity rather than for body-building competition. Orthopedic surgeons often see men who have focused on very heavy lifting for super strength and body building who end up with broken-down arthritic joints from years of overuse. For the most part, muscle strengthening, when done properly, is a safe, low-impact activity. Anything from free-weights, machines, and body-weight-type exercises can be done with safety. With the advent of routines such as Crossfit, we have seen an emphasis on functional weight lifting, which incorporates several muscle groups at once. The key is to maintain a moderate, gradual approach to the exercises so that muscles have time to recover and adapt to the load and exercise. This again is something that we middle-agers can be all too painfully aware of. In our glory years, a few months layoff from the gym might mean a day or two of soreness when we resumed. Now, it may take a week!

We typically think of strength training as the only way to increase and maintain muscle mass, but even here a focus on diet and weight can be helpful. Studies have shown that calorie restriction, for example, can diminish damage to DNA in our cells. Damaged DNA leads to decreased levels of proteins involved in the health and vitality of muscles. Clearly, the calorie restriction should also be accompanied by choosing calories that nourish the body.

Focusing on activities that minimize joint impact and eating the right food in the right amounts are premiere strategies to achieve health and vitality now and into old age.

PAIN MANAGEMENT

Anti-inflammatory supplements. As we age, for some of us it becomes essential to find a way to enhance pain relief and the function of our joints. In these scenarios, one may turn to medications or supplements to help. While most prescription and over-the-counter medications are regulated and cannot be marketed beyond what they have been proven to do, supplements are not so closely scrutinized. The labels may contain claims that aren't necessarily (and often not) backed by science, but it doesn't mean they can't be helpful. Suggested here are key supplements that have some science to support them.

- **Krill oil and other Omega 3 oils**. Krill oil is derived from a tiny shrimp-like animal that whales enjoy eating. It contains fatty acids that are similar to fish oil and can help with inflammation in general, and has been shown to help with inflammation and pain associated with arthritis.

- *Boswellia serrata.* Better known as frankincense, this ancient spice is derived from the resin of a branching tree found in India. It is thought to have anti-inflammatory properties. The Arthritis Foundation recommends taking approximately 300–400 milligrams (mg) of boswellia three times per day to deliver bo-swellic acids to the body. Their recommendation is to look for a formulation that contains 60% boswellic acid as the active ingredient.

- **Curcumin.** This is the phytoactive form of the spice turmeric, the active constituent within the spice that provides healing benefits. Like many other medicinals, it has been used in the far east for millennia and has more recently been adopted as a joint pain-relieving supplement.

A PERSONAL EXERCISE PLAN

Once your diet and supplement game is on point, it is time to scrutinize your exercise plan, or lack thereof. The health benefits of exercise we have already noted, but getting to the right level of exercise so that one reaps the benefits without getting injured is often the trick. While the joints are still healthy and feeling good in middle age, that is the time to develop a balanced plan going forward.

- **Balancing high and low exertion.** High exertion for strength and power (judiciously applied) with low exertion to build and maintain aerobic capacity.

- **Resistance training.** Resistance-type exercise like weights and Crossfit.

- **Endurance training.** Endurance activities like swimming, biking, and running.

- **Low-impact movement.** With onset of disease and joint pain (or even before!) it is critical to still keep the joints moving, but equally critical to minimize impact on the joints with a switch to lower-impact aerobic activity such as swimming, rowing, tai chi, Pilates, yoga, and biking, to name a partial list of lower-impact sports and activities.

The key with all the exercises is adapting to them slowly with time for recovery between activities (read: taking the rest of the day off) to allow our not-so-youthful tissues to recover and repair and be ready for the next onslaught of activity.

Now that you have it *all* under control—proper diet, proper exercise, maybe supplements—is there anything left that the doctor can help with?

MEDICATIONS

Apart from the standard NSAID regimen that aging athletes know all too well—such as Aleve, Motrin, Advil, and ibuprofen—there are a couple of other meds that can be of some help.

- **Topical NSAIDs.** The first is simply a topical form of an NSAID. Think Ben Gay meets Motrin, only the NSAID in the ointment is a prescription NSAID called Voltaren. The specific preparation is Voltaren Gel that can be topically applied to sore joints and works well to temporarily alleviate symptoms. It is particularly good for those who get an upset stomach when taking NSAIDS, as Voltaren is not ingested orally, but rather rubbed on the skin.

- **Platelet-rich plasma (PRP).** In addition to medications, one area that is showing increasing promise in the treatment of degenerative arthritis is injections that nourish the tissue. Platelet-rich plasma (PRP) is obtained by drawing a small amount of blood from the patient and placing it in a centrifuge to concentrate the healing factors from the blood. This concentrate is then injected into the affected joint, where alpha granules from the platelets release multiple growth factors and cytokines (immune-signaling proteins), which decrease inflammation and support cartilage health and metabolism. Increasingly, our medical scientific literature is publishing studies showing favorable outcomes compared to other types of injections.

MEDICAL INTERVENTIONS

In the event that we have gone through all available options and still haven't gotten the situation under control, there are recent, promising diagnostic and treatment options that have evolved to more precisely correct the damage and ongoing disease of arthritis.

MRI evaluations and cartilage mapping. MRI can now look at cartilage and the quality of cartilage via cartilage mapping. This is a specific sequencing that color codes the joint surface to expose unhealthy areas of cartilage on the otherwise healthy surface. This can allow surgeons to choose from a multitude of options for those with limited lesions to help the body fill the cartilage defects.

Grafting. Donor cartilage and host cartilage options can be used to graft the deficient areas and allow for healing. Some of these techniques are now more than two decades old and are continually being refined. With the help of MRI, we can now identify patterns of meniscus tearing that are amenable to repair, giving the patient the opportunity to undergo a procedure to save the meniscus instead of having it removed. Even in the presence of degenerative change in the knee, the repaired meniscus restores stability and cushioning that would otherwise vanish if the meniscus was removed.

Joint replacement. The endpoint procedure we all dread and want to avoid is total joint replacement. There is good reason for this, as it is a big, painful procedure with some incidence of fairly significant complications. Additionally, several authors have reported a dissatisfaction rate with total knee replacement approaching 20%. Despite this, progress continues to be made in refining materials and techniques. Currently, my patients have the option of receiving a custom-made knee replacement built entirely from a model based on a three-dimensional CT scan of their own knee. The knee replacement parts are made specifically for that individual patient and no other. What's more, the instruments that are used to make the precision cuts necessary to ensure adequate fit and alignment are 3D printed, based on the same CT scan.

While we can do our best to be fit and eat well, sometimes our genetics and life history get in the way of optimal joint health. Choosing to eat well and participating in low-impact activities can help keep the joints working well, but if that isn't enough, a host of supplements, medications, injections, and even surgery can help keep you in the game.

For more information about the medical practice of Dr. William Workman, please see: https://www.calsportsdoc.com/.

Chapter 39
Remember to Stretch
Judson Brandeis, MD, Urologist
& Johnny Jackson, Personal Trainer

Notice that the stiffest tree is most easily cracked,
while the bamboo and the willow survive by bending with the wind.
— *Bruce Lee*

Flexibility is an area of health and wellness that is especially important as a man ages. Flexibility improves poise, posture, muscle coordination, and stability, reducing the risk of injuries.

When you stretch, you are elongating the muscle fibers. If your muscles are tight, this is due to muscle filaments that remain in a shortened state, reducing your flexibility and overall mobility. As you stretch and the muscle elongates, this realigns the muscle fibers. Once the fibers are appropriately aligned and organized, they work better, feel better, and function properly, with a reduced risk of injury.

Skeletal muscles move bones and produce force. Movement of the muscle fibers creates muscle elasticity as well as strength and muscle size (for example, through exercise and resistance training). The unfortunate aspect of muscle tissue is that it's a matter of "use it or lose it." Sedentary men lose muscle size over time unless they are active and exercise regularly.

Tendons are sturdy connective tissue that attaches muscle to bone. Tendons are present at both ends of each muscle where collagen fibers fuse onto the bone, which allows the muscle to provide and withstand tension. Tendons have extraordinary tensile strength, greater than that of steel cable.

Ligaments attach one bone to another and aid in stabilizing a joint (such as the knee). Their role is to allow the joint to move, yet to maintain stabilization and proper alignment. Within the knee joint, for example, four different ligaments keep the knee bones in place and stabilized to prevent injury.

REDUCING THE RISK OF INJURY

As we age, our tissues tend to be less well hydrated (less water is present in our tissues), which can cause a loss of elasticity in skeletal muscle and stiffness in joints and tendons. A daily stretching protocol promotes flexibility and the free movement of muscles, tendons, and ligaments. However, not all stretching is created equal:

- **Active stretching** takes the muscle beyond its normal range of motion.

- **Passive stretching** allows the muscles and tendons to stretch naturally without the use of additional forces acting on the muscle/tendon. However, flexibility improves more slowly with passive stretching.

There are four major types of stretching—static, PNF, dynamic, and ballistic:

- **Static stretching** is a general-purpose technique in which the muscle is slowly stretched and then held for several seconds. This type of stretching allows the muscle to relax, achieving a greater length and more extended stretch. This is the most frequently used and most recommended type of stretching, with low risk of injury.

- **PNF** (proprioceptive neuromuscular facilitation) stretching is a much longer stretching session and requires a partner's help. This type of stretching is the most effective form of stretching, but it is also considered the most painful.

- **Dynamic stretching** is a technique that many athletes utilize. This approach puts the muscles through a full range of motion, while mirroring movements used in a given sport or athletic activity; for example, swinging a leg repetitively.

- **Ballistic stretching** uses the momentum of a moving body or a limb in an attempt to force it beyond its normal range of motion. Here the stretch is achieved by bouncing into a stretched position. Ballistic stretching uses muscles as a spring, but bouncing can stretch ligaments too far.

When should you stretch? Anytime you exercise, you should make sure you take the time to stretch properly. It is important to have a daily stretching routine that will help create lasting improvements in your flexibility and overall mobility. The optimal time to stretch is after any typical physical activity such as cardiovascular training or resistance training. That is the perfect time to work on your flexibility, since the muscles and ligaments are warm and limber.

THE DAILY STRETCH

Need a quick 10-minute morning routine? Not sure where to start with a stretching routine? This daily stretch routine will take on average around 20 minutes to complete if you do four total sets of each stretch.

Hold each stretch for 30 seconds. Many consider 15 seconds "good enough," but as you age, you need a longer duration for the stretch. Research has shown that 30 seconds seems to be the sweet spot, and anything longer usually does not provide further benefit. Additionally, studies have found that if you hold a stretch for more than 45 seconds, that could negatively impact your speed, strength, and power.

- **Don't bounce a stretch.** Holding a stretch is more effective, and there is less risk of injury.

- **Don't hold your breath.** Instead, continue to breathe normally and use the breath to deepen a stretch.

Muscles have built-in sensory receptors—muscle spindles—that protect the muscle from stretching too far and causing injury. As you elongate and stretch the muscle, you will reach a point where the muscle is taut and there is some slight discomfort, but not pain. That is the sweet spot, the point where you should hold the stretch.

Repeat the stretch. You will want to repeat each stretch an additional two or more times for a total of three to five sets and then move onto your next stretch. The reason for repetition is to fully stretch out the muscle spindles, which become accustomed to the stretch. This allows you to achieve an even deeper stretch with each session.

DAILY STRETCH ROUTINE

Stretch	*Duration to Hold The Stretch*	*Number of Total Sets*
Upper Back Stretch		
Shoulder Stretch*		
Neck Stretch*		
Spinal Twist Stretch*		
Quadriceps Stretch		
Hamstring Stretch		
Calf Stretch		

Figure 39.1. A format for tracking your stretching routine.
* These stretches require both sides to be stretched independently.

Never stretch cold muscles. Muscles that have not been warmed up lack proper blood flow, inhibiting their flexibility. If you begin stretching before the muscles relax and have adequate blood flow, that runs the risk of pulling or tearing a muscle.

Don't consider stretching to be a warmup. The current thinking is that stretching cold muscles increases the risk of injury. Before stretching, warm up with light walking, jogging, or biking at low intensity for 5 to 10 minutes. Even better, stretch after your workout when your muscles are warm.

- **Skip stretching before an intense activity**, such as sprinting or track and field activities. Some research suggests that pre-event stretching may actually decrease performance. Research has also shown that stretching immediately before an event can weaken hamstring strength.

- **Performing a dynamic warmup** involves movements similar to those in your sport or physical activity at a low level, then gradually increasing the speed and intensity as you warm up.

- **Strive for symmetry**, since everyone's genetics are a bit different in terms of flexibility. Rather than striving initially for the flexibility of a dancer or gymnast, focus on achieving equal flexibility side to side to prevent injury (especially if you have a history of previous injury).

- **Focus on major muscle groups.** Concentrate your stretches on major muscle groups such as your lower back or neck and shoulders, and stretch both sides.

MUSCULOSKELETAL ISSUES

SIGNS AND SYMPTOMS

- **Muscle cramps and spasms** are whole muscle contractions, ranging from mild to stabbing sensations.

- **Inflamed trigger points** are focal areas of localized muscle spasm and involve no actual damage to the muscle. Trigger points can become exquisitely painful and, surprisingly, can persist for years. Intervention involves trigger point massage with a trained therapist or good self-care (see the excellent self-care guides from New Harbinger).

- **Delayed onset muscle soreness** that men experience after heavy exertion of underused muscles is due to microscopic damage to the muscle fibers, which results in inflammation and pain.

- **Muscle strains** occur when an overwhelming force causes the tissue to tear. This may involve either the muscle itself, the junction between the muscle and tendon (most common), or the attachment of the tendon to the bone. During activities that require explosive movements, such as pushing off during a sprint or quickly changing directions, the force across the connected muscle and tendon can be so great that tissues tear.

- **Muscles that cross two joints are the most susceptible to injury.** They include the quadriceps (the hip and knee joints), the hamstrings (between the hip and knee joints), and the calf (the knee and ankle joints).

Factors that can predispose an athlete to injury. Risk increases when there is less flexibility, lack of strength in the muscle, and/or fatigue, as well as with age or previous muscle injury. Many athletes sustain muscle injuries when they first begin a training regimen.

GRADES OF MUSCLE STRAIN

The severity of a strain depends on how much strength and range of motion are lost, which can determine recovery time. Muscle strains are categorized into three grades, based on severity:

- *Grade 1.* Mild damage to individual muscle fibers (less than 5% of fibers) that causes minimal loss of strength and motion.

- *Grade 2.* Greater than 5% damages, but less than a complete rupture. These injuries present with significant loss of strength and motion and may require two to three months before a complete return to athletics and a full schedule of activities.

- *Grade 3.* Complete rupture of a muscle or tendon. These can present with a palpable defect in the muscle or tendon and swelling. These injuries sometimes require surgery to reattach the damaged muscle or tendon.

When a muscle is initially injured, men often report sudden stabbing pain, followed by swelling and bruising. After this inflammatory phase, the muscle begins to heal by regenerating muscle fibers from stem cells in the area of injury. However, a significant amount of scar tissue also forms in the area of the injury. Over time, this scar tissue remodels, but the muscle tissue may never fully regenerate.

If you strain a muscle or tendon, you should immediately implement the RICE strategy.

R - Rest – Keep pressure off the injured area to prevent further damage and allow the body to start the recovery process.

I - Ice – Apply an ice pack for 20 minutes multiple times throughout the day, but make sure the ice is not in direct contact with the skin.

C - Compression – Wrap the injured area with a compression bandage such as an ACE wrap, but not so tightly that it cuts off circulation. The goal is to manage the swelling, while providing support for the area.

E - Elevation – Place the limb at a level higher than your heart to help minimize inflammation.

Once the swelling has subsided, apply heat (like a heating pad) to the area to help improve blood flow. Typically a strain can last several weeks, and if the strain is more severe, it could take months to return to normal.

As we age, we naturally tend to become less flexible, and our muscles become less elastic. Stretching lengthens and aligns muscle fibers, allowing muscles to function optimally.

This is motivation to emphasize low-impact activity and dynamic movement ranging from walking and hiking to swimming or cycling, and qigong or yoga.

For additional information, please see:
www.TheTwentyFirstCenturyMan.com.

Chapter 40
Yoga for Real Men
Dean Pohlman, Yoga Instructor

Yoga is not about touching your toes, it is what you learn on the way down.
— Jigar Gor

Yoga is a physical, mental, and often spiritual practice that can provide incredible benefit to men at all phases of life. Whether you're a couch potato, an active guy, or just want to be a bit more healthy, yoga can help you perform physically at a higher level, increase your ability to concentrate, and keep your body feeling great throughout the day.

Beyond the benefits of physical fitness, yoga promotes better sleep, lower stress, and improved heart rate variability (HRV). It can also support more satisfying sex.

You don't have to join an ashram or live a yogic lifestyle to reap these benefits. All you need is an average of 10 minutes a day to begin fitting a few yoga postures into your weekly or daily routines. Best of all, it's now easier than ever to practice yoga. You can follow pre-recorded workouts online, join a live class on Zoom, or visit a local yoga studio if you want the in-person experience. Find the teacher and the style that works best for you, and the rest should flow naturally.

Contrary to what you may have heard, yoga is not "just stretching," and you don't have to be flexible to do it. (For the same reason that we lift weights to get stronger, we practice yoga so we can become more limber. Stretching is just one aspect of yoga.)

In fact, far from being reserved for the young and flexible, yoga can be done by men of all ages and fitness levels, as long as you have the proper instructor teaching you appropriate modifications.

While women still make up the majority of attendance at yoga studios, you'll now find plenty of yoga studios filled with more men than women. (Yoga was originally practiced exclusively by men. It wasn't until it became popular in the West that it became a primarily female activity.)

Unique Benefits of Yoga

If I have piqued your interest and you want to practice yoga, there are five aspects of the practice that make it useful for overall fitness and well-being:

1. *Emphasis on breathing.* This deepens your practice, going beyond fitness.
2. *Practicing mindfulness.* Awareness is expanded through the immersion of focus on breath, body perception, and movement.
3. *Targeting core and hip muscles.* Yoga provides strength to address common muscular imbalances and weaknesses. This can help to prevent issues such as back pain, knee and hip problems, sciatica, and other physical conditions that we experience as a result of living a mostly sedentary lifestyle.
4. *Slow, controlled movements.* This is a superb way to develop coordination, body awareness, and strength, regardless of how fit you are at this moment.
5. *Supporting both flexibility and endurance.* The nature of the physical postures (asanas) in yoga facilitates a range of fitness benefits, including balance and mobility. This increased physical capability can provide a solid foundation of fitness for anyone of any age—especially when practiced appropriately.

#1. BREATHING

Yoga focuses on breathing to help you develop the relationship between respiration and your body's physiological responses. Breathing is a natural physiologic process that you can learn to influence and manage with mindfulness.

By paying attention, you develop an awareness of how your body responds to all the sequences of the breath, including the inhale, the exhale, and the space between these actions. Through practice, you'll develop the ability to use your breathing to complement movement, to relax and stretch more deeply into the postures. Breathwork enables you to maintain your composure when exerting yourself physically, and to release muscle tension.

The time spent practicing breathing will translate into your day-to-day life as well. You'll develop the ability to recognize when you are becoming stressed, and how to use your breath to help your body and mind relax. Whether you are driving in bumper-to-bumper traffic, are in the middle of an intense meeting, or are in the thick of a stressful situation with loved ones, you will be better able to stop, pause, and manage the stress.

In sum, the benefits of improved breathing won't just improve your fitness—it will also reduce your overall stress, improve your focus, and help you be more present in your life.

#2. MINDFULNESS—Breath, body awareness, and movement in combination

Most of us are aware of the benefits of mindfulness, but few of us do much to improve our mindfulness regularly. Mindfulness, like your muscular strength, is something to be trained. Yoga is a perfect opportunity to do just that.

One aspect of mindfulness involves being in the present moment. Yoga helps you experience the present without worrying about what happened in the past or what's going to happen in the future. The concentration required to perform the postures (asanas) correctly forces you to engage in the present. By its very nature, yoga is the ideal vehicle for mindfulness practice.

The ability to be immersed in the present moment has been a goal of philosophers throughout history. As Tolstoy wrote: "Remember then: there is only one time that is important – now! It is the most important time because it is the only time when we have any power."

Consider any given posture. A standing mountain pose, for example, requires you to stand with perfect posture, your feet parallel to one another, hips and spine in neutral alignment, palms facing forward, and shoulders relaxed. While doing this, you want to also ensure that your breathing stays consistent, inhaling and exhaling slowly, using your inhales to stand taller and lengthen your spine. Use your exhales to lightly tighten your core, and to make sure your body remains properly aligned. Every posture involves a constant process of checking in with your breath, checking your body positioning, and then checking back in with your breath. This focus creates a tranquil state of mind that is quite extraordinary.

The mindfulness needed when you perform a series of dynamic movements that are physically complex requires you to focus more intensely. When practicing yoga in this way, it becomes impossible to worry about that embarrassing thing you did earlier today or to dread that event you don't want to go to later this week. The movements require you to stay present, and like the breathing work, this mindfulness will carry over into the rest of your life.

#3. CORE STRENGTHENING

Core strength is essential to any type of fitness, and even more so to those of us who spend our days sitting (or standing) at our desks. Although most of us understand the importance of core strength intellectually, almost all of us lack essential strength in this area.

You might think that you're targeting your core and hips with weight lifting sessions, but unless you've done the necessary strengthening to train your core muscles, you're probably just using your knees and your lower back. This is precisely why you hear people say, "I don't do squats – they hurt my knees" or "I don't do deadlifts anymore, because it hurts my back." It's not because the exercise itself is inherently wrong; it's because we don't have the necessary strength in our hips and core.

Drop the philosophy of "No pain, no gain." Similarly, believing that "Pain is weakness leaving the body" just puts you at risk of injuring yourself. Pain occurs when we don't have the proper strength or mobility to complete a specific movement or move a particular load. The preventable injuries or exercise-related pain that the vast majority of us experience can usually be traced back to a lack of strength in the hips or core area.

Yoga is an excellent way to target core strength. Using the proper technique, it's impossible not to strengthen these areas. Beyond improving your yoga practice, you'll notice the benefits of this improved strength in many other facets of your life, including your workouts, the state of your muscles and joints the day after a workout, and even how you feel at the end of an average work day.

#4. CONTROLLED MOVEMENT—Enhanced coordination, muscle activation, and strength

If you think about most typical forms of exercise, few of them move slowly. With running, swimming, and even weight lifting, the goal is to finish laps or reps as quickly as possible, and then move on to the next thing. This objective makes sense when you're trying to elevate your heart rate and work up a sweat, but the lack of slow, controlled movement usually comes at the expense of proper technique. It's only when we repeatedly practice something slowly with deliberate movement and focused attention that we're able to refine the technique. This is critical when it comes to exercising with longevity in mind.

Injury prevention. The majority of exercise-related injuries are entirely preventable with the right training. That starts with slow, controlled movement to develop the coordination and strength that ensures we are using proper technique. Yoga is perfect for building muscle strength because it involves foundational exercises that make up basic human patterns of movement, such as squats, lunges, side bends, twists, and so on.

Body awareness. When we move slowly, we also have the opportunity to practice increased awareness of our body. Moving quickly does not give us this opportunity. Think of this awareness as the ability to notice and feel the different parts of your body.

Muscle awareness. Another major area of emphasis is motor control, (also referred to as muscle activation), which is the ability to control specific sets of muscles to engage and flex. Muscle activation is an issue with most of us. Given our modern, sedentary workstyle, most of us simply don't use our muscles during the day. Maybe you've heard of "dead butt syndrome" or a lack of "core engagement." These are types of muscle engagement issues, and they're much more common than you would think. Without the necessary exercises to develop this muscle awareness, muscular imbalances can develop that lead to discomfort or eventual injury. By practicing yoga, moving slowly with conscious control, and developing the body awareness to engage your muscles properly, you are building the foundation for a healthy, capable body that is injury-resilient.

#5. FLEXIBILITY AND ENDURANCE

One final unique benefit of yoga reflects the comprehensive nature of "asanas" involved in yoga practice. By comprehensive, I'm referring to the many different aspects of physical fitness each of the postures addresses, including strength, flexibility, endurance, balance, and mobility. While many types of exercise work solely on strength (for example: weight training with lower reps), flexibility (passive stretching), or endurance (running), few disciplines combine all of these elements into a single workout. Yoga just happens to hit all of these areas and more. The result is a very well-balanced workout that can serve as a primary form of exercise to create a solid foundation for all your fitness endeavors.

While you may undoubtedly feel sore the day after a yoga workout (or days after, if you're new), you won't feel debilitating soreness as you would the day after you lifted too hard at the gym. Most people finish a yoga workout feeling energized and confident rather than drained and dreading the next routine.

> *As a bonus, there will be an immediate noticeable mood boost following your practice session, which will help you enjoy your day more. That will also help you be more consistent with your fitness because the rewards of the practice are immediately noticeable. This is* **exactly** *how good habits are formed (cue > action > reward).*

GETTING STARTED

No matter what style of yoga you choose to practice, you are likely to experience benefit by immersing yourself in the experience of breath and body awareness paired with movement. Practicing full-body yoga postures provides an opportunity to strengthen your hips and core and to enhance your strength, flexibility, endurance, and balance.

Online programs. To begin, my recommendation would be to utilize an online yoga program, particularly one that is specially created for men new to yoga and that provides detailed instructions on proper technique. In addition to the ease and confidence you'll experience from following an organized system of workouts, you'll be able to follow along at your own pace, in the privacy of your own home, and be confident that you're doing the postures correctly.

Classes. Many yoga instructors cater to men who, understandably, often have different fitness backgrounds from their female counterparts. Compared to women, men are less flexible (especially in the hips) and rely more on their upper-body strength (women use their core and hips more). Men tend to build muscle more quickly. It helps to have an instructor who understands these differences, since men tend to make different mistakes than women when it comes to yoga.

If you prefer the atmosphere of an in-person class, check out the local yoga studios in your area. Most offer an introductory deal of some sort that allows you to try out classes for a week or a full 30 days before joining at a higher monthly price. The type of yoga is important, but I've found that even more significant is the yoga *instructor*.

Some instructors are very focused on the physical fitness aspects of yoga, while others are more focused on the spiritual. Most are a blend of the two. Try out as many as you can; you'll want to explore different approaches to see what—and who—jives well with you. My only word of caution here would be to make sure that you find an instructor who covers the proper technique of the postures. If you find yourself mirroring other people rather than doing the positions according to the instructor's guidance, you may push yourself too deep into a pose and overstretch, which can lead to discomfort or eventual injury.

Starting simple. Before you go out and buy a no-slip, oversized cork yoga mat, I'd recommend getting started with what you have around the house. Instead of a yoga mat, use a towel. For the block, just get something that will bring the ground up a foot or so. And in place of a strap, grab a belt or a dog leash. When you're ready, go out and purchase a real mat for yourself. (The yoga mat you may find on clearance at the bargain store isn't your best bet.)

If you do decide that you want to make yoga a regular part of your routine, then I'd recommend creating a specific space in your home to practice. You'll want this to be a clean, tidy space that is free from distractions and away from your work area. Even a few square feet of space in the corner of a room can work well.

Immediate benefit. One of the remarkable things about yoga is how quickly you notice its positive effects. While it may take months to see the results of your hard work in the gym,

---

An Initial Yoga Sequence

A sequence of eight beginner-friendly postures can provide an immediately noticeable benefit. Between each posture, relax fully, lying on your back:

1. Mountain Pose – 60 seconds
2. Warrior 1 – 45-60 seconds per side
3. Standing Side Bend & Back Bend – 30-45 seconds per side
4. Plank – 30-60 seconds
5. Cobra – 30-45 seconds
6. Child's Pose – 45-90 seconds
7. Reclined Twist – 30-60 seconds per side
8. Reclined Figure 4 (Pigeon alternative) – 45-60 seconds per side

---

you'll feel the results of a good yoga session almost immediately, during and afterward. The combination of strength and flexibility practice inherent in the movements releases tension in your muscles, relieves pressure on your joints, corrects your posture, and helps to activate your parasympathetic nervous system (aka The Relaxation Response), which enables you to wind down and release stress.

Don't let yoga intimidate you. Though you may be accustomed to a certain portrayal of yoga, there are modifications for each posture that can make it accessible at any fitness level. (You can even do chair yoga!) Just make sure you find a resource or instructor with whom you feel comfortable.

As with anything new, it's easier to start small. Try making it a goal to do one to two yoga postures every day, and try to do it at the same time and location every day. Once you start to make that a routine and notice your body feeling better, it will be much easier to do more (if you'd like to). Don't wait—make this happen by the end of the week! The biggest regret most people have when it comes to yoga is not starting sooner, and I'm sure you'll be no different.

For more information on yoga, including a follow-along video routine for the postures, described above, visit: www.manflowyoga.com.

Chapter 41
Why Work with a Personal Trainer?
Johnny Jackson, Personal Trainer
& Judson Brandeis, MD, Urologist

If at first you don't succeed, try doing what your trainer told you to do the first time.
— *Darren Weeks*

Tom worked for Caltrans for 35 years as a structural engineer. One week after he retired, he joined a gym and started exercising. One week after that, he went to the orthopedist and discovered he had torn his rotator cuff and required surgery. A year later, following a three-hour surgery and eleven months of excruciatingly painful physical therapy, he is back where he started.

Often people think that training is just for athletes, but I believe that, ideally, everyone should work with a coach or trainer—a professional who can help them design a program specific to their own needs. A personal trainer can decrease your risk of injury and maximize your results.

We all took physical education in school, and many of us played a sport at the high school or college level. However, training a 20-year-old is vastly different than training for a 50- or 60-year-old. By 50, recovery cycles take longer, and the strength and flexibility of bones and joints are also quite different. The information that you knew 20 years ago related more to the physical specimen you were at that time, rather than the midlife breadwinner you are now.

Today, personal fitness is far more sophisticated than the best practices in sports and exercise from our youth. Clinical research on exercise physiology has become its own scientific field. There are thousands of professionals who have gone beyond being glorified gym rats. Knowledge from the training of professional athletes has trickled down to the weekend warriors. The best and easiest way to tap into this body of knowledge is through a certified professional trainer.

Johnny Jackson: *I played football professionally, and since then I've been working as a personal trainer. I'd like to tell you the story of one of my favorite clients, Rob. I had been at the gym* *for about seven years when I met Rob. I would see him come in almost every day, we would talk, and over time we became friends. One day as we chatted, he told me about the aches and pains he was having in his knees and his back. I suggested an assessment and offered to do it free of charge because we were friends.*

In the assessment, I noticed that he had a lot of imbalances in terms of muscle development. His thigh muscles (quadriceps) were a lot weaker than his hamstrings. His feet and knees turned out (pronated) when he was doing squats. I offered to coach him on balancing the strength and tone of his muscles, knowing that might eliminate some of the pain. I felt that if he continued to do the same workout, that could cause more damage. He opted to work out on his own, but before long, he confided that the doctors were recommending knee and back surgery.

I felt that he should work on strengthening his muscles to protect his ligaments and joints. In an act of faith, he signed up for ten sessions to see if a personalized workout could get him back on track. The first time he came in, we did another assessment. I took his measurements and developed a program that was specific to him. He had been working out on his own for so long, he didn't realize that a lot of what he had been doing was hurting him.

A PERSONALIZED APPROACH TO EXERCIZE

Every individual is unique in terms of their genetics, body composition, motivation, goals, history of injuries, and muscle memory. What works for one person does not necessarily work for another. A skilled personal trainer can design a customized fitness plan that is adaptable to the individual and to their fitness journey. This can be compared to the master tailor's ability to individualize clothing to a customer's style and body type. A good personal trainer can optimize an individual's athletic potential and help them set realistic, achievable goals.

Everyone wants to be fit and look great tomorrow. However, the foundation of fitness takes months and even years. Based on a man's genetics and time constraints, it is critical to set realistic and achievable goals. Not everyone can have six-pack abs or lift 300 pounds. A personal trainer can help set goals that are realistic for an individual, to minimize discouragement and keep him motivated.

NUTRITION

Rob made a real commitment. Yet despite his enthusiasm, there were limits to what he was willing to do: "Johnny, no way am I going to change my diet. This is what I eat. End of story." So I encouraged him to take it one step at a time: "First, let's just get you in here consistently, working out, focused on your cardio."

We started with a workout designed to protect his heart. Once he had lost a few pounds and gained a little muscle, he felt encouraged and came to me for ideas. "If I was going to change my diet, could you help me with that?" I said sure. So we changed his diet.

In Rob's case, he was only eating two times a day in order to loose weight. But the intermittent fasting was giving his body the impression that he was in the middle of a famine. To speed up his metabolism naturally, I encouraged him to eat small meals periodically throughout the day. We also supplemented some of his meals with protein shakes. That way his body was under the impression that there was plenty of food. (When we fast, the message to the body is to turn down the thermostat, conserve energy, and store fat.)

Studies show that it takes almost a month to make a shift. The most effective weight loss happens gradually. We don't gain 20 pounds overnight. If we gain a pound a month, that's 12 pounds in a year. When we are thinking about losing weight, think in terms of a gradual process as well.

For someone who's trying to lose weight, I recommend a protein powder that is low in calories and carbs with all the nutrients that they need. We also want ingredients that promote fat burning, which means a formula high in fiber with herbs to turn up the metabolic rate and to speed up metabolism during training. It is important to be aware of lactose or casein intolerance (sensitivity to the natural sugars and protein in dairy products) and consider hypoallergenic options. Most people know if they are allergic to dairy and therefore should not do whey protein.

In Rob's case, after about four weeks, I developed an entire meal plan for him, and after that he started to feel a little better physically and psychologically. He bought the program, and we just went from there. Over that next year, he lost 28 pounds and gained 18 pounds of muscle. His body fat went from 33% to 18% and now he no longer has high blood pressure. He had also been on meds for high cholesterol. At this point, he no longer needs to take medication.

Achieving optimal weight. "What you eat in private, you wear in public." An essential part of training and personal fitness is completion of a module on nutrition. What you eat and how that affects your physical performance is an entire field unto itself, encompassing genetics, body composition, and lifestyle. A trainer can help to identify nutritional goals and coach you on how to eat to optimize your wellness and fitness.

Here's what I hear from one of my clients, who seems to be really feeling stuck. "Almost every night I tell myself that I am going to wake up early the next morning, make a healthy breakfast, and go exercise. When the alarm goes off, I hit snooze and rollover. Once I'm finally in motion, I grab a cup of coffee and two power bars, which I eat in the car on the way to work." A personal trainer is critical to ensure that you commit to, and stick to, your schedule and fitness goals. If you pay for an appointment with a trainer, you are far more likely to follow through.

Supplements

Once a man begins aging, he obviously loses muscle. When you train, you also break down muscle tissue, but when you're young, the muscles rebuild fairly quickly. The older you get, the slower it is to rebuild muscle.

Many people don't realize that you can still build muscle with the correct nutrition and the right program, even in your seventies like my client, Rob. In my work, I also see the gains you get from taking supplements that enable you to start burning fat instead of muscle. (Rob has made amazing strides. At this point, he is actually one of my best clients.)

- **Amino acids.** *If you take amino acids in a creatine formula, that will help rebuild muscle and help with soreness. Note that creatine is not something that I give to older clients, because it can be harmful to the kidneys.*

- **Protein powder.** *To avoid soreness when you're working out, you need to have the proper amount of protein in your diet.*

- **Glutamine** *is an amino acid contained in protein that is especially helpful with soreness and recovery. The older we get, the more glutamine our bodies need.*

- **A multivitamin.** *A good multivitamin, paired with an amino acid formula, provides a good basis for building lean muscle.*

- **Milk thistle.** *Milk thistle is an herbal supplement that supports liver function and helps your body metabolize nutrients.*

The aminos acids in some form, glutamine powder, and a one-a-day multivitamin are key for older men who want to work out to build muscle and burn fat. I also have clients who are in high school who are 15 or 16, and they take protein, aminos, and glutamine. Lady clients like Miss Verna (who is 81) also take aminos. That's how important they are.

— *Johnny Jackson*

INSPIRATION

Training without a purpose is more difficult. It is always good to work towards a goal, a specific event or occasion. That could be a triathlon, a Spartan race, a tennis club competition, or a high school reunion. The important thing is to put something out there and then work incrementally towards achieving that goal.

Creating good habits. A good personal trainer will help you form good habits from a nutritional, athletic, and motivational perspective. Left to our own devices, many of us do not form good habits.

Many men put on weight when they travel for business. One day of travel, a few fancy dinners, and some sugary alcoholic beverages can set you back a month. A personal trainer can help you find a gym when you travel or design exercises you can do in your hotel room. They also can help you figure out what to eat that will not cause you to gain weight.

One cost-effective way to work with a trainer is to see them for periodic check-ins. I have clients who schedule an assessment, we work out a program, and I get them set up to do their own thing for a few months. A couple of months later, we take measurements. Without the assessments, we don't know if they're getting better or worse. Just because we work out doesn't mean that we're always going to get results. Similarly, if I give a client a new diet and I don't take their measurements, I don't know if the diet is working.

Maintaining mental balance. It is well-established that physical exercise can help with psychological issues like depression, so physical activity is frequently recommended by mental health professionals. A personal trainer can identify exercises that will improve your mental state—whether that means going for a long run, lifting weights, or some other form of vigorous exercise.

Building in variety. Depending on the music, most men have about three good dance moves. However, that gets tiresome after a while. Similarly, most men know know one or two exercises for a muscle. A good personal trainer will know dozens of different ways to strengthen a muscle. This helps prevent injury due to overuse or repetitive motion and prevents you from becoming bored doing the same workout over and over. Training that includes variety allows different areas of the muscle to be strengthened. In addition, muscle building requires periods of rest. A personal trainer will understand how much rest a muscle group requires and create a schedule of exercises that will be most beneficial.

Professional athletes are highly gifted, motivated, and self-disciplined. However, they *still* have coaches and personal trainers. We all benefit from external motivation and encouragement. Professional football teams have cheerleaders. A personal trainer can be both a coach and a cheerleader to help you achieve your optimum level of performance.

KEY TAKE AWAYS

1. *Establishing lifelong exercise habits.* Personal trainers help their clients achieve fitness goals, but they also help them reevaluate how they view health and wellness. For some men, this is a matter of realizing the benefits of fitness and making it a priority (rather than an item to check off on the to-do list). Other men struggle with physical limitations and see exercise as an impossibility. A personal trainer can create a workout routine suited to the client's individual fitness level and specific needs, establishing small initial goals to set them up for success.

2. *Avoiding injury.* Progress is more achievable when there's no time lost due to injury. Using unfamiliar gym equipment or lifting weights without the proper approach is a recipe for serious injury. A personal trainer can teach the right form and course correct throughout the process.

3. *Losing fat and gaining muscle.* Most people who embark on a fitness journey want to lose fat, build muscle, or do both. However, not many know how to achieve that. They may spend too long on cardio and not enough time on strength training or vice versa. A personal trainer can help you strike a good balance in your workout.

4. *Breaking through plateaus.* Even the most experienced gym-goer will encounter the dreaded *plateau*. Once the individual stops seeing results, his incentive to keep going to the gym may dwindle or he may stop working out altogether. A personal trainer can identify new techniques to push beyond the plateau.

5. *Seeing better results, sooner.* Left to their own devices, many men wind up on cardio machines at the gym or listlessly moving from one piece of exercise equipment to another. A personal trainer can ensure that the client spends his time performing the right exercises with the proper equipment. Trainers are also ideal for someone who can only commit a limited amount of time to the gym each week. A good personal trainer can make the most of that time and maximize the results.

For additional information, please see:
www.TheTwentyFirstCenturyMan.com.

Chapter 42
Emsculpt: High-Tech Muscle Building
Brian M. Kinney, MD, FACS, MSME

Obese people now outnumber the underweight population for the first time in global history, making it critically important that we learn how to effectively build muscle and burn fat.
— *The Lancet*

If you're a man over age 30, I've got some bad news for you. Chances are you've already begun losing muscle. Muscle aging is a result of decreased numbers of muscle stem cells, diminished protein absorption, slowed energy production, and a gradual decline in testosterone levels. Growth hormone levels peak in the mid-'20s and after that begin to diminish.

Loss of muscle mass is associated with gradual, progressive weakness that makes daily activities more difficult, eventually leading to inactivity and more muscle loss. As the saying goes, "Use it or lose it," except that with aging, it may be "Use it and still lose it." As sedentary people age, they enter a vicious circle that can involve falls, loss of independence, and premature death.

Muscle is the most abundant tissue in the average human body, accounting for 30% to 40% of its total mass:

- Muscle is critical for breathing, movement, and circulation.

- Muscle is also essential to maintain stable levels of nutrients in the body: stored blood sugar (glycogen), lipids (fat), and protein (amino acids).

- Age-associated loss of muscle mass and muscle quality contributes to the general metabolic dysfunction and energy loss commonly seen in elderly patients.

The good news is that proper exercise can prevent and even reverse muscle loss and weakness. The amount and duration of exercise over time strengthens muscle.

How Muscles Work

Many single neurons make up a nerve. The path of a nerve impulse starts in the brain, travels to the primary motor neuron which is in the spinal cord, and then jumps to the secondary motor neuron which is in the appendage or organ.

In the case of a muscle, the nerve fibers stimulate the muscle to contract, through changes in the charge (polarity) of the cell membranes which shortens the length of the muscle fibers.

Muscle fibers contain hundreds of smaller units (myofibrils), which have two layers of protein filaments: a thick layer termed myosin and a thin layer, actin. When nerves cause muscles to contract, the actin filaments slide past the myosin filaments resulting in shortening of the muscle and the generation of force.

Muscular contractions occur as muscle fibers shorten. Conversely muscle fibers become longer with relaxation.

- Physical activity promotes the health of the mitochondria, which produce energy and increase protein turnover.

- Activity replenishes signaling molecules involved in muscle function, regeneration, and growth.

- Exercise prevents or reverses many age-related changes.

THE LIMITATIONS OF EXERCISE

Workout efficiency: 60% utilization. It is important to understand the limits of muscular contraction. When you go to the gym and have your best workout ever, you likely utilize 60% of your muscle fibers. Elite athletes may be able to increase this by up to 80%. Any more than that would require cross-training, multiple days, alternating sessions, and "hitting" the muscle from multiple vectors at various rates (fast-twitch, slow-twitch).

Evolutionary forces prevent us from overexerting our muscles to prevent injury. If a caveman overextended a muscle and tore the tendon off the bone, he would no longer be able to hunt, to survive, or to procreate and pass on his genes to progeny.

Maximum capacity. Muscles can, however, generate more force under extreme conditions, which is why we hear stories of ordinary people lifting cars or other feats of strength. For example, if you are hiking and become trapped under a boulder in a rockslide, you might as well take a chance on tearing a tendon off the bone if your alternative is to be permanently trapped. A massive surge of adrenaline can allow you to recruit a higher percentage of your muscle fibers in order to survive. The point is that muscles are capable of generating higher levels of force under extreme circumstances.

The most common goal of exercise is to grow big muscles, which occurs through two mechanisms:

- Hyperplasia, which involves making more muscle cells

- Hypertrophy, which refers to the process of making existing muscle cells bigger.

What occurs during exercise is a combination of both hypertrophy and hyperplasia. The relative influence of one versus the other is related to the type of exercise and rate of muscle contraction.

Limiting factors. Several factors influence how well your efforts at the gym pay off, including: the circulatory system, which brings oxygen; the extracellular matrix, which protects the muscle; the cytoskeleton (tubules and filaments that support the muscle); and the mitochondria within each cell, which provide energy (ATP). Working against the strength of muscular contraction are several factors, including biochemical stress, oxidative stress, and inflammation. The amount and duration of exercise over time strengthen the muscles. Depending on the type of exercise (endurance or strength training, for example), the primary emphasis in the workout may be oxygen utilization or bulk.

BEYOND EXERCISE

High-intensity focused electromagnetic technology (HIFEM). HIFEM is an emerging technology that creates an alternating electrical field at the site of muscle and fat tissue. Since the peak of the current density is within the muscle, that allows for extremely intense stimulation of muscle fibers. This supports contractions that are intense, but relatively comfortable. The two important benefits of HIFEM currents are:

- **The generation of supramaximal muscle contractions.** On a cellular level, HIFEM produces contractions that cause micro-injuries to a muscle, just as weight training does, which then triggers muscular growth, reflected in increased muscle fiber size and an increased number of fibers.

- **The burning and utilization of fat.** Fat metabolism occurs through a process known as electroporation.

Muscle Building and Fat Reduction in Tandem

To boost results of muscle building and localized fat reduction, BTL recently created Emsculpt NEO, which combines HIFEM for muscle building and Radio Frequency for fat destruction. HIFEM and RF are applied simultaneously in a synchronized fashion. Due to radio frequency heating, the muscle temperature quickly increases by several degrees. This prepares the muscle for exposure to stress, similar to the effect of a warmup activity before any workout. In less than four minutes, the fat layer below the skin reaches a level that causes permanent damage to fat cells. The fragments of the fat cells are slowly removed from the body through the lymphatic system. Since fat cells do not grow back, the treated area will decrease 30% in size. If you eat excessively, the remaining fat cells will increase in size, but will not increase in number. Additionally, the HIFEM energy of Emsculpt is more effective at the elevated temperature. Clinical studies show muscular growth with the Emsculpt NEO at approximately 25%, as compared with HIFEM alone, which was 16%.

Emsculpt is the first HIFEM device to be used in aesthetics to stimulate muscle and reduce fat in one noninvasive treatment. Studies have shown that one can strengthen the biceps, triceps, abdominal wall, and buttock muscles (gluteus) using this approach. Doctors and patients report that Emsculpt can be used to build muscle in all areas of the body, including hamstrings, calves, flanks, lateral thighs, and quads.

Research. A study of Emsculpt by this author involved four treatments, two per week for two weeks. Each session was 30 minutes. MRI technology was used to document loss of body fat and increase in muscle. Applying HIFEM technology, which generates an electromagnetic alternating current in subcutaneous muscle and fat, four Emsculpt sessions in two weeks can grow muscle 16% and reduce the localized fat layer by 19%. In the study, loose, sagging abdominal muscles (*diastasis recti*) improved by 11%, and abdominal circumference decreased by more than 1½ inches (4 cm). Initial studies utilizing ultrasound, CT scan, and MRI technology have shown that the beneficial effects of reducing fat volume last as long as six months. Further radiology studies found that the effects persisted for up to one year.

EXERCISE VS. LIPOLYSIS

How weight loss occurs with exercise. During physical activity, muscles need energy to produce contractions. That energy is derived primarily from ATP (adenosine triphosphate). In addition, energy to fuel the muscles is derived from glycogen and from creatine phosphate, which is synthesized in the liver and pancreas, stored in the muscle and brain, and converted to creatinine. When these run out, the body breaks down fats into free fatty acids (FFA) and glycerol. These released molecules usually act as an energy source for the needed muscle activity and body metabolism. Exercise is effective, but it is a gradual process. Losing weight means spending at least 5 hours a week in physical activity for each pound lost. An hour of swimming (the crawl or the butterfly) will burn about 680 calories. An hour of weight training and cardio or of cycling will burn on average 600 calories.

Weight loss by lipolysis. During an Emsculpt treatment, the muscles contract to supramaximal levels, greater than is physiologically possible with exercise:

- **The release of epinephrine is acutely increased.** This results in an extreme catabolic (breakdown) reaction and supramaximal reduction of fat tissue, which in turn brings about a dramatic release of free fatty acids. This was confirmed in recent Emsculpt laboratory studies.

- **The destruction of fat cells through the release of free fatty acids at higher-than-normal levels.** This effect, breaking down fat tissue, occurs primarily in the area close to the actual contracting muscles. HIFEM reduces fat by inducing an exaggerated metabolic reaction, thereby creating an excessive accumulation of free fatty acids. This principle of cell death induced by an overflow of free fatty acids has been demonstrated in numerous research studies. Fat cells become intoxicated and initiate programmed cell death.

HIFEM technology generates muscular contractions that go far beyond what a person could accomplish through exercise. Emsculpt creates super muscular contractions that result in growth of muscle (hypertrophy) and the burning of fat (lipolysis).

In sum, the studies of four 30-minute treatments of the abdominal wall showed a 19% reduction in fat, 16% growth of muscle, 11% reduction in diastasis, and 1½ inch (4 cm) reduction in abdominal circumference. These benefits lasted at least six months, and subsequent follow-up at twelve months found that the benefits were sustained.

Electromagnetic Interventions for Weight Loss

Muscles contract in response to electrical impulses. If positive and negative electrodes are placed on either side of a muscle and an electrical current is run through the skin to the nerves that control that muscle, the muscle will contract forcibly. Researchers have found several ways to accomplish this.

Electromagnetic stimulation. The most common, easiest, but generally less effective approach is to use skin patches, similar to those used with an electrocardiogram.

Stimulation via needle. A less common approach that is more effective (but more difficult) uses needles inserted directly into the muscle. However, these contractions tend to be painful, because electrical currents generate heat and trigger pain receptors. Also, this typically affects only muscle without any involvement of fatty adipose tissue. Fatty tissue acts as an insulator and has electrical resistance, altering the strength and path of the current, while partially shielding the muscle from the stimulating current.

Direct current. This approach finds the shortest path between two electrodes. However, most of the energy from direct-current concentrates in the body's superficial layers, the skin and subcutaneous fat, and only a small part of it reaches the muscle. As a result, the intensity of contraction is limited due to pain and the risk of burns.

High-intensity focused electromagnetic energy. HIFEM creates a secondary alternating current, induced by strong magnetic fields, that bypasses the skin. This limits the stimulation of pain receptors, providing an approach that does not cause pain.

KEY TAKE AWAYS

- HIFEM technology is available to safely build muscle at a greatly accelerated rate, even as you age.

- HIFEM technology can be used to reduce localized fat.

- HIFEM (commercially known as Emsculpt) has been shown anecdotally to build abdominal core strength, biceps, triceps, gluteus, and calf muscles which last for at least six months.

- Emsculpt is contraindicated in men with any type of metal implant in the body.

- Emsculpt is excellent for men with bad backs who are unable to build core strength and is also a great way to quickly, safely build muscle strength to get back into shape.

- Emsculpt is used by many men to supplement their routine workout regimen beyond what is normally achievable.

- Many men who are generally physically fit with lower body fat have considered surgical procedures to give those finishing touches that have eluded them in the gym. Now many are using Emsculpt instead.

Research: Kinney BM, Lozanova P. High intensity focused electromagnetic therapy evaluated by magnetic resonance imaging: Safety and efficacy study of a dual tissue effect based non-invasive abdominal body shaping. *Lasers in Surgery and Medicine.* 2019 Jan; vol. 51, issue 1: pages 40-46.

BrandeisMD Physical Rejuvenation Protocol

Within two minutes of trying the Emsculpt machine at the Aesthetic Show, I knew I needed to have one for my practice. In my younger days, I was a competitive runner and triathlete, so my body instinctively recognized the intensity and fullness of the contraction of the abdominal muscles.

After delivery of the machine, I began Emsculpting my abs. I have three daughters and a son, so I serve as both father and buddy to my son (given that we live in a house full of women). We sneak around the house, trying to ambush each other. Early one morning, on the way to make my first cup of coffee, I came around a corner, and my 14-year-old son whacked me in the abs. Grinning from ear to ear, I whispered, "Is that all you got, punk?" My abs felt so strong. A few weeks later, the paddles for Emsculpt arms arrived at the office. Within a month, I had put an inch on my arms by Emsculpting my biceps and triceps.

The patients at BrandeisMD are hard-working, mature men who are too busy to exercise as often and as intensely as they did when they were younger. Even if they have the time, their testosterone has declined, and their dietary habits are typically suboptimal. I found that the Emsculpt (HIFEM) technology provides an opportunity to efficiently regain muscle lost over the previous 20 to 30 years.

As a clinical researcher, I quantify results, so I purchased an InBody body composition scale, and what I observed was fascinating.

Tracking results. It is essential to establish baseline testosterone and body composition so that both the physician and the client can track the results. It is also critical to get a basic lab panel to make sure that there are no medical issues that would get in the way of progress. At BrandeisMD, these include labs looking at the kidneys, liver, electrolytes, protein levels, vitamin D, vitamin B12, thyroid, cholesterol panel, and PSA (prostate-specific antigen). In addition, sometimes, I will order a heart calcium score to make sure that I'm not missing heart disease. I want to confirm that a man's heart is good enough to begin stepping up an individual's exercise level.

BrandeisMD Physical Rejuvenation Protocol:

- *Boost testosterone levels.* Suppose a man has both laboratory results and symptoms that suggest low testosterone. In that case, I prefer to use BioTE pellets to optimize testosterone because there are no extreme highs and lows in the level of T. For men with adequate testosterone, we provide the extra testosterone by creating small increases with a DHEA-based formulation like SupporT from AFFIRM Science. This supplement provides DIM (also found in cruciferous vegetables such as broccoli and kale) to block the conversion of testosterone into estrogen, which is important in maximizing T and minimizing estrogen.

- *Emsculpt abs, glutes, biceps, and triceps* once a week for six to eight weeks and then maintenance every three months. I add Emsculpt for quadriceps and calves as needed, based on physique and goals.

- *Vigorous exercise.* If you are not sweating, you are not exercising. When you actively exercise, you burn an additional 500 calories an hour, and then you can add this to your daily caloric intake. The type of exercise is less important than the consistency and intensity. It doesn't matter to me whether you are running, swimming, playing basketball, or playing pickleball, as long as you enjoy it and avoid injury.

- *Cardio exercise* should be at least 40 minutes four days per week. The Heart Rate Goal for exercise is 220 minus age x 0.75. For a fifty-year-old man, this is (220-50) x 0.75 = 128 Beats per Minute. (To increase your level of exercise, be sure to read chapter 37: Getting Back in Shape, with tips on how to scale up your program while avoiding injury.)

- *Circuit training with weights* 2 to 3 days per week. Hit all major muscle groups, including arms, legs, core, chest, back, and glutes. Use free weights, machines, bodyweight, bands, or classes. It does not matter to me other than that you enjoy it, and you can (and will) make time for it.

- *Stretching or yoga* for at least 15 minutes every morning. Wake up 15 minutes earlier and start the day with better flexibility and circulation.

- *Basal metabolic rate.* You need to know what your Basal Metabolic Rate is to begin the process of losing weight. Daily caloric intake is 500 calories less than BMR plus calories burned during exercise. This formula will give you 1 pound of fat loss per week. Crash diets make you lose water weight, which quickly comes back when you eat salty foods. So the healthiest way to lose weight is one pound of fat per week.

- *Protein intake.* Eat at least 0.5 grams of protein per pound of body weight — a 200-pound man needs to eat at least 3 to four ounces of protein (1/4 cup or 100 grams). The source of protein is less important to me. You can eat red meat, chicken, fish, beans, nuts, tofu, or whey protein as long as you hit your protein goal.

- *Optimal individualized diet.* A diet high in protein, low in carbs, high in micronutrients, and fiber, add healthy fats to reach goal daily caloric intake. I support any diet that follows these principles: Mediterranean, Keto, Zone, Vegan, Intermittent Fasting, South Beach, Paleo, as long as you still enjoy eating and can stay on the diet.

- *Supporting nitric oxide (NO).* AFFIRM nitric oxide booster two tablets twice a day. Boosting circulation and improving blood pressure is mission-critical.

- *Creatine monohydrate* 5 grams per day, half before and half after exercise to increase energy production (ATP).

- *Drink fluids* so that your urine is a light straw yellow color. If your urine is clear, drink less and if your urine is yellow, drink more

I want to share the body composition results of the first two patients to complete three months of the BrandeisMD Physical Rejuvenation Protocol. Both patients had testosterone levels less than 300 and clinical symptoms of low testosterone. I performed an InBody composition analysis to establish initial baseline values for weight, fat, muscle, and basal metabolic rate.

Your Basal Metabolic Rate is the number of calories per day required to keep your body functioning at rest.

Mr. W is 61 with four children and owns an insurance company. When I first met him, he weighed 163 pounds with approximately 17% body fat. He is athletic but never a competitive athlete and has dedicated the past forty years to his family and career. He was on weekly testosterone injections when we first met. As you can see below, in just three months, he added:

- Over 5 pounds of muscle

- Dropped 9 pounds of fat

- His testosterone went from 285 to 986.

When I saw him in the office for his follow up InBody assessment, he had an aura of invincibility.

Mr. T is 66 with two children and runs his own executive consulting company. When I first met him, he weighed 192 pounds with 27% body fat. He had been seeing a talented personal trainer for years but had reached a plateau. He is athletic but never a competitive athlete and has dedicated the past 45 years to his family and career. His testosterone was low, so I started him on BioTE pellets. As you can see below, in just four months he:

- Added over 5 pounds of muscle

- Dropped 21.8 pounds of fat.

- His testosterone went from 301 to 1056.

I was amazed at the progress he had made! He was not just thinner, but much stronger and more confident.

The results from these two gentlemen are astonishing. To build over 5 pounds of muscle and lose more than 10 pounds of fat in a normal 60-year-old man with a demanding job is truly remarkable. Yet, the program I've described is reproducible.

The BrandeisMD Physical Rejuvenation Protocol combines hormones, nutrition, hydration, supplementation, and physical exercise principles with cutting-edge diagnostic and exercise technology. It builds in flexibility of diet and exercise to accommodate all men. Except for Emsculpt and possibly the cost of testosterone replacement, the rest of the program is free. All that is required is dedication and determination.

— **Judson Brandeis, MD**

Mr. W.	Pre	Post	Units	+/-	Change	Percent
Age	61	61	Years			
Testosterone	285	986	ng/dl	+	701	345
Weight	163.3	162.6	Lbs.	-	0.7	1
Height	5'10	5'10"			0	0
Skeletal Muscle Mass	75.6	80.9	Lbs.	+	5.3	6.4
Body Fat Mass	28.2	18.9	Lbs.	-	9.3	33
Percentage Body Fat	17.2	11.5	Percent	-	5.7	33
Left Arm	7.61	8.38	Lbs.	+	0.77	9
Right Arm	7.41	8.16	Lbs.	+	0.75	9
Trunk	58.6	62.5	Lbs.	+	3.9	6
Left Leg	20.64	21.36	Lbs.	+	0.72	3.5
Right Leg	20.50	21.25	Lbs.	+	0.75	3.5
Basal Metabolic Rate	1695	1779	Calories	+	84	5

Mr. T	Pre	Post	Units	+/-	Change	Percent
Age	65	66	Years			
Testosterone	301	1056	ng/dl	+	755	351
Weight	192.0	179.0	Lbs.	-	13	7
Height	5'10"	5'10"			0	0
Skeletal Muscle Mass	78.9	84.0	Lbs.	+	5.1	6
Body Fat Mass	52.2	30.4	Lbs.	-	21.8	42
Percentage Body Fat	27.2	17.0	Percent	-	10.2	38
Left Arm	7.74	8.53	Lbs.	+	0.79	9
Right Arm	8.00	8.77	Lbs.	+	0.77	9
Trunk	61.6	65	Lbs.	+	3.4	5
Left Leg	20.81	21.91	Lbs.	+	0.9	5
Right Leg	20.88	22.11	Lbs.	+	0.77	5.5
Basal Metabolic Rate	1739	1826	Calories	+	87	5

For additional information on the practice of Dr. Kinney, please see
www.DrKinney.com.
For information on Emsculpt and its creator, BTL, please visit
www.BodyByBTL.com.

Chapter 43
Biohacking
Judson Brandeis, MD, Urologist

Don't quit. Suffer now and live the rest of your life as a champion.
— Muhammad Ali

As a generalization, the American healthcare system takes sick people and makes them better. However, what if you've tried to lead a healthy life, but still don't feel your best? How do you go from good to great?

Biohacking is an emerging field that leverages cutting-edge science, discoveries in human biology, and self-experimentation with lifestyle, supplements, and complementary therapies to optimize the physical, mental, and emotional aspects of human performance. Biohacking enables you to upgrade your brain, optimize your body, defer aging, and take your existence to the next level. The vital information provided by physicians and other professionals in this book will give you strategies to dramatically improve your health.

The average middle-aged man wanders through life stressed out, with brain fog, bloating, indigestion, constipation, aching joints, insomnia, and low libido. At this stage, the average man has accumulated excess fat that is constantly releasing inflammation, keeping his body in a state of red alert, and gradually squeezing the lifeblood out of his organs. Amidst all this fatigue and pain, he continues to search for the next big thing, for elusive happiness.

The goal of biohacking is to optimize recovery and peak performance, enhancing lean muscle, hormones, and sleep. The final destination of the journey is to become boundless—the total optimization of body, mind, and spirit.

A boundless mind means you have ideal levels of essential brain chemistry, particularly the neurotransmitters, so your nervous system communicates flawlessly. Your mind is free of inflammation and brain fog, and you develop potent coping strategies to manage stress and minimize destructive cortisol levels. Your IQ is elevated, as are your working memory and executive function. You understand how to effectively use brain-enhancing foods, nootropics (drugs, supplements, and other substances that are claimed to improve cognitive function), smart drugs, and other biohacker's tools. Your sleep is pure, uninterrupted, and efficient, and, ultimately, you feel as though you have power and control over your thoughts, feelings, interactions, and communication.

A boundless body means that you know how to effectively burn fat and get lean. You know how to build muscle in the safest, cleanest, and fastest way possible. You have fixed your gut, eliminated digestive issues, and maximized nutrient absorption. You understand the power of dynamic movement, exercise, workouts, supplements, and foods to build strength, power, speed, balance, mobility, and endurance. You have cracked the code on maximizing recovery and recovery speed. You possess a vital immune system, and you have a potent arsenal of tools to increase your symmetry and physical attractiveness.

A boundless spirit means that you can consciously manage your thoughts and beliefs to affect your health positively. You practice gratitude, love, and joy. You understand how to use new methods, such as sound healing and vibrational frequencies, to enhance your physiology. You have optimized your relationships, friendships, and social connections, and you've maximized the power of love in tandem with the practice of tantra and sexual satisfaction. You have addressed hidden variables that can compromise your health, both mind and body, factors that include air, light, electricity, and water. You have learned from residents of the world's Blue Zones and longevity hotspots how to optimize your life, happiness, and fulfillment, and your daily habits and routines enable you to create the perfect day.

Biohacking is your blueprint to becoming boundless. This mean escaping the modern norm of staggering through life with low energy, brain fog, a sluggish body, and untapped potential—instead, being able to call on the energy you want when you need it, so you can achieve the most adventurous, joyful, and fulfilling life possible. Attaining optimization of body, mind, and spirit requires mindful attention to good self-care.

This involves an extensive body of knowledge, techniques, pharmaceuticals, and medical interventions to optimize performance. These are strategies that are in development, evolving and being tested in real-world situations. The current medical model is disease-oriented, focused on the sick patient and how to get them back to "normal function." Biohacking seeks to go from good to excellent by taking a systems approach, selectively incorporating resources to optimize systems:

- *Athletic recovery* might include cryotherapy, infrared sauna, deep tissue massage, pulsed electromagnetic field, red-light laser therapy, or hyperbaric oxygen.

- *Supplements that support immune function* such as vitamin C, quercetin, CoEnzyme-Q10, PQQ (pyrroloquinoline quinone), zinc, glutathione, colostrum, or melatonin

- *Herbs for immune function* that include echinacea, rosemary, oregano oil, turmeric, or the beta-glucans in medicinal mushrooms

- *Strategies to maximize weight loss*, such as fasting, intermittent fasting, or ketosis, and healthy gut bacteria

- *Complementary therapies* such as acupuncture, lymphatic drainage, or Ayurvedic detox to support your immune function

- *Mind-body strategies* such as the practice of yoga or qigong, and mindfulness meditation, visualization, or gratitude journaling

- *Mitochondrial support* to interrupt the inflammation and free radicals that damage the mitochondria (thousands of microscopic energy sources within all the cells of the body), avoiding the oxidative stress that results in programmed cell death. (Mitochondrial damage is a problem that accompanies aging.)

- *Antiaging supplements* such as nicotinamide adenine dinucleotide (NAD), nicotinamide riboside (NR), astaxanthin (AX), or carnosine, as well as anti-inflammatories such as curcumin or alpha lipoic acid, used by bio-hackers to protect against mitochondrial degradation, aging processes, and excessive immune activity

- *Reducing toxic exposures* in the home could mean installing a HEPA air filter, using natural household cleaners, reducing mold and mold toxins, drinking filtered or spring water, and reducing exposure to common (but harmful) home and garden chemicals.

The world is continuously changing. As new scientific breakthroughs occur, the secrets of our ancestors are revealed. Knowledge once accepted as orthodox and established is replaced by better research. Biohacking is about pushing the boundaries of what is possible to maximize your health using intelligence, observation, nontoxic therapies, and leading-edge strategies.

REFERENCE

The field of Biohacking is too vast to encompass here, given the range of approaches involved. For deep insight and a wealth of practical strategies, I strongly recommend *Boundless*.

Ben Greenfield. *Boundless*. Las Vegas, NV: Victory Belt Publishing, 2020.

For additional information on fitness, nutrition, and biohacking, please see www.BenGreenfieldFitness.com.

PART 6
ADDICTIONS
Introduction
Judson Brandeis, MD

Chains of habit are too light to be felt until they are too heavy to be broken.
— Warren Buffett

Yearly Fatalities Linked to Bad Habits

- **480,000 deaths due to smoking**

- **300,000 premature deaths due to obesity (poor diet and inactivity; for example, sugary drinks alone account for mortality of 25,000 individuals)**

- **88,000 deaths linked to alcohol-related causes**

- **65,000 deaths associated with drug overdose in a single year**

- **28% increased risk associated with driving while under the influence of cannabis**

- **9,000 fatalities due to electronic addiction and distracted driving (and walking)**

- **30 million children have lost their childhood through sexual exploitation over the past 30 years—porn can play a role in this.**

We all have bad habits, myself included. Often these are strategies for coping, strategies that were initially effective. At this point, they probably seem less rewarding and more damaging. The purpose of this section is not to be judgmental or to make anyone feel bad. The chapters in this section describe habits that can have potentially destructive consequences if not done in moderation. We examine the scope of the problem in terms of the number of men affected, the personal cost in terms of health-related quality of life and the economic cost to society. There is a cost-benefit with everything that we do, and my hope is that, after reading these chapters, you will understand what those costs are. Ultimately, the decision that you make should be informed, but should be your own.

He that is without sin among you, let him cast the first stone . . .
Bible, King James Version, John 8:7

Chapter 44
The Truth About Tobacco
Judson Brandeis, MD, Urologist

Tobacco companies kill their best customers.
— The 21st Century Man

Everyone knows that smoking is bad for you, but millions of men still smoke. So many men try to quit and fail. As a urologist, I know first-hand that cigarette smoking can also be a major factor in men's sexual health. By impairing circulation, smoking can restrict blood flow, cause leaking veins and ED, and wreak havoc with your sex life.

Recently I had a patient, a medical professional, who had been smoking since the age of 16 when he immigrated to the States. He drove a taxi at night to support himself through college and medical school, so stress was always an issue. He had tried several times to quit without success. When I saw him in the office, our discussion included his enthusiasm for his kids, which prompted me to point out that smoking a pack a day could cost him 13 years of his life expectancy and time with his family.

At that point an idea came to me, and I told him that I wanted him to make a sign with "13 YEARS LOST" in big letters and post it on his daughters' bedroom doors. It wasn't long after that when he quit smoking for good.

Tobacco use is the leading *preventable* cause of mortality in the United States and worldwide, contributing to at least 480,000 deaths per year in the U.S. alone:

- 40% from cardiovascular disease

- 35% from cancer

- 25% from lung diseases.

RISK FACTORS

Being male. In the U.S. tobacco use is more common among men (26% vs. 14% for women), younger adults, and the less affluent. Worldwide, the prevalence of daily smoking is 25% among men and 5% among women.

Genetics account for more than half of the addiction. When it comes to tobacco, genetics are estimated to account for about 75% of a person's inclination to begin smoking, reports University of Pennsylvania psychologist Caryn Lerman, PhD. Genes also account for 60% of the tendency to become addicted and more than 50% of one's ability to quit.

Consuming tobacco in the form of cigarettes increases the risk of addiction. Tobacco smoke contains more than 7,000 chemicals, including added nicotine, which causes and sustains the addiction. At least 75% of cigarette smokers smoke daily, an indication of the power of the addictive chemicals in cigarettes.

Starting young means it will take more effort to overcome. Almost every adult who smokes started smoking by the age of 18, and the earlier the age at which a person begins smoking, the more likely they are to continue smoking into adulthood.

WHY MEN STILL SMOKE . . .

Smoking is highly addictive. Nicotine is the drug primarily responsible for addiction to tobacco products, including cigarettes.

Nicotine addiction is driven by dopamine. This response in brain chemistry is also an aspect of heroin and cocaine addiction. (Nicotine is present naturally in the tobacco plant, but tobacco companies intentionally design cigarettes to contain a level of nicotine that creates and sustains addiction.)

Tobacco companies spend $10 billion a year on marketing. The profit of American tobacco companies is $35 billion a year.

SIDE EFFECTS AND HARMS

Effects on the heart and blood vessels. Studies have shown that smoking causes heart and blood vessel disease. The more and longer one smokes, the higher the risk for acute myocardial infarction. The cardiovascular risk of the use of noncigarette tobacco products, such as pipes, cigars, and smokeless tobacco, is less significant than that of cigarettes.

The incidence of heart attacks is three times greater in men who smoke at least a pack of cigarettes per day.

Smoking even one cigarette a day is associated with a 50% increased risk for coronary heart disease and 25% increased risk for stroke.

Smoking causes an estimated 20% of deaths due to heart disease, because it:

- Increases LDL, the harmful form of cholesterol

- Activates a low-level stress response, causing increased heart rate and blood pressure

- Causes inflammation in blood vessels and damages blood vessel walls, preventing them from opening fully and causing them to narrow

- Raises carbon monoxide levels, inhaled in cigarette smoke, which reduces the oxygen level in your blood stream and interferes with its effective delivery

Cancer. Contains at least 250 chemical additives known to be harmful, including 70 known to cause cancer.

Types of cancer known to be caused by smoking include:
- Mouth
- Throat
- Larynx
- Esophagus
- Lungs
- Stomach
- Colon
- Pancreas
- Kidneys
- Bladder
- Liver
- Cervix
- Rectum
- Acute myeloid leukemia.

Smoking is also a causal factor in:
- Chronic obstructive pulmonary disease (COPD)
- Emphysema and asthma
- Diabetes
- Osteoporosis
- Rheumatoid arthritis
- Age-related macular degeneration
- Cataracts
- Higher risk of developing pneumonia, tuberculosis, and other airway infections.

Cigarette smoking is the most crucial risk factor in the development of lung cancer, the number one cause of cancer deaths in the U.S. and in the world.

Less ability to fight infection or disease. Smokers with any form of cancer tend to respond less well to treatment and have more recurrences and complications from treatment compared to non-smokers. Tobacco use leads to problems with infections, wound healing, cardiovascular complications, and the development of recurring cancers.

QUITTING

The benefits of quitting cigarette smoking, regardless of whether it is early or late, are well-established. The cardiac risks associated with cigarette smoking diminish within a few years after smoking cessation and continue to decline over time.

The increased risk for lung cancer is 30 times higher for smokers than for non-smokers.

Stopping smoking reduces this risk, especially for those who stop smoking for more than 15 years, in which case, the incidence of lung cancer is reduced by 80%.

Adults who quit smoking gain six to ten years of life expectancy depending on the age at which they quit.

After 10 to 15 years of abstinence, the rate of heart disease is equivalent to that of non-smokers.

The benefits of quitting:

Within minutes: Heart rate and blood pressure, which are abnormally high while smoking, begin to return to normal, and circulation improves.

Within a few hours: The level of carbon monoxide in the blood begins to decline, and oxygen delivery in the body improves.

Within a few weeks: Those who quit experience less phlegm and don't cough or wheeze as often.

Within a few months: Lung function improves.

Within a few years of quitting: People have lower risks of cancer, heart disease, lung disorders such as emphysema, and other chronic diseases than if they had continued to smoke.

Although it is never too late to benefit from quitting, the benefit is greatest among those who quit at a younger age. Regardless of age, people who quit smoking have substantial gains in life expectancy, compared with those who continue to smoke. Data from an NHANES federal survey show that:

- Those who quit between ages 25 and 34 live about ten years longer

- Those who quit between ages 35 and 44 live about nine years longer

- Those who quit between ages 45 and 54 live about six years longer

- Those who quit between ages 55 and 64 live about four years longer

Despite a drop in cigarette use over the past 50 years, smokers' risk of developing lung cancer or COPD has increased. The type of lung cancer smokers develop has changed from squamous cell carcinomas to adenocarcinomas, with potentially worse outcomes. Changes in cigarette design and composition, tobacco composition and toxicity, and depth of inhalation have created this unfortunate shift.

KEY TAKE AWAYS

Globally, an estimated 1.3 billion people smoke cigarettes. Globally, tobacco and tobacco products are a $663 billion industry that will grow to $1 trillion by 2026. Tobacco products include cigars, pipes, chewing tobacco, and electronic cigarettes.

The United States wastes over $300 billion a year on the effects of smoking, including $170 billion on direct medical care and $156 billion in lost productivity due to chronic health disorders.

- Tobacco use is the leading preventable cause of mortality in the United States, resulting in 480,000 deaths a year.

- Approximately 40% of this mortality is from cardiovascular disease, 35% is from cancer, and 25% from lung disease.

- Less than one-third of adult smokers who try to quit seek help, and even fewer use the most effective treatments.

For additional information on stopping smoking, please see:
https://tobaccofreeca.com/ and
https://www.lung.org/quit-smoking/smoking-facts/health-effects.

Chapter 45
How To Quit Smoking
Adriana Bustamante, PhD, Researcher
& Lucia Romo, PhD, Professor

The best time to quit smoking is the day you started;
the second-best time to quit is today.
— Anonymous

If you smoke, is quitting simply a matter of willpower? The short answer is yes. Quitting takes willpower, but that alone is not enough. Most smokers have already tried to quit at least once in their lives. They are also aware of the harm that tobacco can cause to their health and that of their loved ones.

Yet the desire to quit smoking is often accompanied by the opposite drive as well—the basic urge to satisfy cravings. Someone in the process of quitting is likely to hear two inner voices—one that says, "I really want to quit smoking," and the other that says, "I really want a cigarette." Each voice represents a different area of the brain.

The first is an area of the brain that is capable of logic and able to rationalize (the *prefrontal cortex*). This is the aspect of personality that is aware of the dangers of smoking and is associated with the conscious decision to stop.

The second voice comes from our primitive reptilian brain (located in the brainstem), which keeps us informed of our primary needs (hunger, thirst, sleep). As an individual consumes tobacco (and cigarette additives), the brain changes. With the onset of addiction, this primal brain is automatically activated whenever the body is in need of nicotine.

When a craving arises, the negotiations between the two voices (the desire to smoke and the desire to quit) can consume a great deal of time and energy, especially when there is no well-defined strategy for dealing with cravings.

Smoking is an automatism, so it does not reflect free choice, nor is it proof of freedom. Nevertheless, smoking is associated with a degree of pleasure, satisfaction, and even relief, although disgust is sometimes a factor in the equation as well. Moreover, it is precisely the degree of pleasure that makes abstinence difficult. Emotionally, the smoker may be likely to confuse "quitting smoking" with "quitting enjoyment." Therefore, it is important to redefine who we are, what makes us happy in the short and the long term, and how the mechanics of addiction affect us.

Quitting smoking is a personal journey that is most successful when it is supported. Willingness is necessary, but not enough. The will is the starting point; it provides the necessary energy to take the firsts steps in the quitting journey. Indeed, we are not all equal when it comes to tobacco, and several steps may be needed to overcome dependency. We need to address the biological, psychological, and socio-cultural factors of addiction. Ignoring their impact is counterproductive.

QUITTING, STEP BY STEP

Different types of assistance may be needed to get through each stage of smoking cessation You need to prepare for quitting by calibrating your compass, anticipating obstacles, and by recognizing your internal and external resources. The goal is to be prepared, so when a craving emerges, it won't determine your actions.

THE COMPASS—Defining the life you want to live

Every daily action has a consequence. It is true that changing our habits requires effort, whether mental, physical, or economic. Why would we want to change? Because we have a life's ideal, and the way we are living at present does not necessarily bring us closer to that ideal.

As the first step, it is important to ask yourself: What is the life I want to live? What is important to me? What gives meaning to my existence? When you answer these questions, you will find the compass that can ultimately guide your life and help you through difficult situations.

Another approach is to think about your future. Imagine meeting yourself in ten years. What do you want your life to look like in ten years? When we identify what is important to us, we define our purpose and gain clarity on our life path. This awareness leads us to act in coherence with what is important to us. We can then question daily actions that take us away from our "ideal life."

Changing a habit, such as smoking, certainly requires a short-term effort, but at the same time is an additional step towards the meaningful life you deserve.

THE PLAN—Identifying the milestones essential to quitting

Once you have defined your goal, you need to identify the path to reach it. The future non-smoker typically goes through three primary stages: preparation, quitting, and maintenance. In each phase, you will need specific types of support to give yourself the maximum chance of success.

Preparation. In this milestone, first adopt an observer's attitude. About two weeks before your quit date, become aware of situations in which you find it easier to deal with cravings and, in contrast, situations that put you at risk of relapse. Three of the most common examples of an increased desire to smoke are: 1) following an emotional outburst, 2) in social situations, and 3) when you are acting automatically, for example, in the morning with the first coffee or while drinking alcohol.

It is essential that smokers who are planning to quit anticipate these challenges and devise coping strategies to deal with them. This means adopting the researcher's mindset, by brainstorming, testing, and experimenting with new coping strategies:

- For the biological factors involved in smoking, it is possible to use nicotine substitutes or pharmacotherapy.

- For the psychological and socio-cultural factors, therapeutic support can be a real help in developing new skills, such as saying "no" when a friend offers a cigarette.

- Therapeutic and medical support increases the chances of success by 20%, compared to a 5% success rate for those who quit without any type of help.

The best treatment is usually one that combines psychotherapy and pharmacotherapy.

If you have already tried to stop on your own, a tobacco professional can help you identify the psycho-social reasons that led to a relapse (irritability, weight gain, stressful situations, etc.) in addition to the addictive chemistry of commercial tobacco products. This will help you define a personalized action plan to make your recovery a success. For example, adding hypnosis or acupuncture can be helpful, but to date, we don't yet have the research evidence of efficacy.

Quitting. Once you have defined a stop date, you can do it effectively in two ways: either abruptly or gradually. In the preparation phase, you may have already started using nicotine substitutes or other medications. Even though this phase is called "quitting," consider your primary goal to be gaining knowledge about the effect of nicotine on your needs, your emotions, and the circumstances in which you are able to regulate the cravings.

Consider learning the 4D strategy: Delay, Drink water, Deep breath, and Distract. Withdrawal symptoms are numerous and are often the first cause of relapse. They are most noticeable during the first three months of abstinence. Withdrawal symptoms may be unfamiliar and, for some, unpleasant. This is the time to keep your goals in mind. Withdrawal symptoms are proof that your body is clearing itself of tobacco, so it's a good sign! Each time you let a craving go by, applying effective substitution strategies, the next craving will diminish as your body's demand for nicotine decreases.

Maintenance/relapse prevention. The maintenance phase starts approximately three months after the quitting date. At that point you will have fewer symptoms, and you will be increasingly aware of the benefits of your decision to quit. Yet the temptations are often still there. This is a good reason to continuing using strategies over the long-term that have been most effective during quitting. Following your cessation, don't take even a single puff, because that's how a relapse begins.

You'll have ups and downs, but if you stick with it, this phase will end about two years after the quit date. Once you reach that point, your chances of success are 95%.

Case Study: Kwit, a Mobile App

A smoker who wanted to quit tobacco created Kwit as a mobile app that would help him stay tobacco free. Today, Kwit has evolved and has become a subject of academic research at several universities including the University of Pittsburgh, the Royal College of London, and Université Paris-Nanterre.

Changing your habits is an everyday choice. Some days are easier than others, but Kwit is the app that will always be there for you. You can download Kwit from both the Apple and Google stores or from the website: https://kwit.app.

The app was inspired by cognitive behavioral therapy and by game principles. The end result is that the app makes it easier to handle withdrawal. The app provides an opportunity to take a step back from the difficulties you have already gone through and to implement new coping strategies, such as some form of substitution or relaxation exercises. The application is also designed to be a source of motivation. Each stage of progress is recognized, in order to reinforce your efforts and help you move to the next level, because each success achieved depends on your constant efforts.

The app consists of a dashboard to follow progress on your health, a page to record your cravings (whether you smoked or not), and access to statistics to better understand your needs. On the dashboard, you can see motivational reminders such as money saved, cigarettes not smoked, and years of healthy life gained. With each new step taken (a day without smoking, a week without smoking, etc.) the app records your achievements: the benefits to your health, the environment, your bank account, and your general wellbeing.

How a Cravings Management Tool Works

■ To record a craving, click on the "+" at the bottom of your screen and then click on "I feel like smoking" if the urge to smoke is currently present.

■ Select the emotions you feel and the context you are in. This process allows you to understand what situations trigger the urge to smoke, and to respond in accordance with your objectives. This will help you better identify what triggers cravings, allow you to become aware of your automatic responses (automatisms), help you recognize the circumstances in which you are most vulnerable (or not), anticipate risky situations, and choose new strategies for dealing with them.

■ Choose a strategy to manage your cravings. Kwit provides new alternatives, such as breathing exercises, which enable you to alternate strategies according to your needs and to repeat each new strategy until it becomes part of you.

If a craving arises, you can also simply shake your phone and a motivational card will appear! Typically, cravings last for 3 to 5 minutes, so the goal is to keep you busy during this short interval until the craving passes. The aim of the app is to accompany and encourage the former smoker on a daily basis so that they feel supported. If you need advice or want to share your experiences, Kwit also has created a support group for Kwitters in Facebook. Kwit is a pocket coach that will always be at your side through good times and bad.

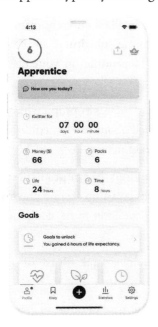

At this point in time, former smokers using Kwit have avoided the use of 1,002,144,082 cigarettes, saved $349,912,580, and gained 20,973 years of life expectancy.

A free download of the Kwit App is available at kwit.app.

RESOURCES

NICOTINE SUBSTITUTES

The chemistry of the brain is altered as a result of tobacco consumption. It gradually becomes dependent on the nicotine from cigarettes in order to function. When the dose of nicotine decreases, strong cravings to smoke emerge, as well as some withdrawal symptoms. Although often unpleasant, they are not life-threatening. Hold on, take the nicotine supplement you need, or use a behavioral strategy. Ask your doctor how to assess your level of nicotine dependence and substitute the right dose for it, no more and no less.

Compensatory smoking. One quitting strategy is to cut down the number of cigarettes or to switch from normal to light cigarettes. However, it is a temptation to use this approach, but consume the same nicotine level; this is called compensatory smoking. The individual inhales more deeply to reach the same nicotine level and therefore consumes the same amount of nicotine and tobacco. In this case, the best approach to successful withdrawal is to supply the brain with the dose of nicotine it is accustomed to by using a nicotine substitute.

Pharmaceuticals. Today, there are three types of pharmaceutical treatments that double your chances of staying smoke-free: nicotine substitutes, antidepressants such as bupropion, and medications designed for smoking cessation such as varenicline.

- *Nicotine replacement therapy* is equally effective in all its different forms, which include patches, gums, and mouth sprays. Nicotine substitutes are used for a minimum of three months to be effective, but, depending on your needs, you may choose to use them for six months or more.

- *An antidepressant* prescribed for smoking cessation such as bupropion has definite pros and cons, so you will want to educate yourself about these medications and then talk with your doctor about what's most ideal for you.

- *Varenicline* is a medication created exclusively to address the symptoms of smoking withdrawal. Both bupropion and varenicline help you stop feeling cravings and double your chances of stopping successfully in the long term, compared with nicotine replacement therapy alone.

Combination therapy. You may also want to combine several forms of nicotine replacement products to enhance their effectiveness.

- You can start using them two weeks before your quit date to improve your success rate.

- After your quit date, continue to use the patches. You can also begin using the gum for cravings.

- If by chance you have a relapse, don't stop using nicotine replacement products. They will protect you and help you get back on track.

- In determining the optimal dose of medication, if you feel like smoking, chances are you are underdosed. No matter what option you choose, don't be afraid to "take too much." Given your smoking habits, the level of pure nicotine in patches or gum will not be toxic to you.

Vaping. Vape has also been used as a smoking cessation tool in many countries. Accompanied by guidance from a health professional, it has been found to be effective. The use of vaping without any form of tobacco helps to reduce the risks associated with toxic substances from tobacco products. At least half of vape users were able to reduce their tobacco consumption by half. Compared with other nicotine substitutes, the vape was used more frequently and for a longer period, helping the user to reduce cravings.

SUPPORT — Self-help tools, online programs, and mobile apps

The journey of smoking cessation is unique to each person, but the future non-smoker is not alone. Several solutions exist today to accompany him or her on a day-to-day basis. The most recognized are self-help books, mobile apps, and self-help groups on social platforms such as Facebook or WhatsApp. These internet-based interventions are useful and effective when compared with a lack of any other type of help.

Using an app. Researchers have found that using an app and/or virtual support can help you foster a sense of commitment to your own personal health. Positive reinforcement is available through nudges from the app, such as tracking habits, messaging, regular feedback, and/or audiovisual support. See page 404 for info about Kwit, a mobile app.

Relapse response. In the process of stopping smoking, it is common for relapses to occur. Relapse is part of the process and is the perfect situation to learn more about your habits and responses associated with smoking. You can join a self-help community to talk with people who understand what you are going through and who can support you. You can also monitor the situation by using an app or journaling to keep track of your experience. This could be of help in the future, because you will be able to step back and recognize your progress.

For additional information on using an app to help you stop smoking see: kwit.app.

Chapter 46
Understanding Alcohol Overuse
Judson Brandeis, MD, Urologist
& Michael Abassian, MPH, Researcher

Sobriety is the greatest gift I ever gave myself.
— Rob Lowe

At the age of 45 I stopped drinking alcohol. I was never a heavy drinker. Like most guys, I binge drank in college and graduate school. As a doctor, I would have a glass of wine or two with my wife at the end of the day. But when our four children started to grow up, we decided that we did not want any alcohol in our house. Even though I was not a heavy drinker, once I stopped, I noticed that I had more energy and a better mood. It was clearly easier to keep off weight, and I was waking up more rested. I recommend to all of my patients that they consider removing alcohol from their lives. I don't judge men for drinking; I just provide them with the data.

Men have been drinking alcohol since the earliest recorded history, and the use of alcohol is thoroughly ingrained in societies around the world. Drinking alcohol has become an integral part of spectator sports, socialization, holidays, and celebrations.

According to a 2015 United States national survey on drug use and health, more than 50% of Americans over the age of 12 have used alcohol at least once in the past month. More than 5% reported heavy drinking, defined as five or more drinks on five or more days in the past month.

Alcohol is clearly big business. Beer is a $114 billion industry in the United States and wine, a $30 billion industry. So, it's not surprising that we are constantly bombarded with positive messaging about beer, wine, and spirits.

What is the truth about alcohol? And what is the impact?
More than 85,000 deaths a year in the United States are directly attributable to alcohol use. Roughly one in ten deaths among working-age adults results from excessive drinking.

RISK FACTORS

Genetics. Genetics are now considered 50% of the underlying reason for an alcohol use disorder. Children with one parent who struggles with alcohol overuse have three to four times the risk of becoming an alcoholic themselves.

Being male. Men are two to three times more prone to alcohol use disorders than women.

History of abuse in childhood. Children who were verbally, physically, or sexually abused are at a higher risk of alcohol overuse.

Mental health problems. Psychiatric conditions, including depression, anxiety, bipolar disorder, ADHD, schizophrenia, and unrelenting stress are associated with alcohol abuse, perhaps as attempts at self-medication.

Drinking at an early age. People who drink in adolescence are more likely to develop alcohol use disorder. This raises the question of whether early drinking creates risk or reflects an existing genetic or family-related risk.

WHY MEN STILL DRINK . . .

Short-term stress relief. Alcohol is a well-known depressant of the central nervous system, which can reduce anxiety, heart rate, and blood pressure, providing short-term stress relief.

Lowered inhibitions. Alcohol reduces inhibition by altering the balance between neuro-transmitters, resulting in reduced attention, alteration in memory, and mood changes.

The debate over moderate use. Alcohol consumption at moderate levels has been associated with *reduced* risk of heart disease, stroke, and diabetes. However, the potential damage to brain cells offsets these benefits.

In a study of 600,000 drinkers published in the British journal *Lancet* in 2018, the threshold for health risks is 1,000 g of alcohol for one week, which is the equivalent of one standard American beer per day (or equivalent alcohol content).

- Drinking 2 to 3.5 drinks a day is associated with a one- to two-year decline in life expectancy.

- Drinking 4 drinks a day or more corresponds to a four- to five-year drop in life expectancy.

IMMEDIATE HARMS

Toxic effects on the liver have an impact throughout the body, making the intoxicated person more likely to be moody, violent, or abusive. As a result, alcohol is associated with negative behaviors.

A tendency to abuse or violence. More than half (55%) of domestic violence is associated with alcohol use and 50% of all sexual assaults are committed by men who have been drinking alcohol.

Fatal accidents. More than one-third of fatal crashes (38.6%) involved drivers or pedestrians with significant blood alcohol levels. Alcohol impairs perception and slows reaction time, significantly increasing the risk of accidents.

LONG-TERM RISKS

Heart disease. The cardiovascular system is affected by alcohol. In the long term, excessive alcohol consumption can lead to high blood pressure, irregular heartbeat, and weakened heart muscles with the potential for heart failure.

Brain and nervous system. In the long term, heavy drinking can cause mental health issues such as depression or dementia.

- *Brain shrinkage.* People who drink just one to seven drinks per week have smaller brains than nondrinkers, according to a 2008 study at Johns Hopkins that appeared in the *Archives of Neurology*. Two drinks a day was associated with three times the risk of brain shrinkage and with lower total brain volume (which means reduced memory and intelligence) by the age of 39 to 45.

- *Impaired memory.* Alcohol has been found to shrink an area of the brain associated with memory, the hippocampus. Having four drinks a day was associated with six times the shrinkage found in nondrinkers.

- *Reduced blood flow to the brain.* Neurologist Daniel Amen, MD, reports that brain scans of heavy drinkers show reduced overall blood flow to the brain. Note that low blood flow is the #1 predictor of potential Alzheimer's.

- *Fewer new brain cells.* Excessive alcohol consumption lowers the generation of new brain cells, especially in the hippocampus, according to animal research. In the study, monkeys that consumed alcohol experienced a 58% decline in the number of new brain cells formed and a 63% reduction in the survival rate of new brain cells.

- *Seizures.* Long-term alcohol abuse increases the risk for epilepsy.

Cancer. The body breaks down alcohol into a chemical, acetaldehyde, that can damage cellular DNA and potentially cause cancer. There is a clear link between heavy alcohol use and malignancies, including cancers of the liver, breast, intestine, esophagus, and throat.

Liver disease. Alcohol is a toxin, and the liver removes toxins, including alcohol, from the bloodstream. However, the liver may not be able to keep up if you drink too much or too fast. Alcohol kills liver cells leading to scarring (cirrhosis). Liver damage can affect the body's ability to clear other toxic substances and metabolize medications.

Digestive issues. Alcohol can irritate and inflame the lining of the stomach, leading to ulcers and chronic inflammation. Alcohol can also make it more difficult to digest essential nutrients. Additionally, alcohol can result in an inflamed pancreas and in pancreatitis.

Diabetes. Alcohol is a simple sugar. Consumed on a frequent basis, like any simple carbohydrate, it increases the risk of diabetes.

Gout. Alcohol increases levels of purines, which result in a buildup of uric acid crystals in the joints, causing severe pain and impairing mobility.

Blood sugar issues. Alcohol is a *fast carb,* so like any fast carb, it spikes your blood sugar. That's one of the reasons you feel so good soon after drinking. However, the flood of glucose is burned quickly, followed by a rapid crash, which can trigger anger, depression, or a sense of exhaustion — and the need for another drink.

Infections. Drinking can interfere with your ability to fight off viruses and bacteria.

Impaired quality of sleep. Alcohol can affect your sleep pattern and lower the quality of your sleep. It has become clear from a study published in 2018 on 600,000 drinkers that healthy alcohol consumption is about the equivalent of one standard beer a day.

On the whole, American men do not drink responsibly. Alcohol kills one of every ten men and costs our economy $250 billion. Drinking is associated with 28% of all fatal car crashes, as well as more than half of sexual assaults and domestic violence. It is clear that alcohol is a bad habit for many of us and that we need to detach from the societal norms and relentless advertising that leads to pain and suffering for many men and communities.

KEY TAKE AWAYS

The annual economic cost of alcohol use is estimated to be over $250 billion. This figure converts to more than $2.00 per drink. Most of the costs result from losses of workplace productivity (72% of the total cost), healthcare expenses for treating problems caused by excessive drinking (11% of the total), law enforcement and other criminal justice expenses (10%), and losses from motor vehicle crashes related to excessive alcohol use (5%). More than 40% of these expenses were paid by federal, state, and local governments, which shows that we are all paying for excessive alcohol use.

For additional information on coping with alcohol issues, see:
https://www.aa.org/ and
https://www.samhsa.gov/find-help/national-helpline.

Chapter 47
Cocaine Is Not Your Friend
Judson Brandeis, MD, Urologist
& Michael Abassian, MPH, Researcher

Cocaine is God's way of telling you that you are making too much money.
— Robin Williams

Used by 18 million people worldwide, cocaine is a stimulant purified from the leaves of a bush-like plant that grows in the Andes Mountains of South America. North America has 5 million users, representing almost 2% of the adult population, exceeded by the United Kingdom and Spain with more than 3% of adults using cocaine. Men are at least twice as likely to use cocaine as women. The primary users of cocaine are men ages 15 to 35 living in urban areas (3.5 million users).

> *Currently, more than half a million of those who abuse cocaine are over age 55, and approximately one million Americans over 65 have some form of substance abuse.*

Cocaine use varies, but more than half of individuals who use cocaine recreationally use it less than 12 times in the year. However, in 2014, almost one million Americans met the criteria for dependence or abuse of cocaine, according to the National Institute on Drug Abuse.

RISK FACTORS

Identifying the underlying causal factors in addiction is an important aspect of recovery. Primary factors in addiction cited by the National Institute on Drug Abuse include:

- **Genetics,** which are estimated to account for 40% to 60% of the risk of addiction.

- **Extreme addictiveness.** At least 15% of people who use cocaine will develop dependence. Those who smoke or inject cocaine are more likely to become addicted because of the faster rate of drug delivery to the brain and rapid onset of psychological effects, associated with a more intensely pleasurable response.

- **Psychological issues** such as a chaotic home environment, abuse, or other forms of chronic stress increase the risk of addiction. When stress or PTSD is the primary risk, counseling, group therapy, or 12-step programs may be of benefit.

- **Mental health disorders** increase the risk for drug and alcohol use and addiction. More than 20% of individuals over age 65 battling substance abuse also suffer from some form of mental illness.

WHY MEN STILL USE COCAINE . . .

Cocaine enhances the activity of neurotransmitters such as dopamine, serotonin, and norepinephrine. Cocaine euphoria, in particular, is due to the enhancement of dopamine activity in the brain. It has a second mechanism of action that produces a local anesthetic effect.

Produced in two forms, base and salt, the onset of action for cocaine depends on the route of administration. Cocaine base, also known as crack or free base, can be smoked because it has a relatively low melting point and vaporizes. Smoked or intravenous cocaine has an onset of action of 10 seconds, and the effects last 15-30 minutes. Cocaine salt dissolves, so it can be injected or snorted through the nose. Snorting cocaine takes effect within three to five minutes and lasts about one to three hours. Regardless of how it is administered, cocaine is eliminated in the urine. Cocaine users may experience poor sleep, anxiety, agitation, restlessness, irritability, depression, or panic attacks. Physiologic effects include elevated heart rate, dilated pupils, sweating, or nausea.

IMMEDIATE HARMS

The body's physical response to cocaine is variable, and fatal cases of cocaine intoxication may present with 100-fold differences in cocaine levels in the blood. Unintended adverse effects occur with increased dose, duration of use, or a more efficient route of administration. Overdose also occurs randomly when the purity of a street drug is greater than anticipated.

Auto accidents. Almost half of drivers from all traffic fatalities tested positive for some type of drug in 2016—double the percentage of 2007.

Cocaine and alcohol in combination. Using cocaine together with alcohol leads to the formation of a new compound, which remains in the body longer and can be more toxic than cocaine by itself.

LONG-TERM RISKS

In the U.S. in 2015, at least 615,000 cocaine users received specialized treatment for their cocaine use, associated medical problems, or withdrawal. Cocaine is associated with 40% of the visits to emergency departments due to illegal drug use.

Possible effects of chronic cocaine addiction:

- Racing heart rate (tachycardia), high blood pressure, and arrhythmias
- Seizures
- Stroke (cocaine use increases the risk by a factor of six)
- Risk of sudden cardiac death
- Impaired kidney function
- Sexual dysfunction/impaired erectile activity.

Overdose. Nearly 600,000 cocaine overdoses in 2016 resulted in hospitalization, according to the CDC.

Suicide risk. Cocaine addiction is also associated with suicidal ideation and suicide attempts. Researchers found that 20% of suicides in New York City among those 60 or younger had used cocaine within a matter of days. Suicide risk is especially high when cocaine use is associated with depression, intense withdrawal symptoms, alcohol or opioid dependence, history of childhood trauma, or family history of suicide.

Heart attack. Cocaine use is a factor in about one quarter of non-fatal heart attacks in persons younger than 45 years old. Increased oxygen demand by the heart, coupled with decreased flow through the arteries to the heart due to spasm and/or constriction can cause an acute heart attack, even in young people with no symptoms of cardiovascular disease.

Stroke. The risk of adverse effects increases with age. In a study of 1,000 individuals who had experienced a stroke while using cocaine, the average age was 40.

Risk of mental illness. Excessive long-term use of concentrated forms of cocaine such as crack cocaine can trigger psychotic symptoms such as delusions or hallucinations.

KEY TAKE AWAYS

- Use of cocaine increases stroke risk six-fold.
- The average age for stroke among people overusing cocaine is 40 years of age.
- Cocaine use is also a risk factor for midlife heart attack. About one-quarter of all non-fatal heart attacks in individuals younger than 45 is associated with cocaine use.
- One of every six people who uses cocaine will eventually develop dependence.
- Concentrated forms of cocaine are associated with suicidal ideation and attempts.

For additional information and resources, please see
www.samhsa.gov/find-help/national-helpline and www.drugabuse.gov.

Chapter 48
The Dark Side of Cannabis
Judson Brandeis, MD, Urologist

When you smoke marijuana, it reveals you to yourself.
— Bob Marley

The call came in around 1 am. As a urologist, I know that it's never good news when the phone rings at 1 am. It was the emergency room at the local trauma center. A 20-year-old man had tried to cut his penis off. As I raced to the hospital, I called ahead to the operating room. Two hours later I had reattached the partially severed penis. It was 4 am, and I was exhausted and irritated when I walked down to the main lobby of the hospital to meet the man's father.

As it turned out, the father was an old patient of mine. He opened up to me about his son's struggles, overusing cannabis, and how it seemed to be triggering schizophrenic episodes.

In writing this chapter, I learned that marijuana is not quite as bad a drug as I had thought it was. What I also learned is that, tragically, the cannabis he had purchased on the street was probably laced with methamphetamine, PCP, or LSD, triggering a psychotic break in my patient.

In researching this, I found that it is common for dealers to combine "weed" with heroin, cocaine, methamphetamine, PCP, or LSD. For example, PCP (also known as angel dust), is very damaging; the damage is clearly visible on an MRI. Methamphetamine is also associated with schizophrenia symptoms. In 40% of users, apparently these episodes are so common they are referred to as "meth psychosis."

Cannabis laced with more highly addictive drugs becomes a gateway drug.

Cannabis, also known as marijuana, is one of the most commonly used psychoactive substances worldwide. According to the World Health Organization, 147 million people, or almost 3% of the world population, use cannabis. A Gallup poll conducted in 2019 reported that 12% of Americans smoke cannabis. In California, 25% of cannabis consumers are said to be Baby Boomers, age 50 and over. Public health concerns associated with cannabis use focus on three primary areas: the potential for auto accidents; the risks of consuming street cannabis laced with hard drugs; and the unknown effects on adolescents, whose brains are still developing.

IMMEDIATE HARMS

The risk of cannabis laced with damaging drugs such as methamphetamine. Street drugs marketed as cannabis can contain additional drugs of unknown origin with potentially devastating effects such as psychosis, brain injury, or fatal overdose.

The risk of traffic accidents. Like alcohol, cannabis slows reaction time and impairs concentration, short-term memory, risk assessment, and judgement.

- Norwegian researchers analyzed data involving more than 90,000 drivers, reporting that cannabis intoxication was associated with a 28% increase in the risk of an accident.

- Yale researchers found that combining marijuana with alcohol results in impairment *"even at doses which would normally be insignificant if they were of cannabis or alcohol alone."*

- French researchers found a delay in the euphoria associated with cannabis. As a result, drivers assumed that they were alert enough to drive hours after they had smoked, not realizing that there was a delayed onset that impaired their reaction time and ability to focus. This effect was more pronounced in those who only smoked occasionally.

LONG-TERM RISKS

Cannabis use disorder. Indications of overuse include impaired function at work, significant lack of motivation, giving up previously enjoyed activities, and the potential risks associated with driving while high. The development of cannabis use disorder likely has a genetic component as well as a social component.

First-line treatment for cannabis use disorder is either cognitive behavioral therapy or motivational enhancement treatment. For patients who were unable to maintain abstinence with psychosocial intervention, no medication has been identified for cannabis overuse.

Unknown effects on emotions, memory, and learning. The area of greatest concern is the impact of stronger cannabis on brain development in teenage smokers. A New Zealand study found that people who started smoking marijuana heavily in their teens—*and had an ongoing marijuana use disorder*—lost an average of 8 IQ points between the age of 13 and 38. The lost mental abilities did not fully return in those who quit marijuana as adults.

Those who started smoking marijuana as adults did not show IQ declines.

THE CHEMISTRY AND USE OF CANNABIS

The discovery in 1992 of endocannabinoid receptors (CB1 and CB2) throughout the brain and human body has shifted the scientific perspective on cannabis. Endocannabinoids occur in three forms:

- *As a type of neurotransmitter produced within our own bodies* with receptors throughout the brain and the tissue of the body.

- *As a natural part of plants of the hemp family,* most notably *Cannabis sativa,* that has been used as herbal medicine for more than 1,000 years, and ritually for more than 3,000 years (for example, in burial sites).

- *As synthetic cannabinoids,* a class of molecules that bind to the same endocannabinoid receptors in the body. Synthetic endocannabinoids come in two forms: those created by pharmaceutical manufacturers as medications and those synthesized in laboratories for recreational purposes.

The psychoactive properties of cannabis plants are primarily due to THC (delta-9-tetrahydrocannabinol).

Recreational Use

The potency of plant-based marijuana (reflecting the THC content) has increased significantly over time. The THC concentration in the 1960s was between 1% and 5%, but today it is typically 5% to 12%. THC content in street drugs is 15% to 20%. Hashish and hashish oil refer to compressed resin with a THC content ranging from 20% to 80%. The major non-psychoactive constituent of the plant is CBD (cannabidiol) and its various constituents, which promote relaxation and sleep, improve appetite, and reduce pain and inflammation.

People who use cannabis experience euphoric and pleasurable feelings with a decrease in anxiety, depression, and tension. Cannabis use can lead to perceptual changes, the sensation that colors are brighter, and music is more vivid. Time and spatial perception may be distorted. Mystical thinking and a sense of expanded consciousness may occur. However, these responses are individual. Some people may experience transient paranoia.

THC activates CB1 receptors in the brain, resulting in enhanced release of dopamine, the brain's reward system. Chronic regular cannabis use reduces the sensitivity of CB1 receptors in the brain, and the effects of the cannabis are slightly reduced. Abstinence results in an increase in receptor sensitivity within several days.

Effects of smoking cannabis include relaxation and the disengagement of mental functions (due to mildly impaired concentration, short-term memory, and decision-making). After inhalation of smoke, the onset of psychoactive effects occurs rapidly, with peak effects felt at 15 to 30 minutes and lasting up to four hours.

Cannabis in edibles becomes effective at 30 minutes to two hours with clinical effects that may last three or four hours. When cannabis is consumed in edibles by unfamiliar users, given the delay, they may be tempted to eat more, resulting in discomfort or even vomiting as the cumulative dose is absorbed and metabolized.

Synthetic cannabinoids are associated with a more intense high that is longer-lasting, apparently accompanied by a withdrawal syndrome in contrast to plant-based cannabis.

Intoxication. Serious cannabis intoxication is rare in adolescents and adults. Most adults presenting for treatment with cannabis intoxication experience mild intoxication with dysphoria that can be managed with a dimly lit room, reassurance, decreased stimulation, and a sedative such as a benzodiazepine.

Statistics on emergency room use. Colorado was the first state to legalize medical cannabis in 2000 and recreational cannabis in 2014. Researchers tracking emergency room admissions for cannabis overuse found that in 2014, visits peaked at a little over 1,000 per 100,000 ER visits. However, ER rates fell in 2015 to approximately 750 per 100,000.

Metabolism and testing. Drug testing for THC, typically in urine, identifies cannabis use, but not necessarily how recently. Because THC has extensive storage in fat tissue, detectable blood and urine concentrations may occur weeks after last cannabis use. The liver metabolizes THC using the CYP450 (cytochrome P450) system. One-third of THC and its metabolites are excreted in the urine and two-thirds in the feces.

Medical Cannabis

Cannabis and its extracts and constituents have been utilized in Europe for the management of a range of debilitating conditions, including AIDS treatment, addiction, cancer therapy, nausea and vomiting, seizure disorders in both adults and children, and severe chronic pain conditions.

Research. More than 400 clinical trials in the world medical literature have shown efficacy for cannabis in the treatment of:

- Anxiety and reactive depression (but not treatment-resistant depression)

- High blood pressure (hypertension)

- Lung conditions, including asthma, COPD, and chronic bronchitis
- Neurological disorders including multiple sclerosis, Parkinson's disease, post-traumatic stress disorder, and Tourette syndrome.

Pain management. Cannabis can be a useful aspect of pain management, by reducing pain to a level where it can then be managed with lower levels of opioids, significantly reducing the risk of opioid overuse and addiction. Specific studies have found efficacy for fibromyalgia pain, as well as migraine headaches, and benefit in reducing inflammation and insomnia.

KEY TAKE AWAYS

- The psychoactive properties of cannabis are primarily due to THC, which is used to measure potency.
- Drug testing for THC is typically a urine test. THC is stored in fat and can remain in the body for weeks.
- Cannabis slows reaction time and impairs concentration, which interferes the ability to drive. Drivers using cannabis are two to seven times more likely to be responsible for accidents, which is dependent on the level of THC content consumed.

**For additional information, please see
www.samhsa.gov/find-help/national-helpline.**

Chapter 49
Health Benefits of CBD
Adam Wenguer, Element Health

The biggest killer on the planet is stress, and I still think the best medicine is and always has been cannabis.
— Willie Nelson

My vocations include martial arts and combat instructor, strength and conditioning specialist, and health coach, with a four-stripe brown belt in jiu-jitsu and Thai boxing. I discovered CBD in 2015 and realized the incredible health benefits after trying my very first dose. I had read stories of people getting exceptionally deep sleep and finding themselves much more capable of dealing with daily stress when they started regularly supplementing with full spectrum CBD oil. However, this came after 15+ years of using medical cannabis, with mixed results in improving my sleep, and helping me relax and recover from daily workouts.

Traditional cannabis (marijuana or "weed") is high in a cannabinoid compound known as THC, which is responsible for relaxation, the "high" or stoned effect, the THC buzz. The problem is that THC may alleviate stress for some users, but in others, it can enhance stress, anxiety, or paranoia depending on the plant strain and the individual's body chemistry.

CBD oil is extracted from strains of the hemp plant that do not produce the large amounts of THC that you would find in cannabis plants intended for the recreational market. Because of this, a vast majority of individuals who use CBD experience only positive effects. There is no high or buzz. There is simply a general calming effect that lowers the "noise" that many of us experience, living in large cities and working in stressful environments. What's more, in this age of 24/7 technology, many of us have lost the ability to stay present. With so much stimulation, we seem to stay on high alert. Stress used to be reserved for students in graduate school and people working long hours with strict deadlines. Now even children are experiencing the adverse effects of an ultra fast-paced society. No one is immune from feeling disconnected. Thankfully, I have found full-spectrum CBD to be an essential tool in allowing me to experience the optimized, healthy, and connected version of myself.

What drew me to CBD supplementation was the idea that I could use a natural plant compound that wouldn't make me high, lazy, or slow me down, but that could allow me to maintain composure in daily high-pressure situations. CBD has also been shown time and again through *studies and individual accounts to vastly improve the quality of sleep. It doesn't cause fatigue, but studies show that it reduces cortisol (a stress hormone) so your body can naturally ease itself into a deeper mode of sleep.*

CBD is, in essence, so benign that even children with intractable illness find benefit. A recent study of medical cannabis by researchers at the medical school of Tel-Aviv University was reported in the Journal of Child Neurology. *The study followed the responses of 25 young people to the use of various concentrations of CBD oil. Study participants were ages 1 through 17, with complex neurological disorders. Researchers reported:* "Significant improvement in spasticity and dystonia, sleep difficulties, pain severity, and quality of life was observed in the total study cohort . . . . Adverse effects were rare."

CBD BENEFITS

Surprisingly, when taken in the daytime, CBD has been found to improve clarity, focus, and overall sense of well-being. This wide range of benefits comes from CBD's effects on the endocannabinoid system (ECS) of the human body.

Discovered in the 1940s, the endocannabinoid system is a fat (lipid) signaling system found in all vertebrates including humans. It helps regulate nearly every facet of our body from our immune, nervous, and gastrointestinal systems to our hormones, metabolism, muscles, and bones. A broad range of basic processes affects memory, appetite, sex drive, and blood pressure. Pain sensation, inflammation, and immunity are all influenced and affected by the endocannabinoid system. Supplementing with CBD optimizes the ECS and gives our body a nudge towards balance.

The world of cannabis culture and consumption has changed drastically over the years. Since the 20th century, the narrative of cannabis has evolved from a drug that is associated with psychosis to a wellness adjunct that can be of great value to overall wellness and performance. Since the discovery of the endocannabinoid system, more research—both observational and outcomes-based—has come to the fore, leading us to conclude that the ECS, and associated cannabinoids, are of paramount importance in human health.

Here, we will differentiate THC and CBD, the physiology of CBD in the body in association with the ECS, identify the benefits of CBD supplementation, offer insight into CBD extraction, and what the future of CBD research has in store. It is useful to understand the context of CBD, its effects, and its mechanisms of action.

The endocannabinoid system plays an essential role in immune and nervous system regulation through a complex network of molecules and receptors. The two primary players in this system are the receptors CB1 and CB2, which are found throughout the body. This receptor system assists and maintains the regulation of several physiological processes. CBD is one amongst hundreds of cannabinoids that interact with the ECS to elicit various changes in the body's physiology and overall homeostatic balance.

Cannabinol (CBD) and delta-9-tetrahydrocannabinol (THC) are both cannabinoids, chemical compounds found within the cannabis plant, but when extracted from the plant and consumed offer varying interactions and therapeutic benefits to the consumer.

When consumed, THC provides a psychoactive effect, otherwise known as the high, whereas CBD does not. THC elicits this psychoactive quality through binding and stimulation of the CB1 and CB2 receptors found within the body and the endocannabinoid system.

Conversely, CBD does not bind to these receptors. Instead, CBD reduces the binding strength and effect of the CB1 receptor, resulting in the suppression and reduced release of several neurotransmitters in the body. This has led researchers to believe that CBD could be playing a key role in treating both anxiety and insomnia.

THERAPEUTIC EFFECTS

Due to this inhibitory characteristic, researchers have proposed CBD as a viable product for treating anxiety (an anxiolytic), improving sleep, reducing inflammation, and treating a host of mental health and neurological disorders, including but not limited to schizophrenia, epilepsy, chronic headaches/migraines, and dystonia (Health Canada, 2018).

Some of the most promising potential therapeutic uses gathered from Health Canada's 2018 review of research in healthcare (intended to guide the legalization of cannabis) include:

- Improving the quality of life in palliative care and those being treated with chemotherapy

- Delaying disease progression and reducing symptoms of tremor and spasticity for those suffering from multiple sclerosis (MS) and spinal cord injuries

- Reducing/treating convulsions and seizures in epilepsy

- Treating chronic pain and neuropathic pain

- Reducing the need for opioids in treating pain ("opioid-sparing" effect)

- Treating osteoarthritis symptoms.

Clinical trials have confirmed the efficacy of CBD and CBD/THC blends for a broad range of conditions relevant to the health issues that many men experience in midlife and beyond.

Favorable research outcomes for physical disorders treated include: asthma, autoimmune disorders, COPD, cancer management, chronic bronchitis, diabetes mellitus, high blood pressure (hypertension), insomnia, psoriasis, rheumatoid arthritis (RA), sports injuries, and workout inflammation.

Positive outcomes for neurological and neuropsychiatric indications include: ADHD/hyperactivity, antiaging benefits, anxiety, bipolar disorder, dementia, depression, epilepsy, fibromyalgia pain, migraine headaches, MS (multiple sclerosis), Parkinson's disease, post-traumatic stress disorder, stress, and Tourette syndrome.

Undoubtedly, the potential of CBD's power to address so many disorders and reduce the need for opioid pharmaceuticals is exciting. Probably the most widely consumed CBD products are tinctures, which are a concentrated solution of CBD bound in an oil base, most commonly hemp oil or coconut oil. This solution goes through a process that extracts the CBD from THC, leaving trace amounts of THC in the solution, and thus providing the consumer with the body-mind benefits from CBD, without the psychoactive effects of THC.

When smoking cannabis, the consumer is taking in both THC and CBD, in addition to an array of several other cannabinoids. The pitfall with smoking cannabis, excluding the combustion process which can have inflammatory and damaging effects on lung tissue, is that the consumer is at the mercy of the psychoactive effects from THC in conjunction with the benefits of CBD. Many consumers of THC enjoy the psychoactive effects, but research has shown time and time again that THC has a biphasic effect in the body, meaning that, depending on the dose, the effect on the body can increase or decrease the desired effect. An example would be, at one dose, THC may provide a calming effect but at a higher dose could actually increase anxiety.

In terms of CBD products, the two primary tinctures available are broad-spectrum and full-spectrum tinctures. A broad-spectrum tincture goes through a process of extraction of all the constituent cannabinoids, leaving the consumer with solely a CBD tincture. Conversely, a full-spectrum product (such as those available at Element Health) go through a process of eliminating primarily THC and leaving the remaining cannabinoids in the tincture. So, the question is which one is better? Nature has a beautiful process of creating natural remedies, and their benefits are most apparent when consuming the natural product as a whole.

Practical, clinical applications of CBD of particular interest include efficacy in pain management, utility in addictions treatment, antiaging benefits, affecting COX-2 pain pathways, and reducing oxidative stress. The consensus among physicians is that CBD does not totally resolve either chronic pain or addiction. However, it does appear to lower pain enough to significantly reduce the risk of addiction. Statistics cited pointed toward a 50% success rate. Since in-treatment success with alcohol addiction and drug treatment has a five-year success rate of about 10%, this is noteworthy. About 20% CBD has been useful in the treatment of both alcohol *and* drug addiction.

The human body is always seeking balance, but unhealthy diets, lack of exercise, overstimulation, and harmful sleeping patterns can cause a loss of homeostasis. When we are under these constant or intense stresses, we don't feel like ourselves. We may experience depression, anxiety, or a general disconnect between body, mind, and spirit. A majority of people will seek out junk food, alcohol, drugs, or entertainment, chasing feel-good endorphins and neurotransmitters. That positive sensation doesn't last very long, and then we may feel even worse than we did before. Unfortunately, this destructive cycle occurs for many aging men bombarded with stress. As we age, body systems begin to feel taxed, and we no longer feel like our vibrant self anymore. For some readers, CBD will be the key that enables them to feel younger, healthier, and calmer. Full-spectrum CBD can serve as a valuable natural tool to make you more productive in each of those endeavors.

For additional information on CBD and CBD products, please see www.ElementHealthSupply.com.

Chapter 50
Electronic Addiction
Judson Brandeis, MD, Urologist

Life was easier when Apple and Blackberry were just fruits.
— Anonymous

On August 6, 1991, the first website went online, followed in 1992 by the upload of the first photo onto the web, which was an image of the CERN house band *Les Horribles Cernettes*. Two years later, Jerry Yang started *Yahoo*, and Jeff Bezos founded *Amazon*. In 1995, *eBay* began reselling consumer goods, and email became more popular than snail mail. By 1998 Sergey Brin and Larry Page had created *Google*, and then in rapid sequence, *Craigslist*, and later *Wikipedia* were launched. Social media took off in 2004 with *Facebook*, *Twitter* in 2006, and *Instagram* in 2010.

By 2019, 317 million Americans were on the Internet, and 80% used social media. E-commerce sales topped $600 billion, equating to 11% of retail sales and rising. Today, the average email user sends 74 emails a day. At least 74% of Americans use Facebook, and on average Americans spend 116 minutes daily on social media—essentially two hours a day. There are 7 billion instant message accounts in the world that send 438 billion messages daily. Netflix consumes 26% of the Internet streaming traffic, and 75% of the music industry's revenue comes from streaming music. PornHub users watched five billion hours of video. Weekly podcast users spend an hour a day listening to podcasts. One-quarter of Americans do some or all of their work online.

The acceleration of the Internet, and the extent of its saturation into our lives is staggering. It is no surprise that more than 10% of the population is believed to suffer from an Internet addiction disorder, a form of behavioral disorder.

According to the Entertainment Software Association, the average age of gamers is 30 years, debunking the myth that only adolescents are interested in gaming. In fact, 68% of the gaming population is older than 18 years old. So, a question: Just because you use the internet often, does that mean that you suffer from an internet addiction disorder?

We are considered addicted when these activities start to interfere with our daily lives. The most common categories of Internet addiction include gaming and pornography (predominantly male), as well as social media and online shopping. These are all forms of escape from the pressures and disappointments of real life, but escapism can be overdone.

Gaming. The average millennial spends $1,000 per year for online gaming, but some men spend $10,000 and up on this preoccupation. In 2017, Americans spent $36 billion on video games. Of this, $6.9 billion was spent on hardware. Midlife male gamers devote an hour a day, on average, playing online games, but this addiction can preoccupy hard-core users for hours on end, forgetting to eat or drink.

Studies link internet addiction disorder to physical changes in the brain structure in the prefrontal cortex, the area of the brain responsible for personality, complex thinking, decision making, and social behavior.

Similar to other addictions, internet addiction also seems to affect the pleasure center of the brain. Addictive behavior triggers a release of dopamine, which is recognized as one of our major feel-good neurotransmitters. As with any other addiction, over time more and more online activity is needed to induce the same pleasurable response, creating a dependency.

The novelty and unpredictability of the web is another lure for the browser. Every time you sign on to your favorite site, whether it is Instagram, Amazon, or Facebook, the site gives you surprising results that keep you entertained and coming back for more. We know that major sites such as YouTube hire scientists to write algorithms whose primary intent is to keep you engaged for longer and longer periods of time.

Biological predispositions such as depression or anxiety are also likely to affect the levels of dopamine and serotonin, intensifying the need for solace. If a man suffers from either anxiety or depression, he may turn to the internet to attempt to elevate his mood. Men who are shy or extremely introverted might be at higher risk of internet addiction since it does not require interpersonal interaction, and it can be emotionally rewarding.

Symptoms associated with internet addiction disorder:

- Emotional issues: anxiety, depression, isolation, loneliness, mood swings, or agitation; boredom with routine tasks, procrastination or avoidance of work; defensiveness, guilty feelings, and/or dishonesty

- Physical symptoms: backache, carpal tunnel, headaches or neck pain, dry eyes, insomnia, poor nutrition, weight gain or loss

Clearly, internet addiction can affect a man's relationships, job, finances, or education. In terms of actual research findings:

- Internet addiction is a global trend affecting young people in the West, in Asia, and worldwide.

- In terms of gaming, males are three times more likely to become addicted to gaming than females. Researchers found that online pornography and online gambling are also more frequent among adult males.

- While data tends to be scarce, studies show that about 10% of young males with an Internet addiction suffer from depression.

Underlying issues. Free time and underlying psychosocial issues appear to be major factors in internet addiction. A study of problematic internet use among two groups found that in those 55 or older, overuse was associated with either an anxiety disorder or OCD (obsessive-compulsive disorder). Among people 25 and younger, ADHD or a social anxiety disorder was associated with problematic internet use.

The first step in treatment is the recognition that the problem exists. In some cases, self-correction can be achieved through self-management. There is software available that controls access to the internet and the type of sites that can be visited. If anxiety or depression are present, treating those conditions (with or without medication) can be helpful. Various forms of cognitive and behavioral therapy are useful as well.

Let's be honest: we are all a little addicted to the internet and to our phones. However, as more and more of our lives transition to business and schooling online, men need to be aware of how much time they are spending in the virtual world rather than the real world.

At this point, technology is changing at a much faster pace than our biology. However, our children, spouses, and communities still crave real human interaction, rather than simply virtual communication. The key is finding the balance between the efficiency and convenience that technology can provide while avoiding the escapism and false reinforcement of the internet.

**For additional information, please see
www.TheTwentyFirstCenturyMan.com.**

Chapter 51
Pornography
Michael Abassian, MPH, Researcher
& Judson Brandeis, MD, Urologist

If pornography releases sexual tension,
then why don't we send recipe books to the starving?
— Andrea Dworkin

**The data: Over $3,000 is spent on online pornography every second.
Why it matters: The more men view porn, the less satisfied they are
with their own sex lives, and the more likely they are to have issues
with sexual arousal and erectile dysfunction.**

The term pornography first appeared in the Oxford English Dictionary in 1842, and if you happen to have an ancient dictionary around the house, take a look and see how the word is defined. You might find it amusing. In fact, if you happen to have a Merriam-Webster's Dictionary from the late 1800s, you'll find pornography defined as: Licentious painting or literature; especially, the painting anciently employed to decorate the walls of rooms devoted to bacchanalian orgies (which in the Victorian era simply meant drunken parties).

Today, pornography refers to material such as books, photographs, writings, or videos that depict erotic behavior intended to cause sexual arousal or excitement. With the exponential growth of the internet and easy access to media, the consumption of pornography has dramatically increased globally. There are over two and a half million porn websites, and over $3,000 is spent on online pornography *every second*. One out of every three Internet downloads relates to pornography. Porn has become so common that researchers attempting to study its effects on adolescents often struggle to find large enough control groups or research participants who do not watch porn.

Pornography influences how companies advertise, the literature we read, the films we watch, our economy, and even our laws. It is an estimated $17 billion-dollar industry in the United States alone. Virtual reality (VR) porn is projected to be a billion-dollar business by 2025, just behind the VR market for video games and NFL content. In 2008, three million Americans purchased pornography online, paying an average of $60 U.S. per month.

Still, one thing for sure is that the consumption of pornography affects men and women differently.

RISK FACTORS

Men 35 to 49 years old are the largest consumer group of online pornography. The thalamus and hypothalamus in men are significantly activated when watching pornography compared to women, which is why men are more stimulated through visuals. The hypothalamus, in particular, influences essential aspects of survival reflected in motivation, hormones, and the desire for sex (as well as other necessities such as water and food). Over time the brain learns to view pornography not just as a stimulant for sexual arousal, but as a need for survival. Studies show that men prefer images and pornographic websites with media content, whereas women prefer erotic stories and sites that emphasize romance.

Statistics to consider about porn consumption:

- Men are more than five times more likely to look at porn than females (543%).

- Happily married men are less likely to look at porn.

- Individuals who are politically liberal are more likely to view porn.

- Individuals who have ever committed adultery are more than twice as likely to look at porn.

- Those with teenage children are less likely to look at porn.

Regions that are more urban, have higher than average household income, have a large number of young adults, and have a higher proportion of individuals with undergraduate degrees have higher rates of porn subscriptions. Getting an accurate estimate of who watches pornography, how often they do, and what kind they watch is complicated: people may not want to admit they watch porn due to stigma and shame. However, researchers conduct many surveys around this topic, and anonymous polls help us get a clearer picture of the scope of pornographic consumption. Research reported by the Barna group in 2014 and 2016 indicates that:

- 67% of 31- to 49-year-old men view porn at least once a month.

- 49% of 50- to 68-year-old men view porn at least once monthly.

- 38% of 31- to 49-year-old men view porn at least several times a week.

- 25% of 50- to 68-year-old men view porn weekly.

One out of every ten adults admits to internet sexual addiction, and 40 million adults in the United States regularly visit porn websites. Two out of every three adult site visitors are men, and on average, men get first exposed to pornography at the early age of 12. A survey of 782 U.S. college students found that 58% of young men view porn once a week or more. Three out of every ten people who have computers at work visit sexual sites at some point in time. Thus, pornography can contribute to indirect costs to society through lost productivity, addiction treatment and management, and the effects it has on relationships. Let's take a closer look at why pornographic consumption is a bad habit and how it hinders optimal mental health.

Self-Esteem, Body-Image, and Sexual Performance

Misinterpreting reality. It is essential to understand that pornography is fiction. Plain and simple. Pornographic films are the creation of adult actors, directors, and staff members who collaborate to produce a body of work that looks and feels erotic. For example, film scenes are often edited to make it seem like men are able to perform longer than they normally do. We usually do not know what supplements or substances adult film actors take to influence their performance. Adult film actress Erin Moore reported that on set, they binged on ecstasy, cocaine, marijuana, Xanax, Valium, Vicodin, and alcohol, indicating the circumstances behind the scenes can be problematic, can be highly anxiety-producing, and are unknown to the viewer.

Then there are cultural figures like John Curtis Holmes from the 1970s and 80s, who is described as a "legendary American adult film actor" and "an icon of Hollywood success," and lived a lifestyle filled with entertainment, money, and sex. His story ended with drug addiction and HIV/AIDS. What constitutes pornography and what society deems acceptable are not always clear-cut and evolve over time.

Effects on intimacy. Excessive consumption of porn can alter the way men view women, influence expectations about what sex and intimacy should look like, how a sexually desirable woman should look, and even change the way men see themselves, contributing to lower self-esteem and confidence.

> *The frequency of viewing pornography correlates with lower satisfaction from sex and relationships.*

The more men view porn, the less satisfied they are with their own sex lives, and the more likely they are to have issues with sexual arousal and erectile dysfunction. It can also be the case that low satisfaction from sex and poor relationships can lead to more porn consumption, but randomized controlled trials and landmark studies in the 1980s show that groups exposed to more porn report less intimate satisfaction with their partners.

"Pornography viewers tend to have problems with premature ejaculation and erectile dysfunction. Having spent so much time in unnatural sexual experiences with paper, celluloid, and cyberspace [erotica], they seem to find it difficult to have sex with a real human being." — Dr. MaryAnne Layden

Pornography and Relationships

Men who excessively consume porn are at increased risk of believing that marriage is sexually restricting and that monogamy is not the norm. There is an increased risk of infidelity, marital distress, separation, and divorce. Psychologist Dr. Gary Brooks describes five symptoms associated with consumption of pornography, which include:

- *Voyeurism.* The obsession with looking at women rather than interacting with them.

- *Objectification.* Women are viewed as objects and judged entirely by physical attributes such as size, shape, and looks.

- *Validation.* The need to validate masculinity through association with good-looking women (or the fantasy of that scenario).

- *Trophyism.* The notion that women are collectibles and reveal how successful the man is (or that type of fantasy).

- *Fear of real intimacy.* The inability to connect with women honestly and intimately is detrimental to a healthy relationship and instills a negative outlook on how to bond and connect with women that is far from optimal.

Pornography and the Brain

Excessive porn consumption increases the release of dopamine and, if used for the sole purpose of ejaculating, can contribute to premature ejaculation as the body is trained to ejaculate more quickly compared to in-person sexual experiences with a partner, which typically takes longer, involves foreplay, human connection, and more intimacy.

Researchers have also seen correlations between excessive porn consumption and decreasing gray matter in the prefrontal cortex. Although more research is needed to establish how this occurs, experts hypothesize that intense stimulation of the brain's reward system degrades gray matter over time. Researchers also see these changes in individuals suffering from substance abuse and other forms of addiction. The prefrontal cortex influences planning and decision making and is normally one of the most active areas of the brain.

Pornography and Addiction

If you look for porn addiction in the DSM-5 (Diagnostic and Statistical Manual of Mental Disorder 5th Edition), you won't find it. Porn addiction is not officially recognized by the American Psychiatric Association, which means there are no official criteria used by mental health professionals to diagnose such a condition. Yet, those who compulsively view pornography exhibit behavioral traits similar to those with substance addiction. Keep in mind that addictions typically involve a lack of control and have significant negative consequences that interfere with daily life and the ability to function.

Among a survey of 800 regular porn users, nearly 90% said they would be willing to seek professional help if it were offered online. When porn consumption is out of control, the user is unable to stop, and it negatively affects their life and those around them.

If porn is an issue for you, there are some things you can do:

- Consider why you watch porn and when. Take note of events or circumstances that may trigger an urge.

- Get rid of any pornographic material in your home and on your computer including magazines, electronic bookmarks, pictures, and the like.

- Keep a journal to track progress, relapses, reminders, and reflections on your journey.

- Choose an alternative activity like sports, travel, or reading.

- Have an ally. Share your concerns with someone you trust such as your spouse, your physician, your therapist, or simply a close friend. Talking helps.

The good news is that compulsive use of pornography, compared to other addictions, is relatively easy to overcome. Specialized therapy, including cognitive behavioral therapy (CBT) and acceptance and commitment therapy (ACT), have high success rates. Studies show that those who seriously participate in ACT reduce porn consumption by more than 90% and maintain these new habits in the long term.

KEY TAKE AWAYS

Pornography is here to stay. Access to the Internet through our phones, tablets, and laptops has made pornography easily accessible and very common in our society.

- The porn industry is a multibillion-dollar global phenomenon.

- Men 35 to 49 years old are the largest consumer group of online pornography.

- Excessive porn consumption increases your risk of poor self-esteem, lower satisfaction from sex with your partner, and lower satisfaction and motivation in your relationship.

- Porn addiction is not an official diagnosis, yet it can be a serious behavioral issue. Seeking therapy, sharing with those you trust, and keeping a journal can help.

Recall that on average men first get exposed to pornography around the age of 12. The earlier we get exposed to porn, the more normal it may seem, and the more we may become desensitized to it. We run the risk of having a generation of children who learn about sex through fictional entertainment. This unrealistic learning can be problematic and counterproductive to sexual education taught either at school or in the home from more trusted and reliable sources. We'd like to conclude by saying that not everyone who consumes pornography experiences adverse effects, and some may believe it has a positive effect on their lives. In moderation, some users see it as just another form of entertainment, a way to reduce anxiety and stress, and an opportunity to add some exploration and curiosity to their sex lives. However, in the pursuit of optimizing your manhood, research favors avoiding excessive porn consumption.

For more information see
www.TheTwentiethFirstCenturyMan.com.

PART 7
LOOKING GOOD
Introduction
Judson Brandeis, MD

The characteristics that men and women look for in potential mates vary widely. In general, men strongly prefer a woman's beautiful appearance over resources, whereas women value a man's resources over his appearance.

The standard biological explanation for this is that men are looking for healthy, fertile women who will bear high-quality offspring for them. Since fertility for women rises in the late teens and peaks in the mid-twenties, men tend to prefer mates in that age range. Furthermore, characteristics of feminine beauty—such as low waist-to-hip ratio, clear skin, and lustrous hair—are all signs of good health, so it's only natural that men would find these attractive.

In contrast, women are at a natural disadvantage when it comes to acquiring resources. They're physically weaker than men, and their mobility and earning capacity is hampered by pregnancy and child-rearing, so women are more dependent on men to provide for them and their children. For this reason, women value resources over looks in a potential mate.

So it is no surprise that men make up less than 10% of the aesthetic market. But in the same way that women have gradually moved into the workforce, men are beginning to focus more on their appearance, perhaps in response to the highly competitive job market. Men are living longer and working longer than ever before.

However, since men and women have different anatomies, the interventions that improve a woman's appearance are not necessarily appropriate for a man. The women's skincare market is ten times the value of the men's, demonstrating that men are less likely to protect their skin from sun damage and windburn. As a result, men develop wrinkles and lose facial volume at an earlier age. In general, men have larger foreheads with prominent brows and protruding mandibles, and their skin is thicker and oilier. Men have more facial blood vessels but less superficial fat.

Unlike women, there is a wide variation in what is considered the perfect look for men. Male aging occurs more gradually, and aging is more socially acceptable in men than in women. Some men refer to their wrinkles as character lines and interpret their graying hair as distinguished. However, you can't go wrong with younger and healthier. As aging men, we should embrace technologies developed to help our appearance stand the test of time.

Chapter 52
Good Grooming
Judson Brandeis, MD, Urologist
& Scott Lu, MD, Researcher

Elegance is not standing out, but being remembered.
— Giorgio Armani

Economists Daniel Hamermesh and Jeff Biddle examined the impact of appearance on a person's earnings. Their research revealed that a person with below-average looks tended to earn 9% less per hour, and an above-average person earned 5% more per hour than an average-looking person, regardless of occupation. That equates to thousands of dollars a year just for looking better. Biddle and Hamermesh assessed the influence of good looks on the wages of lawyers as they began to age, and found that five years after graduating, attractive male attorneys had approximately 10% higher earnings than their less attractive counterparts. Ten years later, the income differential increased to 12%, implying that looks matter more as you age.

Do you put time and effort into your appearance? How often do you shave? How do you clean and take care of the skin on your face? How much do you actually know about the hair on your face and head, and how to properly take care of it? How often do you wash and condition your hair? Most men know almost nothing about these subjects. This chapter will review the basics of shaving, skin care, hair, the chemistry of hair products, and facial aesthetic procedures.

SHAVING

Hair, up close and personal. A hair follicle is a living system that anchors each hair into the skin. The hair bulb forms the base of the hair follicle where living cells divide and grow to build the hair shaft. Blood vessels nourish the cells in the hair bulb and deliver hormones that modify hair growth and structure at different times of life. The actual hair is made of a tough protein called keratin. Hair growth occurs in cycles consisting of three phases:

- *Growth phase* (anagen). Most hair is growing at any given time. Each strand of hair spends several years in this phase.

- *Transitional phase* (catagen). Over a few weeks, hair growth slows and the hair follicle shrinks.

- *Resting phase* (telogen). Over months, hair growth stops and the old hair detaches from the hair follicle. A new hair begins the growth phase, pushing the old hair out.

Hair grows at different rates, but the average is around one-half inch per month. Hair color is created by pigment cells producing melanin in the hair follicle. With aging, pigment cells die, and hair turns gray.

Sebaceous glands, connected to the hair follicle, secrete sebum, a light yellow, oily substance. Sebum is composed of various oils and natural antioxidants that hydrate your skin, including triglycerides, free fatty acids, wax esters, cholesterol esters, cholesterol, and squalene. Before sebum makes its way to the surface of the skin, it combines with cells that are in the process of being sloughed off inside the hair follicle. When the follicle fills up, sebum spreads over the surface of the skin, making it moisturized and healthy. When this process works too well, it results in oily skin and hair, a condition that is known medically as *seborrhea*. When not enough sebum is produced, the skin and hair become dry.

Sebum production is controlled by hormones—specifically, androgens such as testosterone. During puberty, the sebaceous glands enlarge, the hormones become more active, and more sebum is produced. This is why *acne* is such a hallmark of adolescence. During this period, males produce up to five times more sebum than females, but production slowly declines with age. Facial hair grows at a rate of half an inch per month, slower in the winter and faster in the summer.

The lather. Dry hair is difficult to cut and can have the strength of copper wire. When hair absorbs water, it swells, becoming softer and easier to cut. It is better to shave after a shower or after holding a hot washcloth against your face. Warm water or steam help hydrate facial hair and make it easier to cut by up to 70%.

Better still is to wash your face and neck with a mild cleanser before you shave. This will not only soften the hairs, but the rubbing action of your hand as you lather may help to release trapped, ingrown, or low-lying facial hair.

Shaving creams provide a protective anti-friction layer and improve razor glide for a smoother, more comfortable shaving experience. Shaving cream helps to keep moisture in the beard hair during the shave, leaving it softer and easier to cut. When less force is needed to cut each hair, your shave can be more comfortable. Shaving cream creates a thin

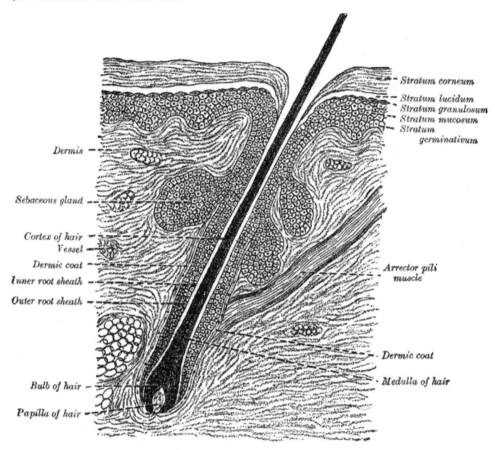

Labels on figure:

Stratum corneum
Stratum lucidum
Stratum granulosum
Stratum mucosum
Stratum germinativum

Dermis

Sebaceous gland

Cortex of hair
Vessel
Dermic coat
Inner root sheath
Outer root sheath

Arrector pili muscle

Dermic coat

Medulla of hair

Bulb of hair
Papilla of hair

Figure 52.1. Cross-section of a hair shaft. (Art by Henry Vandyke Carter, *Gray's Anatomy*.)

layer of protection between the blade and the skin, ensuring less friction and minimizing the risk of redness, razor burn, and irritation—and fewer nicks and cuts.

Most men find that using light strokes and first shaving in the direction of the hair growth and then following up with re-strokes against the grain provides the closest, smoothest shave. However, men's facial hair tends to grow in different directions (especially in the neck area), so this may not be so easy to do. Even if a man shaves with the grain (in the direction of the hair growth), some hair will still unknowingly be cut against the grain.

The shave. Using a multi-blade razor provides a closer shave because the first blade extends the hair out of the hair follicle, allowing the subsequent blade to cut further down the hair before it has fully retracted back into the follicle. A multi-blade razor spreads the load of your hand pressing down on the handle evenly across each blade. Adding more blades equals better load distribution, provided the blades are placed at the right distance apart, and will improve the comfort of the shave.

Facial skin is soft and elastic, and when you press against it with your razor's cartridge, it bulges between the individual razor blades as the cartridge passes over it. This bulging can result in irritation, nicks, and cuts. Additional blades (at the right distance apart) reduce the bulge, which means the skin surface is more even. As a result, you get a close, comfortable shave, and you're less likely to cut yourself. Note that tapping the razor against the sink basin to remove hair/shaving cream can damage the precisely engineered parts of your razor and make shaving uneven and irritating.

Years of exposure to external factors such as sun, smoking, drying indoor air, and weather conditions, as well as the aging process, can lead to dry skin problems. Men average about 170 strokes while shaving, and almost 120 of these are re-strokes. Once you scrape off the shaving cream, be mindful of repeating strokes, as this decreases lubrication, leading to shaving irritation. The skin on your face is sensitive. Shave with the grain and a slight amount of pressure to help avoid razor burn, irritation, and cuts. Razor burn, or razor rash, is skin irritation that can be caused by dry shaving, shaving that's a little too aggressive, or shaving with dull blades. Typically, it arrives a few minutes after shaving, and can be in the form of a rash if bad enough. Skin can feel irritated, tight, hot, and uncomfortable after the shave. Regular use of a moisturizing after-shave product will help to re-hydrate the skin, calm and soothe the skin, and leave it feeling smooth and comfortable. To recap:

- Exposing facial hair to hot water/steam for three minutes prior to shaving makes the hairs 70% easier to cut.

- Shaving creams are essential to reduce friction and keep moisture in the facial hair.

- A multi-blade razor usually gives a closer and smoother shave.

- Shave with the grain, and then reapply shaving cream before shaving against the grain.

Razor bumps. Razor burn and razor rash are not the same as clinical razor bumps, a condition caused by ingrown hairs that is scientifically known as *Pseudofolliculitis barbae* (PFB). PFB (informally referred to as *razor bumps*) is a common, chronic, inflammatory skin condition that develops primarily as a result of shaving. Usually occurring in the beard area in men, PFB is characterized by painful, itchy, red bumps and pus-filled bumps that are typically 2 to 5 mm in diameter. Other areas of the body that are frequently shaven may also be affected, including the armpits, scalp, nape of the neck, and pubic region.

Razor bumps and ingrown hair start with a genetic tendency toward extremely curly hair. The irregular shape of curly hair shafts and the curls themselves make hairs prone to pushing back into the surface of the skin as they regrow after being cut. This genetic factor makes ingrown hair and razor bumps surprisingly common. To minimize razor bumps:

- Use barber-style electric clippers with an adjustable guard or comb attachment that maintains a hair length of 1 to 3 mm (known as a *five-o'clock shadow*).

- Men desiring a closer shave may need to use a razor blade.

- Single-edged razor blades that contain a protective foil guard to prevent the hair from being trimmed too close to the skin are recommended for patients with PFB.

- Multiple-blade razors that cut the hair at skin level or just below the skin's surface should be avoided.

- Do not shave every day.

FACIAL AESTHETICS FOR GUYS

Every spring I bring out my pressure washer to clean the dirt and grime off my concrete pathways. Similarly, the goal of a HydraFacial is to provide the same type of benefits to your skin. The three steps involve 1) deep-cleaning (removing oil and dirt from facial pores), 2) exfoliation to resurface the skin, and 3) hydration with antioxidants. This procedure helps any skin, but especially those with acne, dryness, or wrinkles. An aesthetician uses a mechanized wand to deeply clean and exfoliate your skin while delivering therapeutic serums matched to your skin type. A HydraFacial session typically takes less than an hour and costs about $200.

Microneedling. In the spring, I also aerate the lawn so that air, water, and fertilizer can reach the grass roots and my lawn can grow back healthier and greener. Microneedling aerates the skin. A dermatologist or aesthetician uses tiny needles to prick the skin on the face and neck in order to stimulate the growth of new collagen and skin tissue for smoother, firmer skin.

Microneedling is safe and requires no downtime. Most clients experience minor redness and irritation for a few days after the procedure. Microneedling typically costs around $300, and four sessions are required to treat minor scarring related to acne, wounds, or aging. Most clients notice brighter, firmer skin following microneedling sessions.

Microdermabrasion. Every few years the sun gets the better of the paint on my house, and I have to sandblast the paint off before I reapply it. Microdermabrasion of the skin is a similar process in which an instrument gently sands your skin to remove the thick and uneven outer layer. The benefits of this treatment are to improve light scarring, reduce wrinkles, lessen discoloration, and help sun damage.

Microdermabrasion costs between $100 and $200. Expect some redness and swelling, which should subside within a few hours, as well as flaky skin that lasts for several days. Be sure to protect your skin with sunscreen because it will burn more easily. Microdermabrasion stimulates collagen to grow, which makes your skin more youthful and smoother.

HAIR CARE

How often do you wash and condition your hair? If your hair is healthy, it looks clean, is soft to the touch, untangled, and has a bounce when your head moves. To maintain hair health, use shampoo that cleans both the scalp and hair fibers.

Some men tend to have oily hair, which means that they have excess natural oil, sebum. Produced by the sebaceous glands, sebum's primary role is to moisturize the face, scalp, and hair to keep it healthy. Sebum protects the protein structure of hair so that it doesn't split. Your body constantly produces sebum, potentially leading to oily hair and scalp problems. (For example, if you are not washing your hair often enough, these natural oils will trap dust and pollution, causing your hair to look dull.)

Shampoos are cleansers designed for this area. Most body soaps do not have good lathering ability and are also relatively more difficult to fully wash away, especially with hard water. Shampoo offers a gentler solution to clean the scalp of sebum, dirt, environmental pollutants, sweat, and other residues without removing all the natural oils. Residues you don't want to stay in your hair unnecessarily include hair products such as mousses, pomades, sprays, lotions, or oils.

Shampoos are composed of detergents, conditioners, thickeners, sequestering agents, pH adjusters, preservatives, and specialty additives. Most shampoos include:

- A surfactant or detergent that binds to oily deposits on the scalp and allows for removal via water. Modern shampoos contain precise mixtures to provide optimal cleaning for normal, dyed, or damaged hair.

- Foaming agents are usually added to create a foamy lather.

- Thickeners increase the viscosity of the soap.

- Modern soaps also contain sequestering agents such as chelated magnesium or calcium to help prevent soap scum from forming.

- To maintain an optimum hair pH, which lies around 3.7, pH adjustors are added to the formula. Increases in pH (more basic) can cause hair shaft swelling, damaging hair follicles.

- Preservatives are added to prevent decomposition by microbes.

- Special additives may be included such as vitamins and botanicals. Whether the short contact time shampoo has with hair is long enough for these agents to have a clear clinical effect is questionable, but this is one of the areas of highest variability when it comes to marketing claims.

■ Finally, conditioners may be added to shampoo (2-in-1 formulations), which typically involve silicone droplets suspended in a surfactant mixture. Examples include hydrolyzed silk and animal protein, glycerin, and propylene glycol. The end result is a more manageable, glossy quality to hair, with anti-static properties.

Shampoos are complicated mixtures. Sebum, one of the oily substances cleaned from the scalp, has a protective effect on the hair, so a good shampoo must balance the amount of oil cleaned from the hair without drying out the hair and scalp. Complicating this is the need to leave hair manageable and shiny.

So, who should use which shampoo?

■ Men with normal hair can use normal shampoos. By normal hair we mean men with chemically untouched hair and a scalp that produces a moderate amount of sebum.

■ Men who produce an abundance of sebum may benefit more from shampoo formulated for oily hair.

■ There are also shampoos for men who wash their hair daily. These contain milder detergents and typically don't contain conditioners.

■ Deep cleaning shampoos are useful for those who use strong styling products. These should only be used once weekly.

■ Dry shampoo is useful for those who have undergone chemical treatment or harsh styling procedures. These shampoos are generally milder. Dry shampoo can also be used during illness or following surgery when it is more difficult to shower or bend over a sink.

■ Professional shampoos are used before cutting or styling, or before and after chemical treatments to bleach or color hair. These contain concentrated ingredients to neutralize the harsh effects of the chemicals on the hair follicles and scalp and are not meant to be used for daily hair care.

The choice of hair shampoo and the type of hair also affect how often we should wash our hair. In general, this is by individual preference. Washing hair daily with a well-formulated shampoo should not damage hair, and there is no upper limit to the frequency of conditioner use. Sebum can be seen as the ideal hair conditioner. It will be replenished naturally. Another common issue men develop is dandruff, which causes the skin on the scalp to flake. Treat dandruff with a gentle daily shampoo or periodically with a medicated shampoo specific for dandruff. Dandruff signs and symptoms may include skin flakes in your hair and an itchy scalp. These signs and symptoms may be more severe if you're stressed, and they tend to flare up in cold, dry seasons.

Conditioners. Conditioning agents contain a number of additives to improve manageability. These additives are meant to enhance appearance and fullness of the hair. This may become necessary due to the potential of shampoo to remove too much of the natural oils from your hair. If your hair is too dry after you shampoo, a good first step is to try a different shampoo that's less drying. Avoid using liquid hand soap as shampoo, since they are designed specifically to remove oil residue from our hands and are extremely drying. Another effect of conditioner is to reduce static electricity to hair. Conditioners contain cationic surfactants, providing a positive electric charge that balances the negative charge that hair naturally carries. Conditioners also flatten cuticle scales over the hair shaft, reducing friction between hair fibers and increasing reflectivity of light, improving shininess. Like shampoos, there are multiple types of conditioners to choose from:

- Instant conditioners are applied immediately after shampooing and left in for a few minutes before rinsing. This is the type of conditioner most useful for daily washing.

- Blow drying conditioners are a type of instant conditioner that do not contain oil and can be left on the hair. This is especially useful for men with fine hair and excessive scalp sebum.

- Deep conditioners are more concentrated and left on the hair longer (20 to 30 minutes).

- Hair thickening conditioners coat hair shafts to increase their diameter, giving the view of thicker hair.

- Leave-in conditioners are typically applied to hair after washing and drying. They provide an extra level of moisture and help to detangle strands. This type of conditioner can be left in through a styling routine without having to be washed out.

Ever since COVID turned our lives upside down, facial aesthetics have become a larger part of how we present ourselves. Our hair and facial skin are most of what someone sees on a computer screen. In the pre-COVID days, your looks may have cost you 10% of your expected income. However, in the post-COVID Zoom conference era, it may be even more. In the Zoom-conference era, fortunately, there are simple and relatively inexpensive grooming and aesthetic resources, such as are mentioned in this section, that can take your looks to the next level.

For more information, please see www.TheTwentyFirstCenturyMan.com.

Chapter 53
A Healthy Smile
Paul Scholberg, DDS

Life is short; smile while you still have teeth.
— Mallory Hopkins

What makes a great smile? A smile involves more than just your teeth—it is a facial expression of emotion that reflects positive nonverbal communication and social interaction. Just the right angle of the mouth, a glimpse of healthy teeth, and the symmetry of the face combine to produce an impression of harmony.

The history of creating a smile in dentistry is extensive. The art of constructing replacements for patients with missing teeth dates to at least 700 BC, with animal and human teeth bound together by gold banding. In the 20th century, dentistry developed the appearance and proportions of teeth using the Golden Ratio. Thanks to the Greeks, this design language (applying "the Golden Mean") has led to the creation of the "perfect smile," one that mathematically balances the proportions of the face and the teeth. Comparing the length and width of the face, a formula is employed that is roughly 1 to 1.6. This same ratio is used to create a visual sense of balance in the appearance of the teeth as well. That is the standard that we use today.

DESIGNING A SMILE

During the last decade in my practice, I did nothing but smile solutions—fixing smiles that were not quite right, whether that meant adjusting one tooth or all twenty-eight in order to fix the entire bite and the overall appearance of the smile. These are not inexpensive procedures. There are quite a few dentists who provide smile makeovers, and who do it competently—though this is not true of every provider, given the learning curve involved. So as a consumer, it is important to educate yourself, since typical smile design costs upwards of $15,000 for the usual remake of eight to ten teeth. Thinking in broad terms, three of the most effective strategies for brightening a smile are bleaching/whitening, Invisalign (having teeth aligned), and veneering (applying a laminate to the teeth).

Whitening

Whitening teeth is a cost-effective way to brighten a smile. Whiter teeth are usually associated with a youthful appearance. However, it is important to remember that whitening can be overdone. Periodically, I see people with blinding smiles. This raises the question of how to achieve a natural outcome, an appearance that is not too white, and one that looks age appropriate.

Whitening teeth is a chemical process that reduces external stains on the enamel, but also has an effect on the dentin core of the tooth. The whitening effect is achieved using peroxides in various forms. The peroxides are applied to the tooth surface, and they penetrate the enamel to the underlying layer of dentin.

What works:

- Whitening is effective for most patients.

- Teeth displaying yellow to orange discoloration can be successfully treated.

What may not work:

- Over-whitening can break down the protective enamel on the surface of the teeth.

- Teeth with a grey discoloration will not whiten well due to underlying deep stains. (Tetracycline antibiotics are a common cause.)

- Trauma to developing teeth or a high fever can also discolor the dentin layer and those teeth are then difficult to whiten completely.

I prefer using custom-made bleaching trays to gradually whiten the teeth, but it takes longer than an in-office laser treatment. (Peroxide tends to be nontoxic, since it resembles a substance that is created in our own bodies by the immune system.)

Often people have no patience and are attracted to immediate results. The intense light source (high intensity light or diode laser) used in office treatments acts as a catalyst, creating more heat and more activity for the solutions that create the bleaching process. In-office treatment is effective, but the teeth are going to be sensitive. Patients are sent home with the products necessary to support them through that first week or so. However, it is an instant process, and they walk away four, five, or six shades lighter. Note that aggressive bleaching or laser use can injure the teeth in some cases.

Protective care. Using a bleaching tray is a longer and slower process, but it protects the health of the teeth. An Invisalign tray, for example, is a retainer that can be used as a bleaching tray. The bulk of the whitening is achieved by lightening the dentin core of the teeth. A retainer or a bleaching tray allows us to moderate the strength of the solution that we use, depending on the time the patient is willing to invest.

Lower concentrations and longer application time give the best long-term results. A mild solution of a carbamide peroxide can be used for two weeks or more. Darker teeth can be treated for an even longer period of time with supervision.

Whitening strips. Although quite popular, whitening strips do not seem to be as effective at whitening deep stains. They are particularly useful, however, for mild stains and for the periodic touchups required with all whitening treatments. A limitation to whitening strips is their placement on just the front teeth. They need to extend beyond the front teeth to blend with the posterior teeth esthetically. The bicuspids essentially frame your smile, so you will want to whiten at least ten of the upper teeth.

Invisalign

Invisalign is orthodontic software developed to correct moderate dental crowding in adults. This is a CAD/CAM tool that was invented by orthodontists to improve their practice. It is not useful for children because their bones and teeth are still growing.

With Invisalign, the look of your teeth is designed in the digital software, enabling the dentist to determine where each tooth should be positioned. The technology creates ideal images of the desired effect and then the software predicts the movement and positioning required of the teeth at each week of treatment. The procedure is defined, step by step, whether the teeth are to be moved, rotated, adjusted, or manipulated in some other way. The retainers are digitally crafted so that each of these adjustments is performed incrementally, just tenths of a millimeter at a time. The patient wears a retainer for a week and then is fitted with another retainer that continues the realignment of the teeth. Ultimately, 28 or more retainers later, the teeth have gradually moved into the desired alignment.

Invisalign has been in use since the early 2000s. This technology can create a better outcome, but the consumer must be savvy in choosing an experienced dentist. When working with the right dentist, it can be highly effective.

Who is a good candidate for Invisalign? The short answer is, someone who is not happy with their smile because their teeth are crowded or misaligned.

Most patients may simply need some minor repositioning of their teeth and whitening. Often, restorations are not required. In other cases, restoring a smile may involve a combination of strategies, positioning the teeth more ideally before placing veneers. That can mean maneuvering the teeth a little so that the root position and tooth spacing is more symmetrical and will enhance the restorative outcome.

Men in midlife who are professionals, for example, often work in highly competitive environments. It is understandable that they would want a great smile to keep them looking and feeling attractive.

Veneers

Veneers are a thin layer of ceramic or resin composite material bonded to the underlying tooth surface to reface the outer surface of a tooth. They are commonly used to correct tooth appearance.

One of the technical beauties of veneers is that you can build on the strength of the natural underlying color of the teeth and enhance them with the new veneer, which is essentially a new layer of "enamel" that you are placing over the existing tooth.

Bonding. Adhering a porcelain or composite restoration to the surface of the tooth uses a bonding process. The underlying enamel and dentin are acid etched (typically with a mild phosphoric acid) to create microscopic surface textures, enabling bonding with an enhanced resin material. Bonding greatly enhances the total strength of the restoration and underlying tooth.

Good work takes time. A typical ten-unit smile may involve two to four somewhat lengthy office visits. Then there are prepless veneers, which require a highly skilled laboratory to construct as the veneers may be only a few tenths of a millimeter thick, but that may shorten chairside time.

Prepless veneers. Early in the 1970s and 1980s, there were prepless veneers, essentially "press-on" veneers, which could be bonded over the existing teeth. Unfortunately, they made the teeth much thicker than before and were not very aesthetic. Newer technology provides a more effective process, resulting in more naturally shaped teeth.

There are a limited number of labs that specialize in this type of veneer, but some of the cases I have seen are quite remarkable.

CEREC

CEREC (Chairside Economical Restoration of Esthetic Ceramic) is a computer-aided technology that is widely used in dentistry, a tool for the practitioner that ultimately benefits the patient as well.

Traditional crowns. A crown is a dental restoration that covers and replaces most of the tooth surface. They can be constructed of all-ceramic material or use a metal casting after reshaping the coronal component of the tooth. Crowns are usually provided due to damage from deeper decay or a tooth fracture. Crowns currently average $1500 a tooth, but a highly skilled provider with extensive experience may charge more per crown. Back in the day, your dentist would prepare the tooth, create a mold, send it to the lab, and send you home with a temporary crown that was unattractive and usually did not work very well. The crown was not completed until a second office visit. All that has changed with recent technology.

Creating a crown using software. Today, we can make a crown right on the spot. CEREC, although not new, has gained significance over the past decade. Used in restorative dentistry, implantology, and orthodontics, this approach allows one-visit ceramic restorations.

The entire procedure to create a crown is all done in the office in a single visit. Digital scanning, design, milling, and construction are completed in a single, step-by-step procedure, facilitated by the software. Even the modeling required for construction of retainers or mouthguards is facilitated through a digital intraoral scanner, capturing information required to print the model or appliance on an office 3D printer.

Ultimately, it is both patient-friendly and practitioner-friendly. If the dentist is skilled at this technology, the patient gets a better result than that of the multistep process—they have a crown that is as good as or better than a conventional lab-made product.

That raises the question, how do you find a dentist who is skilled in using this approach? Do you want someone who has done 500 hours or 1,000 hours? The best strategy is to go by referral, either from other patients, dental professionals, or a medical practice.

STATE-OF-THE-SCIENCE IMAGING, ROOT CANALS, AND OTHER SITUATIONS

Dental CT scans. High-quality scanning that minimizes the use of in-office x-rays is now provided in specialty dental imaging centers and is in use in many progressive offices. If you are going to have an implant placed, you will want to get a CBCT (cone beam computed tomography) scan. This incredible tool provides a type of 3D x-ray image that can be manipulated in many different ways, enhancing the ability to identify nuanced pathologies such as deteriorated bone structure. CBCT imaging enables the dentist to view all aspects of the patient's dentition in detailed segments horizontally, laterally, or vertically.

Root canals. A root canal is the process of replacing the inner pulp tissue of a tooth. This is a crisis response to deterioration caused by invading dental caries as the body attempts to wall off advancing decay. If not repaired in time, inflammation will destroy the remaining blood supply to the tissue, eventually causing death of the pulp and ultimately the potential loss of the tooth. The treatment is painstaking, using small file-like instruments that are manipulated inside the pulp chamber within the tooth to carefully clean and reshape the dental canals. An inert filling is used to seal the space to the tip of the root. Often a microscope is used to aid the operator in visualizing the inner structure of the tooth. After this procedure, a crown with internal reinforcement is placed.

When an endodontist performs a root canal, they are dealing with a highly intricate structure. Back in the day, we thought that there was simply a tubular canal within the root of each tooth shaped like a carrot. It turns out that's not the case. These are incredibly complex structures.

Better outcomes. Using CBCT scans allow endodontists to have a higher rate of success with root canals. With access to these images, the dentist knows whether there are lateral canals, what degree of branching is present, and where the branching is located. In the past, when root canals failed, it was due to inadequate sealing of the spaces within the tooth. This single imaging tool has completely changed endodontics because now we can see the complete structure inside and outside the tooth root system. The endodontist can determine whether you can be treated successfully or not. In short, the imaging allows for much more sophisticated root canal treatment.

If you need a root canal and your dentist is not using this type of technology, you are best served by seeing a dentist who is using this newer type of imaging to maximize your chances of success. These digital technologies allow much greater precision and have become the standard of care.

Reduced radiation exposure. The use of CBCT imaging is found in many progressive offices today and is augmenting in-office x-rays. Since radiation exposure is cumulative, the goal is to reduce it to the least amount of exposure possible. Today, a CBCT and four bitewing x-rays have significantly less exposure with far greater diagnostic information.

MINIMIZING DAMAGE TO YOUR TEETH

Immediate care for a knocked-out tooth. Dental avulsion is a true clinical emergency. If the tooth is intact, a gentle rinse with saline and immediate reimplantation is the best treatment. Place the tooth in a suitable storage medium such as whole milk for that trip to the dentist. Typically, 20 to 40 minutes is the window of time if the tooth is still viable, and the timing significantly affects the outcome. A dentist will clean the socket and the tooth and replant the tooth into the socket. Splinting the tooth to the adjacent teeth will stabilize it for a week to ten days, at which point a root canal can be performed. Long-term survival of the tooth depends on the favorable healing of the periodontal ligament. The chance of success is about 50/50 or perhaps greater, but worth the effort.

Using a mouthguard. Impact sports require protection of the teeth. Fabrication of a flexible maxillary mouthguard is a simple, relatively inexpensive level of insurance against avulsion accidents. A mouthguard made in the dental office provides the fit required to keep it in place during activity. Those made on the stovetop do not fit well and usually end up not being used.

Stupid things that break teeth. It happens. Teeth are not unbreakable. Popcorn kernels, ice, hard candy, nuts, inadvertent bits of stuff in your sandwich, or even tearing duct tape with your teeth take a toll. Most coronal tooth fractures occur if previous large repairs have been performed, typically involving fillings of amalgam or non-bonded restorations. These situations are usually repairable, but sometimes fractures can affect the root, with subsequent loss of the tooth.

Medications that damage teeth. Side effects harmful to teeth can occur with any medication that has dry-mouth effects. Other medications that affect teeth at formative stages can also be damaging, as well as:

- Beta blockers, calcium channel blockers, diuretics, and ACE inhibitors

- Opioids, antihistamines, decongestants, and similar medications

- Tetracycline use in children is well-recognized as a cause of damage to forming adult teeth, producing dark stains in dentin.

- Fluoride added to municipal water systems is responsible for a massive reduction in dental caries in these populations. However, too much fluoride can leave white streaks in the enamel, usually seen in well-water communities.

Bruxism. Tooth grinding is a complicated and controversial condition. Typically, it involves nighttime muscular activity leading to excessive wear of the teeth and supporting structures. Awake bruxism also can occur but is thought to have different origins. Both can create significant discomfort in chewing muscles and jaw joints (TMJ). In nighttime bruxism, there is a dynamic in the central nervous system involving sleep arousal and neurotransmitter origins. Our stressful lifestyle is certainly a contributor. Mechanical misalignment of the teeth and jaws are triggers as well. Certain prescribed medications can also exacerbate the underlying triggers.

To control tooth grinding, most dentists rely on a relatively noninvasive appliance that can be worn at night. A night guard (also termed occlusal splint) covers the chewing surfaces, allowing relief from muscle strain, and transferring tooth abrasion and wear to the plastic surface of the appliance. Note that this is intended as a strategy to protect the teeth but is not a treatment for the underlying cause of bruxism.

PERIODONTAL WORK

A bridge. These multiple tooth restorations replace one or more missing teeth. In the past, when a tooth was missing, a bridge was created to span from the tooth on one side of the missing tooth to the one on the other. A single missing tooth, for example, would require a three-unit (three-tooth) bridge.

The bridge is supported by a crown on either end of the bridge structure with the replacement tooth (or teeth) between them. Constructed of all-ceramic material or a metal core with overlying ceramic, the all-ceramic bridges are bonded in place, whereas metal-core bridges are cemented in place.

An implant. In these situations, an implant can be an effective alternative. An implant is a prosthesis for replacing a missing tooth that consists of a titanium fixture (a screw-like, threaded cylinder), placed in the bone to act as the tooth root. Some varying time is required for complete integration into the supporting bone. When the fixture is deemed stable, an intermediate abutment is fitted to replace the tooth core above the bone. A crown is then constructed and connected to the abutment.

With an implant, if a single tooth is damaged, there is no need to affect the teeth on either side. When a single tooth is lost, often the teeth next to it are healthy and we do not want to have to grind them down in order to create a base for the bridge. As a result, implants have become the treatment of choice. Although they are expensive, in comparison with a three-unit bridge, placing a single implant is still less expensive than working on three teeth.

In-office CAD/CAM imaging and integration with CBCT imaging provide precise implant placement, producing intraoral surgical guides printed by in-office 3D printers. When seeking an implant specialist, the professionals most skilled tend to be oral surgeons and periodontists because they are well-trained in managing the supporting structures of the teeth.

Grafting. Some patients have fragile gum tissue, perhaps due to genetics. We refer to that as a thin biotype, in which the gum tissue overlaying the bone is quite thin and very fragile. These are people who tend to have problems with recession, for example. Recession means that the overlying gum tissue and underlying bone is being stripped away from the base of the tooth. An individual with a thin biotype can be a periodontist's nightmare. Grafting is one solution. Periodontists will use tissue from the roof of the mouth by creating an incision, harvesting a very thin layer of the underlying connective tissue, and use that as the matrix to grow new tissue around the denuded area of the roots. Techniques in predictable bone grafting have also improved. The goal of the periodontist and restorative dentist is to create an undetectable outcome. This is ultimately the plastic surgery of dentistry, and there are a number of highly skilled people who provide these techniques.

MAINTAINING A GREAT SMILE

These basic resources will give you the tools to optimize your dental health.

Preventing tooth decay. Dental caries involve the formation of cavities in the teeth due to the action of bacteria interacting with your diet. Acid production occurs in the presence of sugar and other sweeteners, as well as refined starches, by the bacteria of the natural biofilm (dental plaque) in your mouth.

Initial decalcification of the enamel occurs as a cavity develops, then rapid destruction of the underlying dentin, and eventual infection of the pulp at the center of the tooth. Abscesses and loss of teeth are endemic in our world population.

Cavities on the biting surface are usually related to incomplete development of the enamel and are known as pit and fissure caries. Cavities between the teeth are described as interproximal caries and are directly related to lack of proper dental hygiene, particularly by not flossing. Pits and fissures are easily sealed with flowable resins.

Chewing gum. If you are unable to brush after meals, chewing gum can be a refreshing experience after eating and will reduce cavities and dental plaque.

- Gum containing xylitol inhibits acid formation by *Strep. mutans,* which is a prominent bacterium in oral plaque.

- Gum is also helpful in reduction of bad breath (halitosis) because the gum encourages the production of saliva, washing away bacteria.

Brushing after meals. If you are inclined to brush after meals, small portable toothbrushes (half the size of a ballpoint pen) are available that fit easily in your briefcase, backpack, or pocket. Obviously, sweet breath is always more appealing than halitosis.

Electric toothbrushes. There are two major kinds of electric toothbrush: Sonic and Rotary. I have not observed much difference in effectiveness. Ultimately, it comes down to user preference. However, each type has a different feel. Sonic can feel more aggressive, so a soft brush is recommended. All brands have two-minute timers to aid with their consistent use.

- Brushing. Generally, a gentle application to the various segments of your mouth gets the job done. Twice a day should be enough.

- Change the toothbrush head every three months.

- Choose soft brushes with either model since hard brushes can damage teeth and gums.

- Use a sodium fluoride toothpaste as stannous fluoride can stain teeth.

Dental floss. Teflon-coated floss such as Glide is quite easy to use. The key to proper use is understanding the anatomy of the tooth and the gum tissue structure. The contact between the teeth is flat but as you manipulate the floss towards the gum, the tooth structure becomes rounded. At that level, the floss should be gently curved to follow the anatomy at the base of the tooth. There are two spaces to clean, one on either side of the contact between the teeth and the gum on both sides of each tooth.

- Devices. There are floss aid devices such as Glide Gum Care Floss Pics that are extremely helpful and convenient to manipulate to clean these spaces.

- Timing. I floss after every meal. However, you can over-floss and damage the base of the teeth. Work with your hygienist or dentist to perfect your technique.

A tongue scraper. Tongue scrapers are highly effective at removing the accumulations of anaerobic bacteria on the surface of the tongue, particularly the bacteria that accumulate at night. Volatile sulfur compounds form from these bacteria and create bad breath. Use daily at least.

Mouthwashes. At best, over-the-counter mouthwashes do little to eliminate bacteria.

- Prescription chlorhexidine mouthwashes can depress bacteria formation but can also stain teeth.

- Certain systemic conditions such as diabetes create bad breath, which is difficult to control.

Only brush the teeth you want to keep. Brushing and flossing are nonnegotiable. You need to pay attention to all those little crevices and contours that are part of the landscape of your mouth. The alternative is fighting your way through tooth decay repair or gum disease and periodontal bills. You could also end up with an endocarditis due to *Strep. viridans* in the dental plaque. In addition, we now know there is some risk of cancers from forms of *Fusobacterium* that are also harbored in the biofilm.

Dental insurance. Most people have some dental insurance through their employment. Some of these plans can be very generous, but most cover simply essential services such as cleanings and basic restorative care. Be aware of the true benefits your plan provides. In many cases, the return on premium investment in my opinion is a wash. (You simply break even.)

Make life easy. Brush. Floss. Enjoy. Smile.

For more information and resources, please see www.TheTwentyFirstCenturyMan.com.

Chapter 54
Protecting Your Skin
Adam Wallach, MD, Dermatologist

It's a sad man, my friend who is living in his own skin
and can't stand the company.
— Bruce Springsteen

How do I take care of my skin? What are the best products on the market? My patients ask these questions tens of times a day. The answers reside in an interesting mix of science and common sense.

We know that our health and the way we age is a combination of genetics and exposure. There are those of us who pay little attention to the care of our skin, and yet we look great into later life. Conversely, there are younger men who look far older than their chronological age. At the moment, there's not much to be done on the genetic front — you've got the cards you were dealt; however, there are some variables that we can control. Getting adequate sleep, eating a balanced diet low in carbohydrates and sugars, and not smoking are all good general habits that will help your skin look its best. Of all the external exposures we encounter through life, the one that will age us more than any other is ultraviolet light from the sun. Let's look at how this happens. Our skin is a shield against all types of exposures, composed of:

- The outer layer, the epidermis (composed of keratinocytes)

- A second layer, the dermis

- A third layer, the subcutis.

As we age, we accumulate atrophy and damage to all the layers of our skin, but destruction to the underlying dermis from sunlight creates the biggest issues over time. The dermis layer is where collagen and elastin reside, the two key proteins that give your skin suppleness and elasticity. As these proteins diminish, the overlying epidermis no longer has the support it needs and begins to appear thin or crepe-like. The epidermal or surface layer also has an important barrier function and a role to play in youthful appearance, because it is critical to retaining moisture in the skin. Over time and exposure, as the barrier function declines, the epidermis on our face accumulates damage from continual exposure to the elements, and most of us develop blotchy pigmentation and rough skin. The underlying facial bones diminish over time as well, changing our appearance because they support the skin above it.

Most men don't realize that their skin is actually very different from women's skin. Male skin is generally much thicker and is protected from UV by the presence of mature hair follicles (women have fine peach-fuzz hairs). Consequently, male skin tends to age better than that of our female counterparts. Male skin also typically produces more sebum or oil, hence the reason younger men often feel no need or desire to moisturize their skin.

SUNSCREEN AND BEYOND

Sunscreens and Sunblocks

Sun exposure. If you are fair skinned then you have less melanin (the brown pigment that protects you from sunlight), and if you're dark skinned you've got loads of it. Furthermore, if you are fair skinned, even a small amount of UV light will cause much more damage than an equivalent amount of exposure to a darker skinned individual. Although it has never been proven scientifically that sunscreens prevent premature aging or reduce the chance of skin cancer, it makes logical sense to assume that sunscreens help prevent both of these occurrences, given what we know about the damaging effects of UV light on keratinocytes (causing cancer) and on vital skin structures like collagen, elastin, and barrier function (causing premature aging).

Sunblocks actually block UV light, whereas sunscreens are chemicals that absorb UV light, by way of comparison, and convert it to heat (why we sometimes feel hotter after applying sunscreen). Most products on the market are combinations of both, but there are pure sunblock products that contain only zinc or titanium dioxide that are often labelled "sensitive skin" or "baby" products. The use of daily sunblock may seem like elementary advice that most men know, but the fact is that most of us simply do not do it. As men, we are not generally used to smearing cream on our faces like our female counterparts.

The key to getting a sunblock ritual going is first finding a product that feels good to you — not too heavy, not fragranced, one that blends with your skin color and is easy to use. To that end, I often recommend that men try different products, trying two at a time with one product applied on the left side and the second product to the right. Which feels better? In this way, you can quickly sort through various products to find what suits you best. Clearly, a dark-skinned man with oily skin will need a different product than a fair-skinned man with drier skin. Often your local dermatologist can provide you with samples to conduct this trial-and-error approach or simply ask your dermatologist what he or she recommends.

Next, keep the sunblock beside the bathroom sink where you are likely to notice it every morning when you come out of the shower or finish washing your face. (Don't place the tube in a drawer.) Additionally, one needs a simple and reproducible way to apply the product, so it is done the same way with the same amount each day. I like to use a dotting method, whereby I dispense two generous pumps of my favorite product to my palm and then place a specified number of dots to various areas of the face, ears, and neck before rubbing it all in. This will avoid missed areas or globs of unblended sunblock. Most importantly, do this every day, at least on the face, regardless of the forecast or your schedule because weather often changes, as do our plans — a cloudy day is suddenly balmy and that plan of not leaving the office turns into a spontaneous lunch outing.

- Use an SPF of at least 30-50.

- Avoid an SPF>50 since the FDA will be eliminating them soon, and they provide only marginal added benefit, often at the cost of feeling heavier.

Assume that you are getting about half of the SPF on the label as those numbers are predicated on strict laboratory assessment of SPF that doesn't approximate real-life usage. I have a favorite facial sunblock for everyday use when I go to work, in case I step outside for a quick lunch. I also have a weekend sports water-resistant sunblock intended for sports and recreation, used for both the face and body. This water-resistant sunblock has a tackier texture and is designed to withstand the effects of sweating or water. If your total exposure will be more than two hours, be sure to reapply your sunblock. If you're actively swimming, consider reapplying every time you exit the water as even a *water resistant product* will sometime not adhere or be washed away more readily than expected. Note that the tests conducted to attain a water-resistant labelling are performed with sunblock applied in two coats, allowed to dry 20 minutes prior to testing, which is not how most folks apply sunscreen. Finally, don't forget that sunscreen is not a substitute for sun avoidance or sun-protective clothing. Protect your lips with a lip specific product that will adhere better than regular sunblock, don the broad-brimmed hat, and grab your sunglasses.

Ingredients. There has been recent discussion about whether the ingredients within sunblocks are systemically absorbed and potentially dangerous. It appears that some of these ingredients do get absorbed in the body, but there is no good scientific evidence currently that the very small level of absorption is dangerous to our health. If you want to play it conservatively, avoid oxybenzone, a common sunscreen agent. In animal studies, that is the one ingredient that appears to produce adverse effects. In addition, it has an untoward effect on marine life when it washes off our bodies, and consequently has been banned in Europe. If you don't want to get too mired down in which ingredients to avoid, but generally want to play it safer, then simply use sunscreens only during the day when sun exposure may occur and do not use them at night. In terms of vitamin D absorption, rather than not wearing sunscreen, take a vitamin D supplement or simply add wild salmon (rich in vitamin D) to your weekly shopping list.

Moisturizers

Some men, especially as they age, discover that retaining moisture in the skin not only makes the skin feel better, but also makes it look more youthful. To simplify, a good product will provide emollient qualities that smooth the skin by acting like a glue that keeps adjacent keratinocytes (the cells of the outer epidermis) together, will possess humectants (for example, hyaluronic acid or urea), which help retain water, and will have occlusive properties to diminish epidermal water loss.

An important aspect of moisturizers is that they do not moisturize the skin per se, but more accurately, they enhance barrier repair by supporting your skin's natural restorative processes. The best time to apply them is immediately after a shower when the skin has absorbed lots of water. If you live in a sunny climate and routinely shower in the morning, find a sunblock with a good moisturizing base so that you will only need one product to do both jobs. Unfortunately, the product options are almost overwhelming when one begins to look. Your preference will depend largely on:

- The type of skin you have.

- What feels good to you. Try some of the products you already own or borrow some of your spouse's products.

- If the cream feels great when you first apply it, but later in the day your skin feels dry, likely it's too light or lacking occlusive properties that keep your skin hydrated. Try something a bit heavier.

- Most men prefer *oil-free* moisturizers that are silicone based (often containing dimethicone) rather than oil-based because they will feel less oily and are more cosmetically elegant.

- Finally, one of the simplest, least expensive, and most effective moisturizing agents available is petrolatum (or Aquaphor). It is cheap, nonallergenic, and decreases evaporative water loss better than almost anything else. The key to embracing this typically "greasy" product is to use small amounts applied to the palms and then to damp warm areas of the body.

As far as cleansers go, keep it simple, and again use what feels good. Because of that added sebum in male skin, most men can use more typical soaps on the face without feeling dry. Don't over wash or scrub or get overzealous with rotating scrubbing brushes or you will damage the critical skin barrier that retains moisture. If your skin is dryer or more sensitive, consider a lipid-free cleanser like Cetaphil or Aquanil.

Antiaging Creams

What about creams that advertise that they will make me look younger? The sad truth is that cosmeceuticals are a multibillion-dollar market of products with incredibly sexy packaging that primarily have no well-controlled studies to support their use. The number of antioxidants, botanical, anti-inflammatory, peptide, and stem cell products currently available is mind numbing. Although many of these products make your skin feel good, most are probably functioning simply as very expensive moisturizers rather than providing any added benefit.

For example, there has been a trend in the promotion of creams containing certain peptides (also termed neuropeptides) that mimic the effects of injectable botulinum toxin, also known as BOTOX. The companies producing these products are careful to avoid outright claims, although they make suggestions with creative word play that these creams might work as well or similar to the injectable form of botulinum toxin.

However, there is no evidence to support this intimation. In fact, the marketing is incredibly misleading, but the companies producing these products are simply interested in the sales of their product, not truth. Another popular molecule being touted is *matrixyl,* which is purported to produce increased levels of certain types of collagen. These are peptides that are classified as foods and are likely safe, although their suggested effects are questionable.

The unfortunate reality at this point in time is that this immense group of potentially helpful products is treated like an over-the-counter cosmetic and, therefore, is not exposed to the same set of rigorous standards that FDA-approved drugs must traverse, including double-blind controlled studies comparing active to inactive ingredients. Physicians and patients are then left to their own devices to determine if a product is worth using, based on anecdotal evidence and small studies done in petri dishes (*in vitro*), so the product is ultimately released without validated testing. At some point if the evidence is compelling enough, one must take a leap of faith and hope that the effort and cost pay off in some real effect. What makes this vetting process even harder is that "reputable" companies will sometimes produce an inferior product in a new category so they are not left out of the marketing stampede.

Topical vitamin C. One such product that I have been interested in for years and in my experience is worth the effort is the use of topical vitamin C. This is based in part on vitamin C's well-documented systemic importance in collagen stabilization, its critical role in wound healing, and its likely role in base excision repair in mutated DNA. Topical vitamin C possesses some challenges as only the L form is absorbed, and concentrations must be at least 10% to see an effect. Like vitamin E, vitamin C is a potent antioxidant that if placed on the skin beneath one's sunblock may provide added protection from all types of oxidative stress, including UV light. Some of the most popular products contain both vitamin C and vitamin E, which act synergistically, as vitamin C can regenerate vitamin E's antioxidant properties once used.

Stem cell growth factors. This is another exciting frontier in skincare. These products also lack the scrutiny of FDA approval, but the application of stem cell technology in other areas of the body makes this a compelling area to watch. Stem cells are found in all tissues, but those that garner the most attention are found in bone marrow and placenta, where stem cells are used directly to repopulate other cells. In the production of cream, we keep stem cells in culture, collect their protein products, concentrate them, and voila that is the basis of a stem cell growth product cream. We know from some elegant studies that as we age, stem cells diminish more with each decade, everywhere in the body, including the skin. If in theory we could deliver a high concentration of growth signals to the skin as our own stem cells diminish, we may be able to continue providing those critical growth signals. Choose a stem cell growth factor cream that is based on human biology from a highly reputable source, rather than of animal or bacterial origin.

Retinoids. Retinoids are a group of products derived from vitamin A that have been studied for years. The benefit of retinoids to the skin has been confirmed scientifically without question. Tretinoin (also known as retinoid acid or Retin-A) is the best-studied and a well-known product in this group. It has been used for more than twenty years for its benefits in diminishing fine wrinkles, lessening skin darkening, and generally improving the tone of the skin. Tretinoin is a differentiating factor, which means that it normalizes the development of cells, which over time are altered by aging or oxidative damage. In theory, tretinoin returns proper signaling to the skin so that it develops normally. Related molecules to tretinoin are retinaldehyde and retinol which are not quite as potent as tretinoin but still exert the same effects with fewer of the downsides of sun sensitivity and dryness. If you are new to this product category, start with one of these less potent molecules, and you can always transition to tretinoin later as your skin becomes used to it. Nighttime is the perfect time to use retinoids.

PREVENTING SKIN CANCER

The good news is that most skin cancer is highly curable.

Basal cell carcinoma (BCC), the most common form of skin cancer, grows slowly over months to years. It often appears as "acne that won't go away" or as an enlarging red bump. On occasion, it will repeatedly bleed simply from the abrasion of face-washing. When you see such a lesion, skip the DIY treatment and go to your local dermatologist to describe what you noticed. BCC is quite easy to eliminate with simple in-office procedures or even chemotherapeutic creams. There are a few more aggressive variants of BCC that can be locally deforming if, for example, they occur on the nose and were to invade the cartilage.

Squamous cell carcinoma (SCC) is the first cousin to BCC. It often appears as an asymmetric flat or raised pink growth that slowly enlarges and is typically asymptomatic. It, too, is often easy to treat, but can be more dangerous if it invades past the surface or occurs on a mucus membrane. Both BCC and SCC are strongly correlated to sun exposure, although not exclusively.

Malignant melanoma is the most notorious form of skin cancer. Unlike basal cell carcinoma and squamous cell carcinoma, which typically grow radially or along the surface, melanoma can invade the deeper levels of the skin more quickly, and thus has a much more aggressive capability. If caught early, melanoma is highly curable with a simple surgical excision, but if it invades past the surface, the treatment can become more complex, necessitating lymph node removal. The depth of invasion of malignant melanoma correlates strongly with survival. Although sun exposure plays a role in the development of malignant melanoma, there appear to be more genetic underpinnings to this cancer. Hence, the reason patients can develop melanoma, not only in sun exposed areas but also between the toes, on the buttocks or any sun-protected areas of the body for that matter. Melanoma can also occur in the retina so make sure you get your eyes checked yearly.

If you have a family or personal history of melanoma, get your skin checked twice a year by a reputable dermatologist rather than by your internist.

In addition, a good self-exam is a critical aspect of detection because you see your skin daily. I recommend looking at yourself in a full-length mirror with a handheld mirror to help see the backside of your body. What are you looking for? You may have heard about the ABCDE's of melanoma (area, border, color, diameter, and evolving), but that's a tough acronym to use as a practical tool. What I stress is knowing your skin and looking for the lone wolf (the one or two moles that look different from the rest). Anything that is growing rapidly, bleeds, appears asymmetrical, or simply gets your attention should be discussed with your dermatologist. If you're going to have melanoma, you want to catch it early while it is still superficial, and it is easy to treat.

Prevention. The best strategy for avoiding these cancers is to limit UV exposure and to be vigilant about detecting them early. BCC and SCC rarely kill you, but they can leave disfiguring scars. There is evidence to support the use of daily oral nicotinamide (a form of vitamin B3) 500 mg twice daily may reduce your chances of developing BCC- and SCC-type cancers. However, the surest way to reduce your chances of developing all types of skin cancer is to protect yourself and be self-aware. I don't recommend using fun new phone apps to help diagnose your undefined bumps or to distinguish benign moles from melanoma, although I would encourage you to do a bit of study to understand the differences. Visit your local dermatologist, who, hopefully, will spend a bit of time educating you on what to look for. The one app that I can recommend is *Miiskin,* produced by the Skin Cancer Foundation, which helps you track the appearance of a mole or lesion over time and provides some solid educational advice.

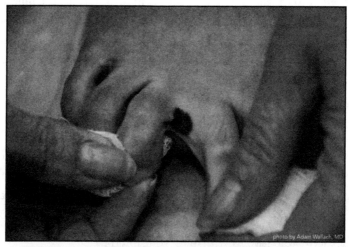

Figure 54.1. Melanomas can show up in strange places.

COSMETIC PROCEDURES

Over the last decade, it has become common for men to seek assistance in the quest to look and feel younger. In my private practice as a dermatologist for more than 20 years, I have seen this trend increase among men of various groups. Some men are just committed to slowing the aging process in all aspects of their lives — they are physically fit, eat healthfully, and generally take good care of their body. Keeping themselves looking young is part of an ongoing way of life. Another group is those aged 50 and above who are still actively employed and who wish to look younger as a way of staying competitive in fields dominated by a younger generation. Divorced men actively dating also want to feel and look more desirable. The list goes on, but we do know that men are engaging more and more in endeavors to create a more youthful version of themselves.

From the physician's perspective, the critical aspect of treating men is keeping the results of any of these undertakings as natural looking as possible. Men have the distinct disadvantage of having no easy way to conceal procedural work, as women do with make-up. Although this may be a double standard, there is cultural acceptance of women engaging in cosmetic or invasive work that makes them look younger and more beautiful. There can be a stigma for men who have cosmetically altered their appearance — consider your reaction to male celebrities who've had too extreme a facelift.

Fortunately for men, many small procedures can be rejuvenating without being obvious. Find a doctor who understands the differences in the male aesthetic and embraces the approach of restoring appearance rather than altering it. You will be duly impressed, as will those around you who will only think you've slept well or are just taking great care of yourself. When you see a less aged and more vibrant version of yourself, that goes a long way toward empowering you both at work and in your personal life.

BOTOX – Neurotoxins

BOTOX has become a household term. Simply, BOTOX is a brand of botulinum toxin, type A (often referred to as a neurotoxin) that comes in various branded forms, BOTOX being the most widely known. Other brands of this same toxin include Dysport and Myobloc, each one differing by a single atom within the larger botulinum molecule. Generally, the effects of different brands are more similar than different, although some patients and doctors prefer one or find that one product lasts a bit longer than another. The main effect of botulinum toxin is to partially *relax overactive muscles* of facial expression.

BOTOX brand has been FDA-approved for cosmetic use for over 20 years, and it enjoys an enormously safe track record, as do the other later-to-market neurotoxins. This impressive safety profile results from using highly purified toxin made in large batches from highly reputable sources. What makes neurotoxins so safe is that the amounts of neurotoxin used for cosmetic applications are so small that systemic absorption is minimal. Rare anecdotes of problems with the cosmetic use of botulinum toxin almost always relate to homemade production of the toxin or indiscriminate use of it. The possibility of a ptosis or droopy eyelid as a result of injecting neurotoxins is uncommon and wears off after two to four weeks.

An important starting point for injecting neurotoxins lies in carefully observing the location and size of facial muscles. As I am talking with the patient, getting to know them, discovering what their concerns are and what they were hoping to achieve, I am carefully observing their expressions, asymmetries, and general use of facial muscles. For men, in particular, the trick to using neurotoxins well is keeping the appearance of the face as unaltered as possible. For example, brow shape in men is typically flat. Maintaining that appearance is critical, because creating any shape or lateral elevation that was not preexisting could be construed as femininizing, unless this is the desired outcome.

Most men appreciate a fresher look, but one that is not stiff or overdone. Especially with patients new to this procedure, one attempts to get a great result without stepping over the line—one can always add more units en route to the desired result. Neurotoxins are mainly used on the upper face, although in some specific circumstances can be used on the lower face and neck by an experienced injector. If you're consistent with its use, neurotoxins can lessen the depth of wrinkles and slow their progression. If you find that you dislike the effect of neurotoxins, perhaps try another practitioner with a better artistic sense.

Neurotoxins are an immediate gratification product whose effect takes place within one to seven days of injection and wears off in three to four months. There is no addiction to its use, and failure to maintain treatments will not result in accelerated aging. Conversely, those who have used it consistently over the years sometimes require less frequent injections to achieve the same result. Neurotoxins are often used at the same time as fillers, and in the same facial areas, resulting in a synergistic effect. Finally, a neurotoxin can be used very effectively for the treatment of excessive sweating, whether it's under the arms or on the palms. There are, however, rare patients with pre-existing neuromuscular disorders such as myasthenia gravis who should not receive cosmetic use of neurotoxins.

Fillers

Soft tissue fillers have also become very popular over the last twenty years. We are relatively lucky in that the filler products available today, when injected into the face, last 8-14 months in my experience (although the claims of some manufacturers are up to 24 months). The products we inject also do not require any sensitivity testing since almost all of the possible contaminants and all allergens have been eliminated. Like botulinum toxin, fillers have an impeccable safety record when used appropriately. However, slight bruising or swelling for a few days is common.

The most widely used fillers worldwide are hyaluronic acid fillers (HA). HA is a normal component of the dermis so, in effect, we are replacing something your body already makes. The ones used most commonly in the United States are Restylane and Juvederm products manufactured by Galderma and Allergan, respectively. In the 1990s, when I was completing my training, we were using bovine or cow-sourced collagen. This product lasted in the face about three to four months, and, before use it required subcutaneous allergy testing done twice, one month apart. In hindsight, it is amazing that so many patients wanted this product, given the short length of time it lasted, combined with the inconvenient delay in allergy testing that had to be done, once the patient decided they wanted it.

A major advancement in the field was the development of genetically engineered HA products identical to human HA, avoiding the animal allergens once encountered with bovine collagen. HA fillers today are an immediate gratification product that one can have injected just as soon as deciding one wants it. There are many HA fillers within the Restylane and Juvederm product lines, each differing in its viscosity and elasticity, giving the injector many tools with which to work in different areas of the face for different effects.

There are semi-permanent and permanent facial fillers, because they cannot be removed if they are placed incorrectly, I believe the risks outweigh their benefits, so avoid them.

When injecting fillers in men, we attempt to restore appearance—rather than augment it — to avoid a look that is feminizing or overdone. Typically men tend to lose facial volume in the cheeks, a noticeable sign of aging. Diminishing this one aspect of appearance goes a long way toward making a man's face look younger, without creating visible alteration. Likewise, softening the vertical and horizontal furrows in the area between the eyes and brows softens a man's face without bringing undue attention. Over time, if one is consistent with the use of fillers, one can maintain a more youthful and natural appearance. In addition to using neurotoxins concurrently with fillers, we often combine other less invasive procedures such as non-ablative laser procedures or microneedling with fillers to optimize rejuvenation. Studies show that using neurotoxins and fillers is associated with improved psychosocial function and even relief from depression. Who doesn't feel better about themselves when they look better?

Other Non-Invasive Procedures

There are many other non-invasive and small invasive procedures that men can take advantage of today. In the laser realm, I often recommend using vascular lasers like KTP or pulse dye lasers to eliminate blood vessels on the nose and cheeks that arise from years of sunlight exposure. Likewise, brown sun spots can be easily eliminated without significant downtime, often at the same time as vessel removal. This alone can make a huge difference without breaking the budget or keeping you from work or social obligations. Non-ablative lasers (meaning non-destructive to the surface of the skin, for example, Fraxel Restore or Cooltouch) generally have less downtime than ablative lasers (like carbon dioxide or erbium lasers, which remove the surface skin), but both stimulate collagen. Most men prefer non-ablative laser procedures because there is some minimal redness and swelling for only about two to four days. Ablative lasers today are almost all *fractionated*, which means that the energy is delivered in tiny dots, making them infinitely safer with less downtime than the lasers of just ten years ago. Both types of lasers translate into thickened collagen, which in turn creates a stronger second layer of underlying skin (dermis), thereby helping to smooth the top layer of skin (epidermis). In case you were wondering — you cannot thicken the collagen in your skin with oral supplements.

- **Microneedling** is basically the delivery of thousands of small needle pricks to the superficial skin. Not all microneedling is the same, so avoid rollers and pens, which are ultimately traumatizing. Rather opt for robotically delivered stamping types of microneedling that do not abrade the skin and deliver radiofrequency energy at the tips of the needles to stimulate collagen, and possibly elastin. The combined effects give the skin a more youthful appearance without much downtime, and this procedure may even diminish enlarged pores.

- **CoolSculpting** can eliminate excess pockets of fat around the waist and chest non-invasively by freezing fat cells that then die over the course of months, translating into a diminished bulge.

- **Kybella** (deoxycholic acid) also causes the death of superficial fat cells, especially for small areas like a "double chin."

- **Ultherapy** can help tighten the skin of the face and neck by delivering hyper-focused ultrasound.

The best results for natural looking rejuvenation occur using a combination of techniques done slowly over time to create a restored you. There are a number of interesting apps that demonstrate how you might look when you age. They are worthwhile in so far as they can motivate you to act sooner rather than later, but they are not necessarily accurate. Look at them as the worst-case scenario of your aged self. Likewise beware of apps that attempt to demonstrate what the effects of certain procedures might be. The best recommendation is to sit down with your doctor to review before and after photos of cases similar to yours and to look in the mirror together, to better understand what you'd like restored or corrected.

For additional information on the services of Dr. Wallach, please see
www.wallachdermacenter.com.
For more resources, please visit
www.TheTwentyFirstCenturyMan.com.

Chapter 55
Removing Unwanted Body Hair
Kevin Wilson, Medical Writer

Dear Body Hair, I've had you removed for the thousandth time now. Please take the hint. Sincerely, Me

Humans evolved from apes covered in fur, which served as insulation from the cold and protection against insect bites and parasites. Although we became furless around 1.7 million years ago, hair does cover almost the entire human body, with about the same number of hair follicles as other primates. Although most of our body hair is wispy, short, and nearly invisible, in some areas it is coarse and curly. Human hair comes in two basic types: terminal hair, which grows on the scalp, eyebrows, and eyelashes, and vellus hair, located everywhere else.

The removal of unwanted hair from the face and body has been a common concern for thousands of years for aesthetic or hygienic reasons. Results were temporary at best, but more recently developed methods such as laser hair removal and electrolysis are FDA-cleared for the permanent removal of unwanted hair. Nowadays, a buff but bushy back can be "treated" to reveal those muscles in all their glory, and the hassles associated with removing or trimming hair on a man's body for cosmetic effect (aka manscaping) can be reduced or avoided altogether.

Body hair. When considering hair removal, typically the emphasis is on body or facial hair that develops with the onset of puberty, when levels of male hormones increase. Androgenic hair tends to be shorter, thicker, and curlier than hair on the scalp. It has a short growth cycle (a few months) with a dormancy period of up to a year before falling out, after which new hair grows to replace it.

The scalp. The hair on the scalp has a years-long growth phase. Male pattern hair loss, or alopecia, tends to be limited to the scalp and comes from genetic or hormonal factors as well as medical conditions. This permanent shutdown of hair follicles is often a sign of aging but may stem from another source.

Aesthetically pleasing body hair (or lack thereof) is a cultural and personal preference. Shaving or removal of armpit or facial hair is a good example. While appearance and self-image are important issues, what do women think? The reality is that confidence and positive self-image in a man are more attractive qualities to women than physical appearance. However, excessive body hair is not considered desirable by many women. On areas such as the chest, arms, or abdomen, body hair may be alluring. Excessively hairy backs, not so much.

For men, the presence and/or length of facial hair and length of scalp hair are often part of the presentation of a professional, well-groomed appearance in business circles. Consumer research has found that beyond shaving or styling head and facial hair, many men wish to remove or thin out excessive body hair on the abdomen, back, chest, genitals, shoulders, or arms and legs to improve their appearance. Advantages beyond appearance include less irritation or itchiness, especially during summer months.

LASER HAIR REMOVAL

Treatments such as *laser hair removal* can also make regular grooming more manageable. This is the only treatment for excessive ingrown hairs due to shaving (*Pseudofolliculitis barbae*).

Laser hair removal to improve appearance or to assist regular grooming is becoming more and more popular among men because it's easy and safe, the results last longer, and treatment discomfort is manageable. Men who regularly shave their body locations can avoid the annoying recurrence of sandpaper stubble (particularly important with pubic hair). Additionally, there is no recovery or downtime associated. Treatment time depends on the size and location, as well as the thickness and character of the hair.

Economics. At several hundred dollars per session (or more in high-demand areas such as large cities) with the recommended six to ten sessions, the procedure may seem pricey, especially for those with significant hair removal needs. However, considering the lifetime cost of alternatives such as waxing, the procedure is more of an investment. There are other aspects to consider as well. Options such as shaving, waxing, or the use of depilatory compounds only provide temporary results. Waxing is painful, especially for large body areas such as the back or chest, and the chemicals associated with depilatory compounds (think Nair) may be harsh to the skin or even dangerous, especially for individuals with sensitive skin. Follicle-by-follicle hair removal via electrolysis, the most effective method, is painstaking, time-consuming, and thus undesirable to many men, especially those with excessive body hair.

Timeframe. For laser hair removal, six to ten sessions are needed on average. Spaced several weeks apart, it takes several weeks to begin seeing results. Hair follicles respond best to treatment during the early growth stage, so hair at other growth stages will be less affected. Overall, a course of treatment takes several months to complete, by no means a quick solution. The downside of laser hair removal is that white and gray hair does not respond to treatment.

How it works. Laser hair removal depends on two main concepts. The first is the principle of selective photothermolysis, based on a theory developed in 1983. The concept is that a substance that readily absorbs laser energy due to its color can concentrate this energy and transform it into heat. The concentrated heat can be focused to damage or destroy the target substance (such as the basal stem cells of a follicle). Nearby tissue is spared because it absorbs less laser energy.

Secondly, laser energy is delivered more quickly than the rate at which heat naturally dissipates from the tissue, which is why the heat doesn't spread to the surrounding tissue. This technique maximizes delivered energy while preventing burns, scarring, or post-inflammatory hyperpigmentation (PIH, increased pigmentation from damage to the skin).

Matching treatment with skin type:

- In individuals with darker skin, these serious side effects are more likely to occur because of the higher concentration of melanin, the pigment responsible for skin color. Darker skin absorbs energy meant for hair, reducing the efficacy of treatment and increasing the potential for side effects.

- Asian skin is also particularly susceptible to PIH, given a higher concentration of melanin.

- The presence of tattoo pigment in the treatment area can attract laser energy, resulting in damage to the tattoo as well as the side effects described above.

The contrast between hair color and skin color is an essential factor to consider, given the science behind laser hair removal.

- Dark hair responds best to treatment.

- Lighter hair is progressively more challenging to treat.

- Blond or gray hair does not respond to treatment.

- Red hair responds with the appropriate laser with the proper settings, but the results are likely to be modest and more sessions will be required.

- Freckles are common and may also make treatment problematic.

- The ideal candidate for laser hair removal is light-skinned with dark hair and no tattoos in the treatment area.

- Darker-skinned individuals can safely and effectively treat with minimal risk by a trained professional using the optimal laser wavelength and settings.

The laser wavelength is a crucial aspect of treatment: different wavelengths serve different purposes. The most popular wavelengths are those provided by the alexandrite, diode, and Nd:YAG lasers.

Light-skinned individuals. For light- or olive-skinned individuals with finer hair and individuals who are light-skinned with freckles, the alexandrite (755 nm) lasers are the treatment of choice because they are fired with high energy in short, rapid pulses. This type of laser is popular because treatment speed is high, which is appealing to those with large areas of unwanted hair.

Light to medium-dark skin tones. The 810 nm diode laser is known to be very effective for these individuals and is recognized as a solid, all-around choice. Treatment is typically more painful, although the risk for skin damage is considered very low.

Darker skin. The long-pulsed 1064 nm Nd:YAG laser is ideal for darker skin. This wavelength is most effective for thick and/or coarse hair. It is the most painful of the three wavelengths and will require measures to maintain comfort during treatment such as topical anesthetic, cooling, or both.

Most modern laser hair removal platforms feature more than one wavelength. An excellent example of this is the GentleMax Pro (GPro) system from Candela Corporation. Combining the alexandrite and Nd:YAG laser wavelengths, the device also features a variety of spot sizes (areas treated with a single laser pulse) to maximize the user's ability to safely and effectively treat any viable laser hair removal candidate. It also features onboard cooling in the handpiece, a benefit to the practitioner as well as the patient. There are significant differences in outcome and comfort levels between lasers, so make sure you know which technology is going to be used.

Before undergoing laser hair removal, shave the treatment area so that only the hair at the follicle remains. Avoid waxing, plucking with tweezers, and bleaching for one month before the procedure because the lack of intact follicle root hair reduces effectiveness, as will the intentionally lightening the color of the hair.

People undergoing hair removal may sense heat and pain (a pinprick or a rubber band snapping sensation) from thermal damage as follicles are destroyed. This is especially true of individuals with sensitive skin. Still, the use of cooling and/or topical numbing cream is enough in most cases. With each session, there is progressively less pain because the patient's tolerance for treatment increases. Plus, there are fewer and fewer follicles to remove after each treatment, so there is less concentration of heat.

When it comes to treatment time, size does matter. The main factor is the size of the area to be treated. Facial hair may take several minutes, and a larger area such as the back (or multiple areas in one session) may take an hour or longer. Some devices have a larger spot size, which may speed things up somewhat, but it isn't a simple matter to make the laser spot bigger. According to laser physics, a wider beam needs more energy to deliver the same effect.

After each procedure, hairs begin to shed over the next several weeks. The treatment may seem to be accelerating growth, when in fact, this is part of the process. Temporary side effects of laser hair removal may include:

- Mild swelling

- Redness

- Irritation with crusting or slight blistering

- Mild transient pigmentation changes.

All of these should resolve within a few days. If not, contact the physician for advice. People should avoid the sun and use sunscreen on the treatment area for a few days because the skin will be somewhat tender and inflamed (a natural response to treatment).

While success levels and patient satisfaction rates with laser hair removal are remarkably high, the actual results are somewhat unpredictable. The procedure is often described as permanent, but the phrase "permanent hair reduction" is probably more accurate. Hair regrowth does occur although the regrown hair tends to be finer and lighter in color. Occasional or regular maintenance treatments will be required, but overall results are usually excellent.

The utility of at-home laser hair removal systems is dubious at best. Because the FDA considers this type of device cosmetic (not medical), they are not as heavily regulated. The science behind their effectiveness is based on theory rather than rigorous research. Additionally, these are subject to the same challenges and limitations as professional-grade devices, such as hair color constraints or issues with hair color versus skin color. The intensity of the laser is less than that of a professional device, and consequently, the results will be relatively modest. This often leads to over-use by individuals trying to get a professional result on the cheap. Aggressive lasering may lead to burns, and accidental exposure to the eyes can rapidly cause permanent retinal damage. These devices must be specifically used as directed for results with maximum safety.

You get what you pay for. The most effective therapy is delivered by a skilled medical professional in a safe, ideal environment.

For more information and resources, please visit
www.TheTwentyFirstCenturyMan.com
and also
www.candelamedical.com.

Chapter 56
Restoring the Hair on Your Head
Miguel Canales, MD,
Robotic Hair Transplant Surgeon

Anyone can be confident with a full head of hair, but a confident bald man,
there's your diamond in the rough.
— Larry David

The goal of this chapter is to provide a background on male pattern hair loss, discuss medical prevention of hair loss, and consider surgical options for treatment.

Balding is a common condition. Common male pattern baldness (MPB) or androgenetic alopecia accounts for more than 95% of all hair loss in men. By the age of 35, two-thirds of American men will experience some degree of appreciable hair loss. By the age of 50, approximately 85% of men have significantly thinning hair. Almost 25% of men who suffer from male pattern baldness begin the humiliating process before they reach the age of 21. Men often say that they look pre-maturely older when they are balding, and many express a lack of confidence due to their hair loss.

Most hair loss in men is genetic. There are many possible reasons people lose their hair, including serious disease, reaction to certain medications, and in rare cases, extremely stressful events. However, the majority of male pattern baldness sufferers inherit hair follicles with a genetic sensitivity to dihydrotestosterone (DHT), a form of testosterone. DHT inhibits the growth of hair. Hair follicles that are sensitive to DHT begin to produce thinner hair, and the life span of each affected hair follicle is shortened. Eventually, these affected follicles stop producing cosmetically acceptable hair, and balding develops.

DHT (dihydrotestosterone) is a derivative or by-product of testosterone. Testosterone converts to DHT with the aid of the enzyme in the hair follicle's oil glands called Type II 5-alpha-reductase. While the genetic process of male pattern baldness is not entirely understood, scientists do know that DHT shrinks hair follicles and that when medications suppress the action of DHT, hair follicles continue to thrive. Hair follicles that are sensitive to DHT must be exposed to the hormone for a prolonged period for the affected follicle to stop growing hair. With proper intervention, this process can be slowed or even stopped if caught early enough.

The development of male pattern balding. Male pattern baldness begins with the onset of a receding hairline and thinning crown. Hair in these areas, including the temples and mid-anterior scalp, appears to be the most sensitive to DHT. This pattern eventually progresses into more apparent baldness throughout the entire top of the scalp, leaving only a rim or "horseshoe" pattern of hair remaining in the more advanced stages of MPB. What is essential to recognize is that the remaining hair is permanent, because it is resistant to the effects of DHT.

Diagnosis. Typical male pattern baldness is usually diagnosed based on the appearance and pattern of hair loss, along with a detailed medical history, including questions about the prevalence of hair loss in your family. An experienced medical hair loss expert should examine the scalp under magnification, using a device called a dermoscope to assess the degree of hair thinning of the hair follicles. This assessment is critical when recommending the proper course of treatment.

TREATMENT OF HAIR LOSS

In the past few years, medicine has made tremendous strides in the treatment of men's hair loss. With the advent of 5-alpha-reductase inhibitors such as finasteride (trade name Propecia) and the evolution of surgical hair restoration, for many, living with noticeable hair loss is no longer inevitable. For the first time in the history of humanity, it is now possible to stop or slow the progression of hair loss and to replace lost hair through surgery with completely natural results. The following two treatments successfully treat hair loss in men to varying degrees.

Finasteride (Propecia)

Finasteride is the generic name for the brand name drugs Proscar and Propecia. Merck originally developed finasteride as a drug to treat enlarged prostate glands (Proscar). During the trials on men with prostate problems, researchers observed hair growth. Years later, Merck received FDA approval for a one-mg dose of finasteride for the treatment of androgenic alopecia in men (male pattern baldness). Propecia is the first drug in history to effectively treat male pattern baldness in the vast majority of men who use it.

Finasteride's success is due to its ability to specifically inhibit Type II 5-alpha-reductase, the enzyme that converts testosterone into more potent androgen dihydrotestosterone (DHT). A one-mg dose of finasteride can effectively lower DHT levels by as much as 60% when taken daily. It is DHT that shrinks the hair follicle, which eventually leads to baldness. This 60% reduction in DHT has proven to stop the progression of hair loss in 86% of men taking the drug during clinical trials. At least 65% of trial participants experienced what was considered a substantial increase in hair growth.

While finasteride is generally well tolerated, as with all drugs, side effects can occur. The most worrisome side effects for men include decreased libido and erectile dysfunction. However, the occurrence of these side effects is low (1%-5%), and clinical trials have shown that these effects are reversible. Finasteride may also cause a decrease in blood prostate-specific antigen (PSA) levels and can affect the PSA blood test. It is essential to discuss these issues with your physician to weigh the risk and benefits of starting this medication.

Minoxidil (Loniten)

Minoxidil was the first drug approved by the FDA for the treatment of male pattern baldness. How minoxidil acts to slow hair loss and stimulate hair regrowth is not well understood. Researchers believe that minoxidil prolongs the growth phase of the hair follicle, increasing the size of the follicle. Positive response to minoxidil therapy (reduced hair loss and hair regrowth) has been reported in various studies as less than 50% to more than 80%, possibly owing to genetic variation in study recipients. A man loses his positive response to minoxidil therapy once he stops the medication.

Minoxidil comes in 2% and 5% concentrations, applied to the scalp as a liquid or foam. All topical forms are sold over the counter (OTC) and do not require a prescription. Maximum efficacy requires application two times daily to the affected area for men. The original minoxidil study results used to gain FDA approval looked at the crown area, so minoxidil is approved for crown hair loss. Most hair experts advise patients to use minoxidil on all thinning areas, both the vertex and frontal scalp. However, patients must be consistent and apply this therapy daily or risk causing shedding.

Some hair experts are beginning to use low-dose minoxidil orally (five mg or less per day) with reported success. Patients irritated by minoxidil topically usually do well with the oral route, which allows physiologic activation of the drug to occur internally. However, oral minoxidil has not been FDA approved for hair-loss treatment. Off-label users must take care to maintain low doses to avoid potentially dangerous systemic effects. Combined with oral finasteride, minoxidil appears to enhance the hair regrowth effect of finasteride synergistically. Hair doctors commonly recommend the combination of these drugs, provided patients are committed to the daily regimen that topical minoxidil requires.

OTHER NEWER TREATMENTS

Platelet-rich plasma (PRP). Platelet-rich plasma is a relatively new addition to the list of hair loss treatments. The theory is that platelets store growth factors to help stimulate wound healing and tissue growth where it is needed. Blood contains platelets in varying concentrations. If you take a patient's platelets and re-inject them into an area that needs healing and growth, the body's mechanisms will improve the regeneration of the tissue.

Most studies have concentrated on using PRP injections to possibly help the growth of the native hair in the areas of hair loss and thinning. What these studies have shown so far is that the treatments help reduce hair loss, make the hair thicker in texture, and help regrow a modest amount of hair (10% to 15% more hair). In my practice, I recommend these treatments for men in the early stages of hair loss. The typical protocol is one treatment a month for four months. The PRP injections in the scalp are painful.

Low-level light therapy (LLT). There are several low-level light therapy devices (e.g., Theradome, Capillus) on the market that have received FDA clearance to promote hair growth. Researchers are not sure how low-level light therapy works to stimulate hair growth, but they believe it has to do with stimulating hair to enter the growth phase (anagen re-entry) and maintaining hair in the growth phase. These devices often come in the form of a cap or a helmet placed on a person's head. They are to be used for 20 minutes two to three times a week to be effective in promoting hair growth and increasing the diameter of the hair.

SURGICAL INTERVENTION—HAIR TRANSPLANTATION

Hair transplantation or hair restoration is the only means of restoring permanent hair to an area of baldness. The modern techniques of hair transplantation provide natural results and are performed in a way that makes the surgery undetectable.

Hair in the scalp grows in groups called follicular units. Follicular units can have one, two, three, or more hairs in the grouping, and during hair transplantation, each cluster becomes a follicular unit graft. The length of the session depends on how many follicular unit grafts are transplanted.

The surgery involves three main steps known as harvesting, recipient site making, and implantation, all completed in one day. Hair transplantation involves removing follicular units from the back and sides of the head—the area of the scalp where the hair is permanent and not affected by DHT—and relocating them to the areas of baldness such as the hairline, anterior scalp, or crown. Therefore, hair transplantation is really a re-distribution of healthy hair into areas of need. Surgeries can take six to twelve hours and can cost between $10,000 and $20,000 in total, depending on the length of the hair transplant sessions. The recovery time after the surgery is seven to ten days.

There are two main approaches to hair transplantation: follicular unit transplantation (FUT) and follicular unit extraction (FUE); each may be equally effective in achieving the hair restoration goal. The principal difference in the approaches is in the harvesting of follicular units. In FUT, an elliptically shaped incision is made in the back of the head to remove a piece of hair-bearing skin. A team of highly trained surgical assistants, using microscopes, then dissect out all of the follicular units from the strip of the skin. The surgeon sutures the incision, and a linear scar of a width of one to two mm remains once the incision heals ten days later. Long hair covers the linear scar. The drawback to this technique is that the patient won't be able to wear short hairstyles (hair length below a clipper guard size #2) or tightly faded haircuts without revealing the linear scar.

The FUE technique involves removing the follicular units individually one-by-one directly from the patient's scalp using tiny needles (needle diameters range from 0.70 mm to 1.20 mm). The team shaves the patient's head to less than one mm in length (clipper with guard size #0). Short hair allows the surgeon to visualize the follicular units and microsurgically remove them individually. Upon completion of the extraction, the patient has thousands of pin point dots distributed throughout the back of the head.

These wounds heal on their own without any sutures or stitches. Therefore, the technique is considered to be minimally invasive. There are several heavily marketed surgical technologies such as the ARTAS Robotic System, the Neograft System, and SmartGraft products that assist the surgeon in removing the hair. Patients should know that these technologies, although sophisticated, are surgical tools, and they do not automatically perform the surgeries themselves. Ultimately, the skill and experience of the surgeon will determine the success of the operation.

After harvesting, surgeons make small incisions (recipient sites) using small blades or needles throughout the area to be covered with new hair. The patterning of the incisions and the density with which they are made on the areas of baldness will determine the natural aesthetics of the results. Each graft is then inserted or implanted into each recipient site.

Hair transplantation is like planting a seed. The implanted follicle becomes rooted in the scalp within seven days of the procedure. It then goes through a dormancy phase (telogen) for four months. Newly implanted hair starts growing at six months in a significant way to reveal a new hairline and density in the implanted areas. The final result is at twelve months after the surgery, with more density growing from between six and twelve months after the surgery.

Choosing Your Hair Transplant Surgeon

Hair transplant surgery is a highly specialized field. Few clinics in the United States devote their entire practice to the art and practice of hair transplantation. When choosing a surgeon, some questions to ask are:

- How long have you been performing hair transplantation?

- How many procedures do you do a year?

- How did you learn how to do hair transplantation? What is your training?

- What can I expect on the day of my surgery?

- What hair restoration techniques do you offer, and which is the right one for me?

- Can I see before and after photographs of cases that look like me?

- If I'm not satisfied with the results, how do you address that?

- Do I need to keep taking hair loss medications if I have hair transplant surgery?

- How will you track my hair transplant result?

- What are the follow-ups after surgery? How do I contact you if I have problems after surgery?

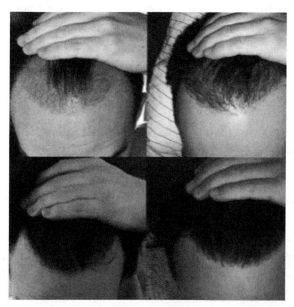

Figure 56.1. Hair transplant. (Miguel Canales, MD)

In general, a surgeon and a team of assistants perform hair transplants. The most experienced hair transplants clinics perform more than 10 cases a month, have a full-time hair technician staff, and offer different approaches to hair restoration. Experienced and dedicated surgeons should be able to show you their catalog of aesthetic results, explain to you their recommended plan, and educate you on the surgical process. Hair transplantation is sometimes a life-changing procedure, so take the time to get to know your surgeon and develop trust, as the results can last a lifetime.

For more information on hair transplantation and the work of Dr. Canales, please see www.siliconvalleyhairinstitute.com.

Chapter 57
Plastic Surgery for Men
Eric Mariotti, MD, Plastic Surgeon

She got her looks from her father. He's a plastic surgeon.
— Groucho Marx

Middle age is often unkind to our bodies. With midlife can come increased career opportunities (and accompanying stress) as well as a reduction in time, motivation, testosterone, and muscle mass. These can lead to changes in our body that defy "looking good, feeling good, and having great sex!" Where once we may have had a trim, narrow waist, broad chest and shoulders, and an overall athletic-looking appearance, we may have succumbed to a larger waistline and loss of chest and shoulder muscle definition. With time, our athletic build becomes a thing of the past.

Ultimately, plastic surgery is not a first-line defense for the aging male. Still, as an adjunct to a proper diet and exercise, plastic surgery can be very successful in addressing stubborn issues with our physical appearance that can't be addressed otherwise.

According to the 2019 Procedural Statistics report by the prestigious Aesthetic Society, the most sought-after plastic surgery procedures by men are:

- Liposuction—32,800 performed in 2019 (unchanged from earlier use)

- Male chest reduction or gynecomastia reduction—21,400 (a 15% decrease)

- Eyelid surgery—18,750 (a 7% increase)

- Tummy tucks—5,830 (a 15% increase).

Plastic surgery is still a form of aesthetics elected primarily by female patients, and they accounted for 93% of plastic surgery procedures performed in 2019. However, over the last five years, we have seen more and more men looking for a little magic from their plastic surgeons. Slightly less popular are facelifts and hair transplantation. Whether it is an eyelid lift that makes you look and feel less old in the boardroom or liposuction of the love handles that helps you look and feel younger in the bedroom, plastic surgery can help many men slow or reverse the hands of time that come with middle age. Everyone has heard the term Mommy Makeover. Now we are hearing more and more of the Daddy Do-over.

AESTHETIC PROCEDURES

Liposuction

By far, the most requested area for liposuction among men that I see in my practice is the flanks (love handles). With age comes constraints on time, as well as a natural decrease of testosterone, resulting in the accumulation of unwanted fat. While women tend to accumulate fat in the hips and thighs, men tend to collect it in the upper body, such as the abdomen and flank.

While liposuction cannot eliminate the fat around internal organs, it is effective in removing fat from love handles. Even with more physical activity, this area tends to be one of the last places a man can lose unwanted fat. The first step is to inject the area to be reduced with a combination of saline (to loosen the fat), lidocaine (for anesthesia), and epinephrine (to minimize bruising). A cannula, the size of a small straw, is then used to remove the extra fat and sculpt the area, restoring a narrower waistline more like that previously seen in our younger years. Variations on standard liposuction can include:

- Ultrasound-assisted liposuction (VASER)

- Laser-assisted liposuction (SmartLipo), which melts fat to make it easier to remove

- CoolSculpting, a device that uses fat-freezing technology to reduce pockets of fat in trouble spots such as the abdomen, flanks, or under the chin.

Cautions—CoolSculpting. This procedure is not for everyone. When performed on the wrong candidate (someone with a lot of loose skin), it can make future treatments with standard liposuction or tummy tucks more difficult or challenging.

The importance of sustainable weight loss. No matter what type of surgical fat reduction method used, subsequent weight gain means the results just won't look as good, and the money and recovery time spent on the procedure could be wasted. For maximum success, maintain a reasonable and nutritious diet and exercise program *that can be sustained.*

Liposuction should never be used as a means of weight loss.

Building on the foundation of a healthy lifestyle leads to better, longer lasting results from the surgery that you have chosen. For those stubborn areas where diet and exercise just don't do the trick, it can be effectively used to give a more masculine appearance.

Male Chest Reduction

Causes. Gynecomastia (abnormal enlargement of the male chest/breast) is either genetic or due to an imbalance of hormones: too much estrogen, too little testosterone, or a combination of both. Whether male or female, every person has a combination of both breast (glandular) tissue and fat within their breasts. In the typical male, the amount of glandular tissue is minimal, while females have considerably more. Genetic factors cause most gynecomastia. Some men are just born with more breast tissue or more fat in their chest.

Although this is predetermined, it does not mean that it is not treatable. Gynecomastia is a fairly common occurrence in teenage boys as they move through puberty. For the vast majority of these young men, the mild fullness of the breasts will dissipate as hormone ratios level out. In this age group, it is best to simply watch and wait until past puberty.

Contributing factors. The other predisposing factors to gynecomastia in addition to genetics and puberty include hormonal imbalances, steroid or marijuana use, overall fat accumulation, and age. Just as in female breast development, both female and male hormones are required for breast growth in males as well. Since a balance exists between those hormones in males, disease, a tumor, or even some medications increase estrogens or decrease testosterone and can cause gynecomastia. Unfortunately, as we age, we tend to rely on some of these medications to assist with the aches and pains of growing older. These can include medicines used to treat an enlarged prostate, prostate cancer, heart conditions, anxiety, depression, or heartburn. Certainly not all, but some of them can. Sometimes other substances or medications outside of the medical realm can be the culprit. Anabolic steroids (used illegally by athletes), heroin, methadone, methamphetamines, and alcohol can all cause gynecomastia and even shrinkage of the testicles. Correction of the imbalance, either with medications or surgery, can sometimes reduce or reverse the growth of male breasts.

Age and weight gain round out the list of potential causes. Being overweight means that your body has to store fat somewhere, and the chest is one of many places it can accumulate. With time, hormone changes and the decreased skin elasticity that occurs with aging can cause gynecomastia, especially in men who are overweight. So, if you are someone who has bigger breasts than you want, make sure you avoid alcohol, don't use drugs, review your medications, and consider losing that weight you've always wanted to lose.

Gynecomastia treatment. Talk to your doctor about the possible causes and medical treatments in your specific case. This may be medications, adjustment or change of medication, surgery to remove a tumor, or weight loss. When you have tried these solutions without success, a consultation with a board-certified plastic surgeon may be appropriate. Depending on whether the issue is too much fat, too much breast tissue, skin laxity, or a combination of the three, your plastic surgeon may recommend liposuction, removal of glandular tissue, excision of extra skin, or a combination procedure.

Liposuction by itself is appropriate if the breast is primarily comprised of fat rather than breast tissue. Remember, every one of us, male or female, have both fat and glandular tissue in our breasts. Glandular breast tissue is what enlarges with pregnancy in order to produce milk for the new baby, while the amount of fat within breasts can change with weight gain or weight loss. In men, glandular breast tissue will never function as it does in women, but is a leftover vestige of embryology. Some of us have more, some of us have less. However, all men have fat in our chest/breasts and that fat can contribute to the size of a male breast. Liposuction does not perform as well for men with fibrous and firm chest tissue, but it may do well for those whose skin elasticity is adequate, and whose fat can be removed more quickly.

The procedure. Removal of breast tissue can take on various forms. In mild cases, a small incision around the circular areola (nipple) can be used to remove the excess glandular tissue, leaving an invisible scar. However, in more severe cases, an incision can be made in the fold of the breast/chest, and the excess breast tissue and fat are removed. In severe cases, or when there is a great deal of extra skin, often seen in massive weight loss, not only the glandular and fat tissue is removed, but excess skin will be removed. This can give the chest a very flat appearance but the resulting scar on the chest may be easier to see. In my experience, men who have lived with the embarrassment of large breasts for many years would usually rather have a scar (that eventually fades) if that means they are able to wear normal shirts without having to hide their chest.

Recovery. The recovery period is generally between a few days and several weeks, depending on the activity level of the patient after surgery.

Eyelid Surgery

Eyelid surgery is among the most popular plastic surgery procedures for men and by far the number one most common surgical facial procedure. With age, our eyes seem to look "older" for a variety of reasons. It is true that over time the amount of actual eyelid skin increases, leading to excess skin that may droop or hang over the upper eyelashes. Compounding this, our forehead slides down slowly, over decades, and exaggerates the appearance of having too much upper eyelid skin.

The appearance of the lower eyelids is a matter of gravity as well. The eyeballs sit on a pad of fat in order to cushion the eyes. Over time, this fat pad can slide forward, and this bulge often results in the appearance of "bags" under the eyes. This can be further worsened if cheek fat drops lower, leading to the appearance of dark circles under the eyes.

Although non-surgical treatments such as Botox or fillers may slow the aging process, they are no match for Father Time. In short, having puffy, tired-looking eyes tend to make a man look older and tired. Has anyone ever told you that you look tired, or that you need a vacation? In some cases, it is our eyes that may be making us look tired or older, and our appearance does not always match how we feel on the inside. Some men seek eyelid surgery to look more refreshed, and younger, and in some cases, to compete for jobs against younger counterparts in the workplace. Eyelid surgery, otherwise known as blepharoplasty, is available in various forms:

Upper eyelid. The most common of these is surgery to remove excess skin from the upper eyelids. Before your surgery, your plastic surgeon will mark the excess skin to be removed, estimating the amount of skin to be removed while positioning the scar right in the fold of the eyelid to make it as least visible as possible. In many instances, this scar can be nearly impossible to see. In some cases, a small amount of fat is removed near the corner of the eyelid to enhance the surgery and the appearance of a more youthful upper eyelid. Although much less common in men than in women, sometimes a surgical lift of the eyebrow can be performed. However, this has the potential to feminize the upper part of the eyes.

Lower eyelid. Bulging of the lower eyelid fat (lower eyelid bags) gives the appearance of age for several reasons. The bulging fat alone is a sign of aging but is made worse when that bulging fat casts a slight shadow below it, giving the appearance of dark circles under the eyes. Surgery of the lower eyelids can be as simple as a small incision behind the lower eyelids (transconjunctival approach), allowing your plastic surgeon to remove only the bulging lower eyelid fat. In other cases, the procedure may involve an incision just under the eyelids (subciliary approach). This will allow your surgeon to remove or reposition the fat, and also to remove excess skin and tighten the appearance of the lower eyelids. It is not uncommon to combine both the upper and lower eyelids for a complete rejuvenation.

Recovery. The recovery can vary, but the upper eyelid surgery and the transconjunctival lower eyelid surgery can come with just a few days of discomfort and bruising, while lower eyelid skin and fat (subciliary) surgery may add several more days to the recovery.

Male Tummy Tuck

Tummy tucks are one of the most popular procedures for women, but its popularity among male patients is continuously on the rise. For women, the most common reason is pregnancy, with associated weight gain, as well as stretched skin and muscle that does not always snap back after having babies. With men, it is a bit different. The most common reason for men seeking a tummy tuck is weight loss, whether that is achieved through diet and exercise or with weight-loss surgery. Losing 30, 40, 50, or more pounds is a gratifying accomplishment, but it can leave a man with excess abdominal skin that just won't get any better on its own. This can leave a man self-conscious or just plain frustrated. The loose skin detracts from the accomplishment of losing the weight in the first place.

In many cases, when a man is overweight or just with getting older, the mons area, or suprapubic fat pad just above the penis, can become large enough that it makes the penis appear smaller. This can interfere with a man's satisfying sex life. Besides removing excess abdominal skin, most male tummy tucks will lift and tighten the pubic area and that often leads to improved appearance, improved self-esteem, and often a better sex life.

Caveat. Not every person, male or female, will be a candidate for a tummy tuck. While almost every woman who has had children and is seeking a tummy tuck will be a candidate for muscle tightening, that is not always the case with male tummy tucks. Men, having not experienced the sudden stretching of the stomach wall experienced with pregnancy, will only need the excess skin removed, and not the muscle tightening.

Being significantly overweight or having a lot of visceral fat around the organs is best treated with diet and exercise first. There is no surgery, liposuction, tummy tuck, or muscle tightening that can get rid of this fat. Your plastic surgeon is the one best fit to evaluate and discuss this aspect of the surgery with you.

Other Procedures

Rounding out the list of other aesthetic procedures that men seek are neck lifts, rhinoplasty, ear surgery, chin augmentation, and lower body lifts. Women seek facelifts more frequently than men at a 13 to 1 ratio. Although an older-looking gentleman may appear wise and distinguished, a facelift is still one of the ways to turn back time for many men. The scars are placed inconspicuously around the ear, although for men with very short hair, or those who are balding, it can be a bit more difficult to hide the scar.

The dreaded double chin, or the turkey neck, can be addressed with a facelift or, in some cases, with a neck lift alone. A neck lift has a shorter recovery time than the normal two to three weeks needed for a standard facelift.

If you are considering this type of facial procedure, you should look for a plastic surgeon experienced in male facial rejuvenation, as the techniques are subtly different so as not to "feminize" a man's face. If you are not yet ready for surgery, neurotoxins (BOTOX, Dysport, and Jeuveau) and fillers (Juvederm, Voluma, Restylane, Radiesse, Sculptra, and many others) can be used in many instances for the younger man and for the older man who is not ready to undergo surgery.

Having surgery does come with scars, some small, some longer. However, there are several strategies you can use to minimize scars, whether they are on your face, your chest, or your abdomen. The classic recommendations to minimize scars include avoiding sun exposure, getting massages, and using topical treatments. Covering a scar with silicone has been shown in research to decrease scars noticeability. Silicone comes in physical strips of silicone as well as in creams or ointments that dry into a silicone covering.

FINDING THE RIGHT PLASTIC SURGEON

With more than 60,000 physicians (including dermatologists, otolaryngologists, ophthalmologists and oral surgeons) performing cosmetic surgery in the U.S., how does one go about finding the right surgeon for you?

Of those 60,000 physicians, only about 7,000 are board-certified plastic and reconstructive surgeons, which means they have high standards of training and adhere to a strict code of ethics. Most, but not all, of the board-certified plastic and reconstructive surgeons belong to the American Society of Plastic Surgery, and roughly 2,600 of them belong to the Aesthetic Society, whose primary mission is education and research in aesthetic surgery. This does not mean that your only choice for surgery is from a board-certified plastic and reconstructive surgeon, but I would strongly suggest that you have a discussion with your surgeon about the procedure you are interested in, and how their training and experience have prepared them for the procedure you are considering.

The term "Mommy Makeover" is a well-known term describing aesthetic surgery to restore feminine contours after having children. The "Daddy Do-Over" is the male equivalent and reflects a growing trend in aesthetic surgery as more men are embracing ways to improve their physical appearance, enhance their self-confidence, compete in the job market, and perhaps along the way, give a little boost to their sex life.

**For additional information on the services of Dr. Mariotti,
please see www.DrMariotti.com.**

Chapter 58
Medical Fat Reduction
Kevin Wilson, Medical Writer

I found there was only one way to look thin, hang out with fat people.
— *Rodney Dangerfield*

Unless we're talking about steak, the word "fat" can bring up a lot of unpleasant feelings regarding our bodies, such as aspects of our appearance we don't like, the food we shouldn't have eaten last night, or the belly that doesn't seem to go away no matter how many hours we labor in the gym. Fat, however, is essential to our bodies.

Animals (including us) rely on fat to protect internal organs and insulate the body. Fat is a macronutrient that serves a wide range of cellular messaging and functions, is a component of key compounds generated by the body, and stores fat-soluble nutrients such as vitamin D. As a source of energy, there are nine calories per gram of fat versus four for protein and carbohydrates.

The problem is that we've become sedentary animals and can consume much more food than we need. The body stores extra calories as fat if carbohydrates and other reserves are full (which they usually are). Thanks to evolution, our bodies are incredibly good at this. Prolonged physical activity necessary for living, long periods without adequate nourishment, and similar situations we rarely encounter today were once facts of life, but no longer. Today, we just get fat, and we're more overweight than ever as a society.

The obesity epidemic is the result of two key components: sedentary lifestyle and an abundance of high-calorie, nutrient-poor food. Processing has made food easier to transport and store, but robs food of its nutritional value. Genetic manipulation, through sophisticated science or simple cross-breeding, has led to improvements to the look, taste, and other qualities of food, but again, at the cost of nutrition. Most fruits and vegetables were more nutritious 50, or even 30, years ago. The skyrocketing incidence of the following is a national crisis: type 2 diabetes, hypertension, stroke, dementia, sleep apnea, and cancer.

While a healthier, more active lifestyle is essential for maximum health and wellness, unwanted pockets of fat, large and small, come to plague most people eventually. At stake, beyond our health, is our appearance, wellness, and sense of self. For men, unwanted fat tends to settle in the middle. Love handles, lower back, and abdomen are the most likely candidates, but it thickens us everywhere. Jiggly thighs and upper arms, sagging chest ("man boobs"), and the double chin don't boost self-esteem. One region not too often discussed, but universally understood, is the pubis. A more prominent pubic mound is less attractive, and worse, it hides the shaft of the penis and reduces its visible length, and when men look in the mirror, every inch counts.

PROCEDURES FOR FAT REDUCTION

While there has been much debate about the role of different factors and the associated details, the fundamental reality is apparent: how we live and what we eat have made us fat. Liposuction is the best method for fat reduction, but has drawbacks. Aside from the risks always associated with surgery, there are long recovery times and high costs. Weight gain after liposuction may not look natural or uniform in the treated areas. There are many other minimally or non-invasive options available, and while they do not replace liposuction, they are safe, effective, and relatively hassle-free in comparison.

The ideal patient is already slim and healthy, but has stubborn regions of fat that don't seem to be responding to the work you put in at the gym and the willpower you show when you sit down at the table. More recent technologies will do more as well, but in the end, the closer you are to your goal, the more likely you'll get the result you want.

One major issue with any fat removal technology is that even after the fat is removed, there still will be extra tissue/skin. This tissue will naturally contract, depending on the health, youth, and genetics of the patient, but often not enough. Synergistic technologies to tighten skin are an essential component of therapy.

Energy-Assisted Liposculpting

Energy-assisted liposculpting is often a less invasive, more superficial version of liposuction, using a laser (Smartlipo), ultrasound (VASER), radio-frequency (RF, BodyTite), or some other form of energy to improve the process. The energy at the tip of the suction cannula emulsifies fat so that the cannula rod can pass through the fatty tissue more easily, with less trauma, and allows the physician to "sculpt" rather than just remove fat in bulk.

Laser and radio-frequency (RF) treatments, due to the thermal effect created, often cause some tissue contraction beneath the skin's surface, but are more likely to cause unwanted damage, especially if not performed correctly.

Ultrasound does not provide this contraction, but it is safer. The overall result is often more natural-looking than straight liposuction, but a skilled surgeon can do better.

Laser or ultrasound liposculpting is costly, but in conjunction with other methods, liposculpting can transform your body—bearing in mind that treatment with additional technologies adds to the cost.

Some surgeons can accentuate underlying musculature to bring out definition and create attractive washboard muscles. Ultrasound is the most popular method for this application. Though expensive, liposculpting is exceedingly popular among men because, well, why wouldn't it be? Who doesn't want washboard abs and a flattened pubis for an attractive stomach and more visible, longer-looking penis?

Energy-Based Non-invasive Techniques

In some ways, these techniques seem very "Star Trek." Reducing fat without an incision or other skin damage? It's true. The past two decades have seen unprecedented devotion of research time and money into this kind of technology, and the last ten years have revealed the fruit of this research: truly non-invasive therapies scientifically proven to reduce fat. What's more, about one in eight patients are men, and the gender gap is closing as more and more men are losing their fear of being stigmatized. Presented with the facts and seeing the results available with minimal to no discomfort, men are coming around.

CoolSculpting. Almost everyone has heard of cryolipolysis under its brand name, CoolSculpting. A unique applicator is placed on the desired body location and draws tissue into itself via vacuum suction. It then chills the tissue significantly for about thirty minutes. This irreversibly damages fat cells but not the skin and nearby tissues. The fat cells die, and the fat itself is processed by the body naturally, slimming down the treatment area. Though strange, the process is comfortable enough, and the side effects are minimal—redness and tenderness in the treatment area lasting a week or two, and diarrhea are the most common. Rarely, though more common in men than women, the fat cells grow larger (paradoxical adipose hyperplasia). Occasionally there is a "shelving" effect—instead of slimming an area, it creates a divot requiring additional treatment to smooth out. Safety, effectiveness, and a good marketing campaign have made cryolipolysis extremely popular. There are different applicators to treat different areas (arms, thighs, back, and abs).

Non-invasive laser lipolysis (SculptSure) is similar to cryolipolysis, but rather than cooling fat, this method heats fat using a penetrating laser wavelength. Efficacy and safety are similar, and side effects are fewer. After strapping the laser emitters onto the region (or regions) to be treated, the laser raises and maintains the temperature of underlying fatty tissue without harming skin for about 30 minutes. Side effects are limited to redness and tenderness in the treatment area that goes away within hours. Treatment is painless. While cryolipolysis treats a single area at a time, non-invasive laser lipolysis can treat multiple sites at once—arms, legs, abdomen, love handles, chest, or any similar area.

Focused-field RF (Vanquish ME). The previously discussed non-invasive methods are great for directly reducing pockets of unwanted fat, but not for de-bulking an area entirely. They're certainly not going to provide a worthwhile, visible result for heavier patients. Focused-field RF (radio frequency) (Vanquish ME) is a different animal entirely. While not as suitable for specific areas of the body, nothing reduces fat in an overall region like focused-field RF. Emitters for legs, arms, and/or the trunk are positioned over the desired areas, and after about 45 minutes of comfortable warmth, you're done—until the next session, and four to six sessions will be needed. But there are no side effects or downtime. Of course, the need for skin tightening will be greater as well. Focused-field RF doesn't replace a liposuction, but it has been proven effective on heavier patients.

Of these three safe, effective methods for fat removal, none of them deal with the laxity in overlying skin, so expect to need additional treatment with a laser- or RF-based device to contract the tissue for a truly satisfying result. Science has also shown that manual or device-assisted massage enhances these results, and many doctors recommend this as an adjunct to non-invasive fat reducing devices.

Non-invasive RF (TruSculpt) delivers the energy deeper into the fat than a laser will, to damage fat cells for later removal by the body, as with other methods. The heat component also promotes tissue contraction, so it's great by itself or with the therapies mentioned above. Only about two sessions are required and the results are similar to non-invasive laser and cryolipolysis.

Non-invasive RF plus ultrasound (Exilis Ultra 360) is a more superficial technique, applying the heat and sound energy through the skin to disrupt fat cells. It can be used in larger areas, but is not ideal. For smaller areas, especially ones the others cannot easily treat (such as knees), this is excellent. Non-invasive RF plus ultrasound is an ideal combination therapy with cryolipolysis, non-invasive laser lipolysis, or focused-field RF, because it not only sculpts fat away in specific areas to enhance the overall outcome, it was designed as a skin tightening technology.

One thing all of these treatments have in common is that the result manifests over time. It takes a few months for the body to entirely remove all the fat and adjust to the new normal, so you will not see results right away. However, another thing they have in common is that they are all safe and effective. A reputable physician will give you an honest appraisal of what to expect.

Injection Lipolysis

Injection lipolysis (Kybella) is becoming more and more popular because it works. The practitioner deposits a unique acid into the treatment area from several injection sites, and, after about two treatments, the fat fades away over several weeks. As with the energy-based alternatives, the destroyed fat cells and their constituents are removed naturally by the body over time. Swelling and redness will last about three days. Skin contraction with this modality tends to be reasonably good. This therapy has limits, with the main one being cost. While you could, technically, treat an abdomen using this technique, it is too expensive. This injection therapy is being used off-label safely in other areas because it is so effective, but larger body areas are just not suited for injection lipolysis. Overall, this is a reliable niche therapy; it has its place, but when most people are thinking about fat reduction, they're thinking bigger.

The safer, easier, less complicated procedures may be available at a medspa (medical spa— usually less expensive), and for some therapies, this isn't a problem. You can never go wrong, however, by placing your trust in a dedicated physician whose direct involvement promotes your best interests—even if the staff is performing some of the treatments. Physician involvement means the highest safety profile, the best education about options, the most realistic assessment of your needs with honest expectations, and above all, the best outcomes.

Any physician will tell you that once you've undergone a course of treatment, a healthy lifestyle will maximize the results you get and help you keep them. It is less expensive, healthier, and better overall to eat healthier and exercise to maintain what you, and your physician, achieve.

For additional information and resources, please see:
www.TheTwentyFirstCenturyMan.com

PART 8
MAKING LIFE FUN
Introduction
Judson Brandeis, MD

According to the National Institute of Mental Health, coping with the impact of chronic stress can be challenging. Because the source of long-term stress is more constant than acute stress, the body never receives a clear signal to return to normal. With chronic stress, the life-saving reactions of the stress response can begin to degrade major systems of the body—compromising the immune, digestive, cardiovascular, and/or reproductive systems, as well as our sleep. Some people may experience mainly digestive symptoms, while others have headaches or develop hypertension (high blood pressure). Over time, continued strain from stress can contribute to serious health problems, such as diabetes, heart disease, or mental disorders like depression or anxiety.

Music has a profound effect on our emotions and our physical health. Electronic dance music boosts alertness and concentration. Upbeat rock and roll or country music makes you feel optimistic and positive about life. Slower tempo jazz will quiet your mind and relax your body, making you feel soothed while releasing the day's stress. Music is good medicine that can heal your mind, body, and soul.

Spectator sports provide psychological benefits by creating a sense of community—spectators bond with people from different walks of life over shared devotion to a team. Becoming engaged with the game allows men to take a mental break from the problems they may be dealing with in their lives. Feeling part of a larger community helps create a sense of belonging that may be missing in other aspects of their lives, like work or neighborhood. A sense of community can boost a person's mental well-being.

Mindfulness. What is mindfulness, and how do you practice it? For a lot of people transitioning from weight lifting, sports, or a sedentary lifestyle, mindfulness may not be something you've ever practiced. To put it simply, mindfulness is being fully in the present moment without judging or criticizing your experience. This is a great coping tool. Mindfulness enables you to take a step back, allowing you more mental clarity and focus to connect with the present moment.

Design. Another boost to a man's mental and emotional health is a sense of place. The Chinese concept of feng shui is the invitation of positive circulating life energy into your home, so you feel more energized and balanced. When a man enters his space, whether at work, at home, or some other special place, the design should resonate with his mood and intention. When I created the medical offices at BrandeisMD, the goal was to develop a comfortable, guy-friendly place where men can come to discuss intensely personal (and often embarrassing) issues. To that end, we used masculine colors, heavy woods, manly music, and masculine imagery to create a relaxing, male space. In this environment, a man would feel comfortable enough to open up about his physical and emotional issues.

Retirement. Many men work hard for decades to reach a level of financial security that will enable them to take well-deserved retirement from the working world. As a urologist, I have seen thousands of men in retirement, and I can confidently say that some men are deliriously happy in retirement, and some are miserable. Retirement can mean identity loss, boredom, and/or financial insecurity for those who don't plan properly. But for the men who retire intentionally and purposefully, it can mean the realization of life goals and time to do what they want to do.

There are many aspects of lifestyle that bring men happiness and the reduction of stress. This section of the book covers a few of them, including music, spectator sports, creativity, and design. Make sure that you have an outlet that will give you a sense of accomplishment. It is time for you to do something for yourself.

Chapter 59
Listen to the Music
Brad Robinson, DJ & Electrical Engineer

*Music is therapy. Music moves people. It connects people in ways that no
other medium can. It pulls heartstrings. It acts as medicine.*
— Macklemore

Imagine walking into a party and all you hear is the low murmur of conversations and subtle clicking of glasses. The situation feels strange, like something is missing, but you can't put your finger on it. The answer may be that there is no music playing, and the absence of that music is something that makes us realize its importance in our lives.

As an audio-visual engineer, music is an integral part of my life, as it is for so many other people. I have made a conscious decision to surround myself in music because I recognize the positive effects that it has on my life and how it provides me with hope and optimism for my future.

As a DJ, I have been playing at festivals and events for over 25 years and they all have one thing in common: people are united by the feeling they share from the music. The Burning Man festival in the Nevada desert stands out, because you have the unique experience of a collective community inspired through art, culture, and music. On our dance floors at the festival, there are thousands of people choosing to unite under the music and opening themselves up to the positive feelings that it can bring.

THE SCIENCE OF MUSIC

Two researchers who study music and the brain, Sugaya and Yonetani, have confirmed that "music impacts at least twelve areas of the brain." It is fascinating to know that almost all of the brain is affected by music. Of those twelve areas, there are five regions that are especially relevant to your present and future mental, physical, and emotional health.

Keeping your edge. "Music affects the frontal lobe of your brain by enhancing your thinking, decision-making, and planning." The playlist during your morning run or on the commute to work is helping to shape your outlook on the world and your future. We choose music to fit our mood, but we also choose music to help inspire us, support our struggles, and help us to get through them.

Dopamine plays a role. "The part of your brain that plays a role in addiction, the nucleus accumbens, releases dopamine to make music feel addictive, like a drug." When you feel a connection to the music, your mind will start to crave more, so your body can continue to feel its effects, boosting your mood and positivity.

Music is primal. "The amygdala [the most ancient, primeval region of the brain] is the part of the brain that increases pleasure." While we often think of pleasure as physical, our brains take immense pleasure in music. "When you are listening to music and feel shivers go down your spine, the amygdala is activated."

Uppers and downers. "The hypothalamus is the part of the brain that maintains the body's status quo, links the endocrine and nervous systems, and produces and releases essential hormones and chemicals that regulate sleep, mood, heart rate, body temperature, metabolism, growth, and sex drive." Depending on your mood and what you are listening to, music can influence this part of the brain to calm or excite your body.

Intimate ties to memory. "The hippocampus is the part of the brain that creates and recalls memories associated with music. Music may increase neurogenesis in the hippocampus, allowing production of new neurons and improving memory." While this allows us to connect with memories associated with music from our past, it also importantly allows music to stimulate the creation of new memories in our lives. While the hippocampus is helping us to create new memories through music, it is also keeping track of the memories from our youth that are associated with music. In fact, according to Lenc, et al., "studies of people with memory disorders, such as Alzheimer's disease, suggest that neuronal memory traces built through music are deeply ingrained and more resilient to neurodegenerative influences." So music leaves quite an impression on us, so much so that those memories are more resilient in our brains than others. Music memories have the power to keep us young, and by keeping music in your life, it will continue to help you hold an ageless mindset.

CREATING THE ENVIRONMENT

Where you listen to music may be just as important as what you are listening to. As an audio-visual engineer, I am frequently thinking about spaces in terms of acoustics and sound isolation. While there is a lot of math that goes into designing a space, the end goal all distills down to creating a calm and quiet space: a space where you can read, reflect, watch movies, and, for many of us, enjoy music. Creating a space of your own to listen to your music will change the effect it has on your mind and your body. Your other senses are just as important as what you hear, and paying attention to them will enhance the music you are listening to. There are some simple things you can do to create your own space, while focusing on your senses:

- **Sound.** Choose a space where you can isolate from the rest of the world. A room or an area where you can close doors and windows will help to dampen outside noise. The acoustics of a space are important and the wrong acoustics can have a very negative effect on your music by reducing clarity and making it sound muddy. One way to reduce reflections that can muddy the sound of music is by softening hard surfaces in your room, using area rugs, plush furniture, and wall hangings.

- **Feel.** You are going to want to be comfortable, so find the best chair or couch that fits your space and budget, to allow you to sink into your music. When your body is relaxed you will be able to focus your attention on the listening experience.

- **Sight.** In this space, you are connecting with your past, present, and future through your music. The environment you are in and the things you see should remind you of where you have been, ground you in your current place, and excite you for what the next chapter in your life has in store.

- **Scent.** How a space smells is obviously a very personal preference, and there are an abundance of candles on the market that turn any room into the aroma of your choice. That said, your mind and body are going to be most relaxed and present in a space that is feeding them. Pick up a couple of plants that can help bring some oxygen into your room and are enjoyable to look at.

- **Taste.** This one is totally optional, but for some people music connects to their soul when food or drink is involved. So, if you fit this description, make sure that your time to enjoy music includes your favorite refreshments.

EXPLORING GENRES

The world is full of so much music to appreciate, and with the advent of apps that offer suggestions for music based on your taste, there has never been an easier time to discover new music. Some apps even allow you to choose from a list of "moods," helping you to set the tone for your day.

Spotify and Pandora apps are current favorites among people wanting to expand their music horizons. Start with songs, artists, and albums that resonate with you and let the app find associated music that has the potential to inspire you in the same way. When you discover a new artist, song, or genre that you love, create a new playlist based on it, and let the journey continue.

TECHNOLOGY

There are so many types of technology today that allow you to enjoy your music. While traditional hi-fi speaker systems are still available, the market also features a range of smaller speaker solutions, including wireless, integral streaming, earbuds, noise-cancelling headphones, and smart devices. Many of these solutions are very good, and there really aren't any wrong choices that you can make as long as your technology meets your needs. So, no pressure when you are ready to make some decisions, but here are thoughts that may be helpful:

- **Stereo, 5.1, 7.1—what's right for me?** For listening to music, you are going to want something that will reproduce the audio that the artist originally recorded, which is most commonly stereo. Both 5.1 and 7.1 surround sound systems are designed to reproduce the audio mastered for movies, and while they will play your music as well, make sure to select the "stereo" option on the device when you do. Otherwise you are listening to an "enhanced" version of the music vs. what the artist originally intended you to hear.

- **Mono.** Mono sound is a sound field coming from a single source, and there are a ton of audio speakers on the market that play audio in this format. This occurs because the drivers are physically too close together to perceive the left and right sounds from the recordings. While many of these products sound very good, and it has become a common way for us to listen to music, be aware that you may be missing out on the stereo mix that the artist intended you to hear.

- **Streaming audio solutions.** There are a number of products on the market that allow us to enjoy our favorite streaming music services (Spotify, Pandora, etc.) as well as to play our own music. Sonos is probably one of the more popular products on the market, and I am a fan of their hardware and software solutions. If you don't want to sacrifice the stereo audio experience that I describe above, check out their AMP product, which allows you to connect your own speakers, enabling you to place them appropriately in the room. That product also allows you to connect your TV to further enhance your experience.

- **Wire it up.** If you are setting up a theater or listening room, make sure that every speaker in the system is wired up to your equipment. There are many manufacturers that offer "wireless" speakers and subwoofers to allow you to avoid having to run wires. While there are a few products in this market that hold up, in general you are compromising the quality of your system by using them.

- **Music on the go.** Using earbuds or headphones can be a great way to enjoy your music when you are out and about, but also at home. My one recommendation with earbuds is to make sure that they fit properly in your ear. Ill-fitting earbuds can result in poor audio quality. Many of these earbud solutions will include optional "tips" to accommodate different ear sizes and shapes. Try them all out and choose the one that sounds the best and stays in place when you are active.

The importance of warmth/bass. A key component that affects how we relate to music is the bass—or low frequency—sound of the music. Lenc et al. found that "typically, people are attracted to move to music in time with a periodic pulse-like beat—for example, by bobbing the head or tapping their foot to the beat of the music. However, specific acoustic features such as bass sounds seem particularly well suited to convey the rhythm of music and support rhythmic motor entertainment."

When we refer to music as having warmth or depth, we are often referring to the bass. It is the part of the music that we feel inside, that penetrates our body. At concert halls and nightclubs, engineers spend a lot of time building audio systems that will reproduce these frequencies, making it easy for you to connect with the music being played. When you are at home or on the go, it can be more challenging to duplicate this experience. Because technology has trended toward compact portable speakers in our homes and earbuds for listening to music on our portable devices, we are often missing out on these low frequencies that allow us to better connect with the music. While these technology trends are convenient and help us to have more music in our lives, it may be worth upgrading your gear to enhance your home listening experience. This can be achieved simply by adding a subwoofer to your speaker system at home or purchasing a set of over-ear headphones that will expand the frequency response of your experience. Check out Velodyne Acoustics for some of the best subwoofers on the market, and Sennheiser for their over-ear headphones.

MEDIA

MP3 and MP4 audio files have become a convenient and compact way for us to share music with each other over the internet, but they are literally and figuratively compressing the heart and soul out of our music. If you are searching for the deepest level of connection with your music, here are some suggestions to help get you there:

- **Rediscovering vinyl.** Some people think that this is just a hipster trend, but there is a good reason why you should check out vinyl. Vinyl records are straight analog and there is an undeniable sound that comes from a turntable that cannot be reproduced on a digital level. You can get a decent turntable for less than $500, but you will also want to invest in a good quality preamp (the device that converts the phono level to line level) and a good cartridge.

- **Reclaiming your favorite music in an uncompressed format.** At some point you probably ripped your CD collection into your computer so that you could carry that music around with you on a portable device. What most people don't realize is that there was a setting option to choose what quality level to rip that CD, and the default was not the best. If you still have those CDs in a box in your garage, it might be worthwhile to pull them out and repeat that process, making sure that your music software is set to rip using an "uncompressed" audio format (WAV, AIFF, or FLAC). This will ensure that your audio file is an exact copy of the original CD quality.

HOW MUSIC CAN ACTIVELY REDUCE STRESS

Stress is something that most of us carry with us, in both a physical and an emotional sense. While there are many options for us to help manage these types of stress, music is something that you can include in your toolkit. Thoma et al. found that "music listening has been suggested to beneficially impact health via stress-reducing effects." Their findings indicate that "music listening impacted the psychobiological stress system. Listening to music prior to a stressful event predominantly affected the autonomic nervous system in terms of a faster recovery." From this, you can see that making music a part of your daily routine will better prepare you for stressful events in your life and allow your body to recover faster from those events, more so than only listening to music when you feel stressed.

Finn and Fancourt noted, "Several studies have demonstrated that listening to music reduces increases in blood glucose. Because blood glucose can increase in response to stress, this provides a further biological marker of the impact of music on stress." This further shows how incorporating music into your life can actively reduce stress and increase your quality of life in the present moment.

KEY TAKE AWAYS

As you search for ways to improve your mental and physical health, moving music from background to foreground will aid you in your journey. The music that you choose is individual and subjective, so take time to find genres and artists that speak to you. Ultimately, the goal is to get the most enjoyment from your music so that you can let it help maintain your wellbeing.

For a glimpse of the musical world of Brad Robinson, check out https://djbradrobinson.com/.

Chapter 60
The Bond of Spectator Sports
Joe Starkey
Hall of Fame Sports Broadcaster

Sports do not build character. They reveal it.
— John Wooden

Want to create an instant bond with a man you've never met before? It's easier than you think! For example, if you live in Texas, any conversation that starts with "How about them Cowboys!" is almost sure to draw an emotional response. Most likely positive, but if the stranger is from Houston, it will be animated in a different way.

As a play-by-play sports broadcaster with four decades of experience in pro and college football, hockey, and basketball, I've watched fans reach the heights of joy and excitement over a victory and the depths of despair in defeat. Win or lose, offering one's heart and soul to a favorite team creates an all but unbreakable bond.

Cold War Hockey Upset

On a national level, no sporting event reached deeper into the souls of Americans than the United States hockey victory over the Soviet Union in the 1980 Olympics at Lake Placid, New York. This was still the era of the Cold War, when the Soviets dominated Eastern Europe, enslaving countries like Hungary and Poland and engulfing others, from Latvia, Lithuania, and Estonia to Armenia and Chechnya. You got the sense that their leaders weren't being sarcastic when they said, "We will bury you."

In 1980, hockey in America was a second-tier sport. Most teams in the National Hockey League could fill the stadium, but television ratings were rather weak. Baseball, football, and basketball all seemed to draw wider national interest.

In an exhibition game at Madison Square Garden a week before the Olympic Games officially began, the powerful Russian team, featuring players who supposedly were amateurs, humiliated Team USA with a final score of 10-1. Actually, they were all professionals claiming to be members of the Russian military who had spent several years together playing hockey and little else.

At that point, there was no expectation that the USA could win a metal, and certainly not the gold. The USA team consisted almost entirely of college amateurs and minor leaguers who had failed to reach the National Hockey League. Even when the Americans reached the semifinal round, earning the dubious right to play the four-time defending Olympic champion Soviet team, the Americans were so lightly regarded that ABC did not even bother to televise the game live on Friday night. That date is forever etched in the consciousness of those who saw it: February 22, 1980. The game began at 5 pm East Coast time, but was not shown on television until 8:30 pm in the East, when the game had already concluded. (Al Michaels, the broadcaster, got the ABC TV assignment primarily because he was the only one at the network who knew the rules!)

When Mike Eruzione made the lead goal to bring the score to 4-3 in favor of the U.S. with exactly 10 minutes to play, the arena went into a frenzy. Packed with Americans among the 8,500 spectators, the chanting of "USA" and the waving of American flags dominated the final 10 minutes. When the match was over, the crowd and everyone throughout the tiny hamlet of Lake Placid continued their celebration deep into the night. As Americans began to hear of the victory, the audience grew dramatically for the delayed telecast. Cries of "USA! USA!" rang throughout the entire country.

This was more than a game. It was the United States prevailing over our most dangerous enemy at the time. (This was eleven years before the fall of the Iron Curtain, before Germany was reunited, before countries like Hungary and Poland regained free nation status.) People of all ages all over America cheered, hugged strangers, and celebrated our pride in being Americans. The frenzy and excitement continued to build for the weekend because there was still one more game to play. But, suddenly, the only topic of importance on American radio and television was how proud we all were of what our underdog hockey players had done for the entire country's morale.

When the Americans beat Finland to clinch the gold medal on Sunday afternoon, it created a shared joy that seemed to make every American swell with pride at what our country could accomplish if we work together. When goalie Jim Craig wrapped an American flag around his shoulders as the game ended, a simple sporting event created a connection that made total strangers embrace one another in a truly unique and unforgettable American event.

The Bond Created by Sports

My experience has led me to believe that that the key to developing and nurturing male friendships is often a shared connection through sports. Men are often less likely to have a wide range of close friends. Women seem to connect through their children, their lunch partners, perhaps through a game of bridge, a walk in the park, or an intimate conversation.

For men, an attachment to a sports team is often multi-generational. My grandfather loved the Cubs, so by the time his two sons were 6 or 7, he would take them to Wrigley Field. When my father took me to see the Cubs as a kid, those outings created memories and shared experiences I remember to this day. My son and grandson have never lived in Chicago, but through my stories, they love cheering for the Cubs with me, and that has become part of our family bonding that now extends five generations.

For many men, even happily married, the attachment to a particular team is critical for their emotional wellbeing. There's a similar motivation for men working in a repetitive job, meeting the same responsibilities day after day, with the same work uniform (whether that's Army khakis, work pants, or an Armani suit). They have limited self-expression at the office or the factory. So where do they turn? On game day, they dress up in team colors, stomp and yell right along with the rest of the fans in the stadium. As a collective group with one united voice, they can boo the referee and their team's opponent while laughing, shouting, cheering, and letting off steam in a way they can't do anywhere else.

The Ultimate Upset in College Football Rivalry

In each of our lives, there are rare events that seem to reach into the soul of an entire community, impacting even those who rarely acknowledge any interest in sports. In Northern California, the annual college football competition between the University of California at Berkeley and Stanford University in Palo Alto attracts students, alumni, and faculty members who otherwise would pay absolutely no attention to sports at Berkeley or otherwise. But Cal and Stanford began their gridiron competition in 1892 and there are professors, coaches, players, and multi-generational families who have deeply rooted connections to both schools. It is not unusual for someone to earn a degree from one school as an undergraduate and then a graduate degree from the other. Nothing illustrates the intensity of the rivalry more than the now legendary 1982 football game at Berkeley, which will forever be known as "The Play."

With four seconds remaining, a Stanford field goal put them ahead of California 20-19. The victory would have guaranteed senior quarterback John Elway an opportunity to play in a postseason bowl game for the only time in his college career.

However, with just four seconds left in the game, on the seemingly routine final kick-off, the Cal Bears brought the ball back into play close to the 50 yard line. At that point, six deft lateral hand-offs between five different players zig-zagged the ball all the way down the field for the game-winning touchdown, just as time expired. To reach the end zone, the last two Bears to touch the ball had to run through the Stanford marching band, which had poured onto the field believing that the game was over and that Stanford had won.

The last Bear to touch the ball was Kevin Moen, who slammed it into the endzone, crashing into Stanford trombonist Gary Tyrell for a final score of California 25, Stanford 20. (Tyrell later joked that it was going to take more than that to keep him down.) Stanford has never admitted that they lost, claiming the officials shouldn't have allowed that crazy play to count. So each year that they win the annual battle, they change the score on the symbolic game-winning axe which is passed to the most recent winner. Talk about an axe to grind, — to this day, among Cal and Stanford alums, "The Play" will always instantly produce intense, but good-natured, bantering over the game's bizarre outcome, creating a shared and indelible memory.

The Unexpected Hero

Nobody in recent memory has been less likely to emerge as an NBA superstar than Stephen Curry. Not recruited out of high school, Steph played for lightly regarded Davidson in college. There was no great scramble by teams to draft him into the pro game. So he found himself a member of the Golden State Warriors, which had been incredibly consistent in their ability to stay out of the playoffs for nearly two decades. Yet suddenly, somehow, this skinny kid and the Warriors evolved into greatness. Curry's story of success and his remarkable leadership in a wide range of charities and humanitarian causes has made him a symbol and a benchmark for how we should all live our lives.

A father can now tell his son: you can be great in your own way. It's OK to dream of greatness, to aim for the stars in sports or business or medicine. Curry did it, so can you!

Sports provide the whole range of human experience, from thrilling victories to gut-wrenching disappointment. But above all, it can provide the shared joy of a common bond. Sports have the unique ability to make us feel better about ourselves and the world around us. What man doesn't want that?

You can watch the footage of The Play between UC Berkeley and Stanford in 1982 on YouTube.com. Simply enter "The Play" in the search box.
The wildly enthusiastic voice calling The Play, second by second, is Joe Starkey.
For a bio of Joe Starkey, please see:
https://calbears.com/honors/california-athletics-hall-of-fame/joe-starkey/1322.

Chapter 61
Practicing Mindfulness
Dean Pohlman

Remember then that there is only one important time, and that time is now. The most important one is always the one you are with. And the most important thing is to do good for the one who is standing at your side. For these, my dear boy, are the answers to what is most important in this world. This is why we are here. — *John Muth, The Three Questions*

What is mindfulness and how do you practice it? If you're like most men, mindfulness might not be something you've ever tried. To put it simply, mindfulness is the practice of focused awareness, being fully in the present moment. This doesn't mean that you're purging your mind of thoughts or thinking of nothing, but rather that you are detaching yourself from your thoughts and feelings.

This involves the practice of being present in the changing moment, letting thoughts and feelings arise and pass away without reaction. The foundations of mindfulness are living and appreciating the current moment (both physically and mentally), without letting anxiety or stressors consume or control your thoughts. That might sound difficult, and it is at first, but it is a skill you develop by practicing it on a regular basis. Happily, activities such as yoga are an amazing way to practice mindfulness, to bring yourself more fully into the present.

THE BENEFITS OF MINDFULNESS

In a state of mindfulness, regardless of what you are doing, you are mentally focused. You are aware of the task at hand, the sensations of the physical world, and any thoughts or feelings that might enter your mind. You become the observer of your external and internal worlds, allowing you to truly live and connect with each moment of your life, no matter how seemingly mundane. In this practice, apparently ordinary events can take on a rather profound significance, which enhances your quality of life:

■ **Coping.** Mindfulness is a great coping tool, designed to reduce any immediate anxiety or stress, a tool that enables you to guide your mind away from destructive or invasive thoughts.

- **Better sleep.** The mindfulness practice of letting go of intrusive thoughts and emotions can improve the quality of your sleep.

- **Reducing stress.** Research has found that mindfulness and yoga can help move your body out of the stress response into the relaxation response.

- **More even emotions.** An empirical review of the research on mindfulness found that it decreases emotional reactivity.

- **Enhanced mental clarity.** Mindfulness allows you to take a step back and calm yourself, supporting greater mental clarity and more rational decision making.

The practice of mindfulness allows you to experience your feelings and thoughts without judgment or self-criticism.

Mindfulness in the everyday world. Mindfulness as daily practice can help manage stressors and relieve the anxiety or feelings of depression that can built up throughout the day. Maybe you're stressing over a deadline at work. Mindfulness can be a tool to help bring you back to the present and gain the insight that will make the task manageable.

Coping with big life changes. For more drastic events such as career changes, a divorce or breakup, the death of someone you're close to, or a serious illness, mindfulness can be an incredible tool to calm anxiety or runaway thoughts. When these extremely stressful events happen in our lives, it's inevitable that we'll have self-doubt, regrets (what if's), criticism, or other forms of negativity.

What consumes your mind controls your life. If we let our thoughts get out of control, we tend to lose ourselves.

We may be tempted to envision an absolute worst-case scenario. But if we let those thoughts take hold, we'll sink deeper into them until they overwhelm us. We may be drawn into decisions we will later regret. That's why mindfulness is so important, especially during critical times in our lives.

Pairing mindfulness with yoga and breathing techniques and being in the present moment can help us pull ourselves out of toxic thoughts. This gives us time to destress, feel better, and actually think constructively about the events that are transpiring. Practiced over time, mindfulness can be life-changing. This could involve informal mindfulness or the practice of focused awareness.

INFORMAL MINDFULNESS

Mindfulness can be practiced throughout the day without having to set a particular time to focus our efforts.

This can be as simple as focusing on how the water feels as you wash your face in the morning, how your feet feel while you stand and wait in line, or even how the wind and sun feel on your skin outside. You're bringing your attention to one particular experience in the present moment. Using this approach, you can practice mindfulness every day.

Another useful way to incorporate mindfulness is by paying close attention to a task and focusing on the experience and the sensations it involves. When we are working, we give the task at hand our total, undivided attention. Engaging in informal mindfulness as we perform our daily activities can help significantly reduce and manage the stress that most of us experience every day, leading to higher quality of life.

FORMAL MINDFULNESS

A formal practice means setting aside time to practice mindfulness, which entails both peripheral awareness and focused awareness.

PERIPHERAL AWARENESS

Practicing peripheral awareness means experiencing the totality of your body without any particular focus. Although this might sound difficult at first, it's relatively easy to do in a practice like yoga. If your peripheral awareness shifts to a particular sensation or discomfort in your body, then you've shifted to focused awareness.

FOCUSED AWARENESS

Single-point focus is often referred to as an anchor. Since your mind can only truly focus on one thing at a time, anchoring provides an opportunity to guide and focus your thought pattern. An anchor could be your breath, or a particular sound, sight, or physical sensation.

For those multi-taskers out there, know that you're not actually hardwired to focus on multiple things at one time. The reality is that your brain is actually switching focus, very quickly back and forth (in some cases, effectively, but in others, not so much). This is not the point of mindfulness or focused awareness, so try to bring your attention back to your anchor.

Finding a balance between these two types of awareness is the goal of a formal mindfulness practice. I recommend practicing the two approaches separately at first, before trying to find the balance between the two.

This type of mindfulness can be done as part of a yoga practice, as an aspect of guided meditation, or learning to guide yourself through the process on your own.

Anchoring Mindfulness

There are a number of ways to practice focused awareness, using the process of anchoring. I'm going to list a few here that aren't entirely yoga-based.

Breath as an anchor. As the saying goes, "Control your breath, control your body." But we can take this one step further, because controlling your breathing can also help you control your thoughts and feelings, and your mind, to some degree.

To practice mindful breathing, focus on how the breath enters your body as it travels down your nostrils, expands your chest, and then exits your body. Notice the cool sensation as you inhale, the feeling of the incoming breath, and the warmth as it exits.

In some practices, the breath has five stages, and noticing each one of those stages can also be very anchoring:

- The inhale
- The pause as the inhale finishes
- The hold
- The exhale
- The pause at the exhale finishes.

As your mind starts to wander, focus on thoughts or emotions that arise, simply observe them, and then bring your attention back to your breathing, anchoring you.

When you first start practicing mindfulness, it can be remarkably difficult to focus on your breathing without the intrusion of other thoughts. Your attention will wander. It does for everyone. Just bring your attention back without judgement. Start with five breaths and over time, work up to longer periods. As you improve, you will begin to experience an inner calmness.

Sound as an anchor. Sound can be a great tool for anchoring your awareness. This practice is often a feature of meditation practice or classes. You can also practice this effectively on your own, if you know what you're looking for in your execution. The key is to patiently bring your attention back every time it wanders.

We hear sounds all day: music, people talking, and ambient sounds, but using sound as an anchor requires active listening. The most common practice using sound as an anchor involves singing bowls, quartz bowls, or bells to guide the listener. As you listen to the sounds, try to focus on them without labeling them, commenting on them, or judging them. Examples of other sounds you can use are:

- A recording of simple sounds in nature

- A repetitive sound like a drum or a gong

- A simple chant

- Repeating a word whose quality you'd like to bring to your awareness

- Music that is simple and designed for meditation (for example, with no lyrics).

Hear the sounds, manifest not only through hearing, but also the tactile nature of the physical vibrations of the sounds. This is all part of your anchor. Using music as an example, a review of more than 400 published scientific articles on music as medicine found strong evidence that music has physical and mental benefits in reducing stress and improving mood.

Sight. Sight can also be an effective anchor. Because our eyes can only focus on one thing at a time, we can use this attribute to our advantage, when it comes to experiencing focused awareness in the present moment.

In this practice, try to focus on a single visual point. This could mean focusing on a simple object such as a symbol, an apple, or a flower.

Don't let your eyes wander; just be fully aware of that one object. The challenge is to let the object of your focus fully saturate your awareness, without labeling it, or judging it. You are simply observing this one focal point with undivided attention.

YOGA AND MINDFULNESS

Yoga at its core is a physical and mental practice, blending movement and breathing in both a workout and a mindfulness practice.

Postures and movements help you experience and connect with your peripheral (non-specific) awareness, while your breathing helps anchor you and channels your focused awareness, leading to a calm, beneficial state of mind.

Mindfulness in yoga means anchoring yourself to the present moment and using movement and breath to bring full awareness to your mind and body. You can apply mindfulness in yoga using a number of different approaches, ranging from Hatha yoga or Yin yoga, to Vinyasa yoga. These are all examples of mindful yoga practices, but this is by no means an exhaustive list.

Yoga for Men

Mindfulness and yoga designed for men combines the physical practice of strength-based yoga with breath work in an approach that is most closely related to Hatha yoga. Yoga practice can be paired with elements of weight training and Pilates to create a well-structured, comprehensive workout that targets strength, mobility, and flexibility.

This is practiced in tandem with breathing to enter a state of mindfulness.

As you go through the postures you'll notice that your breathing changes. With every inhale and exhale, you can deepen each pose a little. Focus inward: notice each breath and how it affects the sensations of your body.

Even if you're holding a difficult pose for a long time you can always bring your awareness to both your breath and body, leading to mindfulness. If your mind wanders, use the anchors of breath and movement to re-enter the present moment.

As you practice this double awareness more and more, it becomes easier to enter a state of mindfulness. Being conscious of what you're trying to achieve and your intentions for the day can also help you focus.

The Body Scan (Yin Yoga)

A more restorative and meditative approach to yoga and mindfulness, Yin yoga involves holding restorative poses for several minutes. As you do this, you're asked to focus on deepening your breath and scanning your body for sensations.

As you hold a posture, focus your awareness on your breath to deepen, relax, and sink into the posture more and more. Scan your body from head to toe and notice how your body feels in that position, in correlation with your breath, rooting yourself in the present moment. Eventually, you will be able to achieve a state in which you focus on deep breathing. being aware of how your whole body feels in its totality, leading to a strong sense of mindfulness.

The Flow State (Vinyasa Yoga)

The most popular type of yoga in the United States currently is Vinyasa yoga, in which you smoothly flow from pose to pose. Practicing mindfulness in this type of yoga is also centered around using the breath as an anchor.

As you move from pose to pose, you will either exhale or inhale to trigger the next movement. Usually, your instructor will cue you on the sequences and the breathing. Notice how the breath works to smoothen the transition to the next posture. Note how your body feels as you move from pose to pose. Bringing awareness to the breath helps to strengthen your core, but also helps you soften into other poses.

For some people, this integration of movement and breathwork results in a flow state, which is a form of mindfulness. It is a mental state in which you are fully immersed in the feeling of energized focus, fully involved in the present moment, and enjoying the process.

Final Thoughts

There are many ways to approach mindfulness ranging from informal practices to meditation, and, of course, yoga. If you're not used to the practice of mindfulness, practicing yoga is a great way to start. You can try a yoga class, pick up a video, or tap into a wealth of resources online.

Happily, activities such as yoga are an amazing way to practice mindfulness, to bring yourself more fully into the present.

For more resources on yoga for men, please see Chapter 40 in this book, by Dean Pohlman, as well as his book from DK Publishing, *Yoga Fitness for Men*, and his website, ManFlowYoga.com.

Chapter 62
Creating a Masculine Space
Michael Tebb,
Landscape Designer

Design is not just what it looks like and feels like. Design is how it works.
— Steve Jobs

Empowering a man through his home environment is at the core of masculine design. Good design has a definite, personal appeal. You know it instinctively, when you find yourself in a room or an outdoor space that speaks to you. It is not just one specific element—everything flows together, and there is a sense of unity. Whether your project is an apartment or a grand estate, the principles and process remain the same.

As a generalization, men understand from the start that design should be practical. There are four primary steps in design, whether you are creating a large backyard, a tiny balcony, or an interior living room. First, put together a portfolio of ideas, then define how the space will be used, and do some research. Lastly, pull it all together in a plan.

BUILDING AN IDEA FILE

Starting your planning process can be intimidating. It's hard to envision how your space might look without input. Fortunately, you don't have to start from scratch. Even experienced designers rely on inspiration from other sources. At this stage of the process, you'll be creating an idea board or a file of photos and screenshots. If you're designing an interior, save images of rooms and furniture, paint swatches, and samples of wood, tile, metal, or fabric. Designing an outdoor space, your clip file might include images of landscapes, plants or trees, furniture, and even activities that appeal to you.

Begin by spending time online on Google, Pinterest, Houzz, or other search engines. Add snapshots of rooms or exteriors you like: a friend's home, an AirBnB you stayed at, or your favorite restaurant. Tear pages from magazines and/or take screenshots of TV programs (set designers can be surprisingly inspiring). Any environment that you find appealing can prove helpful in defining your style.

Set up files to contain your collections and enjoy the process. Allow yourself to daydream. At this step, anything goes. Don't filter while you gather photos. You may be attracted to an Italian villa and find that the stonework is something you can emulate. Or pictures from a Hawaiian resort may inspire you to put in a flowing fountain, a fan, and richly scented vines to remind you of the tropical breezes.

In gathering information for your portfolio, you will start to notice trends appearing in your choices. Perhaps you are drawn to a particular style, or specific materials. Maybe you find a bold Mediterranean garden appealing or prefer a manicured English lawn, or a clean contemporary garden with smooth concrete and steel. And notice the activities that seem to fit in your life: large gatherings, dining at a table, small groups visiting around a fire pit, swimming parties, tending a garden.

Notice any colors that recur in your files—some men enjoy primary reds, blues, and yellows while others prefer muted tones. Do you like high contrast or blended shades? Every piece of information will be useful in creating your personalized space.

Now that you have some ideas to inspire you, it's time to move on to the next phase.

Developing a comprehensive plan puts you firmly in control of your project. When you consider your choices carefully in advance, you avoid impulsive and expensive mistakes and can create a project you will enjoy for years.

Men may find the process of designing to be a foreign concept. In the past, you may have been discouraged from getting involved in the aesthetics of your home. Indulging your imagination may be the most important investment you make in your project.

Divide the planning process into four classic steps: Function, Form, Research, and Development. Each stage will be developed in order, but also revisited throughout the project, to adjust and adapt the plan.

DEFINING HOW THE SPACE WILL FUNCTION

Think about how you are going to live your life in the space that you are creating. How is it going to function? What features and furnishings will you need so that it looks good and makes you feel good? Factor in what you respond to, in terms of your personality and your taste.

Consider Your Stage in Life

The career man. At this phase of a man's life, many men defer the decision-making on home design to their wives. Often, the lack of male involvement is a function of time. They

514 THE 21st CENTURY MAN

head off to work, and although they will look at the final design, they are not going to be involved in the blow-by-blow decisions. In the case of landscape design, this is true of 80% to 90% of male clients. There is no time, but still, they care. A good designer will make an extra effort to include aspects of design that are appealing to the men in the household. In some cases, their partner is very empathic and can express for the man what he would enjoy.

Midlife. Once the kids are a little older, this is an opportunity for a man to take part in designing his personal space, in creating an area of the home that reflects who *he* is. By midlife, many guys have gone through the stage in their life when they were attracted to status symbols. This time is an opportunity to do something a little different.

The thinking is, "This is my chance. I don't have to work quite so many hours now. Maybe I could get more involved in the design of my home, in defining what I want."

Men in transition. A transitional state is an ideal time to rethink the home environment. This is true whether the man is moving from one home to another, in a new relationship, empty nesting, downsizing, or welcoming grandkids. During a transition, your home space may assume greater importance. A choice that is static or boring is not the ideal next step. It's not going to feed your soul.

Retirement. Designing for retirement can take many different forms. It might include an outdoor cooking area, for example, a pizza or bread oven, or space for home brewing. In an affluent community, it might mean a home vineyard or a bocce ball court.

DIY. Good design with forethought is just as critical for a man who is doing the work himself as it is for the man with resources. If it's your time, your labor, and you're on a budget, you certainly do not want to waste your money on a do-over. You want to get it right. You can spend the same amount of money on good design or bad design, so it's essential to take the time to figure out how you're going to use that space and what you want it to look like.

Defining Elements

Substantial design. Masculine furniture tends to be big and bulky—it's square, it's heavy, and it's comfortable. There's a favorite chair. In general, men tend to like color, clean design, and bold, strong lines, without a lot of clutter. In some cases, the overall design is relaxing, and some men prefer a quieter look. Visually, male preference runs toward more texture and natural materials like brick, stone, and wood.

Communal spaces for entertaining. For men who are still active in their careers, in their forties, fifties, and beyond, areas tend to be more about entertaining clients, colleagues, and friends. The thought is, "When I bring home a client or a colleague, I want to feel proud of my home. I want the space to have an open-door feeling where friends can stop by, with social spaces for lounging."

Fire: fireplaces, fire pits, and barbeque. Although cooking is usually an activity one or two people perform, in a communal or outdoor space, this can become a collective effort. Similarly, with a fireplace, the fire draws people in and creates a sense of community. Fire adds a primordial aspect, whether it takes the form of a barbeque, an outdoor kitchen area, a fireplace, a pizza or bread oven, or a fire pit.

The home gym. Today, home design may include an interior or exterior area that serves as a home gym, with shower or sauna. The idea is to be able to come home and work out. Consider the exercise equipment you will use in the planning process.

Doing the Research

You don't have to be wealthy to create a masculine space that you are happy to call home. How can you get in touch with what you want? How can you get a good design? Whether you are investing a great deal of money or time and effort, the goal is to create a space that you love.

Getting inspired when you travel. As men travel, their taste tends to broaden, to become more sophisticated. They gain ideas from the places where they have traveled, and they bring that back home to their benefit. Interesting design is everywhere, in hotels, at other people's homes, at resort areas, even in films, and these are all excellent sources of ideas.

Discovering your sensibility. Ten people may say they love a design, but if it doesn't feel right to you, then it's not right. You are the one who is going to have to live with it. It has to feel right on a gut level, or else every time you walk into that space, it will be an irritant instead of a pleasure. Although you want to create an environment that pleases your friends, colleagues, and associates, at the end of the day, it's your home.

PLANNING

Now that you have gathered ideas, inspiration, and lists, you're ready to apply it to your space. First, develop a plan on paper—measuring it carefully and drawing it to scale. Research online to learn how to create this. Next, draw dining, lounge, kitchen, small sitting areas, and any other features to scale. Cut out furnishings, appliances, and other aspects of the design so you can move them around on the floor plan to find the best possible arrangement. Pay attention to available space, traffic flow, shade and sun patterns, views, and other considerations.

A man wants to come home to a place he can feel proud of, whether it is a bachelor studio or a grand mansion. After working all day, when he walks in the door, he wants to feel that he has gotten something for his efforts, that trading his time for his lifestyle was worth it. Men want to be able to come home and spend time with their kids outside, playing ball, teaching them about insects, or helping them construct forts. They want to connect with their partner, sit by the fire, eat outside, or soak in the spa, in an area that is relaxing and personal.

Ultimately when a man designs a space, he's envisioning *home*. It's not just about some furniture and some pictures on the wall. It's not just about a lawn and some plants. It's a feeling. It is an environment that's talking to your soul, that relates to who you are. It has to feed that piece of you that makes you feel good. This feeling tends to be challenging to put into words, but when you experience it, you know it.

CASE STUDY: DESIGNING AN OUTDOOR SPACE

Here outdoor spaces and landscaping serve as a case in point. Planning for function involves two parts: exploring the purpose of the space and understanding the parameters needed for each activity. Based on your idea files, you have some sense of the activities you'd like to include.

A masculine landscape that supports individual passions. That may involve golfing, growing vegetables, woodworking, or just lounging under a tree or by the pool. Do the work to plan your space before starting to build, so all the work you put in will bring you closer to your goals.

How would you like to spend your time in your garden? Here are a few ideas to get you started:

- *Living room.* Take your living outside with comfy sofas, cushioned chairs, and low lighting.

- *Dining on the patio.* Will you need room for the family or for large gatherings? Will you be cooking in the kitchen and bringing the food outside on trays, or firing up the grill?

- *Outdoor cooking.* Barbecuing, boiling up a pot of corn, or flaming a pizza? Would you consider a full kitchen or simply an area to park a portable BBQ with some counter space and maybe storage for utensils and plates? Do you want to grab some drinks from an outdoor refrigerator, have an area to prep food outside, do some wine or beer tasting, or serve cocktails at a well-appointed bar?

- *Decorative edibles.* Will you be slapping a fat tomato slice on your burger, adding a handful of herbs to baste the steaks, or creating botanical cocktails with fresh herbs? Would you like to include fruit trees so you can grab a crunchy apple straight from the tree?

- *Socializing.* Perhaps you envision hanging out with your friends around a fire pit with chilled beers, watching a game, handing around plates piled high with delectable grilled meats and veggies.

- *Quiet space to recharge.* A place to get away by yourself, to rest or read could be as simple as a hammock or a table and chair for your morning coffee or as elaborate as a pavilion.

- *Creature comforts.* Create an outdoor room with a rainproof roof or shade, heaters, comfy furniture, and possibly a fire pit.

- *Time with kids.* This could mean tossing a ball with the kids or grandkids on an expansive lawn, teaching kids how to train a dog or how to grow vegetables in your outdoor classroom.

- *Staying fit.* Fitness might involve swimming laps or playing sports, and afterward soaking in the spa with your significant other.

- *Entertaining.* Whether you're entertaining one person or one hundred, you can set up your outdoor rooms to have luxuries on hand. You'll be appreciated for keeping cold drinks filled, plates brimming, towels by the spa.

Practical Matters

A checklist for landscape design. Most of my male clients share common goals: they like bold lines, clean shapes, and neat spaces. They want their landscape to be easy to maintain so they can spend their downtime doing what they want and not mowing lawns or pulling weeds. They appreciate neat, clean lines and wide spaces. Hardscape (patios, walks, and other features) must be carefully laid out and constructed to last. Infrastructure, such as grading, drainage, wiring, and water delivery, should all be in place before you plant anything.

- *Lighting.* Extend your entertaining into the evening with mood lighting, giving the garden a soft glow. Include safety lighting for more active areas.

- *Roofs and arbors.* This includes both shade and rain protection.

- *Paths.* Do you want to go efficiently from one place to another, or is the design intended to engage the viewer by creating a series of vistas, which will make the garden feel larger?

- *Maintenance area.* Include space for trash cans, maintenance tools, and a compost bin.

- *Drainage.* Be sure rainwater flows away from the house foundation, and from hardscape surfaces. It is not necessary to remove the water from the site. It is better to allow water to sink into the ground in predetermined low spots (swales) to recharge the groundwater.

- *Irrigation.* Even if you think you will enjoy hand-watering your garden, it's always a good idea to build in an automatic system. Consult with an irrigation designer or visit a professional supplier for information. Installing a quality system will save time and money.

Style. The aesthetic considerations of a project are essential. Men may discount this step of the planning process, but it is necessary to create a consistent look. If you don't pay attention to style, you could end up with a mess, pouring your money into a disorganized living space.

Unifying visual themes. As you review the images in your portfolio, look for a theme or a style that makes you feel at home and that looks the way you imagine your home to look. You also want to be open to unifying visuals that tie everything together, such as:

- Mediterranean, with natural sunbaked stone, cozy nooks, generous dining tables, Italian pots, and herbs

- Traditional styling, with a manicured lawn and shrubs, lots of greenery, and practical spaces

- A natural look with curved spaces, boulders, neat but voluptuous shrubs, flowers, and grasses

Color schemes:

- Bold primaries
- Purple with crisp shapes
- Muted olives and burnt oranges, rusty reds, and powder blues
- Pale green, buff, grays, lilac, and magenta
- Jewel tones in deep burgundies, purple, black, and silver

Research. Knowledge is power. Gather information about all the pieces that will go into the implementation of your concept. Learn all you can about the construction materials: that includes flooring (concrete, pavers, decking), walls (retaining walls, fences, trellises), out buildings, and accessories such as furniture, lights, prefab structures, and appliances.

Working with professionals. Often the best option is to hire a professional designer. A professional will have worked with all of these factors over many projects. They will have the resources and experience to pull together an optimal layout and create a beautiful space that serves your needs. Make sure you see images of their previous projects and check their references.

PUTTING IT ALL TOGETHER

Now that you have invested the time to gather information and explore your options, you are ready to create the space of your dreams. Whether you build it all at once or phase it in over time, with this level of planning, you can be confident that your project will reflect your needs and your style to give you the best value for your investment. You can look forward to a space where you can recharge, entertain, and be active for years to come.

Indeed, a man's home is his castle, but castles come in all shapes and sizes. With some effort and thought, you can create a comfortable and inspiring environment. If you plan and construct your living space well, it will give you years of relaxation and enjoyment.

**For more information on the work of Michael Tebb see
Michaeltebbdesign.houzzsite.com**

Chapter 63
Retirement?
Point Counter Point
Jack Graham, Retired Businessman
& Michael Abassian, MPH, Researcher

Often men work hard for decades to reach a level of financial security that will enable them to take well-deserved retirement from the working world. As a urologist, I have seen thousands of men in retirement, and I can confidently say that some men are deliriously happy in retirement, and some are miserable. Retirement can mean identity loss, boredom, and/or financial insecurity for those who don't plan properly. But for the men who retire intentionally and purposefully, it can mean the realization of life goals and time to do what they want to do.

— Judson Brandeis, MD

Retirement is a time of transition and a significant milestone. It is a period that many of us look forward to, to do the things we've always wanted: check off items on our bucket list, travel and socialize with family, grandkids, and friends we may not have seen in years. A survey of over 1,000 retirees in 2019 found that 40% found the transition "not at all challenging."

THE CHALLENGES OF RETIREMENT
Michael Abassian

Today, the grim reality is that many men are not financially prepared for retirement. As a country, what we can expect from retirement and what it may look like for us is going to be very different from what it was even just a few decades ago. Currently:

- A quarter of 65-year-olds will live past 90.

- Over half of baby boomers will keep working in some form after they retire, either for financial reasons or to stay active and busy.

- Social Security is responsible for keeping 27 million Americans out of poverty.

Year after year, surveys find that the concerns of pre-retirees stay consistent. Men are especially worried that their savings won't keep up with inflation, and that they may not be able to cover health and long-term care expenses. In fact, over half of men (54%) are worried that they will deplete all of their savings in retirement, and 60% are somewhat or very concerned that they won't be able to afford good healthcare.

Recap: A Review of Retirement

Today, the average man retires at 65, whereas the average woman retires at 63. By 2035, the number of Americans 65 and older will increase from 56 million to over 78 million. The life expectancy of a 65-year man in the 1940s was just about 13 additional years of life, whereas now men at 65 are expected to live more than an additional 18 years beyond retirement age. This means more time spent in a retirement phase, additional savings needed, and more healthcare costs anticipated as chronic diseases associated with aging rise. The Social Security Administration provides a quick online tool (https://www.ssa.gov/cgi-bin/longevity.cgi) that will tell you how many additional years you can expect to live on average, based on your gender and date of birth. This is a resource you can use in making retirement decisions, such as the age at which you intend to retire and draw Social Security benefits. Claiming benefits at age 62 or before your full retirement age can result in lower benefits (as much as 30% lower). Therefore, consider your goals, health status, and context when making such decisions.

Men are a little less likely to give serious thought (53%) to how life will change in retirement compared to the proportion of women who think about this topic (62%). That means only half of men are thinking ahead to retirement. This type of planning is an essential aspect of psychological wellbeing, and once we reach retirement age, having an economic base is clearly essential to our physical wellbeing.

Men are also less likely than women to have a relative who will care for them in retirement, and an astonishing four out of ten retirees do not have someone to count on to take care of them as they age. Experts recommend that you start planning for retirement at least five years in advance. These are aspects of reality that cause men distress, but they are important considerations that we need to be thinking about earlier rather than later, to experience optimal aging.

The Role of Social Security Benefits

The impact of Social Security as a safety net is tremendous. Nine out of ten Americans 65 and older receive Social Security benefits and every year, 65 million Americans receive over one trillion dollars through the program. The Social Security Act was signed by President

Number of Retired Male Workers (as of June 2020)
Receiving Social Security by Age and Benefit Amount

Monthly Benefit Amount	Annual Benefit Amount	Total Number of Retirees	Percentage	Average Retirement
<$499-$1,499	$6,000 - $18,000	9.5 million	39%	39% of retirees live on less than $1,500/month social security
$1,500-$2,999	$18,000 - $36,000	13 million	59%	Another 59% receive less than $2,500/month
>$3,000	>$36,000	600,000	2%	
TOTAL		22,722,983	100%	

Figure 63.1 Number of retired male workers (as of June 2020) receiving Social Security. (Source: ssa.gov.)

Roosevelt in 1935 with the intention of creating a program that would give monthly benefits to retired workers starting at age 65 and older. This fund is financed by payroll taxes withheld from employee wages. By the end of 1967, there were more than 7 million retired men receiving an average Social Security Benefit of $95 ($735 in today's value). By the end of July 2020, there were almost 23 million retired men receiving an average Social Security payout of almost $17,000 each. See the table to determine how benefit payouts differ by age among men.

Recent Social Security reports indicate that the trust fund is in danger of depletion by 2034. If a scenario like this occurs, a 23% cut in benefit payouts is projected, since incoming payroll taxes will only be able to sustain 77% of benefits. This is especially troubling because one out of five married retired Americans and two out of five unmarried retirees are completely dependent on Social Security. Our safety net is in danger.

Savings and Retirement

Average retirement savings for 56-to 61-year-old pre-retirees is $17,000. This means half of Americans in this age group have less than that, and half have more. Additionally, median retirement savings for the overall population is a mere $5,000, and for workers 32 to 37 years old, median retirement savings is a depressing $480. What's more, the data tend to be misleading.

It is clear that income level has an impact on how one retires. Half of pre-retirees with household incomes of more than $100,000 have a retirement plan that will be their major source of income, compared to 14% earning a household income of less than $50,000.

A Kaiser Family Foundation report found that only 23% of large companies (200+ employers) that provide health benefits also currently provide retiree coverage. This number has decreased sharply and places an additional financial burden on retirees. The average age at which men start contributing to some form of retirement plan is 26 years old, but the data indicate that half of men do not. The earlier you begin saving for retirement either through an employment program (such as a company pension plan) or an Individual Retirement Account (IRA), the more flexibility and security you will be able to achieve.

As with any emerging chapter in our lives, retirement brings opportunities to try new things. This could mean travel or spending more time with close friends or family, or it could involve a second career or meaningful volunteer work. When thinking about what lies ahead, manifest your purpose by realizing that you are a valuable member of your community simply by virtue of your experience and knowledge. There are many challenges in all of our communities, and rest assured that there is a way you can contribute and make a positive difference. But just as importantly don't forget to pat yourself on the back, kick up your feet, and celebrate the enormous impact you've already had on your family, friends, and community.

THE JOYS OF RETIREMENT
Jack Graham

After graduating from college at 21, like most Americans, I worked hard throughout my 45-year career in two different professions—first at the local newspaper as a sportswriter, and then the last 34 years building a successful insurance agency. I always knew that we would retire at some point, but I just didn't know when. It wasn't until my wife and I met with our financial planner six years ago that the word retirement finally came into focus. Until that time, retirement was just a pipedream, as I continued to work long hours in hopes that someday I could walk away from it all.

Many people have a fear of retirement because they don't know what they would do with their lives if they didn't work. I never had this fear—I relished the idea. I knew in my own mind that I could keep busy and enjoy a stress-free life. Shortly after retiring, I spoke to a dear friend about retirement. He told me that the key to retirement is to stay busy – sort of. Do the things you enjoy doing and don't worry about things you can't control.

What does retirement mean to you? What do you want most out of it? I had to do some serious soul searching to find the answers to these important questions in order to make this thing work. To me, retirement meant living a happy retirement, a healthy retirement, and just as important, it meant living a financially comfortable retirement. To achieve these goals, it was also important to have a sense of purpose and meaning. After I answered all those questions in my mind, the rest was easy. Having a successful and loving relationship with my wife, spending more time with her, and spending more time with our children and our grandchildren gave me this purpose.

Volunteer work. Throughout my career and even today, I have always been active in organizations. For the past 31 years and counting, I've been involved in Rotary, including service as past president. I truly enjoy the people and the opportunity to help make a difference in both our local and international community. I do this because my time is now my own, and I can choose what to participate in, spending time on various projects that I enjoy.

Hobbies. I have several other interests that keep me busy. This is so important. If you don't have a hobby – find one! Personally, I have a great passion for travel, for golf, and for fitness. When I am not on the golf course, my wife and I try to take daily walks around our neighborhood as part of our cardio workouts. These are normally 2- to 3-mile brisk walks that allow us to talk or listen to music. In addition, we have also been doing strength training together twice a week, working with a personal trainer. Being healthy is so important as you get older, especially if you want to enjoy your retirement. And if you have health issues (we all do), don't be afraid to seek medical advice and treatment.

Exceptional role models. I was fortunate growing up, in that I had great parents as role models to look up to and give my life direction and purpose. They were both from the "greatest generation" of people who grew up during the Great Depression, lived through World War II and the Korean War, and raised successful families. They were our role models, which we have tried to emulate in raising our own children. For us, things could not be better. Everything we do, we do for each other, as a team.

Nurturing the next generation. We love spending time with our family and grandkids! Nothing gives us greater joy and satisfaction than being with them, loving them and making a difference in their lives just as our parents did for us. My wife and I have two grown children who are both happily married, and three grandchildren. They give us purpose, the intent that we will always be there for them in every way possible, because they mean the world to us.

Intimacy. One of the best things I love about retirement is being able to spend more time with my wife. We have a healthy and loving relationship and have been happily married for nearly 50 years. That said, one of the big issues we discovered as the years progressed was sexual intimacy. We have always had a deep affection for each other, and our love grows stronger every day. However, it's just not the same as when we were first married. Thus, we sought medical help through a couple of physicians and discovered the revolutionary bioTE hormone pellets. The results have been amazing, increasing testosterone and estrogen levels, bringing back our libidos as if we were in our 20s again.

Managing stress. We are truly blessed to have a great life and great friends, which brings me to another point. We both decided several years ago to get rid of toxic relationships with friends, and instead surround ourselves with friends who are like us, who have similar goals and positive lifestyles. This has made a huge difference for us and allows us to enjoy life to the fullest. Also, don't be afraid to be social with people outside your age group. In fact, some of our best friends are 20 to 25 years younger than we are.

I now look at my life as an adventure. As Mark Twain once said, "Twenty years from now you will be more disappointed by the things you didn't do than by the ones you did do. So throw off the bowlines, sail away from the safe harbor. Catch the trade winds in your sails. Explore. Dream. Discover." That's what retirement is all about. Embrace it and enjoy it.

**For resources and more information, please visit
www.TheTwentyFirstCenturyMan.com.**

PART 9
MENTAL HEALTH
Introduction
Judson Brandeis, MD

If you are not nervous, then you are not paying attention.
— *Miles Davis*

Every stage in life involves psychological stress. In adolescence, young men are forging an identity separate from their parents and beginning to understand who they are as individuals. In their 20s, men determine their life path, learn the craft that will support them, and try to find their mate. In their 30s, men are starting their families and establishing themselves professionally and in their community. When men reach their 40s, the dreams they had when they were younger begin to fade, and the reality of the life they have created begins to set in. At this stage, professional and family responsibilities increase. At the same time, men begin the long process of physical deterioration. They also start to come to terms with who they have become relative to other men they know. Social media has made this even more traumatic because it has falsely raised expectations. A man, and sometimes, more importantly, his spouse, sees the persona that other people project through social media, rather than the reality. It is a temptation to make comparisons to these fictional images.

The intense pressures of midlife have led to soaring alcohol and opioid abuse and suicide rates among middle-aged men. In this toxic environment, the necessity of finding a balance of work and personal life is critical. Too many men are falling victim to depression and anxiety. So many of us have lost the vitality of life.

The chapters in this section are critical to living a fulfilling and joyful life. Know that every man struggles with mental health in some form or another. The experts in this section provide a range of perspectives and resources for optimizing your mental health. I hope you take this opportunity to learn about the issues that affect so many of our brethren.

Chapter 64
Work-Life Balance
Robert Buonfiglio, PhD, Psychologist
& Executive Life Coach

*The human dilemma is the struggle between what we want to do
and what we have to do.*
— Rollo May

As a psychologist and life coach, every day I see hard-working men who want to provide a good life for themselves and their family. As the demands of their profession, the needs of their family, and the pace of their job increase, they begin to lose balance and eventually lose sight of themselves. This occurs across industries, in every economic niche, and in every possible job title, from laborer to cardiologist and from solo entrepreneur to Fortune 500 CEO. How do we unwind this unfortunate reality? Let me tell you a story about one of these men. . . .

John was a happy-go-lucky guy on the fast track to success. At 29, with a degree in finance under his belt, he started a weekend MBA program. A highly skilled auditor, his understated charisma and his dedicated work ethic made him a favorite with clients. His firm ear-marked him for a position in management.

At 33, John had his first child. He loved being a father, but he had trouble juggling his priorities, so pick-up basketball games on the weekend were the first thing to go. At 35, his second child was born, and he was also promoted to vice president. The birth of his second child and his promotion were a double whammy for John. Over the next few years, he took on more and responsibility at work and eight-hour days became ten-hour days, plus the commute. That left him with less and less time for his kids, his wife, and for himself. Something had to give, so he started skipping his regular gym workouts on his way home.

No longer working as an auditor for preferred clients, John was now in charge of massive projects, constantly putting out fires, and being pulled in ten different directions. By the time he got home, the kids were often in bed, and he had little juice left for his wife. He was easily agitated, less social, and his diet was terrible. Comfort food and booze were his primary coping mechanisms.

Seven years later, John has achieved all the markers of success. He's made partner, and traded his cramped city apartment for a suburban three-bedroom with a big yard and great schools for the kids. But at a cost. John now works twelve hours a day, usually six days a week —plus an hour commute each way. At the office, his coworkers and direct reports used to look up to him and see him as a role model. But today, he's running on fumes. He and his wife quarrel more and more. He's withdrawn, edgy, and struggles with depression. And just when everything seems at its worst, he learns that his son needs heart surgery.

John's son's diagnosis is a wake-up call that compels him to take a long, hard look at his life. After years of paying little attention to his family, John is realizing how important they are to him, and he wants to be a more involved father and husband. He doesn't know exactly how to make that happen, but he knows he needs to change. John is lucky enough to have a boss who sees that John is struggling. The boss recommends that John work with a life coach and provides him with the phone numbers of three coaches, including me.

OPENING THE DOOR TO CHANGE

Over the next few pages, I want to take you through important aspects of the process I use to help clients like John. We begin by identifying the issues in the client's life that aren't working, prioritize the changes that need to be made, and create an action plan to work toward achieving the life they want to live.

Willingness to change is an important prerequisite to any type of adjustment. But there's an important step that comes before willingness, and that's *awareness*: before you can change anything, you must first acknowledge that something's not working and that you want to do something about it. At that point, the next step is to figure out what kind of resources and support you'll need. (These insights are gleaned from the work of Kirk Schneider, PhD, a thought leader in the field of existential-humanistic psychology.)

RESOURCE—THE POWER OF ACCOUNTABILITY

As a psychologist and life coach, I'm a believer in the coaching process. But I recognize that coaching can be expensive and not everyone can afford it. And even those who can may prefer to work with a friend or on their own.

- Can you make the necessary changes on your own?
- Do you want assistance from a psychologist or a coach?
- If you're on a tight budget, what about working with an accountability partner?

To translate your vision into action, you will want to build in some form of accountability.

Setting goals is usually a lot easier to do than achieving them. And while it's certainly possible to achieve your goals on your own, I strongly recommend that you work with someone who can encourage and support you.

Some people choose to hire a coach to get them through, but you could also work with a trusted friend or a loved one. In that scenario, you both establish goals and each of you takes the role of holding the other accountable by checking in and making sure that you're on track. It's a *lot* harder to hold yourself accountable. But keep in mind that being an accountability partner is a big job. So, if you opt to have a non-professional help you, be sure that he or she has the time, energy, and organizational ability to do the job. The same is true if you're taking on that role for someone else.

However you decide to proceed, it's important to understand that change is a long-term process. Each person and each situation is unique, and there's no way to predetermine the length of time it will take. Change happens by investing in the process of change, and I urge you to aim for progress, not perfection.

MAKING CHANGE HAPPEN

At this point, the first step is to take inventory of what you are experiencing, what's working, and what isn't. This provides a context for envisioning your future. What does your best life look like? What actions will you need to take to put together a program that will get you there?

RESOURCE—JOURNALING

Most men don't spend a lot of time reflecting on the issues that are bothering them or the challenges they're facing—especially if they are emotionally laden. They just try to overcome them.

However, reflection creates the possibility for new insights that can foster change. That's why I often start by having my clients write the story of their life in as much detail as possible. I ask them to walk me through the different stages of their life (childhood, high school, college, professional life, and significant relationships.). We discuss all the important events that have been influential (both successes and challenges). The point is to have the client reflect on their life and consider what's working, what isn't, and what they want to change. (Note that not all coaches do this. If writing works for you, great. If it doesn't, that's okay too. That said, even if you're reluctant or uncomfortable with the idea of journaling, I recommend that you give it a try—most men I work with are amazed by how much they learn about themselves in the process.)

John was hesitant to journal, but once he got started, he found that he actually enjoyed it. He told me that this was the first time he had reflected on his life in years. Writing seemed to be an easier forum for expressing his feelings than talking, and it became a pathway for deepening his awareness and better understanding his emotions.

RESOURCE—THE FIVE PILLARS (OUR PRIORITIES)

The next tool I provided John focuses on four or five of the most important areas of the client's life. I describe these focal points as "pillars," because they provide the basis of a person's wellbeing. Identifying one's pillars helps to clarify major priorities. I often find that clients truly value things that aren't getting their time and attention. The exercise helps to bring this to the forefront, creating a new level of awareness that makes change possible. In John's case, he chose to focus on four pillars in order to simplify his life and free up the time he needed to make anticipated changes:

- Family dynamics (spouse/partner and children)
- Career
- Health (mental, physical, and economic)
- Friends and community

For each of those areas, we ask a series of questions:

- What are the most challenging issues I'm facing?
- What's working and what's not?
- How much time am I spending nurturing this area of my life?
- Am I happy with the way things are right now?
- What do I want to do differently?
- Where do I want things to be in six months? A year? Five years?

For John, this process was eye-opening. In the Family pillar, he realized that at some point he had essentially checked out, becoming withdrawn, not spending time with his children, and no longer participating in his marriage. Work had consumed him. He talked about his as-yet-unfulfilled dream of coaching his son's baseball team or being more active at his children's school. He also missed watching football with his friends. We worked on trying to make time for these important things. Keeping the goals realistic, he chose a weekly activity involving his son. In the Friends pillar, he has set time aside one night a week to play poker or watch football with his buddies. In Health, he talked about missing gym workouts and recognized the need to cut back on junk food and alcohol. Some weeks are better than others, but he continues to work to improve.

Exploring the Career pillar, John came to realize that in his drive to make VP and then partner, he'd lost sight of what mattered to him. Although he valued his job and had wanted to play a leadership role in the firm, the management workstyle was brutal. Overall, John saw that as he became overwhelmed with responsibility, he lost his relationship with himself. The life he was living wasn't the one he had envisioned. It no longer aligned with his core values and wasn't making him happy. The existential-humanistic psychologist, Rollo May, has said, "The human dilemma is the struggle between what we want to do and what we have to do." John was living solely in the "what I have to do" sphere and just going through the motions.

RESOURCE—ASSESSING HOW YOU SPEND YOUR TIME

There are 168 hours in a week. And in one session, John and I broke down how he spent those hours. Between work (6 days at 12 hours each day) and his commute (6 days at 2 hours), he was gone 84 hours.

When he wasn't working, John spent a lot of time thinking about work, so we conservatively added 10 hours of psychological time. (Psychological time is the time we spend preoccupied, lost in thought. Actual time is the time when we are actually engaged in the present moment.) We can spend a lot of time in our head, preoccupied and and not really present.

We also added another 10 hours to account for getting ready in the morning and unwinding in the evening. That means 104 hours of John's waking hours related to work.

Then we added in time for sleep (6 hours a night, clearly not enough). This brings us to 146 hours, leaving only 22 hours a week (most of them late at night) to eat, exercise, be with his kids, spend time with his wife, call friends, and anything else. (Arriving home in the dark, he had become a stranger to his kids.) It's no wonder John's life was unraveling.

Taking an inventory of how you use your time can be an effective tool for assessing your life and seeing opportunities for change.

RESOURCE—USING AN APP

Another approach to self-exploration is to do an inventory of your values, goals, and lifestyle using a template I call an APP, short for Awareness, Pause, and Pivot. I've found it to be a very powerful way to focus and clarify thinking in every area of your life, whether it has to do with your job, your partner, your children, your friends, or your community.

Here's how it works:

Awareness. Our awareness keeps us attuned to what's truly coming up for us, in terms of our inner reality and our intentions, as well as our external environment.

- Do I have the sense that I'm slipping out of balance?

- Is it time to re-examine my values?

- At this point in my life, what matters to me?

- How am I spending my time?

- Am I nurturing what matters to me?

- How do I *want* to spend my time?

- What are the current obstacles to living a more balanced life?

Pause. With newfound awareness, we need to take a step back, slow down, and reflect. By slowing down, we can gain further insight, building on the awareness we have developed. This provides the opportunity to consider different perspectives, options, choices, and alternatives.

Pivot. Having deepened our awareness, developed insight, and explored our choices, it's now time to take action. What will you *do* to act on your insights, to live out your values, and what matters most to you?

Applying the APP

Here's what the APP process looked like for the Family pillar of John's life:

Awareness. John loves and values his family. His son's heart condition has made him realize how deeply he cares for the child, and he feels very fortunate that his son is well on his way to a full recovery. John has become keenly aware of his lack of involvement with his kids. He also feels that there is a lack of intimacy with his wife.

Pause. John slows down and sits with these feelings. He doesn't like the way things are. The feeling is incongruent with his values. He begins to explore his choices based on his values.

Pivot. John becomes more active in his children's lives. He makes it a point to be home in time to help his kids with their homework, and on Sunday they go to the park or watch movies together. John has also realized that his wife was not happy and that he was not showing up in the relationship. This caused him to initiate couples therapy with his wife. They are working on things and although it isn't easy, they are trying to heal, learn, understand, and make things better.

Remember—The goal is progress, not perfection!

John is using the APP as a compass to help him live more aligned with his values. This is a tool that can be useful in all areas of your life, although it takes some practice to hone this skill. Remind yourself that when you apply it, the goal is to examine your current situation non-judgmentally, with compassion. You may find it helpful to use the APP in your day-to-day to check-in with yourself.

RESOURCE—UPKEEP AND MAINTENANCE

To prevent relapse, we need to consider the concepts of maintenance and restoration. Maintenance refers to upkeep on the things that are working well. This is like getting the oil changed in your car every three months. Restoration is a more complicated project, involving repair that requires additional time and work, like getting an entirely new engine. When we are negligent with maintenance, our lives require much more restoration.

THE PATH TOWARD CHANGE

RESOURCE—LIFE COACHING

The goal of coaching is to help the client discover, explore, and live what has meaning for them. The coach provides support for step-by-step change and utilizes homework assignments. Coaching also encourages the client to draw on their own internal resources to move forward and effect change.

Coaching sessions generally happen weekly or every other week for about an hour and can be conducted by video, phone, or in person. We spend the first few sessions taking a look at the challenges you're facing in your life, what you want to change, and your specific goals. Once we've done that, a typical session has three phases.

To open the conversation we check in, talk about how things are going, what steps you've taken toward achieving your goals, what's been working, and what hasn't.

In the second phase of the session, we focus on next steps and fine tune the strategy. We talk about what's making the successful things successful and what needs to happen to turn around the less-than-successful aspects of your life. The beauty of this process is that even though there's accountability, there's no judgment. We keep chipping away at the problem, so you feel supported. We keep the focus on the positive, working in increments. What did you do that worked? What modest step could you take in the coming week that would make that strategy a little more powerful?

Change is hard, and the coach becomes a supportive companion on the client's journey. During each session, the coach champions wins and helps the client develop new insight and strategies for issues that need to be addressed.

- What did you do that worked?
- What obstacles got in your way?
- What would you like to do differently next time?
- What is the next step?
- What can you do in the coming week that could make your strategies a little more effective?

At the end of session, we identify the steps that will take place in between sessions. The purpose is to build on successes, take more positive steps in the right direction, and keep the momentum going. Sometimes the goal is self-exploration, using a tool such as journaling. At other times, the emphasis is on practical problem solving, for example researching job opportunities or applying for a new job.

We are not human doers—we are human beings. We have wants, needs, and desires and need to give ourselves permission to live them out while also being mindful of our responsibilities. Reflection and awareness are central to this mission. Identifying and then living your values and priorities will enable you to live a happy and healthier life. I encourage you to explore living in this way.

STRATEGIES FOR CHANGE

Maintaining Work-Life Balance

Meditation. Awareness is the key to ongoing balance. It helps us to slow down and be more intentional and present. Finding time to meditate provides a useful component in an effective self-care routine.

Apps. Mediation apps such as Headspace and Calm can teach you more about the process and how you can integrate it into your life.

Reading. Useful books on meditation include classics such as *Breath Sweeps Mind, The Power of Now,* and *Practicing Mindfulness.*

Videos. YouTube is one of many sources that provide videos on learning to meditate and on deepening your practice. Enter the search term "how to meditate."

Audio recordings. SoundsTrue.com is an excellent source of recordings that coach you through guided meditations and mindfulness practice.

Group meditation. If you find doing things in a group motivating, group meditation can ground, deepen, and reinforce your practice. Many religious traditions incorporate group meditation, including various branches of Buddhism such as Zen, the Christian Quaker tradition, and Vedic meditation and yoga.

Movement. Walking meditation can be useful if you tend to be highly active and find it challenging to slow down enough to do sitting meditation. Simple practices include mindfulness (simply walking with heightened consciousness), and Qigong walking meditation, which coordinates breath with each step.

Deepening Your Relationships

Date night. Dedicated time with your significant other can help keep the spark alive and provide the space to nurture your relationship. This should just be fun. Once a week is the classic date-night template, but it's always important to tailor any approach to your own needs.

Family meetings. How are we doing? Are you happy? Am I happy? What do we need to do to stay on track? Perhaps once a week, you can also raise the question of balance: How are we doing? What is working well, and what needs an upgrade?

Family dinners. Consider having one night a week that is committed to the people with whom you spend your life, to maintain these relationships and a sense of balance.

Family counseling. If these strategies don't help foster the relationships you seek, consider seeing a family therapist to find common ground and understanding. The incentive here is to nurture and improve the things that matter to you.

Hobbies and avocations. What do you enjoy? What do you want to spend time learning? Joining a sports team, an interest group, or an educational program can create enjoyment and counteract the stress of work and other responsibilities.

Taking Time Out

A vacation, a retreat, or a workshop. An annual vacation or a retreat can help you recharge your batteries. Although this requires some planning, creativity, and resources, this is another tool for re-establishing a reservoir of calm in your life and the opportunity for re-evaluation. (For example, Yuval Harari, the historian, spends a week in silence at a Zen monastery once every three months.) The key concept here is that you set time aside to have a change of scenery and to evaluate how you're doing, to help you remain closer to your balance point.

If you are a parent, we acknowledge that it will probably require additional planning and collaboration to make this happen, whether that means your young people are with your significant other, with family, close friends, or attending camp. For a weekend retreat, supervised sleepovers could be a resource, if your kids have friends whose parents hold values similar to yours.

One day a week off the grid. Consider taking one day a week when you don't work, turn off your cell phone, and get off the grid in order to reconnect with your own psyche, with those around you, and with the natural world. Unplugging enables your mind and body to recover from the constant stimulation (mental, media, and electronic stress) that bombard us all. If you don't have space to take a day, take half a day and, again, build it right into your calendar, and let colleagues know that you're available six days a week, but not seven.

Working with a Professional One-on-One

Coaching. As we've discussed, coaching can help you create change in your life. It can also be a highly effective strategy if you're not making the progress you'd like. However, if you're experiencing frequent anxiety or depression that's negatively affecting your ability to function, you may want to seek therapy. To find a good coach, get referrals from friends or family, or use online resources, such as the website of the International Coaching Federation (coachfederation.org) and Berkeley Executive Coaching Institute (berkeleyeci.com/coaching-services).

Psychotherapy. If you're struggling with frequent depression or anxiety, therapy is likely to be a more appropriate resource than coaching. Therapy can be particularly effective when issues seem to reflect patterns of stress that repeat in one's life, which may have begun in childhood. Listings for licensed psychologists are available at psychologytoday.com/us

If you're dealing with anxiety or depression, see chapters 66 and 67 in the book. There are many different approaches to therapy. Two of the most common include:

- Cognitive behavioral therapy (CBT) is a method that can help you challenge your thought patterns and reduce negative, critical self-talk. CBT is available one-on-one and in group settings.

- Humanistic psychology is a perspective that is useful in exploring the meaning in your life, to develop a deeper awareness of who you are and how you want to live.

To get a sense of the approach that's right for you, read through the websites of therapists you are considering. Identify several whose experience and style resonate with you. Then contact them to set up a time to talk, to see if they are a good fit for you.

Psychiatry. In some cases, therapy in conjunction with medication can be beneficial. Working with a psychiatrist can be helpful if there is an imbalance in body chemistry that results in frequent depression or anxiety. These conditions can have a genetic origin, reflected in emotional characteristics that may present randomly within a family over several generations.

Functional medicine. Research has shown that as much as 50% of mental and emotional symptoms have a physical cause. This is true of familiar conditions such as depression, which in some cases responds well to exercise, and in others, resolves with improved nutrition, eating small, frequent meals that include a little protein.

Family therapy or parenting classes. Our relationships with our partner and our kids are usually the first casualties when we start slipping into a workaholic lifestyle. The goal is to be proactive, addressing the issues before the relationships are damaged. PsychologyToday.com is a good source of family therapy referrals.

Group Work

Group therapy. If you enjoy interacting in a group, this approach can be quite effective, and tends to be more affordable. Most people are surprised by how universal their challenges are. Group therapy offers you the opportunity to process your concerns and develop skills to address those concerns, to see how others are solving these problems, and to contribute your own solutions as well.

Mastermind or men's group. Exploring work-life balance in a group setting enables you to address that issue with peers. If money is a concern, consider creating your own men's group that meets periodically. That can provide you with a forum to hash out problems, share resources, and support each other. Your life and your goals are not a matter of "set it and forget it." All of us need to periodically check in with ourselves to see if we are maintaining a reasonable balance in our lives.

Key Take Aways to Help You Assess and Maintain Work-Life Balance

- How motivated are you to change?
- Do you have the capacity and willingness to change?
- What resources and support do you need?
- Take inventory: Write the story of your life, reflect on what you've written, and then write the *next* chapter of your life.
- Explore the concept of actual time and psychological time.
- Set aside an hour on the weekend to do something with total mindfulness, whether that's savoring every bite of a superb meal or taking a walk.
- Identify the five most important areas of your life. Rate yourself from 1 to 10 on how you are doing.
- Use the APP format (awareness, pause, pivot).

- Assess what needs to be maintained and what needs to be restored.

- Set boundaries with work and create space and time for the other important areas of your life.

- Live aligned with your values.

- Remember, you can't take care of anyone else if you don't take care of yourself.

The Work-Life Pendulum

Work-life balance is a constant struggle in my life. The cellphone has made it even more difficult, because work can intrude into family life in an instant. The pace of life seems to have accelerated, and it seems like local and global competition have become more intense. I do not have any easy answers. Dr. Buonfiglio has done an admirable job addressing this subject. I view the work-life dichotomy as a pendulum. Those sparkling family images everyone posts on Facebook are just a highlight reel. There are times when work is going to take precedence, and hopefully there are times when you can leave the office, physically, mentally, and emotionally, to focus on your family, friends, and yourself. My advice:

- *Give yourself a break, even if no one else does. How many celebrities put up a façade of family bliss only to get divorced or embarrassed years later.*

- *Do the best you can to take care of yourself, because this will enable you to handle the challenges in life.*

- *Avoid self-destructive habits and time-sinks. I stopped binge watching professional sports and found five to ten extra hours of productive time every week.*

- *Make a list of your life priorities and goals, and focus on these first. In the end, life is short. So many men lose track of what is important to them.*

- *Understand that everyone struggles with this, not just you.*

—Judson Brandeis, MD

For more information on the work of Robert Buonfiglio, please see www.drrobertjbuonfiglio.com.

Chapter 65
Diseases of Despair
Judson Brandeis, MD
& Michael Abassian, MPH

Life begins on the other side of despair.
— *Jean-Paul Sartre*

Richard is a 59-year-old North Carolina native with two sons, Jake and Daniel, and a daughter, Jessica. He has worked as an HVAC technician, in business with his father replacing air conditioning units in homes and apartments, since he was 16 years old. He has made an honest living and put his children through college. He is especially proud of his youngest child, a senior about to graduate from the University of Florida. His wife, Nancy, has been an elementary school teacher for 25 years. They're both looking forward to the day when they'll be able to retire.

Unfortunately, that doesn't seem soon. Richard and Nancy lost their home to foreclosure in the Great Recession of 2007, and the financial demands of raising three children have put significant economic and emotional stress on Richard as the breadwinner of his family. He's increasingly worried about the outlook for their retirement. The residual effects of foreclosure and other money issues have made it difficult for Richard to recover financially and emotionally.

Richard has diabetes, high blood pressure, and progressive arthritis worsened by the physical demands of his job. His wife has noticed his increased alcohol consumption and remembers her mother-in-law's struggles with alcohol addiction. Nancy has tried to talk with Richard about seeking help for his increasing health problems. The conversations typically lead to a dead-end, with Richard promising he'll be able to turn things around. Even though he is 50 pounds overweight, he's defensive and assures his wife that he's in good health and looks better than his friends. As the months roll by, Richard's dependence on alcohol becomes increasingly apparent, and the level of conflict in the household reaches a tipping point. Two weeks before Jessica's graduation, Nancy finds Richard collapsed and unresponsive on the bathroom floor with a broken bottle of whiskey. An ambulance rushes Richard to the hospital, but it is too late. The emergency room physician pronounces Richard dead that night. The cause of death is listed as suicide by alcohol poisoning.

Richard's downward spiral is increasingly common in the United States. This chapter will explore trends in mortality from suicide, drug overdose, and alcoholic liver disease, and what you need to be aware of to protect yourself.

AN EPIDEMIC IN DISEASES OF DESPAIR

Life expectancy, which is the average number of years you can expect to live after birth, began to plateau in the United States in 2010 and declined from 2014 to 2017. What has caused this decline? The trend is not due to the typical culprits you might think of, such as cancer, cardiovascular disease, or motor vehicle accidents. It is because of an extraordinary rise in suicides, drug overdoses due to opiates, and alcoholic liver disease. In 2015, economists Anne Case and Angus Deaton of Princeton University reported that middle-aged white Americans, especially those with limited education and limited job opportunities, were suffering from "diseases of despair," referring to an epidemic of deaths due to suicides and stress-related disorders.

Given the current advances in medicine and public health, we would expect life expectancy to continue to rise, just as it has for much of the history of the United States. However, between 2000 and 2017, the death rate from stress conditions has doubled, jumping from 22.7 persons to 45.8 per 100,000 individuals. Similarly, from 1999 to 2013, the white

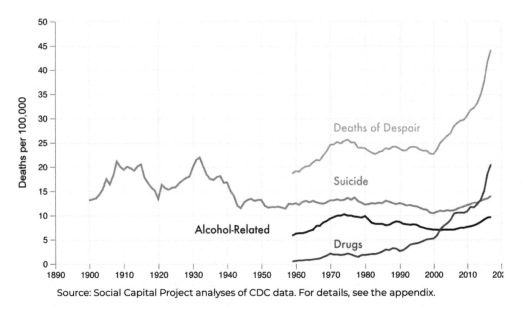

Source: Social Capital Project analyses of CDC data. For details, see the appendix.

**Figure 65.1. Deaths of despair, 1900-2017. Age-adjusted death rates.
(Data source: CDC and senate.gov)**

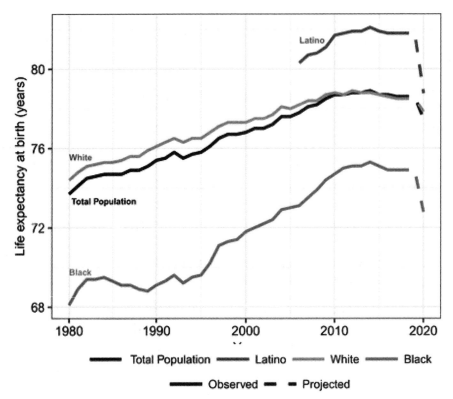

Figure 65.2. Life expectancy, U.S., 1980-2020
(Source: Proceedings of the National Academy of Sciences.)

non-Hispanic mortality rate rose by 34 per 100,000; in contrast, the mortality rates of other groups improved. Awareness of this trend and the underlying issues that drive it will help to empower you and those around you to better address these risks.

CHRONIC PAIN

Chronic conditions are on the rise in the United States, and our population is aging, which means that Americans are living longer with a range of chronic diseases, including chronic pain. These chronic pain disorders have devastating effects on individuals, their families, and the community. Overall, nearly 50 million adults in the United States experience painful conditions that last for at least three months. Over 20 million adults have chronic pain that interferes with daily and work-related activities. Older adults, veterans, and individuals who live in rural areas and high-poverty communities are more likely to develop a chronic pain condition.

Deaths resulting from these conditions often occur because people want to escape either the emotional or physical pain they are experiencing. Physical pain is increasing because more Americans are developing chronic conditions due to poor health and aging. However, another aspect of this picture is emotional stress due to lost economic opportunity, failure in business, bankruptcy, loss of the family home or farm, and the effects on social relationships and family ties. The purely economic costs of chronic pain management in the United States total $635 billion a year, a figure that does not include the incalculable human cost.

ADDICTIONS

Opioids

The growing opioid epidemic in the United States over the last several decades has had a tremendous impact on the quality of life for two generations of Americans, as well as the public health system and the economy. Opioids claimed the lives of over 70,000 people in the U.S. in 2017. The cost is massive: $78 billion in 2013 alone. Every day, 130 people die from an opioid overdose. How we got here is complicated, but the epidemic is divided into three stages. Opioids were introduced on a large scale in the early 1990s to deal with pain management. In the early 2010s, deaths from heroin overdose rapidly increased as heroin became less expensive and more concentrated. Finally, an increase in deaths from synthetic opioids began in 2013 with the availability of more powerful alternatives to heroin such as

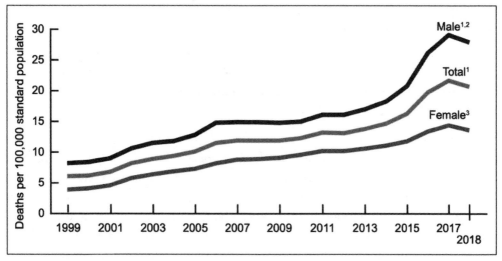

Figure 65.3. Age-adjusted drug overdose death rates, by sex. U.S., 1999-2018 (Source: cdc.gov)

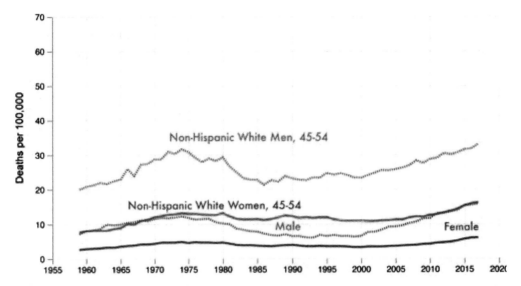

Figure 65.4. Alcohol-related deaths by sex, overall and non-hispanic whites ages 45-54, U.S., 1959-2017.

fentanyl. The opioid epidemic has taught us that anyone can become a victim of substance abuse. Addiction now affects men of every economic class, religion, age, education level, and from every size community in the country.

Drug overdose death rates for men have more than tripled, increasing from 8.2 in 1999 to 27.9 per 100,000 in 2018 (see Figure 65.3). A higher percentage of men age 55 and older are falling victim to opioid overdose deaths, which is also the age group most likely to suffer from chronic disease and pain.

In public health, a common concept used to determine the impact of a disease or epidemic is to calculate disability-adjusted life years (DALY), which reflects a year of healthy life that is lost. This measure takes into account years of life lost and years lived with a disability. For example, if a 45-year-old man, expected to live to 78, has a fatal overdose from heroin, the years of healthy life lost (DALY) would be 33 years. In 1990, men lost 900,000 healthy years of life to drug abuse, and by 2017 this number reached 3.4 million years. If you or anyone you care about has opioid abuse issues, the Substance Abuse and Mental Health Services Administration (SAMHSA) provides a free and confidential service, available seven days a week. You can reach them at 1-800-662-HELP (4357).

Alcoholic Liver Disease

Mortality related to alcohol consumption is at levels that were last seen over a century ago. Chronic liver disease and cirrhosis account for 35,000 deaths every year in the United States, with many people dying from liver damage in their 50s and 60s. Over 2% of men in the U.S. have liver disease, with men 45 to 75 years old having the highest prevalence. The age-adjusted death rate due to chronic liver disease and cirrhosis in men has increased from 12.4 in 2005 to 14.5 per 100,000 in 2017. These rates are drastically higher for non-Hispanic white men 45 to 54 years old (see Figure 65.4).

SUICIDE

More than 123 people die by suicide every day in the United States. Men die due to suicide at 3.5 times the rate women do, and rates are highest among middle-aged white men. To put this another way, eight out of every ten lives lost due to suicide are men. Over half of those suicides involve a firearm. Notions of rugged individualism, that men should be tough or should just get over economic or emotional obstacles, lead to the underdiagnosis of mental health issues. Musician Kurt Cobain, professional wrestling star Chris Benoit, and, more recently, the world-renowned chef Anthony Bourdain are just some of many examples of very talented individuals who have lost their lives to suicide. Depression and suicide can affect anyone. Issues with legal and financial challenges, concerns about physical health, and intimacy in relationships all contribute to depression. Warning signs of

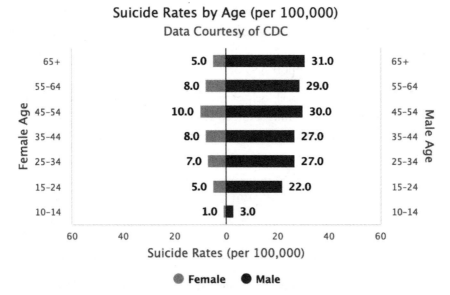

Figure 65.5. Suicide rates by age and gender, U.S.

potential for suicide include increased alcohol or drug use, loss of interest in physical appearance, withdrawal from work, or social and family-related activities, difficulty eating and sleeping, and drastic changes in behavior.

Suicide rates have been on the rise in the United States since 1999, increasing from 10.5 to 14 in 2017 per 100,000 people. Contributing factors include increased economic stagnation (particularly for those without higher education), increased alcohol and drug abuse, and other addictions. Social isolation due to decreased family, community, and social ties has also contributed to this rise. If you or anyone you know may be at risk for suicide, know that there is a free and confidential resource available seven days a week, 24 hours a day. Call the National Suicide Prevention Lifeline at 1-800-273-8255 to speak to professionals who can assist.

EXPLAINING DESPAIR IN THE 21ST CENTURY

People in the baby-boomer generation are currently entering retirement, and many of them are facing a daunting economic reality. Wage stagnation since the 1970s has left many adults unable to retire with economic security. Many older men have chronic medical conditions and inadequately controlled pain, which can result in poverty. Disengaged from communities and social networks, these men turn to alcohol, prescription pain medication, or opioids, which increase the risk of alcoholic liver disease, drug poisoning, and suicide. This is a societal tragedy and a public health disaster.

Overcoming these trends will require individuals, families, communities, and local, state, and federal governments to work together. Men who are financially vulnerable are at higher risk, and safety nets to assist those with these challenges are crucial. We must help one another by creating social support networks.

As individuals, it is important to seek help when needed. Over 80% of people who seek therapy for depression are successfully treated. The human and social costs to families, neighbors, and coworkers and to our country from these issues are too high to ignore.

For additional resources, please see www.TheTwentyFirstCenturyMan.com.

Chapter 66
Anxiety in Men
Bret McLaughlin, PsyD, MBA
Psychologist

Anxiety is a thin stream of fear trickling through the mind. If encouraged, it cuts a channel into which all other thoughts are drained.
— *Somers Roche*

DEFINING ANXIETY

Fear is a response to a threat, while anxiety is the anticipation of a future threat. As primates, we are hardwired to label and categorize the elements in our environment into broad categories of safety or danger. For many animals, this system works well because their levels of anxiety and stress are directly tied to immediate threats. But humans can imagine scenarios, and as a consequence, many live with high levels of stress and anxiety as they anticipate future threats to their person, family, or livelihood.

For example, imagine that you have been working on a report for your boss. It has taken weeks, and you are quite proud of the result. But after you hand it in, the boss calls you into her office. She is irate. It turns out that you misunderstood the report's scope and audience. You leave the office dejected and worried. Will you no longer be up for promotion? What will your colleagues think if you are taken off the project? Could you be fired? Each of these questions is the mind's attempt to anticipate how the report could be a future threat to your employment. While the possible ramifications could be serious, these thoughts are often catastrophic and do not take into consideration mitigating factors. You might have been with the company for decades, your previous work was stellar, and the boss may be known for not giving clear directives. However, when you leave the office, and possibly for days to come, your mind has categorized the result of the meeting as a future threat. Until the situation is resolved, you may remain in a physical and emotional state of anxiety.

THE STRESS RESPONSE

The ramifications of our ability to fabricate worst-case scenarios were studied by Stanford biologist and neuro-endocrinologist Robert Sapolsky and described in his book, *Why Zebras Don't Get Ulcers: The Acclaimed Guide to Stress, Stress-Related Diseases, and Coping.* He was particularly interested in the effects of high stress on the body, focusing on the steroid cortisol. Cortisol is a necessary hormone in the body that helps with blood pressure, metabolism, sleep, and blood sugar levels.

Cortisol is critical to the fight or flight response because it signals the release of glucose to power our muscles so we can defend ourselves or make a dash for safety. However, continuous, high levels of cortisol (a natural steroid) can have harmful effects on the body, including fatigue, muscle weakness, high blood pressure, decreased sex drive, and impaired memory.

Dr. Sapolsky confirmed that animals experience spikes in cortisol periodically throughout the day whenever they are confronted with danger. A zebra's cortisol level will spike when he hears a lion approaching. The zebra's autonomic (automatic) nervous system is activated, preparing him for the massive effort of outrunning a hungry lion. Cortisol goes up. If the lion gets too close, the zebra will take off running. One of two events will conclude this scenario: the zebra escapes or he dies.

If the zebra escapes, the act of running will rapidly circulate the cortisol throughout his body, dispersing it and returning the level to normal. Similarly, levels of adrenaline, which will spike along with the cortisol, will be cleared from his body in the same manner, returning the level of stress chemistry to normal.

Once the zebra escapes, his autonomic nervous system switches into the relaxation response (rest and digest). He returns to eating grass. During the relaxation response, if he has been injured during his hasty escape, his immune system will be activated, healing him as much as possible to optimize his survival.

To the best of our knowledge, zebras do not live in a constant state of worry or anxiety, anticipating the next lion attack. Humans, on the other hand, have been found to have consistently high levels of cortisol for extended periods of time as we anticipate the future threats that we may face in our lives. The result of this pressure is that many of us live in an almost constant state of stress. Additionally, because we work in sedentary jobs, and live a sedentary lifestyle, we are far less likely to work off stress physically. Like the zebra, many of us experience the spike in cortisol and adrenaline, but rather than going for a run after a confrontation with our boss, we may sit and stew at our desk, bathed in stress chemistry.

COPING WITH ANXIETY

Anxiety disorders are pervasive. In any given year, an estimated 19% of adults in the U.S. experience an anxiety disorder. Psychologists estimate that as many as 31.1% of adults in the U.S. will experience an anxiety disorder in their lifetimes. The severity of anxiety disorders vary with 43.5% of cases being mild, 33.7% being moderate, and 22.8% being severe. A survey of primary care physicians indicated that one-third of office visits were due to some form of anxiety.

Anxiety and stress-related disorders account for over 31% of the total costs of psychiatric disorders in the United States, making it the number one mental health problem for patients.

Over 10% of the population will experience either generalized anxiety disorder, panic, or phobias in their lifetime, a higher percentage than those who will experience drug or alcohol abuse.

Reducing Anxiety

Anxiety appears to be an almost constant companion to modern life, but some techniques can be used to both mitigate stressful situations and provide a buffer against future occurrences.

It has become fashionable to talk about mindfulness, meditation, and deep breathing. Many of my patients initially balk at being asked to focus on their breathing, an action that they have taken for granted most of their lives. But there is a reason that diaphragmatic breathing can reduce physical stress reactions. Imagine that you are a caveman wandering near your home when out of the bushes leaps a saber-toothed tiger. Your initial response is fear, since you are presented with a real and true threat to your existence. The autonomic nervous system kicks in, and your body prepares for fight or flight. In our fictitious example, let us assume that you have chosen to fight.

Your body is now working overtime to supply blood to your major muscle groups. Your arms and legs need fuel for the coming fight, so blood flow is reduced to your brain and your digestive system. This makes sense as you are not likely to pause for a snack or review your taxes while a saber-toothed cat is on your heels.

However, the problem occurs when the threat is not immediate, but instead the anxiety is a response to an *anticipated* threat. Have you ever prepared for an important presentation only to find minutes before that your stomach is tight or queasy, and your thoughts are not coming as quickly or clearly as the night before? You are understandably stressed, and your body has shifted blood away from your brain (stage fright) and your digestion (butterflies) in preparation for fight or flight. Unfortunately, sharp cognition is typically necessary to avoid a potential disaster during the presentation! This is a situation in which our physical reactions to stress and anxiety may have been good for our ancestors, but they have not caught up with current societal demands.

In the scenario at the cave, our ancestor, having decided to fight, must try to harm the saber-toothed tiger while protecting vital portions of his body. Where will the animal attack? While limbs or ribs protect most areas, the neck and abdomen are easy targets for a predator. So, the cavemen may instinctively raise his shoulders and bring his arms across his body. The next time you are in an interview, watch the applicants sitting across from you. Are their shoulders raised? Are their arms crossed over their stomach, or are they resting comfortably on the chair?

Have you ever wondered why you finish a particularly stressful day, and your shoulders ache? Perhaps it is because as we go about our standard workday, we are anticipating future threats, assuming a self-protective stance, with raised shoulders and stomachs in turmoil.

To begin counteracting the effects of anxiety and worry, we must tell our bodies that there is no real, immediate threat or danger. This exercise starts with deep breathing.

Strategies for relaxation. Follow the procedure below to bring a state of relaxation:

- Stand up straight and try to relax your shoulders.

- Have someone else come behind you and place both of their hands on your hips so that their thumbs are meeting at the center of the small of your back.

- Now take a deep breath. If you are breathing to reduce stress, the thumbs of your partner will separate. With diaphragmatic breathing, your stomach should extend, and your back expand.

When starting this exercise, most people find that instead of their breath filling out their torso, their shoulders come up and they breathe from the top part of their chest.

- If the thumbs of your exercise partner aren't separating, have them place their hands on your shoulders. Allow them to push down and feel the urge and tension build as you try to stop your shoulders from rising.

- If you are fully engaged in deep breathing, your shoulders won't move.

If you do not have anyone willing to help you with this activity, lie on the floor with your shoulder blades flat against the floor, which prevents them from moving up to your neck. Look down your body. If you are doing this right, your stomach should visibly move up and down.

The relaxation response. While deep breathing comes with some practice, the beneficial effects are immediate. In 1974, cardiologist Herbert Benson and colleagues released a paper called "The Relaxation Response". He found that meditation and deep breathing activated the parasympathetic nervous system and resulted in relaxed skeletal muscles, decreased blood pressure, and decreased respiratory rate. If we go back to our saber-toothed cat example, this makes sense. Instead of protecting the stomach, you are sticking it out as you perform relaxed abdominal breathing. Instead of raising shoulders in defense, you are keeping your neck exposed. These actions tell your body that there is no threat and your defenses can relax.

Progressive muscle relaxation. Another method often used to reduce stress and relieve anxiety is a technique pioneered by psychiatrist Edmond Jacobson called progressive muscle relaxation. In 1929, Dr. Jacobson was studying the connection between anxiety and tension in major muscle groups of the body. He determined that if muscles were willfully tightened beyond normal tension levels, upon release the patient felt great relaxation.

Shorthand muscle relaxation. While the initial protocol included over 20 distinct steps to engage in progressive muscle relaxation, psychologist Matthew McKay found that the process could be reduced to four steps, focusing on major muscle areas in a process which he termed shorthand muscle relaxation. This abbreviated protocol can be employed quickly and throughout the day as feelings of anxiety and stress emerge:

1. Bunch your hands into tight fists while keeping the rest of the arms loose. Hold the tension, then relax.

2. To relax your head and neck: Press your head back. Then roll it in two complete circles both clockwise and counterclockwise. While rolling your head, wrinkle your face as if all its muscles were trying to converge at your nose. Dr. McKay has asked patients to visualize that their face mirrors the surface of a walnut. Next, tighten your jaw and neck muscles while pulling your shoulders up. Then relax.

3. Arch your back while taking a diaphragmatic breath. Hold this position, then relax. Now push out your abdomen as you inhale, then relax.

4. Tighten shin and calf muscles while pointing toes upward. Relax. Now tighten buttock, calf, and thigh muscles while curling your toes before relaxing.

Limiting self-medication. Quite possibly the most critical step you can take in anxiety prevention is the limiting of self-medication, which means avoiding drinking, smoking, and using drugs (illicit or otherwise). Even legal substances can cause significant problems for those that are either anxious or depressed.

More than 12% of men have alcohol problems. Alcohol is a depressant that lowers inhibitions, two effects that at first glance would seem to help those with anxiety. But alcohol does nothing to address the underlining causes of anxiety and comes with the potential for abuse and addiction.

Stimulants (unless they cause an atypical reaction as in those with ADHD) will elicit further feelings of excitability and anxiety. While some who use nicotine claim it calms their nerves, it in fact does the opposite. The reason that people feel initially calm after having a cigarette is that the body is reacting with relief at receiving the addictive substance. This is in part why alcohol and cigarettes have traditionally been paired together: one acts as a stimulant while the other a depressant.

Also, be aware that there are illegal drugs that fall into the stimulant class, including cocaine and methamphetamine. While these drugs can provide temporary relief of symptoms, they are a means of avoidance. Instead of examining the causes of the anxiety, the symptoms are masked and, in many instances, made worse by the use and abuse of these substances.

WHEN TO SEEK PROFESSIONAL HELP

Some of my patients have asked when they should seek professional help. My answer is always the same: when the anxiety is impacting your activities of daily living, and your previous coping strategies are no longer effective. Keep in mind that there are many versions of anxiety. In some cases, anxiety may manifest as a phobia, obsessive-compulsive tendencies, difficulty socializing and interacting with others, neurosis, or a general and pervasive sense of worry. Each of these conditions can be handled differently, and your mental health provider will be able to determine the severity of the situation. From a patient's perspective, the level of symptomatology is not as important as the effect it is having on one's life.

> *Remember that short, mild bursts of anxiety can have a beneficial effect, heightening performance, increasing concentration, and narrowing focus. The question is whether anxiety is having a beneficial, neutral, or adverse effect on your life.*

You may be an extreme arachnophobe, but if your work and personal circumstances cause limited interaction with spiders, your life may not be greatly impacted by the condition. On the other hand, your job may necessitate frequent public appearances, and the mild anxiety you feel in front of people is impacting your performance. If anxiety is affecting your needed life activities, then it may be time to seek further help.

TREATMENT

Medications

When basic methods of stress and anxiety reduction do not have the desired effect, it is time to turn to a professional. You may initially go to your primary care provider who will rule out specific physical ailments. They may also prescribe medication.

Antidepressants. These may be selective serotonin reuptake inhibitors (SSRIs), serotonin and norepinephrine reuptake inhibitors (SNRIs), tricyclics, or monoamine oxidase inhibitors

(MAOIs). These medications typically take between four and six weeks to reach therapeutic effect, so plan on taking the prescribed regimen for at least two months. If the physical effects of anxiety are the primary cause of the discomfort, your doctor may prescribe a beta-blocker.

Antianxiety drugs. Anxiolytics often provide a fast, quick-acting solution when the patient is having an immediate, short-term bout of anxiety. Buspirone is a commonly prescribed drug in this grouping for older adults. Benzodiazepines are another class of medications that are very effective but should be used with caution. I knew a psychiatrist who used to say, "I can make anyone into a drug addict. I'll just prescribe a benzo." The reason these medications are typically prescribed as a short-term or as-needed solution is that a person feels immediate relief that lasts for several hours. For those who have panic attacks, this may be exactly what is needed: short-term relief until the episode passes. The same can be said for those with social or performance anxiety. I had a patient who was employed by a symphony, and while he was excellent in rehearsals, when he got in front of a live audience, his anxiety became so great that his performance suffered. He would take a benzodiazepine before a concert, and that medication would get him through the show. But the very reasons that these medications are so effective are the reasons that can lead to addiction. The drugs can provide almost instant relief but wear off quickly, and if the person is still experiencing high levels of anxiety, they will need to take another dose. The other reason that this class of drugs must be used in close consultation with a medical professional is that benzodiazepines have been shown to cause some memory impairment and falls in older adults.

Seeing a Mental Health Professional

In conjunction with or as an alternative to medication, you may be referred to a mental health professional. While medications have been shown to be more effective in the short term for relief of anxiety symptoms, therapy has been shown to be as effective in the long run. For those experiencing short-term bouts of anxiety, medication may be a more cost-effective and rapid solution. However, these psychiatric medications do not *cure* anxiety. This is not like taking an antibiotic for an infection. Instead, these medications are alleviating the symptoms without addressing the cause. For some patients, that is enough. For those that want a long-term solution to their anxiety problems, therapy is an effective choice.

When deciding on a therapist, it is important to consider the training and background of the individual who you will be seeing. The following is a list of licensed mental health professions who can assist with anxiety and stress-related issues:

Psychiatrist. Psychiatrists attend four years of medical school where they receive a generalist education and, if they are in the United States, earn their doctor of medicine or doctor of osteopathic medicine degree. They then attend a four-year residency program specifically focused on the specialty of mental health and psychiatry. These professionals are physicians and, as such, can prescribe medications. Their focus is often biological, and they work closely with the primary care physician, particularly if the case involves complex medical issues. Most have some knowledge of psychotherapy, though this is typically not their primary means of alleviating symptoms.

Psychologist. Psychologists typically attend five years of graduate school where the focus is on the therapeutic treatment of mental health disorders and earn a doctorate in philosophy or psychology. During these years, they treat patients in practicums and undertake an internship. They will also have at least a year of post-doctoral training. Psychologists specialize in human behavior and are taught a variety of therapeutic approaches. They are also trained in assessment and may give the patient testing before determining the best course of therapy. There is a particular class of psychologists who can prescribe medications in individual states. These professionals are called Prescribing or Medical Psychologists who have taken an additional two years to earn a degree in psychopharmacology and prescribe under the supervision of a physician.

Social worker. Social workers attend a two-year graduate program in which they learn to treat and diagnose mental health disorders with a particular focus on social policy. After they earn their master's degree in social work, they spend an additional two years accruing direct clinical experience. There are also doctorate-level social workers.

Marriage and family therapist. Marriage and family therapists (MFTs) diagnose and treat a variety of mental health disorders with a particular focus on couples and family systems. After two years of graduate school, they earn a master's degree in marriage and family therapy and then have an additional two years of clinical training before receiving licensure. There are also doctorate-level marriage and family therapists.

Professional clinical counselor. Professional clinical counselors (PCCs) are also trained to diagnose and treat mental illness, but while the MFTs focuses on the patient's role within their families or relationships, the PCC focuses more heavily on the individual. After spending two years in graduate school, they earn their master's in clinical counseling and spend an additional two years in clinical training before licensure.

Regardless of the mental health professional you choose, you should look up their license. If you are planning to use a psychiatrist, verify their credentials through the state medical board. If you are going to use a psychologist, look up their license with the state board of psychology. If you are going to use a social worker, marriage and family therapist, or a professional clinical counselor, their licenses can be housed in separate state boards or together at one agency such as California's Board of Behavioral Sciences. By verifying a license, you can often see where the clinician went to school, when they were licensed, if their license is valid, and if they have had any legal actions against their license. When dealing with serious mental health issues, think very carefully before choosing to go to an unlicensed individual or a professional with citations against their license.

Resources. While various therapies can be used to treat anxiety, some helpful resources include:

- Division 12 of the American Psychological Association: The Society of Clinical Psychology. There you can find a list of empirically valid (also called research supported) treatments sorted by diagnosis. For example, under Generalized Anxiety Disorder, CBT or cognitive behavioral therapy is listed as having strong empirical support (For more detail regarding CBT, see the following chapter on Depression). https://www.div12.org/psychological-treatments/

- There is also a list of evidence-based psychological treatments at the National Institute for Health and Care Excellence (NICE) based in the United Kingdom. https://www.nice.org.uk/

- There are additional treatments found at the Evidence-Based Practices Resource Center, part of the U.S. Department of Health and Human Services, Substance Abuse and Mental Health Services Administration. https://www.samhsa.gov/ebp-resource-center

Though not necessary, these websites provide information that you can use when initially interviewing a prospective therapist. Regardless of the professional you choose or the theoretical orientation of the clinician, the most critical factor in determining success or failure in treatment outcomes is the relationship between the clinician and the patient. Because there is still a stigma around seeking mental health treatment, friends and neighbors might not be open about their therapeutic experiences. Without a referral, it can be difficult to cold call a professional. Make sure that you ask your primary care physician about therapists they have referred in the past and ask about the responses from patients.

The way you can find a therapist is the same method you would use to find a good mechanic. You ask people who you trust, including your physician, family, or friends. The difference between finding a therapist and a mechanic is that almost everyone has had a car in the shop, and the only shame that might be felt is inferiority if you are talking to an amateur grease monkey. Mental health issues still have a high degree of stigma, especially for men. If you ask a buddy whether or not they have seen a therapist, you have opened yourself up to questions and possibly ridicule.

The good news is that in the U.S. views on therapy are slowly changing. Current statistics show that 42% of the population have seen a counselor at some point in their lives. During the past year, 13% were seeing a therapist, and 36% said that they would be open to going to therapy. Unfortunately, 23% said that they would never go to a counselor, and only 8% of baby boomers and 1% of older generations worked with a therapist in the past year.

Of those that have seen a therapist, 39% found one through their primary care provider, 19% though a family or friend, and 12% through the internet. The two most important elements used by patients in determining which professional to see were affordability and expertise. People in the U.S. who attend therapy find the experience positive: 47% found that therapy was very positive, and 29% that it was somewhat positive. Only 6% found the experience to be negative.

If you go to a clinician and they don't seem like a good fit, try another. Don't be afraid to fire the therapist; just make sure it is because of the relationship and not because you have entered a particularly difficult phase of therapy. The relationship is paramount, and if something is not working between you, let the clinician know.

KEY TAKE AWAYS

The bottom line is that anxiety is a common disorder in the United States, affecting over 31% of the population. Stress is almost a daily occurrence in our lives and is the direct result of actual or perceived threats. Preventative measures include deep breathing exercises and progressive muscle relaxation. If anxiety is affecting your activities of daily living, it may be time to consult a professional. The two most common forms of treatment are antianxiety medication and therapy. One heavily studied form of therapy used to treat anxiety disorders is cognitive-behavioral therapy. This treatment is effective and will provide concrete tools and techniques to reduce, help eliminate, and manage future bouts of anxiety.

For more information about the work of Bret McLaughlin at California Northstate University, please visit: cnsu.edu.

Chapter 67
Depression in Men
Bret McLaughlin, PsyD, MBA
Psychologist

Depression is not a sign of weakness —
it is a sign that you were trying to be strong too long.
— Sigmund Freud.

DEFINING DEPRESSION

Depression is a prolonged feeling of sadness, emptiness, or hopelessness. Symptoms include:

- A diminished interest in activities
- A gain or loss of body weight (5% over a month)
- Changes in sleeping patterns
- Fatigue
- Feelings of worthlessness and guilt
- Difficulty concentrating
- Possible thoughts of suicide.

While statistics vary, some reports indicate that depression is twice as likely in older adults as their younger counterparts. Much like anxiety, it occurs with greater frequency in women. While the annual prevalence rate of depression in the general population is 5% to 7%, it jumps to 8%—to as high as 16%—in older adults.

The likelihood that someone will have major depression in their lifetime is estimated at 13% to 18%. People with depressive symptoms lose one day or more per month of productivity, and depression remains the fourth leading cause of disability worldwide. The cost to the United States was estimated at $210 billion in 2010.

Temporary, Situational Depression or Major Clinical Depression?

Depression ranges in seriousness from mild, temporary episodes of sadness to severe, persistent depression.

Clinical depression is the more severe form of depression, also known as major depression or major depressive disorder. It isn't the same as depression caused by a loss, such as the death of a loved one, or a medical condition, such as a thyroid disorder.

Situational depression (also referred to as reactive depression) is a short-term form of depression that occurs as the result of a traumatic event, change, or loss in a person's life. Examples of triggers include divorce or the death of a loved one, loss of a job, major life changes such as retirement, or the stress caused by a serious accident or illness.

Subclinical depression that occurs below our level of consciousness (and therefore often goes undiagnosed) is also a significant risk factor for developing depression later in life.

Older adults have almost a 14% increased risk of experiencing mild to moderate depression or having a major depressive episode. These increases in depression later in life may occur because those who experience the traumatic loss of a spouse or a serious physical illness have the highest rates of depression.

Even those who do not have symptoms at the severity of a major depressive disorder are at higher risk for physical ailments. Patients with depressive symptoms are at two to four times higher risk for a new cardiovascular disease and are at two to four times higher risk of dying after a cardiovascular event. A sobering fact is that of those with cardiovascular disease, 17% to 27% also have depression.

> *Over 44% of older people with depression are also medically ill, and it is estimated that nearly half of the adults admitted for psychiatric care are depressed. Depression in older adults is associated with an increased risk for dementia, physical disease, and a reduced quality of life.*

Situational Aspects of Depression

To better understand the causes of depression, let us return to the caveman discussed in the previous chapter. A large saber-toothed cat has jumped out of the bushes, and our caveman is now facing an immediate threat to his life. He must decide if he is going to fight or run. But what happens if he knows that he cannot beat the beast in a fight? What if he is also sure that it will run him down should he decide to flee? There is a third option, and that is to *conserve energy*. While humans do not have the instinct to fall down and play dead, we do have another set of emotions that immobilize us—depression.

Let us imagine that the caveman has just enough strength to dash into a narrow cave. The saber-toothed tiger gives chase but is not quite small enough to follow. Safe, and given a moment of reprieve, the caveman is able to rest and restore his strength. After some time, he is ready to leave his sanctuary. But as soon as he starts to place one foot in the direction of the cave entrance, a thought comes nagging at the back of his mind, "What if the saber-toothed cat is still out there? If you leave now, he might be waiting to kill you!" The caveman decides it is safer to wait and curls up in the back of his shelter for some needed sleep. The next day he wakes up determined to leave the cave. He starts to get ready when the voice returns, "You can't leave. You don't have a weapon. You couldn't fight the saber-toothed tiger before, what makes you think you can fight him now? Best to conserve your energy and wait for the perfect moment to attack." The caveman sees the sense in this argument and curls up on the dirt floor of the cave. Similar thoughts continue to haunt him throughout the day, and by nightfall he is disheveled and hungry but safe in his cave.

This scenario can happen to any of us. As with anxiety, the threat does not have to be immediate, or even real, but if we perceive or imagine a future danger to ourselves or those we love, our minds can respond with the desire to conserve energy. This can happen if we get fired from a job or break up with someone. Each one of these events can feel like a major blow to the flow of our lives and the future that we have planned for ourselves. Often they are reminders of our own mortality or the time we have left to accomplish our goals. The mind is doing its best to protect us from a threat, but depression can disconnect us from sources of pleasure and the people who care about our wellbeing. It tells us that as long as we roll over in our sheets, we won't need to confront the threat. This creates a feedback loop in which a single event can keep a person depressed for weeks or even months. It can also prevent dealing with the depression. The caveman needs to get up and poke his head out of the shelter. He may be surprised to find that the threat is no longer there, that the saber-toothed cat has long since moved on.

COPING STRATEGIES

Because depression is an attempt to conserve energy, the most effective strategy to counter feelings of hopelessness, guilt, or sadness is active engagement. This is not easy to accomplish, particularly if your mind is fighting to keep you in bed and safe. One of the means to help people overcome depression is to rely on the assistance of friends and relatives. They can provide the incentive that you lack and help you reengage with the world. Yet how many times have you confronted a moping colleague with cheerful words or a compliment, only to receive a halfhearted smile in return and the feeling that your words have increased their sadness?

By examining core beliefs (*schemas*), we may gain insight into how we can mitigate depression in ourselves. Schemas are a set of core beliefs that are formed to help us survive in

Psychosocial Factors in Depression

The following illustrative example many be difficult for some readers, but it is a concise way to illustrate this point.

Jack is a young boy living in an intact family. His father drinks heavily and has been known to abuse Jack and his mother. Jack is confused by these experiences and uses his five-year-old mind to rationalize his father's behavior. Why would his dad hurt him? From television shows, movies, family gatherings, and the times in which his father is sober, Jack has been taught that parents are good. If parents are good, there must be a reason that he is hit by his father. Jack comes to the conclusion that he must be bad. Over time, these thoughts solidify into the belief that he himself must be flawed or unworthy. While this core schema might at first seem irrational, it is protective. Because Jack has placed the blame for the abuse on himself, he is able to protect his internal conception of his father as good. This allows Jack to interact with his father in a positive manner, ensuring the young child of continued food, shelter, and a possible reduction of violence.

These core beliefs, that he is flawed or unworthy, continue to stay with Jack into adulthood. What started as a protective mechanism for a child does not serve Jack as an adult. At work, colleagues often compliment him on his excellent writing and easy way with customers. But Jack is unable to hear positive reports about his behavior and instead immediately thinks, "They must be lying," or "I sure fooled them." These thoughts allow Jack to hold onto his core beliefs, often at the cost of relationships, promotions, or a general sense of accomplishment and wellbeing. These thoughts can also be presumptive, allowing Jack to make quick, categorical decisions about what he should do or how he should respond. If a new friend asks him out on a date, his core beliefs jump into play, telling him that he will just disappoint her, that he may be able to convince her that he is a good guy for a little while, but she will eventually discover the truth, and that he should save her pain and turn down the date.

Jack's core beliefs act like a filter or, as McKay describes, like a puzzle piece. Only stimuli that confirm his thoughts about himself match his puzzle piece and are allowed to connect. Those stimuli that do not match his internal picture do not latch on and are disallowed. In the above example, when Jack's colleagues compliment him on his work, those words of praise do not fit his "I am flawed" or "I am unworthy" schema. They do not fit his puzzle piece and are rejected. However, if his boss were to tell him that he has shown up late to work three times this past month and a record will be placed in his personnel file, that would confirm his beliefs about himself and the reprimand would connect perfectly to his schema. The negative review would be considered true, while compliments would be discarded as false. In this way, unexamined core beliefs become self-perpetuating.

uncertain environments and cope with various situations. They help us to place experiences in appropriate categories and allow for rapid interpretations of facts and events. They form a personal monologue that not only interprets external stimuli, but often evaluates our own actions and performance.

Examining Core Beliefs

The examination of core beliefs is important in being able to fend off depression and to assist in your ability to receive help and encouragement when it is offered. The first step in identifying and confronting your schemas is to follow the procedures outlined in the book, *Prisoners of Belief* by Matthew McKay and Patrick Fanningo. For a week, take note of any time you have a powerful emotional reaction such as anxiety, depression, guilt, anger, or embarrassment. Then fill in a quick chart with the following headings:

- Feeling
- Situation
- Monologue.

Using our previous example of Jack receiving a compliment, his feeling might be shame, the situation an interaction with colleagues, and the thought might be, "They don't know. My report was horrible." As you fill in the chart you will see themes emerge around roughly a number of central tenets:

- Your worth
- How safe you feel
- How competent you believe yourself to be
- How in control of your life you are

- The level of nurturance you feel

- Your level of independence

- Whether you believe your life is fair

- How connected you are with others, whether you trust people

- How compassionate you are toward yourself and others.

Once you have your chart and have examined your internal monologue, it is time to test some of your core schemas. Although you may have a few, choose one of the categories described above and match it to a monologue statement. Now imagine a scenario in which you can test your assumptions. Try to conceive of a low-risk situation where you can make a definitive prediction about the outcome.

It should be understood that the challenging of core beliefs is an incremental and purposeful activity that can produce temporary anxiety or deep feelings of pain. The mind will attempt to hold onto strategies that worked at one time but are no longer useful. Despite the difficulty, the outcomes can free a person from years of sadness, shame, and self-doubt.

Jack chooses his belief that he is incompetent. His girlfriend has explained to him that her son wants to join a local little league team but doesn't have the basic skills. She has asked Jack to take her son out and show him how to catch and hit a ball. Jack used to be pretty good at baseball but has been avoiding her request because he believes he will screw up this opportunity by being a lousy teacher. He will only disappoint the young boy. He is also afraid that the boy will reject him. While working with a boy who he cares about might stir up old feelings for Jack, taking someone to the baseball diamond presents little real risk and very little threat to his relationship with his girlfriend. He makes a specific behavioral prediction: his girlfriend's son will refuse to go with him. If he does agree to go, they will leave the field within a half an hour because the boy will realize how incompetent Jack is at throwing a baseball. These predictions are concrete and behavioral and allow for easy confirmation or disproval of his core beliefs. This is one of a variety of techniques that can be used to directly confront negative schemas and start to develop new belief systems. As we can imagine, the boy was happy to have someone show him how to catch, throw, and hit. Both stayed at the park for the afternoon, and Jack had to confront his predictions with reality.

Over time this process could dramatically change the way Jack sees himself in the world if he becomes attuned to these beliefs and compares them with his experience. He may learn to understand that he is not fundamentally flawed and that he is worthy of the attention of his peers and girlfriend.

TREATMENT

Episodes of reactive, temporary depression will typically abate on their own after an interval of between eight and twelve months, as long as new threats do not emerge. However, no one wishes to live through months of depression. If you are experiencing situational depression and your own efforts and those of your family and friends have not provided relief, it may be time to seek professional assistance.

Due to issues of stigma and shame, only about 50% of individuals with major depressive disorder receive treatment and only about one in five receive treatment commensurate with accepted guidelines. Patients come to their primary care physician seeking help, but 69% do not initially report that they are experiencing depression. They instead tell their doctor about multiple physical symptoms and when directly questioned about their feelings, studies show that at least 11% deny depression.

Once depression has been diagnosed, the most researched interventions used by mental health professionals are medication and cognitive behavioral therapy. Both have advantages, but their effectiveness correlates with the severity of symptoms.

Antidepressant medication. Fournier examined the effects of a placebo against the benefits of antidepressants for patients experiencing depression. If patients had mild to moderate depression, they received minimal benefit from medication, while those who had very severe depression gained substantial benefit. Patients with severe depression also gain greater benefit from antidepressants combined with psychotherapy over therapy alone. However, when depression was at a mild to moderate level, therapy and medication have comparable treatment results, not only with each other, but also with those who have received combined treatments. So, *with severe depression, the additive strategy is helpful, but with mild to moderate depression, all three types of treatment have the same rates of effectiveness.*

Cognitive behavioral therapy. While cognitive behavioral therapy (CBT) and antidepressants are comparable in effective rates, therapy has a substantial advantage over pharmaceuticals in that patients retain the benefits they gained while in therapy, whereas relapse is common for those who stop medication. It may require two years on an antidepressant before there is a substantial reduction in patients who relapse, while short-term CBT interventions have stronger maintenance of treatment gains for both anxiety and depression. Patients who receive CBT are over two and a half times less likely to relapse than those who discontinue their medication. CBT for anxiety and depression also offers a significantly better cost benefit ratio than pharmacotherapy. Patients who receive CBT treatment have been found to experience almost double the response relative to the usual care they receive when not referred to a mental health professional.

Suicide. There are a few other topics that should be covered in a discussion about depression: suicide and substance abuse. Suicide is not a diagnosis but a very serious behavior. Depression is a risk factor, along with being of middle age, male, not having strong family connections (or being divorced), and being Caucasian. Women attempt suicide with greater frequency, but men are more often successful. Older adults make fewer attempts but die at higher rates than younger adults. Most people who are contemplating suicide

Managing Automatic Thoughts and Reactions

There are many versions of cognitive behavioral therapy, but most rely upon a similar construct. Throughout our lives *there are events that happen to us, we have a thought about those events, and then we experience a feeling.* The order here is very important. In CBT there are no emotions without thoughts and thoughts always occur before emotions. Since we have little control over many events in our lives, and we have no real control over emotions themselves, CBT focuses on the one area in which we have control—our thoughts.

Let us imagine that you are late for work. You have a presentation to give to the department, but you feel you are unprepared. You go into the garage, get in the car, and turn the key. Nothing. You turn it again and receive the same result. You look over the dashboard and see that the lights had been left on. How do you feel?

The event is the car not starting. If your thought is "That daughter! I told her to check before getting out of the car!" you might feel angry. If your thought is "Great. Now I have an excuse to take half a day off work and refine my presentation," you might feel relief. If you think, "This is just the excuse they have been looking for to put me under review," you might feel anxiety. If you think, "This might buy me another half an hour with my wife before AAA arrives," you might feel the stirrings of passion. The car not turning on can produce a different emotion depending on the thought that races through your mind.

This is also true on a physiological level. Have you ever wondered why the Tunnel of Love was full of props designed to frighten people, why horror movies are a common date night outing for teenagers, or why your partner might want to cuddle up after a thrilling rollercoaster ride? The reason is that different extreme states of emotion are treated the same way by our bodies—triggering the stress response. Pupils dilate, pulse quickens, perspiration starts, and the heart thumps in our chest. Is this a description of someone watching the latest zombie flick or preparing to make love? What tells us if we should be feeling passion or fear? The decision is not based on the feelings themselves (both emotional and physical), but on our examination of the environment and the accompanying thoughts. As your date is going through the tunnel of love, they know they should not be scared by the cardboard devils or red lights. But their pulse has quickened and there is a fluttering in their stomach. They look toward you and think, "Maybe I am falling in love."

The immediate thoughts following an event are often so fast that most people do not realize they have occurred. You get into your car, turn the key, car doesn't start, and you get angry. Wouldn't everyone be angry in that situation? The surprising answer is no. During CBT the therapist helps the patient to develop space between the event and the feeling so that they can examine the accompanying thought. Often called automatic thoughts, they are usually brief, short phrases that tell the mind how you should feel about a given situation. By identifying and ultimately uncovering the schemas behind these rapid ideas, the patient begins to recognize and ultimately control them. Thoughts are no longer automatic but conscious decisions by the patient that they can use to shape their feelings. For those who are depressed, the CBT therapist will take a two-pronged approach to treatment. They will confront the physical effects of depression by having the patient reengage with life. They will encourage pleasurable activities and stress the need to leave the house and interact with others. (They will help the patient leave the cave.) The other approach will involve confronting the patient's automatic thoughts to determine the schemas that have led to self-reproach, guilt, or depression.

will let others know, either through their behaviors or conversation. The riskiest time for those contemplating suicide is not when they are severely depressed. As we have discussed, depression is about conserving energy and the taking of one's life requires effort. The highest risk presents itself when a person is slipping into deeper depression or when they are just coming out of depression. This is when the feelings of hopelessness are still present, but the patient is starting to gain energy. In many cases of completed suicide, friends and family have been left devastated and confused, "But he was doing so much better. He was getting out of the house. I really thought we had turned the corner."

Warning signs for suicide include mood disorders (including depression), hopelessness, lack of social connections, physical illness, and/or feeling like a burden. Fortunately, there are many resources for those who are considering suicide or those who are worried about a loved one.

Substance abuse. Even legal substances can cause significant problems for those who are either anxious or depressed. While the rates of alcohol abuse diminish as people pass 65 years of age (1.5%), 8.5% of adults in the United States qualify for an alcohol abuse disorder (almost 25 million individuals). The rates are greater in men, at 12.4%. Estimates place caffeine addiction at 7% of the U.S. population, and tobacco is used by between 13% and 20% of adults with use declining in those over 65 to 4%. Those who are depressed should stay away from alcohol as it is a depressant. It might make you temporarily feel better, but in the long run it will make your symptoms worse. While some who use nicotine claim it calms their nerves, it is in fact a stimulant and does the opposite. The reason that people feel initially calm after using a cigarette is that the body is reacting with relief at receiving the addictive substance. This is in part why alcohol and cigarettes have traditionally been paired together: one acts as a stimulant while the other is a depressant.

Temporary, situational depression is a serious, but manageable condition that is our mind's way of telling us that we need additional resources to handle some event in our life. While depression will naturally abate over time, no one should have to live in misery. For those who are experiencing major depressive symptoms, medications can help alleviate negative emotions, allowing them to reengage with life. For those experiencing mild to moderate depression, the research indicates benefit in working with a mental health professional trained and knowledgeable in treating depression. Supportive therapy can provide you with the skills and strategies needed to reduce current symptoms and modify your thought patterns, increasing your ability to cope when confronting threats in the future.

The National Suicide Prevention Lifeline is open seven days a week, twenty-four hours a day and can be reached at
1.800.273.8255.
They have counselors available trained to address crises and can also help connect the caller with resources in their community.
For more information about the work of Bret McLaughlin at California Northstate University, please visit
cnsu.edu.

Chapter 68
Living with Vitality
Robert Buonfiglio, PhD, Psychologist
& Executive Life Coach

Vitality shows in not only the ability to persist, but the ability to start over.
— *F. Scott Fitzgerald*

As a psychologist and coach, I am passionate about helping men find deeper meaning in life, working diligently with them to help them effect change and live the life they genuinely want to live. This effort also deepens the sense of purpose in my own life and informs the path I have personally strived to embark on.

Mental health is not just about reducing symptoms—good mental health goes beyond that and is about choices that we make (or don't make) each day to function at our optimal capacity. Life can be stressful, and without reflection and self-care, we may experience difficulties that have an impact on our attitudes, moods, behaviors, and state of mind. As we age, we may lose focus periodically or become stagnant at times, bogged down with responsibilities, routines, and norms. Ultimately, we can lose sight of ourselves.

Just as some physicians focus on wellness and performance enhancement, my professional focus is on living with vitality, rather than focusing on problems or pathology. I want to inspire you to live with passion and purpose, to be fully engaged and not living robotically, to live fully in the present moment.

Deferred living . . . *Bob ("The Electrician") was a good man, hardworking and diligent, a loyal provider. He defined himself by his work.*

Yet as he trudged through life, it was clear that he wasn't happy. He neglected himself and used alcohol as a coping mechanism. He enjoyed his job but became a workaholic, throwing himself into work as another way to cope (unconsciously or consciously). Numbed, distant, too busy for his family, he existed in a kind of waking sleep, wishing for retirement when he could finally begin living his life.

At the age of 48, he stopped drinking. He began to develop insight and could be heard saying things like, "You have to have gratitude in your attitude," and "You can curse the darkness or light a candle." He began to change. He started to live life in a new way, and his relationship with his son deepened and grew stronger.

But he still deferred his dreams, planning to someday buy a boat and a summer house, to start really living once he reached 65. Tragically, about the time Bob turned 52, he was diagnosed with Parkinson's disease. This was definitely not in The Plan.

That distant, preoccupied man was my father. I am that son. *My dad's illness had a profound impact on me. His life choices made me start to consider my life and take inventory. In my twenties at the time, I realized that I was not taking full responsibility for myself and my decisions. I had allowed the external world to drive what I did and how I did it. Quite often I conformed to the norms of the society around me, and I lacked attention to my own inner awareness.*

At the age of 26, I started to change, and continue today to strive to align my life with who I am (strive is the keyword here). I was able to make changes by shifting my attention to my inner awareness. When I began not just to hear but to listen actively to my own thoughts, feelings, emotions, and values, a more congruent life path began to emerge for me. My newfound awareness enabled me to take responsibility for my life by honing in on who I am, what I want, and how I truly want to live. I became more conscious of what I felt. I began to realize that, with effort, I could live more aligned with my values, be myself, and do many of the things that I desired.

My dad's illness caused me to reflect on my life and sparked an awakening and a call to action. Over the next three years, I completed a master's program and started on a PhD to become a clinical psychologist. I also traveled extensively throughout Europe, Asia, Australia, and North America. I felt like I was finally living. In response to my dad's challenging circumstances, I have attempted to live my own life with greater vitality.

LIVING WITH VITALITY

Abraham Maslow suggested that a self-actualized person has childlike qualities. I take this to mean that a self-actualized person living with vitality embodies curiosity and wonder. Can you recall a time in your life (perhaps in your youth) when you were living this way? How did you feel? Think of a time when there was a quality of magic to your experience. What was the source of that magic—your own inner state, some effort you were making, or unique opportunities in your life? Let's work to bring this way of being back to the forefront! Take on the challenge to live with vitality! The goal is to listen to your inner voice, and make choices that are congruent with how you really want to live your life.

Taking inventory provides the opportunity to take a closer look at your life and assess how things are going. What is going well, and what could be upgraded? What would you like more of, and what would you like less of? Are you happy? Are you living your best life? Begin with reflection:

- ***Does it feel possible to live with vitality? If not, what is standing in the way?*** Be mindful of how external influences are playing a role in your life. Take inventory of your wants, needs, and desires, and work to overcome obstacles that are impinging on your life.

- ***Are you living robotically or as a human being?*** Assess your current situation and decide whether you're living the life you want to live for yourself or if you're merely going through the motions. Can you recall a time when you were living passionately? What did that feel like? Consider journaling to define that situation and the aspects of your life that made it possible.

- ***Are you making choices that are aligned with your values?*** We have choice in relation to the constructs and limitations in our life. Are you making the space to explore choices that have you feeling energized?

- ***Are you living a balanced life?*** What are you doing too much of and what are you doing too little of? Are you too cognitive or too feeling-oriented? Do you work too much or play too much? Assess your extremes and take steps to live more in balance.

- ***Are you mindful of your destiny and limitations?*** Acknowledge your destiny—your given traits, abilities, life circumstance, and history—and use that information to consciously exercise your freedom of choice.

- ***Are you living what has heart and meaning?*** What matters to you? Who matters to you? What are you passionate about? Are you willing to take steps to live aligned with the answers to these questions?

This is a tough task, requiring motivation and courage, but it has the potential to culminate in your discovery or rediscovery of living with vitality. I know from personal experience that it's a worthwhile proposition. Join me in the journey to live with passion; you can create positive and significant change that will make a profound difference on your life and the lives of those around you!

I was living with vitality, until I wasn't. *My attempts to live more fully worked well for a while, but once I immersed myself in my career, I started living robotically again. At some point along the way, I had reverted to living like my dad, falling into a workaholic pattern as my newfound awareness slipped away.*

I was breaking down. The thirst for truly living had taken a back seat. I finished my degree and my internships, trained with top people in the field, developed a successful private practice, took on leadership roles, and worked for a startup. I trained hard in the gym and would do 200 pushups on my off day. I was working 60-plus hours a week. When people asked me, how do you work all these hours and train like that in the gym? I would respond proudly, "because I can." I was proud of reaching my potential.

But maybe a better reframe is, I had reached the point where I took pride in running myself into the ground. I had diverticulitis, was diagnosed with degenerative discs, and experienced adrenal fatigue. My romantic relationship suffered. I didn't see friends as much. Unfortunately, I was living as a human doer, *not a human* being. *So, what had happened? I lost balance.*

AWAKENING TO BALANCE

The challenges of maintaining balance and exercising conscious choice in my life have caused me a certain amount of suffering. This past year, before turning forty, I attended Berkeley's Executive Coaching Program. I originally participated in this program for professional development, but to my surprise, I experienced the beginning of a personal transformation. The program required that we examine ourselves and our own lives as an aspect of the curriculum.

This started me on a road of reawakening. I began again to take inventory, examine my values, and consider what I wanted in my life. I ask you to consider what has heart and meaning for you. How do you want to live your life? How are you willing to live your life?

I had to face these questions and doing so was uncomfortable. I spoke at length to my fellow attendees of my expansive travels and learning, in contrast with the constrictive aspects of my professional development.

I wanted to live a more balanced life. I started back in therapy, have been mediating most days, making it a point to eat well, maintaining boundaries in my work, working less, and exercising more. This practice means staying attuned to my inner awareness, with the intent to live with vitality. What do you need to do to live your hopes and dreams?

Rollo May, one of the founders of humanistic psychology, felt that at the heart of the human dilemma is the struggle between what we want to do and what we have to do.

By living a balanced life, we can move beyond our struggle to ease or mitigate it. A balanced life is one that encompasses pleasure and responsibility. That means living your life today, in the moment. To make that possible, we need to maintain boundaries with work, in order to maintain self-care and reasonable work hours. Ideally, this is a life that enables you to have time for yourself, time for your partner, and time for your children. This means showing up and being present, not running on fumes, and not just going through the motions. The pathway to such living is through awareness, making space for reflection, and then acting on your insight.

Considerations

Living with vitality has a different meaning to different people. Each person is unique and will have different responses as they define what living with vitality means to them. I have had the fortunate opportunity to train with some of the best existential humanistic psychologists in the world. I have read a great deal of their work, as well as the work of founding existential thought leaders. In my own quest to live with vitality, I have used the following concepts from their work as a compass to help guide me on this journey. Consider how each of these concepts is relevant to you and how you can integrate them into your own life to set yourself up for success.

Holding these concepts in your consciousness has the potential to shift you toward a life of greater meaning and purpose, aligned with your values.

Awe. This encompasses the thrill, wonder, and anxiety of living. It requires curiosity, openness, appreciation, noticing, and discovery, while being mindful of the need for safety, structure, and support. In short, awe is humility and wonder — a sense of adventure — toward living.

Example — You are on vacation. You are taking in everything. You are aware of the sights, the sounds, the smells, and the people. You are fully engaged. You are not taking 200 photos; you are not on your phone. You are noticing the wind and how it's making the leaves dance and move. You are truly present, appreciating the people, the food, the natural environment, the architecture, the sky, the weather. Noticing the details of life around you can help you connect more deeply with your passion for living.

Being. To live a fully engaged life means living in accordance with your values and your purpose. *Becoming* is the constant evolution of living fully engaged, shaping our life according to who we are. We are in a constant flow of being and becoming.

Example — You are a school counselor. You love your work and are engaged in helping students grow and develop, and you realize that you want to further your education and become a psychologist. "Being" implies working in an engaged way in the here and now. "Becoming is working on developing yourself to where you want to be.

Lack of control. Your partner makes all the decisions for you. You never choose where you go to eat or what activities you do. In this dynamic, you are then allowing the external world (your mate) to run your life. This does not reflect living with meaning and purpose.

Adapting. Your current work environment does not support your values, and you are becoming uncomfortable with the toxic culture at your company. You have always dreamt of becoming a photographer, and you have been freelancing and doing side work in this area for a long time. You decide to listen to your gut and leave your position. You start your own wedding photography company, and you utilize your business and marketing background as well as your photography skill set. Listening to your inner awareness has helped you to create more meaningful work and the opportunity to do what you love. You are no longer down and irritable. You have more free time, and you jog most days and see your friends more often.

Tuning in to inner awareness. To connect to our subjective inner world — inner aware-ness — we must actively listen to what is coming up for us. We need to develop the skill of periodically shutting out external distractions, so we can continue to be aware of our own feelings, our responses, and the state of our wellbeing. Be aware of thoughts, feelings and sensations, values and preferences, anticipations, fantasies, and dreams. This is the inner, intimate, and distinctive realm in which individuals live most genuinely.

Example — You are 43 years old and stuck in a job that doesn't align with your values. In order to change your situation, it is useful to set time aside and ask yourself some helpful questions. If we don't explore this sense of dissatisfaction, that could lead to symptoms of depression or anxiety. What would I rather be doing? For example, should I go back to school and get a master's degree that will provide me with a credential to work in a differ-ent field? Are there other resources available to me that might expand my options?

Finding balance. We humans live on a constrictive/expansive continuum, and our polar-ities can promote dysfunction or extremism. Confrontation with or integration of our extremes promotes optimal living (living with vitality).

Example — If you are all work or all play, that generally does not constitute a fulfilling life. We need to balance our responsibilities by doing what makes us happy. This might mean taking on more household responsibilities, being mindful of your partner's needs, and managing work deadlines to free you up so you have time to play basketball with friends, watch movies, and get to the beach on a warm summer day.

Presence. Living in the present moment creates a state of heightened awareness that is grounded and attuned to the here and now.

Example — Your partner is telling you about their day at work. In this moment, you are not thinking about *your* day at work or the basketball game *you* want to watch later. You are fully engaged. You notice that her words are not matching her facial expressions and body language. You ask more questions to clarify and understand what is going on for her. Your partner is happy to see how attuned you are to the conversation. You learn that she is struggling with a problem and is grateful to have your support. This is a moment when you feel genuinely connected, and that makes you feel alive. To live with vitality is to be truly engaged, and that is the pathway to greater connection.

Destiny. Our limitations define physical, psychological, and cultural limits and influence our decisions. Destiny implies that many aspects of our life cannot be chosen. We do not choose our parents, the neighborhood where we grew up, the religion that we were born into, our race, eye color, height, or intellectual potential. However, we can make choices within these constructs.

Example — Your dad is a plumber. He wants you to be a plumber, too. However, your skill set is not in the trades. You are not handy. You realize you are good at math and decide to become an accountant. Your choice is grounded in the construct of who you are, your capabilities, and what you want from your life.

Freedom and Destiny

I'd love to play center for the Knicks, but I'm just over 5'10". True, I have a good post-up game, am able to knock down open jumpers from the elbow, and can make successful bank shots from the wing. I played for a year in high school and then had to settle on men's league basketball.

Freedom and Destiny. These concepts encompass the choices that we have in our lives—freedom within limitations. My height, athletic ability, and speed capped me as a pretty good rec league player. Since I wasn't NBA-bound, I had to make different choices for myself that were more in line with my abilities, characteristics, values, and skill set. I am empathic, reasonably intelligent, and caring. This awareness led me to choose to become a psychologist and, as time went on, a life and executive coach. These choices came from a balanced and pragmatic place. I searched within myself, listened to my awareness, and did research to substantiate my choices.

The Importance of Choice

You may have a mortgage, three children, and work responsibilities. You may want to coach your son's basketball team and feel that you can't because you work a sixty-hour week. Yet within this construct, you still have choices. When we feel stuck, bogged down,

Living with Vitality

What interferes with your ability to live with vitality?	*Conditions that promote living with vitality:*
Overworking and working on the weekends	Awareness
Polarized thinking/extremism/narrow or rigid thinking	Setting boundaries at work
Not listening to your mind or your body	Living that has heart and meaning
Not addressing suffering or mental health issues	Living in line with your values
Poor diet	Being curious
Not exercising	Taking inventory of your needs, wants, and desires
Over-committing yourself	Taking time for yourself
Substance abuse	Scheduling fun and reflection
Stubbornness	Exploring your choices, options, and alternatives
Living in the past	Making a list of things you enjoy doing and doing them
Ruminating/living in your head rather than the present	Living in the present moment, in the here and now
Deferring all pleasure and happiness to some future date	Exercise, whether that means getting to the gym, playing sports, or walking the dog
Living based on other people's values	Eating healthily, even if you have to work with a coach or join a group
Negative self-talk	Eating smart, rather than starving yourself
Losing touch with your one and only precious life	Living with balance and moderation
	Being willing to change
	Having empathy toward yourself and others

Figure 68.1. Factors that promote or deter living with vitality.

and are living in a waking sleep, our choices can feel limited or nonexistent. What choices can you make within the construct of your life that could help you to feel more alive?

Sometimes we get in our own way. We don't see the portals of opportunity. We need to explore these obstacles so that choices, alternatives, and perspectives emerge.

It is a startling fact that freedom has been considered, throughout history, so precious that millions of human beings have willingly died for it. However, the question we might ask is, How many are willing to *live* for freedom? How many have made a strong effort to live with vitality, to live one's hopes and dreams?

> *In loving memory of Bob "the Electrician" Buonfiglio: may his life*
> *and realizations help you to live with passion and vitality.*

For more information on the work of Robert Buonfiglio, please see
www.drrobertjbuonfiglio.com.
For additional resources, please see
www.TheTwentyFirstCenturyMan.com.

PART 10
RELATIONSHIP SKILLS
Introduction
Judson Brandeis, MD

Some people are so poor, all they have is money.
— Chance the Rapper

Humans are social animals. The survival of the species depends on humans working together, so we instinctively connect with others from the time we are babies. Before, during, and after pregnancy, women go through phases in their lives when they are more dependent on others.

Men do not routinely go through a similar experience. However, the enjoyment of our lives still depends on the quality of our interactions with others, especially with our spouse. Every time you forget that annoying phrase, "Happy wife, happy life," it comes back to haunt you.

The first step in a relationship is finding the right partner, which is depressingly difficult to do. In India, the divorce rate for arranged marriages is less than 5% compared to 40% for "love" marriages. One of the aspects of a successful union is evolving with your partner. Listening is a critical aspect of this evolution. When communication is challenging, which normally occurs during a marriage, a therapist can be an essential tool to improve the quality of the relationship. Half of all marriages end in divorce, and family law attorneys have a unique perspective on why marriages fail.

Male physique changes as we age, but the physical and hormonal changes in a woman's body during menopause are much more dramatic. Understanding menopause is *critical* to the health of a relationship, and the way a man handles this difficult time for a woman can determine the trajectory of the relationship.

Biology drives us to have children, but little ones can be a blessing or a curse. Fatherhood is a gift, but also a responsibility. How we handle the communication and balance between spouse and children determines the joy in our family life. As family blossoms, the growth and quality of the intimate relationships in life directly impact health and happiness.

Chapter 69
Find Yourself a Partner Who Can Be Your Best Friend
Nancy Faass, MSW, MPH
Medical Writer

Motivate and support your partner.
You are both a work in progress, so grow and build together.
— Anonymous

Robbie had just gone through a rough divorce. He'd been attracted to his ex, Amber, by her spontaneity and love of adventure. But as the years passed, he found himself with less and less patience for his wife's "creative lifestyle." Over time, her casual approach, her irresponsibility, and her frequent fliers became inconvenient, given his commitment to his career. Robbie was grounded, practical, and hard-working, which Amber came to experience as constricting. His love of order and routine, which had initially provided Amber with a haven from the wildness of her own life, became boring, hum-drum.

Although they tried marriage counseling, it became clear that if they wanted to make things work, they would have to learn to negotiate their differences. Given the amount of conflict, that was going to require more time and emotional energy than either of them had. Rather than invest more effort, Amber found another partner whose personality was closer to her own and moved on. Fortunately, Robbie and she hadn't had children, so the separation and divorce were much less brutal than they could have been.

Robbie poured himself into his work, with time at the gym on his way home every night, and gradually began to heal emotionally. About 14 months later, he was at a conference when he spotted an old friend, and they hit it off immediately. As they chatted, it dawned on him, "This could be The One." So without further ado, they went out for coffee, and he figured out her temperament. Bingo. A match across the board.

Being with her felt like coming home. Although she wasn't quite as exciting as Amber had been, he felt a deep sense of peace, a rightness to the relationship. This one was a keeper.

Temperament theory can be an effective tool for gaining a sense of the people around you and what makes them tick. The core ideas of the theory are based on the work of the psychologist Carl Jung. But the idea that there are four basic personality types goes back to the Greeks. Hippocrates, Plato, and Aristotle described them as the four humors, and Shakespeare included these ideas in his cosmology. Today, temperament theory is used in Fortune 500 companies for hiring, staff development, and team building.

The temperaments are easy to understand and remember; once you know them, you will see them everywhere in the people around you, and in yourself. (Note: Spontaneous Adventurers are put off by the idea of categorizing people, but for the rest of us, the temperaments help us understand people a little better.)

- **Deepening personal insight.** Temperament can be useful in helping you define (and understand) your core values and your personality. This is a tool that you can use to sort out what's most important to you and why.

- **Making sense of those around us.** These snapshots of human personality help us tune into others more quickly, to gain a sense of how they see the world, what makes them happy, and how to work with them more effectively.

- **Gaining a greater understanding of a potential partner.** In love, opposites tend to attract. There's an excitement in getting close to someone that you admire, but who is perhaps quite different than you. Short-term, this can be heady and intoxicating. Yet for the long-term, living with someone very different from you can be wearing, or even exhausting. Partnering with someone of a different temperament means really committing to the relationship in order to bridge the gaps in how you see things.

THE FOUR TEMPERAMENTS

Most people tend to be a combination of two temperaments, or sometimes three, so you'll also want to determine your secondary temperament. And some highly evolved souls have all the bases covered. If temperament theory rings true for you, it could be one of the tools you use to get greater clarity in your own life.

CITIZEN / TRADITIONALIST / WORKER

These people are the doers of the world, and they tend to be highly organized, focused, hardworking, and punctual. They emphasize order and understand its value in providing harmony and stability. Data from the Temperament Research Institute suggest that these folks are in the majority, making up more than 40% of the U.S. population. They are managers and businesspeople, visible in administration, government, and industry. In the corporate world, research shows that more than 85% of leadership has this temperament. Men and women almost equally identify with these values (about 8% fewer men than women). Ultimately, for these people, order is the highest value, and they appreciate how easily order can be lost.

FREE SPIRIT / ADVENTURER / SENSUALIST

Folks with this hardwiring live in the moment, tend to be spontaneous, and are attuned to the pleasure of experience. They bring life to any party, and are the athletes, entertainers, and rock stars of our culture. Adventurers have been described as inventive, pragmatic, and self-reliant, and are attracted to jobs that range from fire fighter, paramedic, or pilot to investor, entrepreneur, or sales rep. They are skilled at trouble shooting and problem solving, adaptable, and able to think on their feet. These folks make up about one-third of the population and 15% more men identify as Free Spirit.

STRATEGIC THINKER / RESEARCHER / VISIONARY

The world of ideas is the realm of these people. They tend to be analytical, rational, focused, and inventive thinkers who are found among writers, entrepreneurs, analysts, engineers, professors, researchers, and scientists. The life of the intellect is where they find their greatest satisfaction. Thinkers tend to be pragmatic and strategic, and they value a logical, realistic world view. About 10% of Americans have this temperament, which is found about twice as frequently among men.

NURTURER / HUMANIST / DEVOTEE

These are the helpers of the world, who serve humanity—nurses, teachers, psychologists, and social workers. People who share the values and emotions of a Nurturer also include those drawn to spirituality or religion, so their number includes ministers, priests, gurus, and devotees of every faith. For Nurturers, fairness is the highest value, so they are found in greater numbers on the liberal side of the spectrum. People with this temperament tend to be imaginative, intuitive, and idealistic. Generally speaking, this temperament is found in a little more than 10% of Americans, and about twice as many women identify as nurturers.

Temperament at a glance. Put a check by all the qualities that describe your personality, workstyle, and lifestyle. Once you know your temperament, do the same for your partner, your children, or coworkers. Given the tremendous variability due to genetics, people in the same bloodline sometimes have surprisingly different personalities.

We can use temperament to better understand the people we love and how to best interact with them by becoming attuned to their values, biases, and personal goals. Understanding more about our own style and the style of others can make it easier to live and work in harmony and to make the deep connections that bring joy to our lives.

CITIZEN		FREE SPIRIT	
Workstyle	*Lifestyle*	*Workstyle*	*Lifestyle*
organized	practical	independent	adventurous
factual	realistic	creative	spontaneous
dependable	traditional	skillful	charismatic
logical	creature of habit	inventive impulsive	
orderly	cooperative	adaptable	fun-loving
punctual loyal		energetic playful	
reliable	responsible	alert	entertaining
industrious	painstaking	observant	outgoing
efficient	prepared	pragmatic	self-reliant
conscientious	decisive	easygoing	tolerant

THINKER		NURTURER	
Workstyle	*Lifestyle*	*Workstyle*	*Lifestyle*
analytical	independent	humanistic	compassionate
knowledgeable	decisive	fair-minded	open
theoretical	pragmatic	conscientious	idealistic
objective inquisitive		empathic altruistic	
intellectual	intelligent	insightful	imaginative
competitive	rational	nurturing	intuitive
focused	reserved	progressive	introspective
strategic	truthful	creative	authentic
inventive perfectionist		verbal	devotional
competent	complex	persuasive	harmonious

Figure 17.1. The Four Temperaments: We can use temperament to better understand the people we care about and how to best interact with them, by becoming attuned to their values, biases, and personal goals. (Source: © 2021 Nancy Faass with thanks to a number of innovators in temperament theory.)

For more on the work of Nancy Faass, see www.HealthWritersGroup.com.

Chapter 70
How Counseling Can Help Build A Lasting Relationship
Brett Beaver, LMFT
Marriage and Family Therapist

Marriage does not guarantee you will be together forever; it's only paper. It takes love, respect, trust, understanding, friendship, and faith in your relationship to make it last.
— Anonymous

Most men have heard the quote "Happy wife, happy life," but how do we achieve this mythical goal. Studies show that a good relationship with a primary partner helps us to stay healthy. The challenge is, what are the pieces of the puzzle that will enable us to sustain a healthy relationship? This section of the book offers tools you can use to support and deepen your relationship beyond the initial romantic phase. It's a fact that a successful marriage tends to support good health.

Lower risk of a heart attack. An analysis published in the journal *Heart*, of studies involving more than two million people found that marriage lowered the odds of having a heart attack or a stroke. In contrast, never being married raised the risk of heart attack by 42%.

What about cancer? In a study from the National Cancer Institute, scientists focused on the ten most important factors in cancer. They found that marriage (or a relationship with a primary partner) was a significant variable influencing survival. Men and women who were married at the time of diagnosis lived longer than those who were single.

And what about stress? Researchers have measured the presence of the stress hormone cortisol. Studies found lower levels of cortisol in married people when compared to those who were never married or were previously married.

REALITY CHECK

Health benefits meet divorce statistics. Statistics from the 2014 United States Census suggest that a primary partnership is difficult to maintain. Researchers estimate that on average 50% of all marriages will end in divorce. but what they really mean is that:

- 41% of all first marriages end in divorce

- 60% of all second marriages end in divorce

- 73% of all third marriages end in divorce.

Can counseling make a difference? Although traditional marriage counseling is rumored to have a success rate of 70% to 80%, more recent research reported that 38% of couples who receive marriage therapy got divorced within four years of completing therapy. That's the bad news, but the good news is that 62% of couples stayed together.

Definition of a healthy relationship. A working definition of a healthy relationship emphasizes a partnership that is a respectful, mutually satisfying, balanced connection with another human that allows for discussion of differences, and is built upon a foundation of trust, communication, and understanding.

> *Nice definition, but have any of us experienced many truly healthy relationships first-hand? Maybe, to a limited extent, but not often.*

Limited reference points. Who did we see that hinted at the presence of a healthy relationship with their primary partner? If we scan the usual suspects, our parents, their family friends, etc., what did we notice that would suggest their relationship was healthy? The reference points we observed were often about what *not* to do. Hence our limited experience of role modeling of day-to-day communication and caring. Many of us feel that we are on our own, learning through trial and error. What's more, the concept of what others expect of us has changed drastically.

EVOLVING EXPECTATIONS

Another challenge is the changing role of men in society. For more than 500,000 years men fed their families by hunting wild game. (We know that the Neanderthals, for example, brought home dinner by spearing huge animals like bulls and mammoths at close range.) So what *was* expected of us?

- Bravery—don't share vulnerability

- Fortitude—stay strong and carry on, handle pain without complaint

- Silence—avoid unnecessary conversation

- Toughness—never admit a mistake

- Maintain your turf

- Clear role definition by gender (he hunts, she gathers)

All the traits that are stereotypic of men are those essential to a successful hunter. A cowardly man would have been a deficit on the hunt, spooking the other hunters and stoking their fears, reducing the chances of success. A talkative hunter would have scared away all the game and the men would have gone home empty handed, unable to feed their families. By natural selection, men today are the descendants of the most successful hunters—understandably the strong, silent type.

Things are different now. In the Paleo, humans lived in small clans of ten to twenty-five individuals, primarily blood relatives. Over an entire lifetime, we might have only encountered a few hundred individuals. Today now most of us live in metro areas of five million or more. In a city like New York, if we commute on the subway and work downtown, we may have crossed the paths of a few hundred individuals before our workday even begins. Urban life requires skilled communication, good cooperation, collaboration, and compassion. Many of us work in teams or manage staff, further intensifying the need for these skillsets.

These heightened expectations are also an aspect of homelife. As a matter of practicality, we need to communicate around highly charged issues such as money, division of labor, childrearing, chronic health issues, and emerging crises (before they become crises).

Rugged individualist or empathic listener? As men, we're still expected to be rugged individualists, highly competitive in our career, someone who stands on their own two feet and is self-reliant. However, we need to have the skills to carry on a conversation with *emotional content*. Our partner wants us to be a sounding board, someone with whom they can share their frustrations of the day. They want us to actively listen, to reflect the content and the emotion of what they are saying without stepping in and giving advice too soon. (In other words, the exact opposite of the strong, silent type.)

Silent and stoic or insightful and sensitive? We are expected to know ourselves—to be in touch with our emotions—and to share our vulnerability. As a hunter, it likely would have been counterproductive to be in touch with our emotions. The choices were clear-cut—the family needed to eat. Repressing fear in order to be a successful hunter seems logical. The message conveyed to little boys today is still, "Be brave, don't cry. If it hurts just suck it up."

Clearly defined gender roles have become outdated. With 57% of women in the workforce, working outside the home, today more men participate in child-rearing, and not only the "fun" activities. Our partners also expect us to do our fair share of the housework.

With all these changes, how are we supposed to know what to do without blowing it?

CHALLENGES

Our world is one of constant overstimulation. The norm is to keep our minds active 18 hours a day. At night, our workday infringes on time with our family, as we respond to work-related texts, phone calls, and e-mails. The only time this is not true is when we sleep. Yet how many of us keep our electronics close to us when we're asleep?

No wonder we struggle to create the space to connect with others. When we do stumble into each other, like ships passing in the night, we scramble to become present, attempting to set aside the remnants of the day bouncing around in our heads. We try our best to align ourselves with our partner, still distracted. We make half-hearted efforts to listen and respond, pretending to listen until we lose focus or our partner recognizes that we are distracted, and they become frustrated and give up on the attempt at communication.

When things start to unravel. There is a saying that when a divorce happens, men replace and women reflect. Men typically do not take the time to look at their role in the demise of the relationship. We focus on moving on to something else. We do not examine what we need to do differently, to avoid making the same mistakes. The divorce statistics would suggest that many of us employ this strategy. The research shows that talking with a trained professional about these challenges can make a difference and can increase the chances of building a stronger, more lasting relationship. This is how men learn about what we need to do differently to stay connected to a primary partner.

Common challenges that prompt one or both partners to seek help include:

- Conflict, arguments, criticism
- Infidelity, betrayal, jealousy
- Lack of process for effective problem solving and accumulated unsolved problems
- Loss of passion
- Emotional needs that are not met
- Differences on parenting in the current relationship or in a blended family
- In-laws and extended family
- Adult children or parents living at home with a couple
- Finances and money issues
- Loss and grief issues
- Unfair division of labor
- Health challenges that inhibit intimacy.

THE EXPERIENCE OF COUPLE'S THERAPY

As a family therapist, I find that often, it is the women who drag the men kicking and screaming into my office. Guys don't want to be there: Their train of thought is something like, "This is useless. What is a therapist going to suggest that we haven't already tried? All they are going to do is gang up on me. My partner is just looking for someone to support their position."

Couples' therapy is not a death sentence for your relationship. It is a forum for discussion where each person's side of the story is given space, where we can practice listening (really listening) to increase the possibility of hearing each other and being heard.

Yet we carry a dire sense of trepidation when entering the therapist's office. True, this is unfamiliar territory where most men feel at a disadvantage.

So yes, there will be moments when you feel unfairly accused or judged. Yes, you will feel out of control. Yet we need to face our fears.

If you are working with a compatible therapist, this is a safe space.

The therapist is not judge, juror, and executioner. They are a human being with their own relationship history who has specialized training in communication skills. Yet we protest, mostly out of fear. Fear that we will feel out of place (maybe), uncomfortable about the intensity of the emotion connected to our relationship issues (probably), fearful that going to a therapist is punishment for all of our relationship mistakes (unlikely, though the feeling is real).

The therapy process is about finding common ground in the relationship and modifying our communication skills. Effective therapy is about looking at recurring themes that manifest in conflict, and collaboratively working together toward effective problem solving. The goal is to find pathways for understanding and connection that affirm the relationship.

Our reluctance, while understandable, simply keeps us in a holding pattern until we find support or end the relationship.

The goals of effective couple's therapy. There are at least eight to ten different evidenced-based philosophies of marriage and family therapy, but the majority of these approaches seek to accomplish similar basic goals:

- Improving communication skills
- Identifying strengths in our partner and in the relationship

- Creating a comfortable environment that allows for an honest, respectful discussion of the challenges each partner is facing

- Increased self-awareness and understanding

- The opportunity to discover the themes and narratives that all of us carry from previous relationships and from our family of origin, which tend to manifest in our current relationship

- Improved communication skills, which turn out to be beneficial to other relationships as well

- Creation of a pathway for connection that invites both members of the relationship to re-engage with their partner.

SEEK HELP EARLIER

Most humans desire a connection with others. We want to be seen, heard, understood, respected, and touched. The inability to achieve this in a primary relationship can have a negative impact on our quality of life and health.

One way to increase our level of connection is to overcome our fear and seek help earlier in the relationship.

The longer we wait to get help with unresolved issues, the more entrenched the cycle of unfulfilling interactions is likely to become. Communication patterns become ingrained and more difficult to adjust. At some point, the path back to each other may be so fraught with levels of pain, reconciliation may feel insurmountable. The couple may opt-out of the relationship (see divorce statistics) rather than re-engage.

Don't wait! Seek support sooner rather than later. Early intervention often leads to more mutually satisfying patterns of communication, affirming the connection to each other.

Be patient. Understand that it took time to arrive at this point in your relationship, and it will take time to experience the full benefit of family therapy. The sooner you get help, the less damage there will be to undo, so don't wait to get help.

FINDING A GOOD THERAPIST

Ask a friend, colleague, or a therapist for a recommendation (someone to whom they would send a member of their own family). Do follow-up research online, reading the reviews (focus on the experience of most clients, not just a few outliers). Contact a local university, training center, or agency that provides psychotherapy. Meet with the therapist, ask questions, and look for a match, a partnership that coincides with your wants, needs, and what you feel will help your relationship.

What to look for in a therapist?

- Do they have the credentials to practice in the state/country where you reside?

- Does the therapist (and the office) intuitively feel comfortable and safe?

- Do you feel welcomed, heard, and understood?

- Is their communication style consistent with what you need?

- Do you feel they have a genuine interest in your well-being and success?

- When explaining a concept or presenting an intervention, do they make sense?

- If they provide homework, are the tasks relevant to your work in the therapist's office?

- Do they have a sense of humor?

- Do they find the balance between nudging you to change and supporting you?

- When you have a dissenting opinion, do they make room for your perspective?

- If they use self-disclosure, does the information further your understanding?

- Do you feel they collaborate with you to support positive change?

- Are they experienced? (While not a firm rule, look for a therapist with at least seven to ten years of experience.)

- Do you feel value derived from the session is commensurate with the fee?

Maximize your experience. Show up on time. Stay present during the session and attuned to how you feel. Engage and share how you really feel, not as an outburst, but more as a willingness to invest emotionally. If the therapist gives you homework, do your best to follow-through. Homework moves the process along further, just as discussion leads to improved understanding and necessary changes.

Avoid defensiveness. Do your best to recognize that the therapist is not singling you out as the problem. Therapists understand that each of us has to take 100% responsibility for our 50% of the challenges in the relationship. Often men opt-out of couples therapy because we feel unfairly and repeatedly singled out. Before you leave therapy, engage the therapist in your perception of the discrepancy. The goal is improved communication and connection, not a 50/50 split of who needs to change what.

Couples' therapy is a place to set egos aside, take a discerning look at what each of us can change to improve the relationship, and consider our willingness to do that. A good therapist will make the effort to be nonjudgmental. Approach the process as a learning experience. Ultimately, therapy can be a genuine opportunity for growth.

For more on the work of Brett Beaver, LMFT, please see:
www.brettbeaver.com.
For additional resources, please see:
www.TheTwentyFirstCenturyMan.com.

Chapter 71
Couple's Counseling: What Works?
Brett Beaver, LMFT
Marriage & Family Therapist

Couples wait an average of six years, being unhappy in their relationship, before seeking help.
— John Gottman, PhD

I'm a marriage and family counselor who sees couples in crisis every day. If you are wondering how I decide which approach to use with a particular couple, I start with the science and the research. In psychology, as in medicine, we ultimately want to know what works.

THE WORK OF THE GOTTMAN INSTITUTE

John Gottman has become one of my favorite theorists. With his wife, Julie Gottman, he cofounded the Gottman Institute in Seattle. To our benefit, he has brought more of a research perspective to the assessment of relationship skills. He came to the work initially as a family therapist with a background in mathematics, so he wanted to do more than simply collect anecdotal stories.

Dr. Gottman developed a lab that was essentially a completely tricked out model home. Couples would come and stay overnight for a long weekend, and he would film their interactions and evaluate their communication. Based on their interaction, he identified patterns (both negative and positive) in the way they related. He became able to predict whether a couple would remain together or part ways. The rumor has it that his average was close to 90% accuracy.

In order to apply what he was seeing in those interactions, he distilled his observations into trends, insight, and guidelines describing various aspects of human relationships. Drs. Gottman have been actively doing this research for more than 40 years and have produced a series of excellent books on this work, written for consumers.

One of the important concepts the Gottmans identified was what they describe as conflict management, which they differentiate from conflict resolution. The term conflict resolution gives you the impression that it's one-and-done, that you can talk about an issue once and it's over, as opposed to the insight that there will be recycling and recurring issues over the life of a relationship.

The couples that stay connected are those who are able to navigate that territory effectively. They can talk about emotionally laden material in a way that furthers the relationship, in contrast to couples who communicate in ways that create barriers and distance them from each other.

> *In every relationship, there are usually four or five issues that are high stakes. How you deal with those issues makes all the difference in how you feel about your relationship.*

The Four Horsemen

Another perspective Gottman is known for is a series of concepts he calls the Four Horsemen. These are four communication patterns that create barriers and get in the way of human connection.

Criticism. The first is criticism, which is defined as blaming or attacking the other person, rather than focusing on the particulars of the issue. Sometimes we get so frustrated (and ultimately so hurt) that we resort to pointing the finger at the other person. We are no longer focusing on the issue itself or what is underlying the issue. Instead of working things out, working them through, we blame the other person. Clearly, that gets in the way of feeling connected.

Contempt. This reflects an escalation of criticism in which the intensity of the attack goes to the essence of who the person is. I call it a scorched earth policy, acting with impunity, in which the angry partner no longer observes any boundaries to their communication. It's all bets off and one of the partners is going for the jugular vein. That often leads to major consequences in a relationship, so I heavily caution people about this emotional habit. (A surprising number of people also do this unconsciously with their kids.)

Defensiveness. In a partnership, there are days when people bring things to our attention that they don't like. If we're defensive and we don't make room to hear what they have to say, that can block communication. In other cases, they may feel upset, slighted, or have hurt feelings. We need to hear how they experience the situation. In sum, defensiveness in and of itself does not lend to reciprocal exchange of communication and dialogue.

Stonewalling. When one partner remains distant and refuses to engage at all, Gottman refers to that as stonewalling. They may be on their phone, not saying much, and not bothering to engage.

Underlying Patterns

Emotional flooding. Human beings can sometimes become flooded with emotion (this seems to be especially true of men). That can happen in a way that makes it difficult to communicate. Understanding emotional flooding and giving the other person a moment to gather themselves is essential to communication. That means creating a compassionate space so they can gather their thoughts, their ideas. A relaxed pause keeps the opportunity open for a shared exchange of emotions and feelings so that the relationship can continue to move forward. I view this as an essential piece.

Balancing positive and negative: 5 to 1. Gottman suggests that for every negative comment, there should be at least five positive comments or interactions so that the dialogue and vibe are predominantly positive. Holding that thought creates the opportunity for you to reverse a tendency toward negativity and work toward a more positive focus. It can totally change the dynamic in a relationship. That also creates new communication pathways and new opportunities for problem solving.

Developing the habit of positive communication. We are creatures of habit. In most couples' theories, communication is one of the key components. The approach may be different, what you communicate about may be different, but communication is central. Changing the way in which we communicate with each other can improve the relationship.

Delicate subjects. When a subject is emotionally laden and it is a difficult conversation, the way you bring that topic to the attention of the other person is important. A useful approach might be something easygoing, such as, "Hey, you know, I was thinking that we might follow up the conversation we had earlier. I want to be open to hearing what you have to say, and I'm hoping that we can find a way to communicate that makes it easier for us to talk about this subject, because it was a bit tough the other day."

Try something as simple as that, an openness when you approach your partner as opposed to saying something like, "Well, do you want to talk about that again?" That is not going to be helpful. Often in couples therapy, the therapist ends up being a bit of a traffic cop, running interference, or stopping the couple before they move on to engage in negativity or conflict.

In Gottman's approach to therapy, emotions are important and there is an acknowledgement that they need to be heard and understood. Communication is seen as important, especially in creating the shared vision of the relationship. But in his work, he doesn't tend to refer back to childhood content or wounds to the degree that other approaches, such as Imago relationship therapy, tend to do.

EMOTIONALLY-FOCUSED COUPLES' THERAPY (EFT)

EFT, developed by Dr. Sue Johnson, focuses on attachment theory. One of her fundamental beliefs is that insecurity causes conflict and that a deep-seated fear of abandonment is often what underlies that conflict. As human beings, most of us carry with us a certain level of insecurity and fear of being abandoned.

The Four Attachment Types

Another of Dr. Johnson's contributions is the identification of four different attachment types.

Secure attachment. It is likely that most of us would like the confidence and sense of security exemplified in the secure attachment type. In that scenario, we don't feel that we need the other person. We like having them in our life. We're able to hear what they have to say without getting too defensive. There is a willingness on our part to share vulnerability. We may know that we have a sensitivity to being abandoned, but we don't fear it incessantly. We know that we'll survive even if the relationship does not. There's balance, there's reciprocity, there's sharing, there's vulnerability, and there's an established way of communicating with each other.

Anxious attachment. With anxious attachment, we value the relationship a bit too much and may feel as though we couldn't survive without it. We all feel this periodically, but the fear of abandonment can reach the point where it becomes the primary preoccupation. We may worry about being more involved in the relationship than our partner to such a degree that we constantly focus on the possibility that they might leave. We may interpret their behavior as affirming the relationship or we may have the sense that they are going to abandon us. Whether one partner or both have an anxious attachment style, that becomes challenging for both people in the relationship. The result is a pattern of being so focused on the other person that they are always worried about what their partner is doing or saying. Instead, it's important to focus on what we need, on what we want, and on the needs of the two of us in the relationship together.

Avoidant attachment. One can be in a relationship and still be avoidant. An avoidant person doesn't really share much about themselves. They don't really invest—they can take or leave the relationship. The feeling that they project is that it doesn't really matter. Often an avoidant partner may feel good about themselves, but they have a tendency to keep their distance, to keep away. It feels as though they're somewhat aloof.

Anxious and avoidant. If you're in a relationship with someone who has this style of attachment, it can feel a bit like you're on a roller coaster. They love you and desperately want to connect. But then they may pull away. At times they act as though it doesn't matter whether they're connected, whether they're in the relationship with you or not. They may feel great about the relationship at one point, and then become triggered or stressed at another point. Periodically, they may get stressed and become anxious and fearful. There are challenges with trust and with depending on others.

While Dr. Johnson focuses intently on attachment type, the Gottman Institute focuses more on techniques that you can use to improve your relationship in the here and now and over time. In contrast, Dr. Johnson looks at the framework of attachment types in the context of the relationship, because that provides an indication of what is needed to improve it.

The Three-Stage Process of Communication

One of the challenges for the therapist is that people come in too late. At that point, they seem to be so far down the road of resentment, frustration, and disengagement that the way back toward each other is too painful and too uncomfortable. As a result, it's really difficult to find a way to create the communication pathways that would make a difference, so they end up opting out.

Deescalating the conflict. With Dr. Johnson's emotionally-focused couples therapy, the first phase in the cycle is de-escalation. The couple may be so hurt, so angry, so frustrated, so resentful that when they engage, the initial step is to find a way to help them relearn how to communicate with each other again in a manner that is positive and compassionate. The goal in the first phase of communication is to avoid escalating to outright frustration or outright anger.

Improving communication. Once you can decrease the escalation, then you begin to look at changing the way the interaction patterns occur. In the second phase, people are calmer, more reflective. They learn to use "I" statements, they're taking responsibility, they focus on feeling states, and they're no longer blaming.

Consolidating gains. In the consolidation phase, the next phase of the communication process, the couple consolidates these learnings. There tends to be an educational aspect in this approach that includes learning about different attachment styles (yours as well as your partner's). The communication pieces consolidate these insights and integrate them into a new form of dialogue that enhances and affirms the reason you were attracted to each other in the first place and chose to be in a relationship.

IMAGO RELATIONSHIP THERAPY

The third approach to couples counseling, Imago relationship therapy, was developed by Harville Hendrix and Dr. Helen LaKelley Hunt. This process is based on the idea that childhood relationship wounds tend to manifest in current relationships. As a family therapist, I would say that there is probably always some truth to that. This approach is especially good for couples who are interested in exploring the ways in which their childhood experiences may be manifesting as some of the challenges in their current partnership.

The ideal couple for Imago therapy. In essence, are you the kind of person who had significant things happen in your childhood? Do you sense that these experiences are showing up in your current relationship? And is this something that you are genuinely interested in exploring in depth with your partner?

Hendrix's premise is that understanding these wounds leads to a more conscious, functional relationship in the present. For example, at times we may unknowingly feel that our partner is treating us in a manner we experienced as a child, or they may unconsciously remind us of someone from our past who was responsible for hurt, harm, or abandonment. These types of unconscious feelings or memories can be triggered and manifest in our current relationships. Note, however, that this form of therapy is not appropriate for individuals with serious mental health issues or a history of domestic violence.

Transitioning from romantic love to a long-term relationship. The focus of Imago relationship therapy is to support the transition from a phase of romantic love to more balanced, reciprocal form of love. In the early phase of a relationship when we open our hearts, everything is so magical, so gorgeous. (To borrow a phrase from Bambi, we are twitterpated.) We can't wait to connect with the other person, and we constantly look forward to spending time with them. This is the romantic phase of love.

Usually, over time, that transitions or abates due to life circumstances, our own intimacy issues, and other challenges that come up.

> *How do you transition from that earlier phase of a relationship to a*
> *more balanced, reciprocal, shared phase of love?*

Hendrix and Hunt believe that this is best done through mirroring, which is basically a form of communication.

Validating our partner's perspective. We want to acknowledge and validate the perspective of our partner. When they bring up something uncomfortable about the relationship or when they share a frustration that they are having in their life, we want to make sure that we take the time to listen and to reflect back or mirror to them both the content and the feelings connected with their experience. We need to take the time to listen to what they have to say. We also want to validate the feelings that they are experiencing. We want to indicate that we've heard the information that they're sharing, even if it's about us and even if we don't necessarily agree with what they're saying.

Engaging with empathy. We also want to bring the empathy piece to the fore, drawing on what we know and understand about them as a person. Here, empathy is expressed by acknowledging our partner's experience, their beliefs, their understanding, their expectations. Even if they don't totally sync with how we see the situation, we want to acknowledge their reality.

In relationships, over time, we develop a history. We evolve an understanding and a perspective on our partner's vulnerabilities and their emotions. It's useful to integrate that empathy in our communication and include it in our responses. Most people are hungry to be understood, to know that someone "gets" them.

Remaining allies. A big piece of this process is engaging with your partner as an ally and not as the enemy. Too often, when we are triggered in a relationship, a line is drawn in the sand, and suddenly the person in front of us becomes the enemy. We may be tempted to attack them, instead of including them. At that moment, we may also be having trouble seeing things from their perspective, just as they may. Ultimately, the goal is a situation in which both partners are trying to work it out. We need to be inclusive rather than shutting our partner out.

Turning complaints into requests. Another useful strategy is to modify complaints into requests. Almost every complaint that we might have about another person or a situation has an underlying request, a desire or a yearning that can be met by a positive action or response. For example, if the complaint is that you never have any time to yourself, rather than complaining, you might open with something like, "I would really like to go swimming once a week. Would you take the kids one evening, and I'll hang out with them on Saturday morning." If you can figure out the nature of your issue and get underneath the complaint, sometimes that transforms the whole situation.

You still need to express what you want out loud. But if you word your issue as a request, rather than as a complaint, that can change the dynamic and improve the tenor of the communication.

Harville and Hunt believe that a partnership based on mutual healing is the most effective form of therapy. If you have childhood wounds that become manifest in the relationship, you can use the process of Imago to move yourself toward healing and improve the relationship.

That involves modifying your communication, employing empathy, mirroring feelings, and providing constructive feedback. This healing process makes it easier for you to stay connected and vulnerable in the relationship, enhancing your reasons for staying together.

Imago tends to be most appropriate for cerebral couples. Both partners need to be open to exploring their feelings. Clearly, there are some people who will never be open to emotional or psychological self-disclosure, whereas in Imago, there has to be the willingness to step into that arena. Exploring one's feelings is inherent in the process.

- The first step in Imago therapy is deciding if the process is right for you and recognizing that some aspect of the relationship needs more work.

- Secondly, there needs to be a willingness on the part of both partners to share their feelings with each other and with the therapist.

To some extent, this is true of all these approaches. There is a humbling aspect of therapy in any form. One of the reasons that people wait so long to begin couple's therapy is that there is so much vulnerability involved. The challenge is that often, the process of disclosure, inherent in therapy, brings back not only childhood experiences, but also the sum total of your relationships to date and their impact on your current relationship. Whether you like it or not, they're all woven into the mix. How do you separate that out? How do you differentiate past and present in order to communicate in a way that makes a difference, that builds the relationship rather than diminishing it?

NARRATIVE THERAPY

A fourth philosophy that has been found to be effective in marriage counseling is narrative therapy for couples by Michael White and David Epston. Basically, their belief is that all of us create working narratives or stories about who we are and who others are. We have working theories, working ideas, working narratives. They are in our minds, they're in our hearts. Often, they are in our souls. They help us make sense of the world. But we don't always identify and recognize what these beliefs are or that these beliefs and narrative are constantly running in the background.

Taking the emotion out of the communication. The process in this type of therapy involves identifying the internal narrative. Sometimes, in a couple's interactions, the emotional intensity of the communication can trigger "internal riots." This can prompt us to verbalize in a way that creates conflict in the relationship. So the goal of this approach is to take the emotion out of the communication or at least set it aside a little. We want to see if there's a larger context, a broader frame of reference through which we can view our own individual story. The idea is not to make the other person the problem but to make the problem the problem. So you don't observe your partner as the source of the problem, rather, you look at the problem as the issue.

Viewing issues from one step removed, it makes the situation a little easier to sort out and not as emotionally reactive. It is the narrative that needs modification, not the other person in the relationship. This is another approach to therapy that tends to be a little more cerebral.

Identifying the narrative. Each of us has developed a personal narrative over the course of our life. We each have a storyline inside our head about relationships, based on our personal history. We want to find a way to separate that out a little, by jointly identifying the narratives that each partner has and understanding those narratives. We also want to identify problems as separate from us and then figure out a way to navigate the problems. This creates an opportunity for people to transition toward easier communication that is not as emotionally laden or overwhelming.

SOLUTIONS-FOCUSED COUPLE'S THERAPY

The fifth type of therapy is a form of short-term therapy that averages five to ten sessions. This approach was developed by Steve De Shazer and Insoo Kim Berg in the 1970s at the Milwaukee Brief Family Therapy Center. While Narrative Therapy is about focusing on the problem without blaming the other person, Solutions-Focused Therapy emphasizes focusing on solutions rather than problems.

Solutions-focused therapy takes the perspective that we don't necessarily need to look at emotionally laden content related to childhood or even the intense emotions triggered in charged situations. Too often, couples focus on negative issues and criticism. Yet John Gottman has found that if the partners say five positive things for every negative, that can have a significant impact on the relationship. Taking a positive perspective also means integrating the solution piece into the discussion.

People usually come into therapy in crisis, at the very least emotionally upset. No one comes to me and says, "Hey, I want to give you this money so I can tell you all about my life and how great things are going." Usually they come in and say, "Hey, here are the challenges I'm facing, and these are all the problems in my life."

What worked in the past? In solutions-focused work, an early step is to acknowledge that the relationship probably wasn't always this way. There were likely times when things were good. Exploring this theme more closely means identifying what was contributing to your well-being—what was the relationship like when things were going really well? This is a shift in focus. Rather than getting bogged down in the problem piece, the emphasis is on recognizing that solutions probably already exist in the relationship. If you identify those strengths and then increase those aspects of the relationship on a day-to-day basis, that will build out the positive facets of the partnership. Essentially, the goal is to co-create a solution, a vision for change that can be agreed on by both partners.

Where is the common ground? As you go through the process, the goal is to find the primary bond in the relationship and the common ground. You're looking for a process that will put the partners back on the same page. That naturally lends itself to better communication and less emotional reactivity. The process also affirms the reason that people became connected in the beginning and the initial core attraction.

Reframing the discussion. In this therapy, reframing or redefining the way in which questions are posed comes down to utmost detail and attention. Open-ended questions are used extensively. The process involves looking for patterns, looking for successes, and how these positive experiences support the vision for change.

Doing the work. Out-of-session homework might be involved, such as practicing using "I" statements rather than "you" statements." With each exercise, the couple rates their success and that of their partner on a scale of one to ten. The therapists actually graph these assessments so you can see where the progress is being made and identify what continues to need attention. That can basically create a map for the therapy as the couple works toward realizing their shared vision of the relationship. The goal is to then scale up that process so that it can be applied more broadly.

The ideal couple for this approach. This particular approach is short-term therapy lasting five to ten sessions, so it's most ideal for people who don't want to delve into emotional issues. The approach is more focused on immediate results with a goal of getting people unstuck, so they don't get bogged down in exploring their childhood or previous relationships. In sum, this approach tends to be more short-term and more practical.

We each have a comfort level that is reflected in how emotionally uncomfortable we're willing to be and for how long. This approach is relevant to those who are more cerebral but want more immediate results, who don't want to feel they have to explore the genesis of their emotional reactivity in childhood or in the relationship.

This process raises fascinating basic questions. What is each of us perceiving? What are we attributing to the other person? What is our own responsibility? How do we find common ground?

To recap these different approaches:

- Gottman basically says that conflict in a relationship can result from patterns that we create, but there are changes we can make right now. Applying these strategies, couples are likely to find some relief and possibly even experience immediate benefit in the relationship.

- Sue Johnson's message focuses on the importance of looking more closely at attachment style. She considers ways in which attachment style may be influencing the communication, and then focuses on modifying that communication.

- Imago therapy connects the present with the past, exploring childhood experiences because the partners seem to be carrying those wounds over into their relationship.

- Narrative therapy takes a closer look at what's happening in the present and then focuses on a larger perspective that concentrates on the problem without blaming each other.

- Solutions-focused couple's therapy is a goal-directed approach that focuses on strengths, skills, coping abilities, and available resources to move the clients toward a future goal.

All these topics are fascinating to me personally. I have been doing this work since I was in my early twenties. What I love about couples therapy are the breakthroughs—those great moments, for example, when a couple looks at each other and just starts laughing. These priceless moments mean that the couple has found their way back to a place of intimacy, when they feel so connected, they know what the other person is thinking. Or they may share an inside joke that warms their hearts and affirms their connection.

In other cases, people will say, "I'm done. I think I'm saturated, I've gotten enough out of this." Or they may acknowledge the complexity of their relationship. In those cases, they may feel overwhelmed and ask for help sorting things out.

In the Bay Area, there is a wide spectrum of humanity and a broad range of styles in how we connect, who we connect to, what is interesting, what is intimate, and what is not. This extensive diversity raises questions of the nature of our agreements and what constitutes a breach of the agreement, what is okay to do and what is not okay. How we navigate that territory, how we negotiate with one another holds an eternal fascination.

For more on the work of Brett Beaver, LMFT, please see:
www.brettbeaver.com.

Chapter 72
How to Listen Better
Brett Beaver, LMFT
Marriage and Family Therapist

There is a difference between listening and waiting for your turn to speak.
— Simon Sinek

If there is one skill above all others that will enhance our opportunities for healthier relationships, it would be listening. Listening is an elusive skill, but worth cultivating because ultimately it is an essential source of power and charisma.

Most couples arrive at my office feeling frustrated about the status of their relationship. Inevitably they are upset with discussions that end up with more discord and less understanding. They feel stuck, angry, stagnant. My role is to create a safe space where they can hone their communication skills and discuss challenging topics with less conflict and more understanding. All couples have core conflicts that pose communication challenges. The key component is assisting them in rekindling their ability to listen to each other. Once this becomes present in their dialogue, the tension decreases, they become more relaxed, and couples remember the connection they are seeking. Listening to each other diffuses conflict and accentuates connection. People feel understood and acknowledged, which affirms the relationship.

QUICK DEFINITIONS OF LISTENING TYPES

DISTRACTED LISTENING

As the name implies, this type of listening happens too often in our relationships. We are engaged elsewhere. Frequently we are intently focused on other than what the person in front of us is saying. We are fleetingly present. We catch pieces of dialogue in our multi-tasking frenzy. We rely on history or previous conversations to assist us with our response.

We probably heard it before—does the conversation merit more focus than a listening drive-by? We reassure ourselves, probably not. And on we go: this becomes the interaction norm with someone we profess to care about—dare we say, love? We have an easier time communicating at work and in other settings. Less hassle, less drama, and no one complains about not being heard. And the topic usually has less emotional content. We have more control in those settings. If it's good enough for others, why is it not sufficient for our significant other?

The cycle repeats. We grow more distant and more frustrated, and suddenly we are one of the divorce statistics, and we wonder how the hell we got here.

What our non-verbal body language looks like to others. When we are listening distractedly, we are looking away from the person, with occasional glances in their direction, probably looking at a technology screen, limited to no eye contact.

What we focus on when listening in this manner. We are predominately focused on ourselves, we are curious about our thoughts and ideas, we are indignant at the audacity of the intrusion, we feel they are impinging upon our right to remain happily self-engaged. We periodically, half-heartedly, toss a comment in their direction that will get them to back off. "Can't they see I am busy"?

What we are communicating to the other person. You are not important, I do not care about you, I do not value you nor what you have to say, I have more important areas of focus that are far more interesting than you, I do not respect you.

Our listening filter calibration. We allow the majority of what is said to pass through without sticking to the listening membrane for further examination, comment, or sorting.

FACT-BASED LISTENING—Focusing on content

We pay closer attention and are less distracted; we may be fully present and engaged (and we may not). We tend to the facts of the conversation, the details. We are interested in the specifics of the story, the content, and this is what we reflect to the person communicating. We share our perspective from what we remember about the details. If we ask questions, our line of inquiry focuses on getting additional facts or clarifying the points we understand. We believe the best way for a person to feel heard is to give them back the information they shared.

What our non-verbal body language looks like to others. We are looking at the person, maybe our body is aligned so our posture mimics theirs, we nod our head in agreement with the receipt of the information.

What we focus on when listening in this manner. We are focused on the details, the specifics of the content shared, we want to understand the details and a bit of the feeling. However, we are less interested in emotions when listening in this mode.

What we are communicating to the other person. We are conveying interest, we want them to understand their value, we want to get the details correctly, and it matters that we reflect the specifics in an accurate fashion. Yet we inadvertently communicate a sense of fear of stepping into the feeling arena with our over-focus on detail.

Our listening filter. We are calibrated to capture the data in the communication, but feelings and other content passes through without retention.

REFLECTIVE LISTENING—Focusing on both details and emotion

This is a more intimate level of communication. In this communication style, we capture the details of the dialogue, as well as the emotions. We listen to the content and endeavor to identify emotions attached to the information. These feelings may be clearly defined by our partner, or they may be embedded in the detail. In that situation, we venture an educated guess as to the feeling state attached to the communication. Our inquiries are open-ended, eliciting additional information from the speaker. We demonstrate a genuine interest in what they have to say, as well as the emotions attached to the words. This approach invites them to divulge more information. When we guess about the emotion associated with the feeling state, we are demonstrating a willingness to engage on a dual level of communication. This listening/acknowledging invitation helps them understand our interest in all aspects of who they are, thus providing a connection that mutually benefits both parties. Even if we inaccurately identify the predominant emotion(s), we are serving notice of our interest in their emotional world.

Words we might use to convey our interest. Yes, I hear you, that makes sense, interesting, fair enough, yup, uh huh, yeah, tell me more, okay, now I understand, I think I am getting a clearer picture, etc.

What our non-verbal body language looks like to others. Our body language conveys interest, our focus is on the person talking, we are all-in with what they are saying and doing. We are looking directly at them; we are watching their lips move, noticing their body movement, and how they communicate verbally and non-verbally. We are aligned with them, in sync, in cadence, and in rhythm with what they have to say. They feel our presence, our interest in what they are saying. We are with them on the journey, interested, attuned, a valued person conveying our interest in them by paying close attention to what they are communicating. We give affirmative head nods, we acknowledge what they are saying with verbal cues, we tend to them, we nurture our relationship through our listening skills.

What we focus on when listening in this manner. We are tracking content, the facts, the emotions connected to the facts, and the implications.

What we are communicating to the other person. We are letting them know they are important to us, what they have to say matters to us, they have value and are worth the energy and effort it takes for us to focus on them. We are letting them know that we are unafraid to step into the emotional arena. We are willing to venture a guess at the emotions attached to the facts. Even if we guess incorrectly, we are serving notice that the feelings they have are important, worth noting, and there is room in the relationship for this type of dialogue.

Our listening filter. We are calibrated to capture the specifics of the content expressed, as well as the emotions connected to the communication. There is more to capture, more of what is communicated adheres to the fiber of our listening settings. We gather the information related to emotions and content, and we feed this back to them in a thoughtful way. At a natural pause in the communication, we let them know what we have heard them by summarizing the content and identifying the emotions expressed during the conversation.

Action steps/hints

- Find a designated time to create space where you listen, in a renewed fashion, to the content and the emotion in conversation with a primary partner. Consistently set aside time one or two times a week for 30 to 45 minutes to listen without interruption. Recognize that you will not feel immediate success (patience). This will take time. Remain patient.

- When talking to your partner to set up the first meeting, approach this with an inviting, open request and a hopeful tone to set the mood. "I was wondering if you would be open to us sitting down for a bit and catch-up, reconnect, chat about". . . . " "Might we catch up with each other for a moment over the next few days to talk?" Less formally, "Hey, wanna talk sometime soon?"

- Set all distracting mechanisms aside to allow for your undivided attention to intently listen to what your partner shares. Try to find a neutral setting.

- *If you are feeling anxious, awkward, nervous, **it's okay to acknowledge these feelings to yourself and then to share them with your partner.*** The ownership of emotion often eases the tension and creates the opportunity for meaningful dialogue.

- In your conversation, once your meeting has been arranged, remember to use clarifying, open-ended inquiries in response to what they share with you: "Let me know if I've captured the majority of what you said. . . . " "If I might take a moment to summarize. . . . " "May I step in at this moment?" or more directly..." "This is what I heard..." When venturing to connect to an emotion: "I think I heard what you said. . . . " and "I sense that the emotion attached to what you are saying is. . . . " "I'm venturing a guess here regarding the emotion you were feeling. . . . ?" "I am new at this and I was thinking you might have felt or are feeling. . . . "

- As the conversation continues, keep track of emotions that may surge inside you. Strong feelings are normal with those we love.

  Do your best not to let the wave of emotion overwhelm your focus in reflective listening skills.

  Let the first wave of emotion roll over you and let it go. See how the second or third, hopefully, less intense rush of emotion feels. Determine if this diminished emotional wave feels eased enough to allow for a balanced response. Usually, the conversation will flow more comfortably if we resist the temptation to retaliate or counterpoint what they say. Even if we disagree with what they are saying or we feel targeted, resist the urge to retaliate. The time for rebuttal and contesting is later, or never, after reflective listening becomes a consistent mode of conversation in our primary relationship.

- Find the internal strength to remain committed to creating the time and space to listen (patience, persistence, and practice). Overcome the desire to give up, especially if the early attempts are not well received. Do your best not to take what they say personally, so you can avoid activating your survival response (fight, flight, freeze).

- Try again. Go back to the top of this list, and remind yourself of the importance of reflective listening. Overcome your frustration that you were not more successful in learning how to listen and communicate. And try again.

Patience, Persistence, Practice

Reflective listening takes time to learn. We must be *patient* with ourselves and our partner, since this will not be easy. You may feel dismayed, and might experience a level of frustration that suggests this is not worth it. Acknowledge the challenge, accept the frustration, and remain patient with yourself and your partner. As a man, sometimes you need to stand up and face the hurricane.

In the middle of it all, call upon your resources to *persistently* step back into the relationship to create new communication pathways. Do not allow doubt to gain a foothold in your thinking. Focus on the goal of improving your quality of life by elevating the connection between you and your partner.

Practice, practice, practice is essential to realize improved communication in your relationship. Research at the University of London College studied 96 participants given the task of introducing a new behavior into their life. The number of days it took for this new behavior to become habit was between 18 and 254 days. The average was 66 days. Change will not happen overnight, it takes time, and we need to practice persistently to live as healthily as possible for as long as possible.

For more on the work of Brett Beaver, LMFT, please see:
www.brettbeaver.com.
For additional resources, please see
www.TheTwentyFirstCenturyMan.com.

Chapter 73
A Guy's Guide to Menopause
Russell Bartels, MD, Gynecologist

For a woman, menopause can fundamentally alter your relationship with yourself and how you relate to other people. When you talk about it, that pulls the veil off, and then it's not so bad.
— *Jane Ordaz*

As men enter their 40s and 50s, guess what else is happening in their lives around the same time? Most of their wives or girlfriends are experiencing the same thing. So, what is the significance of this you may be wondering, and why is this being discussed in a book all about Optimizing Manhood. I am sure everyone reading this has heard the expression, "happy wife…happy life." Understanding what women go through as they age is helpful in becoming a more insightful and knowledgeable human being and in helping you successfully navigate the journey called life. Happiness comes in many forms and means different things to everyone, but optimizing one's health is critical to achieving happiness in its purest form.

You may be going through your own physical, mental, and hormonal changes, focused on improving how you feel and function, but it is imperative to understand the changes women go through, too. For those in a relationship, this awareness can help you understand why you may be experiencing new frustrations with your partner, and for those of you not in a relationship, you may be able to better interact with women at work and in social settings. You could even become a valuable resource to your buddies, who may confide in you that they are having relationship issues and cannot figure out why.

This chapter will focus on the many physical, functional, and emotional issues women go through as they age, their hormones decline, and their bodies change in ways they hoped would never happen to them. Rest assured, I will also discuss treatments and suggest ways of breaking the ice when it comes to discussing these issues. So here goes a guy's guide to menopause.

MENOPAUSE DEFINED

Menopause is the point in life when a woman will no longer menstruate (have periods) and is therefore no longer fertile. Women are generally considered to have reached menopause when they have gone a year without a period. I should point out that a woman's period is the result of a hormonal symphony being played by the ovaries to the uterus, and when the symphony is over, the periods stop as a result. When the ovaries stop producing the hormones estrogen and progesterone, a woman no longer has periods and is considered menopausal. However, many women have had their uterus removed for one reason or another or had a procedure called an endometrial ablation to stop their periods prior to reaching menopause, and therefore will no longer have periods to help them understand when they have entered menopause.

Timeline

Surgical menopause. If both ovaries were removed at the time of hysterectomy during a woman's reproductive years, she will enter surgical menopause at the time of surgery. However, if her ovaries are still producing hormones, at some point down the road, the ovaries will stop producing hormones, and these women will become menopausal.

Ovarian (natural) menopause. Hormonal changes can start as early as the mid to late 30s for some women, but most experience hormonal fluctuations in their mid to late 40s and enter menopause by the age of 52 on average. How these hormonal changes affect a woman is varied, and although there are many common symptoms, each woman has a unique journey through this sometimes-difficult part of life.

One of the first signs of hormonal changes in a woman still having periods is the timing of those periods as well as the amount of bleeding. Eventually the interval between periods becomes longer or shorter and the amount of bleeding lighter or heavier than usual. This irregular bleeding pattern is one of the main reasons women visit their gynecologist. Although most irregular bleeding in the 40 to 50 age group is due to declining ovarian hormone production, it is important to evaluate for other, perhaps more serious, issues such as uterine or cervical polyps, fibroid tumors, or cancers of the uterus, cervix, or vagina. If the bleeding pattern is determined to be the result of hormonal decline and is bothersome due to increased frequency of bleeding or much heavier flow than is tolerable, an endometrial ablation may be suggested. This is a simple procedure, usually performed in the office with sedation and without incisions, which can greatly reduce the amount of bleeding, and in many women, this completely stops the periods. Sometimes a hysterectomy is recommended if the bleeding irregularity is from an enlarged uterus due to fibroids or a condition called adenomyosis. Sometimes the ovaries are removed at the time of hysterectomy, but sometimes they are left in place if the woman decides to keep them after discussing the pros and cons with her gynecologist.

Some women choose to "ride out the storm" and only seek reassurance from their gynecologist that what they are experiencing, although bothersome, is normal and not indicative of underlying medical concerns, while others search for solutions, be that through lifestyle changes, herbal remedies, hormone replacement, or intimate rejuvenation procedures.

Symptoms

As a woman gets further into the years of hormonal decline, new symptoms may arise in addition to an irregular bleeding pattern. Believe it or not, these symptoms of menopause are remarkably like the symptoms of male andropause. So many of the bothersome things you may be experiencing as a man, she may be experiencing, too.

The most common complaints that women report as they transition into menopause are weight gain and fatigue.

As hormones decline, many women report that they gain weight around the midsection and take on a pear shape. They complain of being tired, sometimes due to poor sleep resulting from diminished hormones responsible for healthy sleep patterns or bothersome night sweats that keep them awake. This fatigue can lead to a lack of motivation, which in turn can lead to less exercise and a craving for unhealthy comfort foods.

To summarize and expand on the above discussion, here is a list of common symptoms of menopause. You may recognize them as symptoms you, too, are suffering from as you go through andropause. That is because men and women go through similar changes, but perhaps at different times, with variable severity, and at a different pace:

- Poor quality sleep/insomnia
- Fatigue
- Loss of libido
- Migraines/headaches
- Short-term memory loss or difficulty concentrating
- Weight gain/abdominal fat
- Loss of muscle strength
- Loss of muscle size and tone

- Loss of stamina

- Poor balance

- Arthritis

- Hair loss

- Hot flashes

- Loss of skin tone, sagging, and wrinkles

- Loss of color in facial skin

- Anxiety/irritability/depression

- Loss of motivation and quality of life

- Dry skin

- Dry eyes

- Feeling hot when others are cold

- Loss of sensation in the nipples

- Loss of pubic hair

- Loss of self esteem.

LONG-TERM HEALTH RISKS OF MENOPAUSE

As the hormones continue to decline, other symptoms may pile on, making the experience even worse. Unbearable and random sweating episodes commonly referred to as hot flashes can make life miserable. Nothing says cool, calm, and collected more than a major hot flash and sweating episode in the middle of an office meeting! This can be quite embarrassing, in addition to the sheer unpleasantness of it. Hormone decline has also been associated with the following conditions in both men and women:

- New onset of migraine headaches

- New onset of auto-immune diseases (rheumatoid arthritis, multiple sclerosis, lupus)

- Dementia and Alzheimer's disease

- Parkinson's disease

- Osteopenia/osteoporosis

- Fibromyalgia
- Chronic fatigue syndrome
- Muscle wasting and frailty
- Heart disease and stroke.

COMMUNICATION

Most of us don't realize the vital role our sex hormones play until they begin dropping, reducing our physical strength, mental sharpness, and heart health. So, you can see where all this is going unless corrective action is taken. Perhaps you have recognized some of these perimenopausal and menopausal issues affecting your wife, girlfriend, or friend. What should you do? What is the next step? This can be tricky and must be handled appropriately, with love, concern, and tact.

Self-care. Often, the woman suffering from one or more of these menopausal issues will seek help on her own, most often from her gynecologist. Hopefully that doctor is not just focused on yearly well-woman exams and delivering babies, but has expertise in menopausal management and hormone replacement therapy. It takes a certain knowledge base and skillset to optimize the menopausal woman.

Second Opinion. If a woman is not making progress with that doctor, she should seek out another for a second opinion.

Empathy. If your wife or girlfriend is suffering from any of the symptoms discussed herein and not seeking the help that you know she needs, then you may have to nudge the process along. You must figure out an approach that suits her. I am sure you have been asked by her at one point, "Do I look fat in this outfit?" Well, that scenario can pale in comparison to the can of worms you could open by suggesting that she has been moody, gained 15 pounds, and never wants to have sex with you! So, be careful how you bring this up.

As I have mentioned already, you are most likely going through some hormonal and aging issues yourself at this point in life. One approach is to emphasize what you are going through and how you plan on seeing a hormone and age management expert. Perhaps she will jump in and say that she wants to seek help for what she is going through, too. That would be the easiest way.

Role modeling. If she does decide to wait, you may start the process and make improvements in your own health and lifestyle. Once you start getting in shape and expressing to her how much better you feel and function, perhaps that will get her involved in addressing her issues, too. You may even leave some educational brochures around the house which emphasize the benefits of hormone replacement for men and women and see if she is interested. If all else fails, you actually might have to open that can of worms and say that you have noticed changes in her that seem to be affecting her and subsequently your relationship, and that you want to work on these things with her.

Finding a provider skilled at hormone optimization. Let us now discuss solutions to these many issues. I am passionate about optimizing hormones first and foremost. This is where it is extremely important to seek out an expert in bioidentical hormone replacement therapy. Unfortunately, there are countless uninformed doctors who give bad advice on this topic. They may be great at advising their patients on managing cholesterol, treating a cold, or doing yearly physical exams, but lack training in hormone replacement therapy. Instead of suggesting the patient seek out an expert in hormone replacement, they instead just give bad advice, like bioidentical hormones cause cancer (controversial at best) or that she does not need them (yes, she does).

When asked by a patient about a topic I am not knowledgeable on, for example knee pain, I do not tell them that therapy for knee pain is bad and that they do not need to treat it. Instead, I give them the name of a colleague who can properly evaluate and treat that issue. So please seek out the best hormone replacement and age management doctors you can find, with the following criteria in mind:

- Training and skillset

- Advanced certifications and credentials

- Bedside manner: Is your partner comfortable discussing intimate personal information with this provider?

HORMONE REPLACEMENT

Hormone replacement can mean different things to different doctors and patients. In describing the basic tests that I perform, many are provided by a major laboratory such as LabCorp and Quest and many are covered by insurance. That said, I encourage you to perform due diligence in learning which tests are covered.

Laboratory testing. I suggest checking at least the following lab tests:

- Estradiol

- Progesterone

- Testosterone (Free and Total)

- Thyroid.

Additional useful labs. These are not the only hormones, and some doctors will check others such as:

- Pregnenolone
- Sex hormone binding globulin (SHBG)
- Estriol
- Follicle stimulating hormone (FSH) and luteinizing hormone (LH).

Lab work for vitamin levels and food sensitivities. I am also a proponent of checking vitamin D and B12, but an in-depth vitamin and mineral evaluation along with food sensitivity testing can be extremely helpful in diagnosing certain conditions such as leaky gut syndrome, which can be associated with digestive disorders or frequent fatigue.

- DHEA-S
- Vitamin D
- B12
- In-depth vitamin and mineral evaluation
- Food sensitivity testing.

Thyroid labs. When checking testosterone, it is important to check the free and total values. It is the free form of testosterone that you feel and function on. Similarly, when checking thyroid levels, you want to check free T3, free T4, TSH, and sometimes reverse T3 and thyroid antibodies (not just TSH as so many providers do):

- Free T3
- Free T4
- Reverse T3
- Thyroid stimulating hormone (TSH)
- Thyroid antibodies.

Making Sense of the Lab Tests. Now that the labs have been processed, it is time to interpret them. This is the critical part of formulating a plan. It is imperative that the provider listen to what the patient is suffering from and interpret the lab results with this in mind. For example, not every woman with a low-end estradiol level will complain of hot flashes or vaginal dryness, and perhaps will do fine without supplementing it.

Along that line of thinking, boosting a testosterone level higher than the normal range may be the perfect solution for a woman with low sex drive and fatigue. You read that correctly: women can benefit in many ways from boosting testosterone levels. Testosterone is not just for men, but, when used in women, is prescribed in much lower doses. Hormone replacement comes in many forms: oral pills, troches dissolved under the tongue, topical creams and gels, skin patches, injections, and small pellets placed under the skin lasting 3 to 4 months at a time. Hopefully, the treating practitioner offers all forms to choose from.

Optimizing nutrients. Just being in the normal range is not good enough for many patients. The goal is optimization! Being at the bottom of the normal range is like getting a D-. You can graduate with a D-, but your life opportunities may not be as great as if you got an A. Similarly, you can drag those extra pounds around and get through life, but how about boosting that low (but normal) thyroid level to the top? You are much more likely to feel better and lose the extra weight. If after a few months it does not seem to be the answer, then stop if you want. It often takes some trial and error to optimize your health, as not everyone responds to interventions in the same ways. This is okay because hormone therapy is safe and certainly not a one-size-fits-all type of approach. Whatever the initial hormone recommendation, follow up with labs and discussion. Resolution of bothersome symptoms and possible side effects is imperative to optimize outcomes. If things are not going in the right direction, do not just give up…follow up with the physician for an adjustment in the regimen.

COMPLEMENTARY TREATMENTS

An in-depth discussion of all the hormones and what each is used for is beyond the scope of this chapter, but hopefully hormone optimization corrects many of the bothersome issues. However, there are other treatments and solutions that can stand alone or act synergistically with hormone therapy to correct many of the menopausal symptoms such as bladder leaking, vaginal laxity, vaginal dryness, painful sex, low libido, and/or diminished orgasms. Healthy food and enjoyable exercise cannot be overlooked and are also vital to feel and function the best one can.

Mood swings. It is not uncommon for women to experience moodiness, irritability, anxiety, depression, brain fog, and/or lower self-esteem and confidence during menopause. These psychological issues can be the result of the direct effect of hormonal changes on the brain, and indirectly, they also reflect how a woman feels about her body's physical decline in appearance and function.

> *It is no surprise that many perimenopausal and menopausal women are prescribed antidepressant medications. I would suggest that these women would be better served with hormone replacement instead.*

Bladder issues. As women age and hormones decline, many suffer from bladder dysfunction. This can manifest in several ways, but urinary frequency and urgency are the most common, along with leaking associated with coughing, sneezing, exercise, or just standing up from the seated position. Bladder problems like this can be quite frustrating and embarrassing. Mundane occasions such as long car rides, business meetings, and exercising can become problematic and anxiety-causing events. Furthermore, many women decrease or stop exercising due to bladder dysfunction, which in turn leads to more weight gain.

Decreased libido. Low sex drive is also a common symptom of the perimenopausal and menopausal years. This can be due to a few issues. First and foremost, the decline in hormones leads to an actual physiologic decrease in sexual energy and desire. Secondly, the lack of hormones leads to vaginal dryness which makes sexual intercourse uncomfortable. Thirdly, orgasm can be harder to reach due to reasons one and two. It is not uncommon for the clitoris to shrink and be less sensitive as hormone levels drop. Also, bladder leakage during sex may be embarrassing and messy enough that a woman avoids having sex.

I'm going to offer another reason here, one you may not want to hear, but you may be getting fat and out of shape, suffering from erectile dysfunction, taking longer to orgasm, and just no longer making her feel sexy and wanted. Does it make sense now that a perimenopausal or menopausal woman may not want much to do with sex? Why would she want to have sex when her natural desire is diminished, it physically hurts to engage in sex, she may not experience orgasm, and quite frankly, you may not be the attractive, caring, and loving Adonis you once were! This, and many other issues of aging, are a two-way street. Both men and women need to be participants in the solution.

Vaginal laxity. To be quite blunt, vaginal looseness is another issue menopausal women may suffer from. This issue is not necessarily associated with menopause, and in fact many women in their 20s to 40s may experience this unfortunate, but all too common condition as a result of childbirth. However, as women reach the menopausal years, the natural support of the vagina, which lends itself to a snugger environment, begins to deteriorate. And to add insult to injury, the lack of hormones makes the skin of the vagina less plush and robust.

When vaginal support is compromised, vaginal looseness and diminished sexual friction and pleasure are not necessarily the only problems. Some women may experience a prolapsing of the bladder, uterus, or the top of the vagina if the uterus has been removed. She may feel like something is falling out of her vagina. This can result in pelvic discomfort, bladder dysfunction mentioned earlier, difficult sexual penetration, and a degree of embarrassment and shame. If a woman feels sexually unattractive, she is less likely to want to engage in sexual activities.

This leads into another issue, not necessarily linked to menopause, and possible at any age. That issue is a woman's concern with the appearance of her genitals. In menopause, there can be some visible changes due to a loss of hormones leading to a saggy appearance. Some women are bothered, physically, mentally, or both, by what they perceive to be large labia, or lips. For some women, this can be a barrier to intimacy.

NONSURGICAL TREATMENTS

In-office nonsurgical treatments such as FemiLift (CO2 Laser), Viveve (radiofrequency), Cliovana (low-intensity pulsewave), and the O-Shot (Platelet Rich Plasma) can be excellent options, individually or in combination, to rejuvenate and elevate a woman's intimate health and take sex to a whole new level.

FemiLift is one of several CO2 lasers available for female intimate health. It is performed in the doctor's office three times. Each session is about 10 minutes long and they are spaced a month apart. The procedure is quite tolerable and is performed while the patient is awake. It is used to minimize overactive bladder symptoms and mild bladder leaking that occurs with exertion and to treat vaginal dryness and painful intercourse associated with dryness. Some women report more enjoyable sex from the resulting vaginal snugging effect. This laser can also be used on the external genitalia to impart a more youthful appearance.

Viveve is one of several radiofrequency devices used for feminine rejuvenation. It, too, is performed in the doctor's office and is basically painless. One 40-minute session is done to tighten the vagina (for increased sexual pleasure for both partners), decrease exertional bladder leaking, increase vaginal lubrication, and can be used externally to tighten saggy external labial skin.

As you can see, there is a fair amount of overlap between the Viveve and FemiLift procedures. A discussion about the most bothersome symptoms will help the doctor guide the patient to the right procedure. In certain circumstances, both treatments may be performed to enhance results.

Cliovana uses low-intensity shockwaves to enhance clitoral sensitivity and the orgasmic response. These shockwaves of energy are painless, and the procedure has been described as extremely tolerable. This treatment option takes 10 minutes and is performed twice weekly over two weeks for a total of 4 sessions. (A similar treatment is available for men to treat erectile dysfunction. GAINSWave and Precision ED Solution are brand name examples).

The O-Shot, generically known as an injection of Platelet Rich Plasma (PRP), has several uses. It is done in the office after applying a potent numbing cream in the vagina and over the clitoris. This is also very well tolerated. If a leaky bladder is the problem, the PRP is injected into the anterior wall of the vagina in an area that supports the urethra (the tube through which urine flows). Injecting into this area also rejuvenates the G-Spot for enhanced orgasm. Some of the PRP can also be injected into the clitoris to revitalize sensation, (this does not hurt, I promise). PRP has been found to reduce the symptoms of *Lichen sclerosus*, a painful, itchy genital skin condition that can become disfiguring. The O-Shot can be extremely helpful in improving this situation when injected into the affected areas of the genitals.

All the above procedures can be done as stand-alone treatments, but it is not unusual to combine two or more of them depending on the issues to be treated and the severity of the symptoms. In general, the O-Shot pairs well with all the other treatments in order to optimize results.

Surgery. As great as the above-mentioned nonsurgical procedures are, some women will require surgery to achieve the outcomes they desire. Sometimes there is too much laxity of the supportive tissue of the vagina and bladder, such that surgical vaginal tightening, a bladder lift, or bladder sling is necessary to tighten the vagina and decrease bladder leaking. Furthermore, if a woman is unhappy with the look of her labia, surgical removal of the excess skin can be done. Several weeks of recovery time are required after these surgical procedures.

HORMONE OPTIMIZATION

I strongly recommend hormone replacement therapy when appropriate and have seen firsthand how it has truly transformed my patients' physical health, mental outlook, and personal relationships. In so many ways, how we feel and function is a direct result of proper hormone balance, and as we push through our 40s, 50s, and beyond, our hormone levels can change dramatically. These hormonal changes lead to many of the symptoms both men and women complain about as they age. The good news is that more youthful hormone levels can be reestablished with hormone replacement therapy. However, it is critical to seek the advice of a qualified and experienced hormone replacement provider. For me, one of the most rewarding aspects of being a physician is when my patients tell me how amazing they feel, how their relationship with their significant other has improved both emotionally and sexually, and how their mental focus and outlook on life have been enhanced through hormone optimization.

BEING PROACTIVE

Menopause is a huge topic and impossible to explain in its entirety in a few pages, but hopefully this information has been helpful and provides a strong foundation for understanding what the women in your life are experiencing as they age. Furthermore, it is important to step back from your busy schedule and focus on your health and realize that many of the same changes you are going through as an aging man, the women in your life may be experiencing as well.

Be proactive and seek solutions for yourself and find ways to encourage these women to do the same. Having said that, it has been my experience that it is the women who seek help and need to drag the men in their lives to do the same. Don't be *that* guy. I wish you and your loved ones an optimized life…make it happen now.

**For more on the work of Russell Bartels, MD, please see
www.VitalityMDs.com.
For additional resources, please see
www.TheTwentyFirstCenturyMan.com.**

Chapter 74
Can Avoiding Divorce Improve Your Wellbeing?
A Perspective from a Divorce Attorney
Jonathan D. Larose, Esq., MBA

Wherever you go, there you are.
— *Jon Kabat-Zinn*

How can avoiding divorce improve your well-being? The truth is that divorce could result in your having passionate sex again. Divorce could leave you feeling great and looking good.

You already know that stress can sap your spirit and erode your mental and physical health. Divorce can eviscerate that stress. Divorce can get you back to being the person you were, before you married. Divorce can enhance the quality of your life. The truth is that divorce can save you.

More truth. Marriage can enhance your life. Marriage can provide a nuanced emotional experience that we humans may not be able to duplicate in any other life-setting. Marriage can help you grow as a person. Your mental and physical health can improve. You may be more able to meet your professional and financial objectives. You may live longer, married. Marriage can help you evolve in ways being alone may never achieve.

Great sex and marriage? Let's just agree that only a dumb-ass expects to have great sex throughout marriage. That is, your traditional definition of "great sex." You know, the definition we locked down around 30 years of age. That kind of sex was fortified by the pillars of "passion" and "lust." You know as well as I do—marriage is not primarily about "passion" or "lust," at least not marriages over 15 years in duration. Passion and lust are not emotions marriage can sustain at a high level, long term.

Marriage, however, is much more than that. Marriage is about "connection." It is about "depth" and "intimacy" and "vulnerability." It is about "expression" and "sharing" and "being." It is about "adjustment" and "expectations." The truth is that marriage can provide a transcendent alternative to "passion" or "lust" by offering you different, but sustaining, ranges of experiences.

If you are still reading this, then you are likely married. Great. I am as well, just passing my 25-year marital anniversary.

I am also a divorce attorney. I enjoy what I do and am good at it. Business associations and marriages need attorneys, at times, to unwind them. I unwind marriages.

My clients have already made their decision by the time they come to me. Their reasons to divorce are complex and myriad. To do my job I really do not need to know the minute details of how their partnership went off the rails. Still, I do get to know my clients in ways others may not. That is just the unique nature of the issues that are covered in a divorce.

I have heard a lot in over twenty years of practice. There is rarely one issue that destroys a marriage. Instead, it is usually a combination of issues, some large, some small. Sometimes you can trace problems back to the date of marriage. The longer the marriage, the more complex and nuanced the issues that caused it to die.

I am routinely asked what causes a marriage to end. My answer is usually the same. I have no idea. Every marriage, every relationship, is unique, like a fingerprint. No one can know what any particular marriage really is. The longer the marriage, the more complex the interrelations. That is why offering advice to any person about their marriage can only go so far.

What I have learned is that there are things we can do that may enable our marriages to thrive. Things we can do that may get our marriages through the bumpy times. Nourishment, if you will. Things we can do that could have the additional benefit of improving our overall well-being. What we can do to give our marriages the best shot at success, and additional steps we can take to invest in our marriage:

1. Talk. We need to regularly talk the way we did when we were dating. Deep talks. Long talks. Regular talks. We need dates to just talk. We need to talk aspirations, finances, goals, politics, gossip, friends, family, religion. There can be no excuses not to find time to talk. Children are not an excuse not to talk. Children benefit from seeing us talk. These talks need to happen every week, or more.

2. Listen. Really listen. Active, intense listening. (I know that is not easy. We live in a very noisy world. We have a lot going on in our heads all day long.) Figure out what you need to do to ensure that you are really listening. I try to approach listening to my partner as a form of sexual foreplay. Intense. Focused.

3. Get fit and look good. Get and stay in shape. You will be more confident. You may be happier about yourself and life overall. You may ward off disease. You may live longer. Your partner will be more attracted to you. You will be more interested in sex. Exercise. Eat well.

If you like to eat, exercise some more. Use whatever medicine has to provide including plastic surgery. Wealth is wonderful, but it is not a substitute for taking care of your body.

4. Be financially transparent. Endeavor to share everything with your partner. No financial subject should be off limits. Do not take financial liberties you will not allow your spouse to take. Do not incur material debt without advanced approval by your spouse.

5. Challenge yourself sexually. Live to have sex. Age, health, and familiarity bring challenges. Get over it. Your partner is your chosen sex partner. Don't hold back. Explore. Use whatever medicine or anything else at hand to position you to have satisfying sex. Do your best to be candid with your partner. If it brings you pleasure, nothing should be off limits. If it brings your partner pleasure, nothing should be off limits. Flirt. Compliment. Seduce.

6. Stay fit, mentally. Manage negative emotions like anger with all that will work. Be aware of, and treat, addictions. Never, ever use any form of violence with your partner or children. Narcissism comes in all shapes and sizes: remember that you have a marital partner, so it is about the personal and professional growth of both of you, and not just you.

7. Marital agreements. During marriage, in writing, gift each other something that each clearly owns outright.

8. Vices. Err on the side of caution: If you gamble, assume it's an addiction and approach it as such. If you shop excessively, assume it's an addiction and approach it as such. If you use drugs, including alcohol, more than twice a week, assume it's an addiction and approach it as such.

9. Challenge yourself professionally. Do all you can to avoid work that does not bring you pleasure. Do all you can to help your partner avoid work that does not bring them pleasure.

10. Share a major, regular activity. Golf. Tennis. Working Out. Church. Investing. These are regular activities you can share together. It does not mean you have to golf together. She can golf with her friends and you with your friends. It is the sharing of the subject matter that is vital.

Divorced? If we are married, our well-being is connected to the level of satisfaction we have about our marriage. Avoiding divorce will not improve your well-being. Divorce may be necessary when structural issues, like mistrust, cannot be overcome, or when the relationship just no longer meets expectations.

The truth is that divorce may save your life. Divorce may restore your libido and your interest in sex. If you have children, divorce may improve the quality of their lives. They may even like you more. You will take better care of yourself after a divorce, much as you did before you married.

Or happily married. On the other hand, marriage can provide a sustaining experience that "passion" cannot. Seek ways to maximize all that marriage has to offer. Put yourself in a position for success at every level. That means you need to put in the effort. Marriage is a partnership, and it is best managed, over time, actively, not passively. Active participation is the best way to realize the maximum return on your marital investment. We can invest in our marriage by taking steps to improve it. We can make behavioral adjustments that could enhance the quality of our marriage.

A mutually satisfying marriage can improve your wellbeing. The payoff could well be the attainment of the marriage you expected.

For more on the work of Jonathan Larose, JD, please see:
jdlaroselaw.com.
For additional resources, please see
www.TheTwentyFirstCenturyMan.com.

Chapter 75
Fatherhood
Armin Brott, Medical Writer

Not every successful man is a good father.
But every good father is a successful man.
— Robert Duvall

A man who's just found out that his partner is expecting is clearly very different from the kind of man he'll be when he first holds his newborn in his arms. And, as you might guess, that brand-new dad will have grown tremendously by the time his baby speaks his first words, and he'll keep changing and developing as that same child takes his first steps, gets potty-trained, and starts preschool.

The process doesn't end there—in fact, it never does. Fatherhood is a process that ends only with the death of the father. Fathers continue to change every day, as their children hit puberty, learn to drive, move out, have kids of their own, move back home, and perhaps eventually reverse the roles and care for the father. But no matter how old his children are or where they live, a father is always a father.

So how do dads change over the course of lifelong fatherhood? Many say that being a dad has given their life new meaning and direction. Others say that having children, interacting with them, getting to know them, teaching them, guiding them, being an active part of their lives, and generally dealing with the joys and frustrations of parenthood have made them:

- More patient, understanding, and empathetic

- More aware of their own strengths and flaws and more tolerant of those of others

- More flexible and better able to prepare contingency plans

- More concerned about making the world a better place

- Better able to see and appreciate things from others' perspectives

- A better husband, friend, employee, employer, and person in general

- Emotionally deeper, and better able to experience and express unconditional love as well as many other emotions they'd rarely or never felt

- Restructure their priorities, placing family and children above work and personal advancement

- Proud—of their children's accomplishments and of their own role in helping their children achieve them

- Able to slow down, enjoy life, and have more fun

- Healthier and less likely to engage in risky or dangerous behavior

- Smarter, because it turns out that you can go back and learn all those things you didn't get to when you were a kid.

RECALIBRATING YOUR LIFE

Before I had kids, I worked as a commodities trader, a labor negotiator, and a trade consultant—the kind of jobs you get with an MBA, which I have buried someplace in my attic. But before my first child was even born, I'd already reached the conclusion that being in business and being an involved dad—at least the way I wanted to do it—weren't entirely compatible. I'd published a few articles, and in a moment of feverish optimism, I quit my job to write full-time, which gave me the time with my daughter that I wanted.

I'm certainly not the only father to make dramatic kid-related career moves. Actor Ewan McGregor cut his schedule way back because of his daughter. And former secretary of labor Robert Reich gave up "the best job I've ever had and probably ever will" to spend more time with his family.

Okay, I realize that fatherhood isn't going have as dramatic an impact on everyone's career as it did on mine (and McGregor's and Reich's). In fact, making that kind of career transition isn't practical, or even desirable, for most dads. For some, the changes are more subtle. Here's how a U. S. postal worker, for example, reacted when he was told he'd have to work nights: "I told them I could not work nights because I had a ten-year-old son, and I am a single parent. Being with my son two days a week is not a good way to be a parent."

Not everyone responds to fatherhood by making changes at work. But I have yet to talk to a man who didn't change his life in at least some ways after becoming a father, ways he never would have considered if he hadn't had kids.

WHY BE INVOLVED WITH YOUR CHILD?

Simple. Because the more involved you are in raising your children, the better father you'll be. Being an involved father is good for everyone: your kids, your partner, and even yourself. On the pages that follow, I'm going to dig into some of the specific benefits associated with being actively involved with teen and adult children (I'm focusing on those age groups because most of the guys reading this book are beyond the infant, toddler, and preschooler phase. If you're looking for info on the benefits to being involved with younger children, you'll find a list of my relevant books on my website, www.MrDad.com).

Benefits for Your Teen

- *They're less likely to have sex early.* For example, girls who perceived their biological father as more caring are more likely to postpone their first consensual sexual experience, have fewer male sexual partners before age nineteen, and are less likely to become teen mothers.

- *Increased autonomy and independence.* Fathers are more likely than mothers to encourage teens' independence.

- *They'll go further in life.* Fathers who praise and express pleasure over their children's achievements have children who set their educational goals higher, according to T. E. Smith. In addition, John Snarey found that strong father-child relationships were a big predictor of the child's (boy or girl) later academic and career success.

- *More secure gender identity.* When dads are warm and affectionate, boys grow up with a healthier sense of their own masculinity and girls with a more secure sense of their femininity. Conversely, boys who have little contact may become too dependent on their mothers, says researcher Neil Kalter. That can make them grow up doubting their masculinity. The consequences of this self-doubt are often devastating. A large percentage of boys in prison or involved in gang activity, for example, grew up without a father in the home.

- *Better mental and physical health.* The more their dads are positively involved in their lives, the better kids feel about themselves. Teens who have positive relationships with their fathers (whether they live with them or not) are less likely to have emotional or psychological problems, and are less likely to be sick overall. Adolescent girls, for instance, who are involved in sports are less likely to drop out of school, get pregnant, develop eating disorders, put up with abusive relationships, smoke, drink, or develop breast cancer as adults.

- *Fewer behavioral problems.* Whether kids live with their father or not, a high level of paternal involvement is associated with fewer adolescent behavioral problems, according to Princeton University researcher Marcia Carlson. In addition, adolescents with less involved fathers (or those living with no father at all) are nearly 2.5 times more likely to have used illegal drugs or alcohol.

- *Fewer eating disorders.* Girls with involved, supportive dads are less likely to be bulimic or anorexic. Fathers of women and girls who have eating disorders tend to have an excessive concern about their daughter's weight and body image, to a greater extent than fathers of girls who don't have these issues.

- *They'll be more empathetic adults.* Several long-term studies have found that how compassionate adults (men and women) are and how well they are able to experience others' feelings depends more than anything else on how involved their fathers were during the preschool years.

- *It may make them more popular, assertive, and resilient.* Children (daughters in particular) who are exposed to high levels of paternal play and attention are more popular and assertive with their peers later in adolescence. They're more likely to make friends, and they keep those friendships longer. On the other hand, kids whose fathers are too intrusive and authoritarian tend to be the ones who get rejected by their peers. Studies by Ross Parke and others of extremely successful women have shown that they're more likely than less successful women to have had a high level of paternal support, stimulation, and high expectations from Dad. And other researchers have found that regardless of gender, kids who had warm and loving fathers when they were five years old had longer marriages, were better parents, and had closer friendships as adults.

- *They stay in school longer.* Compared to kids growing up in families without a father, kids with involved dads had half the risk of dropping out of high school. They also had higher test scores, higher GPAs, better school attendance, and higher college expectations.

- *Life is easier for difficult kids.* Hard-to-handle kids and those with learning disabilities have higher feelings of self-esteem and well-being when their fathers are involved in their lives vs. similar kids whose dads aren't as involved.

- *It helps minimize the effects of divorce.* After their parents separate, about a third of children suffer a decrease in academic performance. Even after the divorce, kids with a good ongoing relationship with their father do better in school and have fewer social, emotional, and physical problems than kids who don't see their fathers as much.

What No One Wants to Admit About Fatherhood

One of the horrid little secrets about fatherhood is that sometimes it's just not fun. I know, I know, I shouldn't say things like that, but it's true. Throughout our children's lives, all parents have the occasional why-did-I-ever-have-kids? day. But during the teen years it's not uncommon for dads to watch helplessly as those days sometimes blimp into weeks and then months. Roger Gould found very much the same thing in his landmark studies back in the late 1970s. The teen years, he said, will likely be the least satisfying time of your life as a father. (They're not going to be that much fun for your teen either.) It's nothing to be embarrassed about, I assure you. The only people who don't go through this are those who don't have kids.

Of course, there's all the head-butting that dads and teens do. But at the same time, your child's teen years are a time of real growth and self-examination for you. It's during this stage that the aging process will really sink in. Before now you knew you were getting older because you kept having birthdays, and you stopped getting carded at grocery stores and bars, but you probably didn't feel much different from when you were twenty. But get ready, because this is gradually starting to change—you'll have a few more aches and pains that you didn't before, and it might take a little longer to recover from your weekend basketball game with your buddies. At the same time, you'll watch with envy as your teen steps into a world of unlimited possibilities and choices, and you'll become aware that your options are far more limited. Your teen's largely responsibility-free life is in sharp contrast to your life, which is filled with work, mortgage payments, carpools, and other obligations. They're entering their physical and sexual prime, and you're leaving yours. And as they look toward the future, you can't help but reevaluate the past.

YOUR EVER-CHANGING RELATIONSHIP WITH YOUR CHILD

One of these days, the moment you've hoped for and dreaded is finally going to come. Your child is going to move out. Some researchers have called this the beginning of the "post-parental stage," but I think that's a mistake. Yes, your child is leaving, but that doesn't mean you're going to stop being a parent. In fact, you're just getting started on the longest phase of your fathering experience.

You're going to miss her, and it'll probably take you some time to adjust to your newly empty nest (unless you're in what Craig Roberts and Kaye Zuengler call the "quasi-post-parental stage," which is when you've launched some but not all of your children). It'll also take you some time to get used to your new relationship with your child and with your partner. If you were a very hands-on, involved dad up till now, it may be hard to adjust to your child being gone. If you weren't around that much, having him or her leave home might be even harder because it's unlikely that you'll ever be able to develop that close a relationship.

Overall, having your child leave home will be a good thing for you. (Of course, this could be a case of what you don't know won't worry you. Either way, it's going to be a relief not to have to worry about so much so often.)

As in every other stage of your child's development, his or her struggle for independence is central. But there's a difference between independence at this stage and independence at any other stage. One of the biggest changes in your relationship with your child is that the relationship itself has gone from involuntary to voluntary; as long as she was living under your roof, your child had to live by your rules, and had to have contact with you, whether they wanted to or not. Now they don't. Interestingly, once your child has successfully proven they don't need you, they may feel that it's safe to turn to you for advice again. Asking when they were a teen would have been an acknowledgment of their dependence on you. Now, though, they can do it on their own terms.

Just because the kids have moved out doesn't mean that you're not a parent anymore or that you're not still evolving both as a father and as a man. In a sense you're entering a whole new phase of life. Unless your child has moved back home or hasn't left at all, the years of active parenting are pretty much behind you, the nest is empty, and it's just you and your partner now. This can be a period of great excitement, a second honeymoon of sorts, a peaceful interlude when you and your partner can spend time with each other, get to know each other again, and plan out your future. It can also be a scary period when you'll have to decide what to do with all the free time you have on your hands, an opportunity to wonder who this person is that you're married to and what the two of you have in common now that the children have left home. Most importantly, though, it's a time when you'll be reevaluating who you are. Your relationships with your children have changed, and you're no longer the most important adult in their lives. But you're still a father—it's just a question of figuring out what that means.

Staying Involved with Your Adult Child

The best way to be involved at this stage is to do it from a short distance. Give them the autonomy they need to grow and develop on their own, but make sure they know that the door's always open if they really need you.

- *Don't sell the house just yet.* They may be gone, but they may be back in a year or two. And even if they are not planning to come back, their new place may not be big enough for all the stuff you're going to want them to get out of your basement and attic.

- *Keep in touch.* If you live nearby, try to get together regularly. If you're farther away, set up regular times to talk or e-mail. Either way, make a serious attempt to build a one-on-one relationship with your child that is separate from the one that you and your wife have with her.

- *Ask for advice.* It may seem like a terrible role reversal, but the truth is that your adult kid knows a lot of stuff that you don't. Listen up, and you'll learn a lot.

- *Be a consultant.* If your child gets into trouble, whether it's divorce, bankruptcy, losing a job prospect, dropping out of school, or going to jail, it's going to be incredibly tempting to try to take care of the situation. Don't—at least not right away. There's nothing you can do to keep your child from making mistakes, and if you jump in too quickly and keep them from suffering the consequences of their bad decisions, they'll never grow up.

- *Offer—and let it go at that.* You can't force them to live their life the way you want them to. If they need your help, give them advice, contacts, or whatever they need. But don't do it too often—you don't want them to become (or stay) too dependent on you. Actually, a bigger risk is that if you give too much and are too available, your child may feel that you don't have any confidence that they can do things for themselves. So, ask a lot of questions and encourage them to come to their own conclusions. And whether you agree with the final decision or not, be supportive, not judgmental.

I'm Baaaack . . . When Adult Children Come Back Home

One of the biggest risks to adjusting to a child's leaving is that your young adult might come back. (The title of a book by Stephen Bly, *Just Because They've Left Doesn't Mean They're Gone*, says it all quite well.) All of us have certain preconceived notions about when major life events are supposed to take place, and we have a social clock that rings at the appropriate time. If the clock doesn't go off at the right time, we're likely to feel some stress. Moving out of the house is one of those events, and for most of us, the clock is set for eighteen, which is when the majority of American kids move out.

If a child is going to college at eighteen, we're perfectly content to hit the snooze button and let them hang out at home for a few more years. (You may even be secretly—or not-so-secretly—thrilled to have someone around again who's dependent on you. Or you may be thrilled to have someone around you can be dependent on.) But if they're still home at thirty-five, you're not going to be as happy. If you had plans to retire or to sell your house and spend two years on the road living out of an RV, you may resent them for interfering with your new, more independent lifestyle and for making you be an active parent longer than you wanted to. And you might see them moving back (or never leaving) as a sign of some failure on your—or their—part. In contrast, if the clock goes off too early, say fourteen or fifteen, you might feel that you've done something wrong, that you weren't a caring enough father.

Interestingly, researchers William Aquilino and Khalil Supple found that most parents whose adult children (ages nineteen to thirty-four) live at home are happy with things the way they are. There were, however, two important factors that caused problems. First, the child's being unemployed or financially dependent on the parent increased the chances of parent-child conflict. Second, having a divorced or separated child—especially one with a baby in tow—move back home reduced the parents' satisfaction with the entire living arrangement.

When Your Child Needs Help

As a full-fledged adult, you're in a position to help your child. You've grown up, gotten married (maybe more than once), started a family, had a few jobs, bought a few houses. You've also made a lot of difficult and important decisions in your life; some have turned out well, others not so well. All in all, you can be an excellent resource for your child, especially in one or more of the following areas:

- *General advice.* Things like finding a house or apartment, getting the best deals on cars or computers, and so on.

- *Education and career.* Choice of major, what classes to take, evaluating job prospects, deciding whether to go to grad school, proofreading and sending out résumés, practicing for job interviews, evaluating job opportunities, using your contacts to grease the wheels.

But before we go on, here are a few advice- and help-giving guidelines:

- *You do not have to fix everyone's problems.* It's okay to say, "Gee, that's too bad." Even if you wanted to fix everyone's problems, you couldn't anyway.

- *Your child may not want or even need your help or advice.* Before you jump in, find out.

- *Offer once.* Don't be offended if your advice isn't taken. And banish the words "I told you so" from your vocabulary.

- *Keep your unsolicited advice to a minimum.* If you really think your child needs help, ask. They may not want to call out of fear that you'll think they want something from you, or they may really need something but be too embarrassed to ask for it. The only exception to this is if they're having a real crisis.

- *Keep away from manipulative phrases.* Rather than "You're an adult and you're going to do whatever you want, but I think you should . . ." Instead try, "Here's how I see it," and leave it at that.

- *Be reasonable.* If they don't want to change the oil in their car every 3,000 miles, or they don't eat as much protein as you think they should, it's none of your business.

- *Ask for help or advice if* you *need it.* Your doing so might make your child more receptive.

Embracing the Plan Gone Amok

As we've discussed, your child's growing independence and how the two of you deal with it plays a major role in how you both develop—he or she from a child into an adult, you as you change and grow as a father. Besides that, though, there's another major issue that you've dealt with before and that you'll be dealing with for the rest of your life: the difference between the way you planned or imagined or hoped that your life would turn out and the way it actually is.

The years between about thirty-three and forty are what Daniel Levinson calls the "settling down phase." This is typically the time when fathers (and men in general) focus their energy on taking their place in society: on "making it," on advancing in the workplace, on family and friends, on success. The days of figuring out what you're going to do when you grow up are pretty much gone. You no longer have infinite choices. Any door you open or any choice you make requires closing other doors and missing other opportunities. The worst part about this phase is that each choice makes you grow up a little, and the more you grow up, the more you have to give up. This isn't all bad, of course. For every one door you close, you open a dozen windows—you may lose out on one opportunity, but you'll have all sorts of others you never knew existed.

Are you the kind of über-father you'd imagined you'd be ten years ago?

Had you even planned on being a father at all? Are you able to spend as much time with your family as you want? Do you have the kind of relationship with your kids that you imagined? How does your relationship with your partner compare to the way you thought it would be? Are you living in your dream home in your dream neighborhood? Are you sending your kids to the kind of schools you'd planned on? Are you giving them the life and the things you wanted them to have? Are you keeping the promise you made to yourself when you were a teenager to never, ever raise your kids the way your parents raised you, or have you forgotten and slipped into doing exactly what they did? Do you have the education you wanted? Have you traveled everywhere you wanted to go? And where are you in your career? Are you as far along as you'd hoped? Are you even doing the kind of job you thought you'd be doing?

Your life today may be superlative, or it may . . . not. But no matter what it's like, chances are there are at least a few things about it that have turned out differently than you'd planned—not necessarily better or worse, just different.

The difference between fantasy and reality can cause a tremendous amount of conflict, and there are three basic ways to deal with it. First, you could get absolutely paralyzed and horribly depressed that your life hasn't turned out the way you'd hoped. Second, different or not, you might choose to be perfectly happy with life just the way it is. Third, you can adopt a kind of serenity-prayer attitude: enjoy the things that are going better than expected, accept the things you can't change, fix the things you can, and get clear on the difference between the three options. Life is far from over, and there's still plenty of time to fulfill at least some of those dreams.

BECOMING THE ELDER STATESMAN

Well, it's come to this, the final stage that ends your journey through fatherhood, and your transition from man to husband to father to grandfather, maybe even great-grandfather. To a large extent the relationships you have with your children and grandchildren, and what happens during your grandfather (and great-grandfather) years, will be a reflection of everything that's happened during all of the other stages of fatherhood. But the focus will be a little different.

Whether you're going to be a good father or not isn't going to be as important as whether you've actually been one. Instead of worrying about things like how your kids are going to turn out and whether they'll be able to take care of themselves, you'll think instead about the more distant future, the one that doesn't include you.

So, did you raise decent human beings, people who will do the right thing when they have to? Are you confident that your financial and psychological legacies are safe in the hands of future generations? Will they remember you after you're gone? If so, you've achieved a certain level of immortality. But what if things—and your children—didn't turn out the way you expected or hoped? Will you be able to accept the choices they made, rejoice at their successes, and not feel responsible for their failures?

Why Be an Involved Father and Grandfather?

At this point, you've had about as much influence on your adult child as you possibly can. Your grandchildren, however, are another story—your influence over them is just beginning. In the next few pages, we'll talk about some of the specific ways. Benefits to our children and grandchildren include:

- *Success.* Kids who have close relationships with their grandfathers do better in school, have higher self-esteem, and are more successful at forming and keeping up friendships than kids whose relationships with their grandfathers aren't as close.

- *You can make up for deficits.* If your grandchild's father has abandoned his family or isn't the kind of father he should be, you can provide your grandchild with a positive male role model and teach him—through your own behavior—what it means to be a man in our society.

- *A stronger identity.* As an older person, you have access to your family's history in a way that your grandchild's parents don't. By passing on your family's lore, traditions, and rituals, you're giving your grandchild a link to the past as well as a stronger connection to who he is, where he came from, and his role in the family and the world. This can be tremendously valuable to adolescents during their quest for self-identity.

- *Values and beliefs.* Grandfathers play a key role in transmitting religious beliefs and core values such as the importance of academic and workplace achievement. And by simply being who you are, you'll be teaching your grandchild lessons about things like friendship, loyalty, honesty, and family—lessons they might ignore if they had come from their parents.

■ *A refuge from Mom and Dad.* When your grandchildren hit adolescence, chances are they're going to have a pretty rocky relationship with their parents, which means they'll feel safer talking to you about things they're too embarrassed or angry about to ask their own parents. Just by being there, you allow your grandchild to reject and rebel against their parents while still maintaining an important ally.

■ *Creating respect and empathy for people as they age.* Watching you age (hopefully gracefully) gives your grandchild a great opportunity to see that older people can be smart, active, and engaged. In addition, if you're not divorced or widowed, you're a model to your grandchild of how it's possible to maintain loving relationships over a lifetime.

Benefits to You

■ *A second chance—but with less downside.* A lot of men see grandfathering as a way to compensate for their own guilt over their inadequacies as fathers, says psychiatrist and grandfather expert Stanley Cath. Being a grandfather also gives you a chance to have all the fun of parenting without most of the responsibilities.

■ *A source of pride.* It feels damned nice to know that who your child is and how successful they are in life (and all the other good stuff—none of the bad, of course) is at least partly thanks to you. And it'll feel just as nice to see your child being a good parent and passing along the family values and ideals—just as you taught them.

■ *A connection to the future.* Your grandchild is, in a sense, your legacy. They're your link to the future, the one who will keep a little bit of you alive after you're gone by passing on your philosophy, values, and genes to the next generation.

■ *Reconnecting with your emotions.* Back when your kids were a lot younger, you experienced all sorts of emotions you had never felt before. In the years since then, those emotions have changed and evolved, just as you have. But having a grandchild can reignite those feelings of unconditional love that you haven't felt since your own child was young. You also get a chance to be on the receiving end of unconditional love—something else you haven't felt for a long time. As psychiatrist Kyle Pruett's father once told him:

By this point in my life, I have either made it or not made it, and my grandchildren couldn't care less. They love me without judgment, and I return the favor without a second thought.

CONCLUSION

Although the overall path through fatherhood takes men through some fairly predictable terrain, every man's trip is a little different. Some get started the "traditional" way, having the first of their 2.5 children in their mid- to late twenties, putting the kids through college, marrying them off, becoming grandfathers and possibly even great-grandfathers. Some start earlier, in their teens, while others don't start their families until they're in their forties or fifties. Their experience of the early years of fatherhood will be much different than younger dads', and they'll probably miss out on the grandfather years entirely.

Some men skip the early developmental stages—their own and their children's—and get introduced to fatherhood by step-fathering someone else's children. Some get divorced and raise their kids on their own, while others get cut off from their children's lives. Some adopt, others are widowed; some are married, others not. For a lot of men, the process isn't linear at all; they start off on one trajectory, but may skip and repeat some steps along the way, perhaps even combining two or more at the same time.

All in all, every father—and everyone around him—has a completely unique experience. But whether it's good, bad, or indifferent, one thing is guaranteed: you'll be a father for life, and it will truly be a journey of joy, challenge, and change.

For more on the work of Armin Brott, please see: www.MrDad.com.

The Intangibles of Fatherhood
Judson Brandeis, MD

One summer evening, my wife and I were relaxing with a ginger beer and bag of salt and vinegar kettle chips. Suddenly there was a knock at the door. Bill and Jessica, the young couple who had recently moved in next door, were taking us up on our offer to provide advice. Their question to us really made us think.

An engineer by trade, Bill asked, "I've read a number of studies showing that when couples with children are compared with couples without children, their happiness, quality of life, and finances are all worse than the couples without children. Jessica and I have been thinking about asking you to perform a vasectomy on me. We're thinking about never having children. You have four kids; do you think that it has made you happier?"

Like a typical doctor, I started off talking about biology. "Have you ever seen the movie, The March of the Penguins? Animals are biologically driven to have offspring. Why else would male penguins brave negative 120-degree conditions in the dark for four months with no food to keep an egg warm?"

Jessica leaned in, "However, we're not penguins. We have a choice about whether to have children. We have a good life. We travel, we eat at fancy restaurants, we exercise every day, and we're saving money for retirement. What is it that makes it worthwhile to be parents?"

My wife broached the topic, "Children force you to grow up. They spark memories from your own childhood that can help you reignite your inner work from your youth. Children teach you about yourself."

I nodded in approval, "There is an excitement that children bring to life. We love the joy of seeing things through our kid's eyes. For them, everything is new and interesting. And you get to teach them things like how to read, brush their teeth, and ride a bike. Spending time with kids makes you feel young, and at times brings a unique sense of joy. No amount of money could ever buy that kind of experience.

"I would rather watch my son play 12-year-old basketball than get front row seats to the Warriors. Last year I watched my daughters perform the same dance routine eight different times in one weekend and each time it was a thrill."

My wife chimed back in, "It's just because you see so much of yourself in your children. In fact, my oldest daughter looks so much like me that she can open my iPhone with her face. You want to have children to carry your values into the next generation. You want to see your children make a positive difference in the world. And you are willing to discipline your children and face the repercussions of those difficult decisions to see the seeds of goodness that you have planted in them blossom."

"I agree with everything my wife said. There are some very rough moments that you must suffer through. (We have four teenagers.) Raising kids is like my golf game. I am a lousy golf player, but once or twice every round I hit a perfect shot that keeps me coming back for more. It's those spectacular moments when everything comes together that makes it all worthwhile. I don't think you can achieve those kinds of moments any other way."

I had the sense that Bill and Jessica needed some time to think about our discussion, but my wife and I headed for our children's bedrooms, kissed each of them goodnight, and got ready for another day in the trenches of parenthood.

PART 11
SEXUAL HEALING
Introduction
Judson Brandeis, MD

Some of the saddest patients I see are younger men with prostate cancer who have undergone non-nerve sparing prostate removal. They are potent going into surgery, but they are no longer able to get an erection when they recover. The development of ED can be sudden because, in some cases, the urologic surgeon needs to cut the pelvic nerves to cure a man's cancer. A discussion with one of my patients with ED after prostate cancer surgery prompted me to think about what physical intimacy means to men.

Testosterone's hormonal energy gives a man aggression to pursue his life's work and potential partners. High levels of testosterone drive men toward sexual opportunities, which infuse a man's life with excitement. The instant his partner gets turned on affirms a man's masculinity, and sexual release makes him feel like he is finally home. Sex is a deep and powerful form of intimacy that connects two people beyond the mind and body. A deep and energetic connection that transcends time and space bonds two people when they make love. After dealing with the world's challenges and rejections, physical intimacy embodies acceptance and provides soothing. Making love creates a deep feeling of partner attachment and spurs relational generosity, faith, and optimism. Being desired by a partner can be the single most reassuring part of a man's life.

I enjoy helping men reclaim this aspect of their lives. When grown men come bounding into my office, blushing with a Cheshire Cat grin, and a great story to share with me, I know I'm on the right track. In the sexual healing sections of this book, I reveal much of what I have learned through interactions with physician colleagues and industry innovators. Thousands of discussions with patients of all ages, levels of education, background, and orientations have honed the delivery of my message.

In addition to content on the anatomy and physiology of sexual function, we'll take a closer look at supplements, medications, shockwave therapy, and other regenerative therapies. There is so much to learn beyond the little blue pill! I invite you to immerse yourself in the content provided. It may help you maintain what you already have or reclaim what you once had. Or it may help you go beyond what you thought was possible.

Chapter 76
Sex on the Beach
Judson Brandeis, MD, Urologist

Some of the best moments in life are the ones you can't tell anyone about.
— The 21st Century Man

Jack had been looking forward to this day all year. The first Nantucket lifeguard party of the season was the place to see and be seen. Usually he threw on a crumpled, old T-shirt, board shorts, and flip-flops, but this evening was special. Thinking about the girl in the tangerine bikini he'd seen playing volleyball last weekend, he slipped on a freshly ironed Hawaiian shirt, and he even put some gel in his hair. Finally, at sundown, he could hear a group of his lifeguard buddies drive up, and he raced down the stairs with anticipation.

When they got to the beach, the party had just started, and there was already a line down the block of amped-up summer tourists and locals ready to let loose. Jack and his buddies strutted past the line and slipped into the party. A Jimmy Buffet cover band was cranking out crowd favorites. Within an hour, the party was packed with teens and twenty-somethings. Beer was flowing freely. Exposed skin was everywhere.

Over the music, Jack heard a glass break. He spun around, instinctively looking for the source. It was the girl in the tangerine bikini, looking even more beautiful than she had during the day. Her green eyes shimmered, and her olive skin was flawless. She laughed confidently as several young men scrambled to pick up the shards of broken glass.

Jack felt queasy as butterflies fluttered in his stomach, and what felt like an electric current ran down his spine from his head to his tailbone. Jack was mesmerized. He felt the electricity moving to his pelvis, and his penis started to tingle.

Dr. Brandeis here. Let me put on my white coat so that I can explain what's going on behind the scenes, inside Jack's head and the rest of his body.

An erection—which is where Jack is headed—starts in the brain. Remember how much he was attracted to the gal in the tangerine bikini. The cortex of a guy's brain is 30% visual, so visual cues can be central to getting turned on.

Gracefully, the green-eyed beauty turned her head in Jack's direction. She was so captivating, it took his breath away. Jack could feel his penis begin to grow. The band played "Margaritaville" for the third time that evening, and Jack had to adjust his shorts as he locked eyes with this gorgeous woman. The sexual energy crackled between them.

Getting even more turned on, he awkwardly put his hands in his pockets to reposition his penis so it had more room to grow. This gesture drew a smile from the exotic goddess, as she slowly stood up to reveal her sunbathed, toned body.

At this point, the visual centers of Jack's brain are triggering a cocktail of two potent chemicals—dopamine (the chemistry of pleasure and addiction) and oxytocin (the neurotransmitter of bonding). By pairing the powerful chemistry of pleasure and bonding, nature creates a magnetic attraction that moves two people toward each other.

As Jack's brain is stimulated, dopamine and oxytocin start flowing like ouzo at a Greek wedding. The electrical wave of pleasure that Jack experiences shifts him into the relaxation response. This mode, a state of deep relaxation, is essential for him to get an erection.

The tingling in his groin that he's feeling is the surge of blood into the pelvis, triggered by a release of nitric oxide from pelvic nerves. Nitric oxide is the On Switch that relaxes blood vessels to boost circulation. This increased blood flow into the penis will create Jack's erection.

The surge in nitric oxide leads to the production of another chemical, cGMP (cyclic guanosine monophosphate), in the arteries of Jack's penis. The erection he's about to experience is triggered by cGMP causing a cascade of chemical reactions that expand the arteries in the penis, resulting in a surge of blood flow into the main penile arteries.

The erectile bodies, (the *corpus cavornosa*) shown on the following page, are two cylinders of sponge-like tissue within the penis that fill with blood to create an erection. When Jack's penis is flaccid, it contains just enough blood to stay healthy. An erection increases the amount of blood in the penis by about half a cup.

Watching as she sauntered across the room towards him, Jack took in every step, every subtle movement, every swish of her clothing. In what seemed like an eternity, she was finally standing in front of him. Her perfume was intoxicating, and Jack was at full mast! He could feel his manhood throbbing with the beat of the music.

A full erection can occur in less than a minute. What's more, during an erection, the penis can grow to five times its flaccid size.

The penis is composed of three cylinders nestled together in a tough, elastic sheath of connective tissue (referred to as the tunica or tunica albuginea).

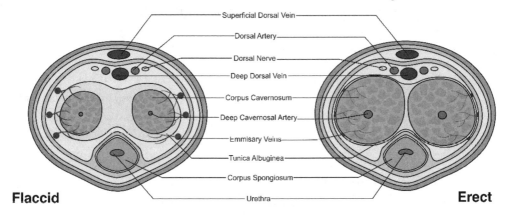

Flaccid

Superficial Dorsal Vein

Dorsal Artery

Dorsal Nerve

Deep Dorsal Vein

Corpus Cavernosum

Deep Cavernosal Artery

Emmisary Veins

Tunica Albuginea

Corpus Spongiosum

Urethra

Erect

Figure 76.1. Cross section of the penis.

Two of these tubes, called erectile bodies (the corpus cavernosa), are substantial in size. Each one is about the thickness of a cigar, and they have an inner structure similar to a sponge. This incredible matrix can absorb and hold a surprising amount of blood.

As the blood flow in Jack's arteries increases, the pressure inside his penis skyrockets. Even the head of his penis (the glans) becomes engorged.

That elevated pressure pinches off the tiny veins that usually carry blood out of the penis. With all the exits blocked, the blood within the penis continues to increase, producing an erection rigid enough for sex.

Jack would vividly remember this night for the rest of his life . . .

Their eyes locked. In a sultry voice, she said, "I'm Stacy . . . . Are you going to stand there, or are you going to get me a drink?" Jack was momentarily speechless. After an awkward silence, Stacy reached out and gently caressed his muscular shoulder. "What are you drinking?" she asked. "I'll have whatever you're having."

An hour later, Jack and Stacy fled the party, seeking the privacy of the Nantucket dunes. Jack grabbed a lifeguard blanket, and soon the two were exploring each other's bodies. Under the summer moon, Jack and Stacy made love on the beach, and soon a tsunami of pleasure cascaded through Jack's body as he achieved orgasm, leaving him in a state of awe, amazed at the intensity of the experience.

Seconds later, Jack's erect penis began to shrink.

Jack's ejaculation originates deep within his body, as the prostate and seminal vesicles contract, resulting in the release of semen.

Simultaneously, waves of contractions of the muscles surrounding the urethra (the fine tube that also carries urine out of the body) push the semen out of the penis.

During an orgasm, the relaxation hormones transition to stress hormones, with the release of adrenaline (epinephrine), which shuts down the erection.

After reaching orgasm, an enzyme (PDE-5) changes cGMP into an inactive form, acting as an Off Switch, which narrows blood vessels and shrinks the penis.

As a result, the Off Switch allows blood to flow out of Jack's penis and return to his body. (That's not a bad thing: at some point, you'll probably want to go to sleep, and in the morning, you'll want to head off to work or school without an erection.)

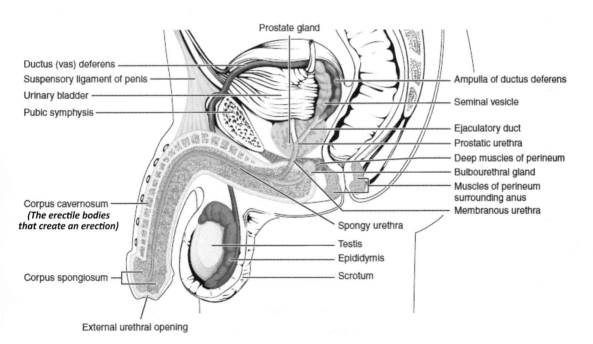

Figure 76.2 Anatomy of the Penis

When we are in our teens and 20s, our system generally works just fine. This whole scenario happens effortlessly. Most of us can achieve an erection within minutes. But as we age, our ability to have erections slowly declines.

The Massachusetts Men's Study followed tens of thousands of men over more than 20 years. This massive dataset revealed that about 40% of men in their 40s experience some degree of erectile dysfunction; so do 50% of men in their fifties, 60% of men in their sixties, and 70% of men in their seventies. However, this loss of function does not occur overnight at age 40. Instead, it's a gradual process. The good news is that with early intervention, it is possible to slow and even reverse the loss of function that tends to occur gradually with aging.

KEY TAKE AWAYS

Over the following twelve chapters, we'll talk about all of that, including:

- What you can do to maintain a healthy, satisfying sex life into your 70s and beyond

- How to improve the quality of your orgasms

- What do to when you run into erectile difficulties

- How your penis is a remarkably accurate indicator of your overall health.

**For more information on Dr. Brandeis's practice in men's health
and sexual medicine, please see:
www.BrandeisMD.com.**

Chapter 77
Erectile Dysfunction Explained
Judson Brandeis, MD, Urologist

See, the problem is that God gives men a brain and a penis,
and only enough blood to run one at a time.
— Robin Williams.

Jack and Stacy were married on Surfside Beach on Nantucket Island five years to the day after they first met. They hired the same Jimmy Buffet cover band for their wedding that was playing when they first hooked up. Jack started work in software sales, and Stacy found a job as a pharmaceutical rep. Life was good, and the sex was great! Then babies (Lisa, Blake, and Diana) came into their lives over the next five years. Life became hectic, and sleep became more important than sex.

Business was great for Jack, which allowed Stacy to stay at home with the kids. Jack was traveling to see customers every other week and then was asked to also take over the corporate sales training program in Texas, which meant one long weekend away every month. To make matters worse, Stacy's father had a stroke, and her parents moved into an assisted living facility 10 minutes from their home. An only child, Jack had to help his parents move out of their home and down to Florida, where they put his father in an early Alzheimer's care facility.

Jack used to be proud of his six-pack abs, but too many sales dinners, plane flights, and corporate golf retreats had led to an embarrassing tire around his mid-section. Gone were the carefree days of summer life on Nantucket. Life in Connecticut had become more stressful, and the years seemed to fly by.

Fast forward to Jack's 50th birthday. Jack and Stacy were finally heading for a well-deserved vacation in the Bahamas. Stacy's mother and the nanny teamed up to watch the kids and drive them to their dance, soccer, tae kwon do, tutoring, and art lessons. Two million frequent flier miles got them first-class tickets and a penthouse room at the Grand Hyatt. (Jack figured there had to be some benefit to being a workaholic.) As Jack and Stacy walked off the plane in Nassau, they could hear the steel drums and feel the balmy sea breeze. After a relaxing day lounging in the sun and a fancy dinner, Jack and Stacy stumbled back to their room, intoxicated with each other once again. And that's when it happened.

Stacy pulled Jack in close and whispered in his ear all of the wild things she wanted to do to him. Eager with anticipation, Jack disrobed and helped Stacy remove her lingerie. He found her as enticing as ever, but to his surprise, his body did not respond. No erection arose to the occasion. "It's not working!" Jack was puzzled at first, and then alarmed... Stacy was worried too, although she knew Jack had been less sexually active over the past few years. "I'll try something else." But nothing seemed to work. Jack tried to laugh it off and blame it on the alcohol, but deep down, he was concerned. Five years ago, he began to notice that he was no longer waking up with an erection, but he had written it off as stress and lack of sleep.

Dr. Brandeis here. Let me take you behind the scenes here to explore what's gone wrong with Jack's sexual function, which used to work just fine.

NIGHTTIME ERECTIONS—YOUR BODY'S EARLY WARNING SYSTEM

Wouldn't it be great if there was an early warning sign to let us know that our erectile function was beginning to deteriorate? Well, there is. It is affectionately known as Morning Wood. During REM sleep, which occurs three to six times a night, men get erections that last for five to ten minutes during each occurrence. Many in the sexual medicine community believe that the purpose of nighttime erections is to periodically stretch the penis and provide it with oxygen and nutrients. Increased blood flow prevents stiffening and scarring of the spongy tissue inside the two cylinders that create your erection (the erectile bodies).

A reduction in nighttime erections is the first sign that blood flow to the penis is beginning to decline. *Do not dismiss or ignore this development!* **Understanding this loss of function is crucial if you want to maintain a lifetime of erectile function and circulatory health.**

Almost every man who walks into my office thinks that they are immune to the effects of aging, but believe me, if you have 50 candles on your birthday cake, you have the physiology and sexual function of a 50-year-old man. The functionality of your penis is a sensitive indicator of blood flow that tells you if your circulation is starting to decline.

So, tomorrow morning when you wake up (or if you get up in the middle of the night to pee), check to see whether your flagpole is at full mast. If it is at half-mast, please pay attention and start eating better, exercising more, and taking care of your health issues.

For Jack, what should have been a second honeymoon had become a nightmare. Two days passed without discussing what had happened. Knowing their vacation was drawing to a close, Jack worked up the courage to try again and took Stacy out to her new favorite sushi bar. After three shots of sake, Jack and Stacy were eager to get back to the room to recapture their youth. But Jack couldn't get the image of his limp penis out of his mind. No matter what they tried, nada. The result was another night of miserable frustration, watching CNN and checking emails. In desperation, Jack tried to call his Kaiser doctor to get some Viagra, but Friday is a lousy day to get a doctor on the phone. Jack ended up at the 7-11 asking the clerk which of the over-the-counter pills was the best seller. In the end, nothing seemed to work. Friday night was a total disaster. Zero for three.

THE MAJOR CAUSES OF ERECTILE DYSFUNCTION

The major causes of ED can all be understood as contributing to either a decrease in blood pressure through the arteries or a reduction in nerve signals.

> *Restoration of erectile function requires the reversal of the conditions that are decreasing blood flow, reducing nerve signals, or creating other health issues.*

Here are some of the common conditions that lead to ED:

- *Decreased circulation,* including narrowing of the arteries, leaking veins, impaired endothelium, high blood pressure, and heart disease. Circulation problems are, by far, the most frequent cause of ED

- *Impaired nerve function,* due to neurological disorders like stroke, Parkinson's, or multiple sclerosis; trauma to the brain, spinal cord, or pelvic area; prostate surgery or radiation; and the effects of aging on nerves

- *Altered body chemistry,* notably low testosterone; reduced nitric oxide production; unbalanced neurotransmitters, which can cause conditions such as depression; low or high thyroid output; medications and drugs that alter sexual function

- *Stress and psychological issues* from a wide range of causes including unrelenting stress, burnout and deep depletion, as well as a range of concerns that include performance anxiety, porn addiction, shaming, or sexual trauma.

CIRCULATION—The Long and Winding Road

Inadequate blood delivery to the penis due to poor circulation causes 85% of cases of erectile dysfunction.

When the heart pumps, the penis and the toes are the last two places in the body to get blood. It is a challenge for the circulatory system to supply those two locations, which is why we get cold feet and a limp penis.

When blood flow decreases to the feet, your toes get cold, and you put on socks, but your feet don't stop working. It takes a substantial loss of circulation for your toes to lose function.

The penis is different. This is the only organ in the body that is entirely dependent on blood flow in order to function.

NARROWED ARTERIES

An erection can only occur if the penis completely fills with blood. (You might compare achieving an erection to inflating an air mattress. But in this case, it's blood flow that inflates the penis and creates the erection. Like the mattress, if the penis is not inflated with blood, it is floppy and not functional.)

Impaired circulation due to narrowed or clogged arteries or a weakened heart reduces blood flow into the penis, making it difficult to achieve or sustain an erection.

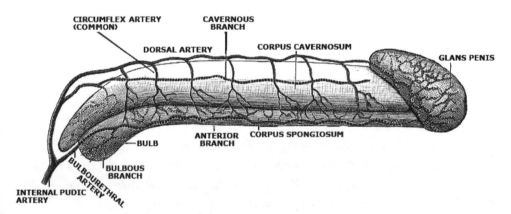

Figure 77.1 This illustration shows the fine arteries that supply the penis. They are so narrow that they are easily disrupted by plaque, short circuiting the ability to achieve an erection.

When the arteries pump blood into the penis, it doesn't immediately return to the heart. Instead, the blood fills tiny chambers called sinusoids (the sponge-like tissue shown in Figure 77.2) within the erectile bodies (corpus cavernosum) of the penis. These tiny chambers resemble the holes in a sponge.

During an erection, as blood fills the sinusoids, localized blood pressure within the penis increases, and the penis expands in length and girth. When the pressure within the penis reaches a critical point, the return of blood to the heart is blocked, so the penis becomes rigid, and rises to an erect position.

LEAKING VEINS

To achieve a firm erection, blood must be sealed within the penis. Here's how that happens:

As the penis fills with blood, the sinusoids expand, and when they are full, the sinusoids begin overflowing.

The excess blood from the sinusoids flows out into small veins and exits the penis.

The veins that exit the erectile bodies are sandwiched between two layers of thick tissue (the tunica) that wrap around the erectile bodies.

As the pressure on the inside of the penis reaches a critical level, these veins filled with exiting blood are compressed. When the veins are sealed off, blood is trapped in the erectile bodies, and the penis becomes rigid, moving it into an erect position for penetrative intercourse.

At this point, there are two major problems that can short-circuit the erection, both caused by poor circulation.

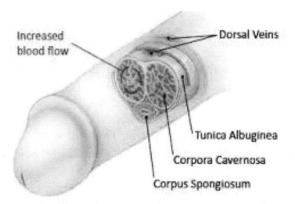

Figure 77.2. Cross section of the penis. Here you can see the sponge-like tissue of the erectile bodies that expand with blood to create an erection. As the flow of incoming blood increases, the veins are compressed against the sheath that wraps the erectile bodies (the tunica). This seals the blood within the penis, resulting in a firm erection.

KEY TAKE AWAY POINTS

Plaque. If the arteries are narrowed due to the build-up of plaque, not enough blood will flow into the penis and an erection may not happen at all.

Leaking veins. In other cases, there may be enough blood flow to fill the erectile bodies, but not enough to fill them completely. Then there won't be enough pressure within the penis to seal off the veins tightly and create an erection firm enough for penetration.

In that situation, blood will continue to leave the penis through the veins, so the penis will be full, but not rigid. It's kind of like jumping from the roof of a burning building onto the top of the neighboring building that is six feet away. If you jump six feet, you're safe, but a jump of anything less than six feet does not make it.

A flaccid penis is a clear indication that there's not enough blood flow (and not enough localized blood pressure within the penis) to do the job. The inability to maintain elevated blood pressure in the penis (to sustain an erection) is often an early indicator of problems within the circulatory system.

I am going to repeat this, because it is a key concept. The swollen and pressurized erectile bodies compress the veins against the tough outer sheath of the penis, preventing the return of blood back into the general circulation. This creates the erection.

Erectile dysfunction is a wake-up call.

The arteries to the penis are fine and delicate, just 1 to 2 mm in diameter. In contrast, the coronary arteries that supply the heart are 3 to 4 mm in diameter.

Any type of impairment or insult to the arteries of the penis can easily narrow, clog, or block any of these blood vessels—whether that's due to plaque buildup, a blood clot, or damage to the blood vessels.

The arteries that supply the penis are smaller than those of the heart, so men get symptoms of a decline in blood flow to the penis long before they experience symptoms of heart disease.

Men notice erectile dysfunction five to ten years before heart disease is usually discovered.

IMPAIRED ENDOTHELIUM

This is another delicate area of the circulation that can become impaired, disrupting erections. The endothelium is a layer of cells, just one cell thick, which covers the inner lining of the blood vessels.

These tiny cells produce much of the nitric oxide used throughout the body.

Nitric oxide is the On Switch that is necessary for an erection.

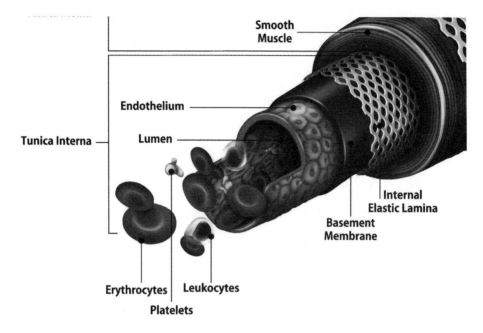

Figure 77.3. The endothelium, which lines every blood vessel in our bodies.

Why Your Endothelium Matters

Endothelial cells are involved in many important aspects of blood vessel function, including:

■ Management of blood pressure throughout the body, by tightening or expanding the blood vessels

■ Production and release of nitric oxide

■ Prevention of blood clotting, because healthy endothelia are coated in substances that inhibit clotting

■ Formation of new blood vessels (angiogenesis) by activation of stem cells

■ In the fine capillaries, the endothelia support the flow of oxygen, nutrients, and white blood cells into the tissue and the release of toxins.

If the endothelium is damaged, its ability to produce nitric oxide is compromised. Major sources of damage include:

- High blood pressure, which causes the erratic rush of blood through the arteries

- Diabetes and associated inflammation

- Plaque buildup in the blood vessels, on the lining and underneath the lining

- Lack of antioxidant nutrients as protection against oxidative stress.

As men age, the level of nitric oxide in the body declines significantly, which decreases circulation and raises systemic blood pressure throughout. By boosting nitric oxide through supplements or a nitric oxide-generating diet (such as leafy greens, beef, eggs, watermelon, pumpkin, and cucumber) men can improve circulation to the brain, heart, muscles, penis, and other important organs.

HIGH BLOOD PRESSURE (HYPERTENSION)

When the heart squeezes and pushes blood into the vessels, blood pressure goes up (systole). It comes down when the heart relaxes (diastole). Blood pressure changes depending on activity, body temperature, diet, emotions, posture, and medication.

The pumping of the heart produces pressure within the blood vessel walls. If blood pressure is high, it strains the vessel walls causing wear and tear on the lining (the endothelium) which can result in plaque buildup and blood clots. When arteries narrow, the resistance within the blood vessels increases. Consequently, the heart must pump harder to deliver blood to the body. As the heart pumps more vigorously, the pressure in the arteries increases, resulting in high blood pressure. In response to the elevated pressures, blood vessels grow more smooth muscle, which makes the artery walls thicker and less elastic, narrowing the channel further and making blood pressure even higher.

Perspective on blood pressure meds. If your primary care physician diagnoses you with hypertension, they will likely put you on a medication to reduce your blood pressure. Unfortunately, many blood pressure medications reduce blood flow to the organs in the periphery like the toes and the penis. It's important to do everything you can to *prevent* high blood pressure such as reducing salt, sugar, and stress and exercising so that you do not need to start blood pressure medications. (See chapter 5, 6, 13, and 14 to learn more about circulation.) When there is less blood flow to the penis, you will be unable to achieve an erection.

HEART DISEASE

Bear in mind that the first sign of heart disease in a quarter of men is sudden death.

Do you really want to be that guy stuck on the side of the highway with a broken-down car because he ignored all the warning signs that the car was deteriorating? But instead of your car, it's your life that's on the line. If you listen to your body and make the necessary changes outlined in this book, you can reverse this decline in function.

> **We can provide you with the information that you need to make a shift, but you are ultimately responsible for your own health and decisions.**
>
> **Erectile dysfunction matters. ED not only deprives you of a healthy, satisfying sex life—it is also a major warning that the cardiovascular system is not working the way it used to.**

HEALTH ISSUES THAT AFFECT CIRCULATION

A decline in blood flow throughout your body (including your penis) can occur due to the damage caused by smoking, high cholesterol, high blood pressure, diabetes, or advanced age.

- **Excessive cholesterol** in a man's blood will become deposited on the endothelial lining of blood vessels, restricting the flow of blood. Smaller blood vessels like the ones going to the penis have lower flow and are more susceptible to cholesterol deposits. This is one of the reasons your primary care physician checks your cholesterol and may put you on a statin medication to reduce your level of cholesterol. See chapters 5, 6, 13, 14 and the sections on food and exercise to improve your circulation.

- **Diabetes** affects both the delivery of blood and nerve signals. This is one of the many reasons that it is essential to control blood sugar. See chapter 18 to understand more about diabetes.

- **Smoking cigarettes** is bad for your lungs and your penis. The smoke you inhale from burning tobacco contains about 7,000 chemicals releasing free radicals, heavy metals, nicotine, cyanide, and carbon monoxide that can damage the arteries that supply your penis. Chapters 44 and 45 explain more.

NERVE FUNCTION

Now that we've looked at the role of blood vessels, let's discuss the nerve signals that increase blood flow, and how a diminished nerve signal affects blood flow to the penis due to:

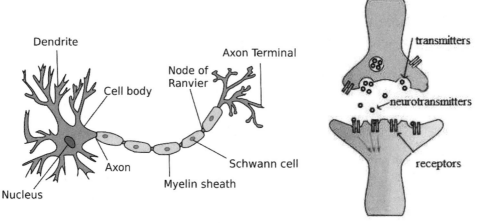

Figure 77.4. Basic components of a nerve cell (neuron).

- Neurological disorder such as a stroke, Parkinson's or multiple sclerosis
- Trauma to the brain, spinal cord, or pelvic area
- Prostate surgery or radiation
- Diabetic neuropathy
- The effects of aging on nerve signaling.

Basic nerve anatomy is key to understanding nerve-related erectile dysfunction. A neuron is a single nerve cell that carries electrical impulses. Neurons have a cell body, dendrites, and an axon, which are the basic units of our nervous system.

- Dendrites are appendages that are designed to receive communications from other cells.

- Axons, also known as nerve fibers, carry nerve impulses away from the cell body.

- Neurons are connected to one another, but they don't actually touch. Instead, there are tiny gaps (synapses) in which chemicals—neurotransmitters—pass the signal from one neuron to the next.

- Receptors on the receiving dendrite transmit the chemical signal along an axon or onto a neighboring blood vessel.

In the circulatory system, axon terminals release the neurotransmitter nitric oxide onto the smooth muscle cells in the wall of blood vessels, causing the muscle to relax and open the blood vessel. Nerve problems can occur in the central nervous system like the brain or spinal cord, or in peripheral nerves like those that carry signals from the spinal cord to the organs.

Nerve signals and body chemistry control blood flow, comparable to the way railroad switches direct trains in different directions. Parts of your body need oxygen and nutrients at different levels, depending on what you are doing. As a result, your circulatory system continually shifts blood around from organ to organ. For example, when you wake up in the morning and exercise, your blood moves to the muscles of your arms and legs. When you eat breakfast, blood flows to your stomach and intestines. After breakfast, you go to work, and blood shoots up to your brain.

Reduction in nerve function can cause a reduction in blood flow or a decrease in the sensitivity of the penis and difficulty in reaching orgasm. Nerve damage occurs due to a range of health issues.

NEUROLOGICAL DISORDERS

Strokes within the brain. There are many ways that strokes can damage the brain by cutting off blood flow to nerve tissues, but a stroke in any of a number of areas of the brain can result in erectile dysfunction.

Diseases of myelin such as multiple sclerosis. Myelin makes up the insulating sheaths of nerves and helps nerves conduct impulses. Multiple sclerosis, Guillain-Barre, and CIPD are all demyelinating diseases that can affect signal transmission.

Problems with neurotransmitters such as Parkinson's disease. Parkinson's disease can reduce erectile function by harming the autonomic nervous system (ANS) which controls both your sexual function and sexual response.

Parkinson's affects dopamine levels which are vital in coordinating, controlling, and promoting movement. Consider how these features of Parkinson's might interfere with sexual function: muscle rigidity and reduction of fine motor control that leads to poor coordination, tremors, slowness of movement, involuntary muscle movements, and failure of the autonomic nervous system to regulate blood pressure.

TRAUMA OR SURGERY

Surgery for prostate cancer can cut the axons of the pelvic nerves that serve the penis. As a result, the brain can no longer signal the penis to fill with blood. These nerves will never grow back.

In 2002 I helped pioneer DaVinci robotic prostate removal for prostate cancer. I recognized that the 3D optics and exceptional control of the surgical instruments gave urologic robotic surgeons like myself the ability to preserve nerve function. Over time the robotic technology and surgical techniques have continued to improve our ability to preserve sexual function after prostate cancer surgery.

Other trauma, such as certain spinal cord injuries and pelvic crush injuries, can have damaging effects on nerves. ED resulting from nerve damage typically does not respond to pills such as Viagra and Cialis.

An example of localized trauma: Bicycle riding for more than 3 hours a week on a rigid bicycle seat can cause damage to both the arteries and the nerves that go to the penis. If your penis becomes numb while you are riding, periodically get off the saddle and then get a bike seat with a drop nose and short beak.

DIABETIC NEUROPATHY

Decreased blood flow and a high blood sugar level cause nerve damage in about 50% of diabetics. Symptoms start many years before diabetes is evident, so some men already have nerve damage when they are first diagnosed. People with diabetes are also at higher risk for other nerve problems. For additional information on diabetes, please see chapter 18.

BODY CHEMISTRY

Issues with body chemistry that affect sexual function include:

- Low testosterone
- Low nitric-oxide production and levels
- Low neurotransmitters resulting in conditions such as depression
- Low or high thyroid output
- Medications that inhibit erections.

LOW TESTOSTERONE

Low testosterone is often present in men with poor erections, but it rarely is the primary cause. Replacing testosterone can resolve ED in only a small percentage of men. Testosterone is more important for libido, so in a sense testosterone is necessary for erections, but it has much less of an impact on blood flow. A comprehensive review of testosterone appears in chapter 89.

LOW NITRIC OXIDE—The effect of nitric oxide on blood flow

The On Switch. Your nerves release chemicals—neurotransmitters—that cause changes in the body. In the case of arteries, nerves release the neurotransmitter nitric oxide (NO), which increases another chemical called cGMP that functions like an On Switch, causing blood vessels to open and blood flow to increase.

The Off Switch. Because you don't want these blood vessels to remain open forever, a series of enzymes called the PDE system functions like an Off Switch and inactivates cGMP. As a result, blood vessels constrict and become narrower which decreases blood flow.

Unlike nitric oxide, which is widely used throughout your body by all the organs, in both men and women and all mammals, there are different PDE enzymes that are specific to the various organs. In the brain, there is PDE-1. In the eyes, PDE-6. In the lungs, PDE-4, and in the penis, there is PDE-5. That is why when you take a PDE-5 enzyme inhibitor like Viagra or Cialis, you specifically dilate blood vessels in the penis and increase penile blood flow without affecting blood flow in any other area of the body.

LOW NEUROTRANSMITTERS

Depression. It is not clear whether ED causes the depression or depression causes the ED, or both. According to a study conducted by the NIMH, men who suffer from depression are likely to lose interest in sex and other activities. Depression is often accompanied by a feeling of worthlessness. It may affect a man's ability to achieve or maintain an erection. Depression results from an imbalance of chemicals in the brain. This means that you may be unable to perform well in bed.

Half of men with depression have erectile dysfunction.

Antidepressant medications. Unfortunately, 40% of men with depression take SSRI medications (selective serotonin reuptake inhibitors), which boost serotonin in the brain. These medications suppress oxytocin, a neurotransmitter that signals both erection and orgasm. There are medications for depression that have fewer side effects on erectile function, and I would recommend that you consult your psychiatrist if you have ED that could be caused by your medications for depression so that you can start a different medication. Chapter 67 reviews depression.

Anxiety. Anxiety can be due to psychological, neurochemical, or physical factors. If there are no morning erections, then it is likely a physical issue rather than a psychological one. Chronic stress can cause the release of stress hormones that shunt blood away from nonessential organs. If this is the case, then you should still be getting morning erections. In that situation, focus on the issue that is causing the anxiety and work with a therapist or a life coach on how to reduce the stressor(s). Chapter 66 addresses anxiety.

LOW OR HIGH THYROID HORMONE LEVELS

Problems in thyroid function, both low and high thyroid output, can cause low sexual desire, erectile dysfunction, premature ejaculation, and delayed ejaculation.

Researchers report that men with sexual disorders related to imbalanced thyroid levels respond well to treatment and quickly show improvement in symptoms. Pursuing assessment and treatment of possible thyroid problems seems to be important in managing sexual dysfunction issues.

Researchers in an Italian study reported, "Most patients with thyroid hormone disorders experience some sexual dysfunction, which can be reversed by normalizing the thyroid hormone levels."

It is not unusual for men to be unaware that their thyroid levels are too high or too low, unless their doctor has recently ordered a laboratory test for thyroid function.

In terms of symptoms, they may simply be experiencing fatigue (if their thyroid output is low) or anxiety or insomnia (if it's high).

In sum, if you have sexual dysfunction, be sure to ask your doctor to check your thyroid function, which is a matter of a simple blood test.

MEDICATIONS THAT CAN BLOCK AN ERECTION

It is beyond the scope of this book to describe how each of these classes of medication interfere with erectile activity. If you are on one of the types of medication listed below, please consult the prescribing physician. (In many cases, there are drugs with similar beneficial effects that have less of an impact on erectile function.)

- 5-alpha reductase inhibitors (finasteride)
- ACE inhibitors
- Acid reflux medications
- Alpha-blockers
- Antiarrhythmics drugs (for irregular heartbeat)
- Antidepressants (SSRIs, SNRIs, MAOIs, tricyclics)
- Antihistamines
- Antihypertensives (drugs for high blood pressure such as thiazides and beta-blockers)

- Antipsychotics (for mental illness)
- Antiseizure drugs
- Barbiturates
- Calcium channel blockers
- Cardiovascular drugs
- Chemotherapy
- Diuretics
- Estrogen
- H2 acid blockers (such as Pepcid, Tagamet, and Zantac)
- Methadone
- Muscle relaxants
- NSAIDs (aspirin, ibuprofen, Aleve)
- Nicotine (found in stimulant formulas)
- Opioid painkillers (codeine, morphine)
- Parkinson's disease drugs
- Prostate cancer drugs
- Psychotropics
- Tranquilizers

Note that recreation drugs can also be a cause of erectile dysfunction. Opioids, for example, tend to reduce not only sexual function, but also blunt interest in sex altogether (low libido).

STRESS—The stress response, penile blood flow, and erections

You might be wondering how your mood affects blood flow to your penis. There are three types of nerves in your body: motor, sensory, and autonomic. Motor neurons enable your body to move. Sensory neurons allow your body to feel.

Your *autonomic nervous system* (think *automatic*) regulates essential body functions like heart rate, blood flow, respiratory rate, digestion, urination, and sexual arousal—all without your conscious input.

How Stress Affects Your Sexual Function
(As Experienced by Paleo Man)

Say you're a caveman hanging out in your cave with your cavewoman. You're both feeling romantic, and you're starting to feel a tingling in your groin. Then, out of the corner of your eye, you notice that there's a hungry, 800-pound saber-tooth tiger pacing outside your cave. You immediately go into full-blown stress response (maximum sympathetic nervous system outflow) because this nasty tiger wants to eat you and your cavewoman. Now is not a good time to get an erection! An erect penis gives the tiger something easy to bite. Seriously, though, while you're in stress response, you're not going to get an erection—your body is going to reroute as much blood as possible to your legs (in case you need to run) and your arms (in case you need to fend off that tiger).

Three days go by, with the tiger pacing outside your cave, and you and your cavewoman start to get hungry. She starts comparing you to her old cave-boyfriend. But, of course, he wouldn't be afraid of a saber-tooth tiger. He would have gone out there and taken care of business. Two more days go by, and your cavewoman is even hungrier and gives you all sorts of grief. At this point, you'd rather take your chances with that vicious saber-tooth tiger than spend one more minute in the cave with your cavewoman.

In a flash, you pick up a sharpened spear, pissed off at the world, and charge out of the cave. With a massive rush of adrenaline, you hurl the spear right into the eye of the tiger. Then, as the beast falls to the ground, you emit a triumphant roar!

Exhausted, with the task completed, your adrenaline plummets (lowering sympathetic nervous outflow), which takes you out of the stress response and into relaxation response (parasympathetic mode). You finally have a chance to catch your breath, to rest and digest, and to repair wounds and bruises you sustained in the battle. Blood drains out of your large muscles and travels to other less essential organs.

You skin the tiger and roll out a velvety tiger-skin rug. Then you light a fire, put a couple of tiger filets on a skewer, and you and your cavewoman enjoy fresh tiger steaks. Blood flow moves to your intestines to digest food and make waste and to the kidneys to produce urine to clean your bloodstream of toxins and balance the minerals in your blood (electrolytes).

Still reveling in your victory, you invite your cavewoman down to the tiger-skin rug to make a baby. You're relaxed (in full parasympathetic mode), so blood flows smoothly to your penis—and stays there.

Nature only invented one stress hormone system. And whether you're running away from a tiger, under a deadline at work, or anxious about whether you'll be able to keep an erection, your body produces adrenaline as one of its stress hormones. Adrenaline prevents an erection by reducing the amount of blood that flows into the penis. That's why when you're nervous or stressed, you tend to lose your erections (or never get them in the first place).

Relaxation produces hormone levels that preferentially shunt blood to non-urgent functions like digestion, waste production, and procreation. Stress causes the release of hormones like adrenaline and cortisol that moves blood to more essential locations like the muscles, eyes, and brain. This is why stress diminishes sexual function.

The autonomic nervous system has two modes: stress and relaxation. The Stress Response or "fight or flight" (also referred to as the sympathetic nervous system) is balanced by the Relaxation Response (the parasympathetic nervous system).

What is less well appreciated is that the Stress Response creates a hormonal outflow of adrenaline and cortisol that works against erections.

The stress response taps into a range of emotions from basic survival instincts to fear, anger, or aggression, all of which can short-circuit your erections. If you don't get erections, your penis doesn't perfuse with oxygenated blood and stretch out.

UNRELENTING STRESS

Chronic stress—whether experienced in the workplace or in personal life—often affects both libido and sexual function. In addition to ruining your sex life, prolonged stress can cause changes in the brain and in the glands that produce hormones. We know, for example, that stress drives down testosterone. Just as erectile dysfunction can be a warning sign of cardiovascular issues, ED due to frequent stress can be a symptom of worsening physical and mental depletion.

BURNOUT AND DEEP DEPLETION

Most of us think of burnout as an emotional or psychological condition. However, the symptoms of burnout often reflect a profound state of depletion. Emotional and physical stress can lead to burnout, which drains hormone production, nutrients, neurotransmitter levels, and energy. This state of physical exhaustion deprives the body of its ability to support non-essential functions such as sex.

I have treated many patients in this state. When burnout is present, reversing this depletion is necessary before even considering the restoration of sexual health.

EMOTIONAL AND PSYCHOLOGICAL ISSUES

Psychological sexual issues that can affect crections include performance anxiety, porn addiction, shaming, and sexual trauma. Excessive pornography causes the desensitization of the brain centers that are important to experience pleasure and intimacy. These areas of the brain atrophy over time and reduce erectile function. Learn more about the harmful effects of pornography in chapter 51.

As a urologist and an expert in sexual medicine, I see men's health through the lens of penile blood flow and erectile function. As men age, all aspects of their health need to be optimized to continue to enjoy their intimate life. Read on to learn about orgasms and what you can do—on your own or with medical supervision—to reduce, prevent, and even reverse ED.

Chapter 78
Orgasm: Too Fast, Too Slow, or Just Right
Judson Brandeis, MD, Urologist

In my next life I want to live backwards.
Start out dead and finish off as an orgasm.
— Woody Allen

While on safari in Tanzania thirty years ago, I came across a male zebra fighting six other male zebras for the right to mate. The fighting was intense and lasted hours. I realized that the right to procreate is a driving force in nature. In the struggle for the opportunity to reproduce, an individual has to out-compete rivals and attract partners.

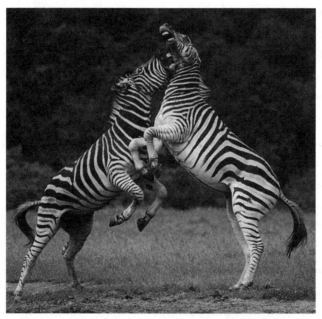

Figure 78.1. Zebras fighting for supremacy in the herd and the right to father the offspring of the group.

Reproduction is the end goal of evolutionary fitness, and sexual selection ultimately dictates who gets to pass their genes onto the next generation, which is why orgasm evolved to be so pleasurable.

Why would you fight other males to the death if sex didn't feel so great? So, you can see why orgasm and ejaculation evolved to be amazing! Reinforcement and reward are the ultimate motivators of behavior.

Orgasm and ejaculation are two separate, but linked, events. Orgasm is a temporary sensation of intense pleasure that creates an altered state of consciousness. Ejaculation is a complex process of semen emission and expulsion that is ultimately responsible for procreation.

In nature, while animals are engaged in sex, they are in a vulnerable position. Rapid ejaculation allows them to get back to protecting themselves quickly. Humans are different because, in many societies, intercourse occurs for purposes other than reproduction.

ORGASM

There is no standard definition of orgasm. However, most of us know one when we feel one. We breathe quicker, our heart races, and our blood pressure rises. We feel pleasurable pelvic floor contractions and pulsation of the muscles located at the base of the penis.

The volume of ejaculate for a healthy man averages about ¾ teaspoon (3.7 ccs). When men are young, they can shoot semen as far as 12 to 24 inches. The ejaculation force gives the sperm a head start in their journey up the vaginal canal to the cervix and the awaiting egg. As men age, the expulsive force propelling the semen diminishes, unless they exercise their pelvic floor muscles.

Major Steps in Orgasm

The human sexual response consists of four stages: desire, arousal, orgasm, and resolution. The orgasmic stage is the shortest but most intense of the four and consists of emission, expulsion, and orgasm.

Emission is the first phase of ejaculation with the passage of seminal fluid from the prostate and seminal vesicle glands into the area of the urethra within the prostate.

- In the prostatic urethra, secretions from the prostate mix with sperm delivered from the vas deferens. Sperm and the prostate secretions contribute about 20% of semen volume. At least 80% of semen is made in the seminal vesicles. These two glands, located behind the bladder, produce a pale-yellow fluid consisting mainly of fructose.

- At the same time, the bladder neck closes to prevent semen from spilling into the bladder.

This entire process is orchestrated by the autonomic nervous system (which performs many functions automatically). Emission of semen requires contractions of the smooth muscles of the prostate, seminal vesicles, and vas deferens.

Note: Given the central role of the autonomic nervous system in emission, any disorder that impairs nerve supply to the smooth muscles of the pelvis can interfere with this early stage of ejaculation.

At the initial phase of ejaculation, the sympathetic nervous system triggers the release of biochemicals that include:

- Noradrenaline (norepinephrine), oxytocin, acetylcholine, ATP (the basic compound of energy), and nitric oxide.

- Oxytocin levels in the blood increase as much as three times normal after male orgasm before returning to baseline 10 minutes after ejaculation. (This is the bonding chemical that brings a couple together.)

- Levels of serotonin increase: this is the brain chemical that gives us the feeling of happiness.

- Prolactin is also elevated, and is believed to promote a sense of sexual satiety, serving to decrease arousal once orgasm is completed.

Expulsion is a spinal cord reflex that occurs as the ejaculatory process reaches a "point of no return." It depends on contractions of the pelvic floor muscles, in addition to the muscles at the base of the penis, the bulbocaverosus and ischiocavnosus.

Orgasm. Rhythmic contractions of the pelvic floor muscles and those at the base of the penis propel semen through the urethral tube. (These contractions occur rhythmically at a rate of about one every second.)

Most of us do not stop and consider the complexity of the coordination of emission, expulsion, and orgasm. However, the survival of a species depends on the perfection of this intricate dance.

PREMATURE EJACULATION

Most of us watch James Bond movies, but we don't assume we can do wild stunts like James Bond. However, many people, especially young men, base their expectations for their sexual performance on what they see in pornographic movies. They eventually learn that professional pornographic actors make these movies, and scenes often require multiple takes. Besides, many of the stars use performance-enhancing medications injected directly into the penis to prolong erections.

The International Society for Sexual Medicine defines premature ejaculation (PE) as a form of male sexual dysfunction characterized by ejaculation within 1 minute of penetration. Other researchers use 2-minute ejaculations as the criterion. Research studies show that this ranges up to 4 minutes—and that one aspect of PE is how the man defines his own performance. To some degree, the conclusion is that PE also reflects the satisfaction level of his partner.

- In a man with no PE, the average ejaculation time is 5 to 7 minutes

- Data suggests that 30% of men experience PE

- It takes women 17 minutes on average to climax, so there's an incentive for men to delay ejaculation.

Types of PE

In the past, PE was considered a psychological condition. However, in this chapter you'll find an extensive list of physical conditions that can cause PE (such as high thyroid, smoldering prostate infections, and low muscle tone of the pelvic floor). Many of these conditions are curable.

Twins studies suggest that 30% of PE incidence is genetically based. There are three main categories of PE: lifelong PE, acquired PE, and variable PE (normal ejaculation at times and premature ejaculation at others). According to these classifications, different physical and mental conditions underlie PE. The most successful treatment involves identifying the underlying condition in order to determine the most optimal treatment. At some point in their life, a majority of men have experienced PE.

The two most prevalent types of PE are:

Lifelong PE. This refers to men who have had PE ever since their first experience of sex, which raises the possibility that it may be genetically based.

Acquired. Men who develop PE due to a health condition or the effects of aging, imbalanced body chemistry such as low serotonin function, or low testosterone.

The inability to delay ejaculation in intercourse can result in distress, frustration, and the avoidance of sexual intimacy. Premature ejaculation affects sexual confidence, relationships, and the satisfaction of both partners. (Please see chapter 88, "How to Please a Woman," for in-depth information on pleasing your partner regardless of any specific sexual issues you may have.)

POSSIBLE CAUSES AND POTENTIAL SOLUTIONS

HYPERSENSITIVITY — NERVE FUNCTION

One of the basic problems in PE is hypersensitivity, meaning that it takes very little penile stimulation to bring about ejaculation. There appear to be several possible causes of this, including:

The number of nerve fibers —The composition of nerves in the head of the penis (the glans) or the frenulum. Interestingly, researchers have actually counted the number of nerve fibers in the tip of the penis. A forensic study conducted in China evaluated the number of nerve fibers in the bodies of deceased men with or without a diagnosis of PE. Researchers focused on the number of nerves on the underside of the penis, which tends to be highly sensitive in many men. Men with no history of PE typically had two large nerves in that area—but those who had experienced PE averaged at least seven nerves. Applying this research in clinical practice, a procedure is now utilized in China (dorsal neurectomy) that severs some of these nerves, reducing sensitivity and curing PE, while enabling men to retain normal sensation.

Sexual lifestyle. Men who are less sexually active appear to have greater sensitivity when engaged in intercourse.

Levels of the neurotransmitter serotonin. Low serotonin activity in men is associated with lifelong PE.

Try This at Home . . .

- *Lubricants.* For many men, the intense friction of intercourse creates a rapid climax. A straightforward solution is to use a lubricant to reduce friction. I recommend a silicone-based lubricant like Überlube, which can significantly cut down on friction. Less stimulation will give you more control.

- *Condoms.* A latex barrier between a man's penis will also blunt sensations and help men stay in control. Several companies also make condoms with numbing medications like Lidocaine or Benzocaine in the inner lining of the condom, which further decreases sensation.

■ *Numbing creams.* The principal ingredient in these creams or sprays is Lidocaine (or similar medication), a skin numbing agent. Decreasing the sensation of the penis makes it more difficult for a man to achieve orgasm. Five or ten minutes before penetration, a man sprays or rubs numbing cream on the underside of the head (frenulum) of the penis. It is essential to wipe off the numbing cream before intercourse so that the numbing cream won't reduce sensation for your partner. It's not uncommon for a man to last one to four minutes longer when using a delay spray such as Promescent.

■ *Sensory therapy.* The start-stop technique is somewhat like sexual teasing that involves stimulating the penis until you feel the urge to ejaculate, then stop until the urge subsides, and restart.

■ *Masters and Johnson's squeeze technique* involves squeezing the head (glans) of the penis until the urge to ejaculate subsides.

■ *Masturbation.* Self-stimulating to climax one to two hours before sex is a common suggestion to take the edge off the drive for ejaculation. (This can be a reasonable solution if you will be able to achieve an erection again in an hour or two.)

BODY CHEMISTY

These are fairly straightforward issues. For example, thyroid levels can be checked by your doctor with a simple blood test, as can testosterone.

High thyroid. At least 50% of men with a hyper-thyroid condition experience PE. The good news is that normalizing thyroid levels brings about rapid improvement. Studies have found rates of PE are as frequent as two of every three men among those with a thyroid condition (low thyroid can also be a problem), and that more than half of them are cured by correction of thyroid levels.

Low brain serotonin. Low serotonin levels associated with PE appear to be due to poor transmission of serotonin (the brain chemistry that promotes feelings of wellbeing and happiness). Recreational drugs, opioids, amphetamine, and cocaine have been found to increase the tendency to premature ejaculation. Researchers have confirmed the specific genes involved, although their interaction is not yet clearly understood. This appears to be an important cause of PE that occurs with very little stimulation. Studies have found that about two of three men with this condition respond well to treatment with SSRI medications or St John's wort, which improves initially low levels and inhibits climax.

Low testosterone. Conclusions on the effects of testosterone have been mixed. While a Finnish survey found no correlation with levels of testosterone, a Turkish study reported that men who received testosterone replacement demonstrated a 4.8-fold increase in the average length of intercourse before ejaculation.

Try This at Home. . . .

- *Herbal therapy.* St. John's wort is a natural anti-depressant that is well recognized as a mood booster, increasing the amount of serotonin available to the brain. In addition to mood elevation, St John's wort improves premature ejaculation without the side effects of pharmaceutical anti-depressants. (There are potential interactions between St John's wort and medications metabolized by the liver, so check a site like drugs.com for possible conflicts.) PreLONG by AFFIRM Science contains a special extract of St. Johns' Wort and is formulated specifically for men with premature ejaculation.

If That Doesn't Work, Seek a Medical Approach

- *Get your thyroid levels checked.* Studies show that 50% to 70% of men with a hyperactive thyroid have premature ejaculation. After men take medication to normalize their thyroid hormones, the rate of PE declines to 15%.

- *SSRI antidepressants* treat depression as well as premature ejaculation. SSRIs (selective serotonin reuptake inhibitors) include fluoxetine (Prozac), sertraline (Zoloft), paroxetine (Paxil), and citalopram (Celexa). An eight-month study involving 480 men experiencing PE evaluated the effects of these four SSRI medications. The resultant delay in climax was similar among the drugs, averaging 70 to 75 seconds. Side effects generally reported include possible decreased libido, fatigue, yawning, nausea, and diarrhea. In addition, men have to take SSRIs every day for them to work.

- *Fast-acting SSRIs.* Priligy, also known as dapoxetine, is an SSRI ideal for PE due to its short half-life. If taken 1-2 hours before intercourse, Priligy results in an increase in control and satisfaction. Unfortunately, the FDA did not approve Priligy for undisclosed reasons, so it's only available outside the U.S.

- *Viagra and other PDE-5 inhibitors* reduce performance anxiety and lower levels of stress hormones, reducing PE in some cases.

- *Penile injection therapy* with medications to dilate blood vessels requires a man to inject a combination of drugs into the penis each time he wants to have penetrative intercourse. This approach does not delay ejaculation, but it allows a man to maintain an erection even after ejaculation to continue penetrative intercourse.

MUSCLE TONE OF THE PELVIC FLOOR

Researchers point out that a significant number of men with PE have low tone in pelvic floor muscles. Lack of awareness of these muscles is apparently also a major factor.

In an Italian study, greater awareness of pelvic floor muscles was increased, using biofeedback training in combination with exercises that developed control and contraction of specific muscles. Half of those who took the training (54%) were cured of premature ejaculation, which was especially significant because the men in the study had a history of lifelong PE.

Try This at Home. . . .

Kegel exercise for men. The first step is to identify your pelvic floor muscles by halting urination in midstream or tightening the muscles that keep you from passing gas. Hold the contraction for three seconds, and then relax for three seconds. Try it a few times in a row while sitting, standing, or lying down. Make sure you are tightening only your pelvic floor muscles and not the muscles in your abdomen or buttocks. Breathe freely during the exercises. Get in the habit of doing Kegels every time you stop at a red light or watch TV. It can also be helpful to do a set after you urinate to get rid of the last few drops of urine.

Pelvic floor training. This approach involves learning pelvic exercises, and once a certain level of control is achieved, practicing that control during sex to delay ejaculation:

1. Greater awareness of the pelvic floor muscles using biofeedback.

2. Learning selective contraction of the pelvic floor muscles in the absence of sexual stimulation

3. Experience the timing and contraction of those muscles during intercourse in the pre-orgasmic phase

4. Ongoing strengthening of control of pelvic floor muscles.

If That Doesn't Work . . .

The Emsella Chair by BTL uses powerful magnetic fields to contract muscles. The chair is FDA approved and can be administered in a protocol for men that strengthens control of the pelvic floor.

HEALTH ISSUES

Chronic infections. Another association with PE is infections of the prostate or the urethra (the tube leading from the bladder). In these situations, effective antibiotic treatment frequently clears up the problem completely. Note that these low-grade infections can persist for years or decades if left untreated and can lead to situations of greater concern.

Prediabetes and diabetes. Two clinical trials on diabetes and PE found that about half of the men in the study with diabetes also had PE at twice the rate of non-diabetics. Although the exact mechanisms involved have not been clearly defined, weight gain and sedentary lifestyle are often associated with diabetes, with potential loss of pelvic floor tone.

Neurological disorders. Disorders of the nervous system that can promote PE include multiple sclerosis, spinal cord tumors, alcoholic neuropathy, and diabetic neuropathy.

Trauma or surgery. Every phase of sexual function is orchestrated by the nervous system, so any type of injury or intervention that severs nerves essential to this function can have an impact on sexual response.

PSYCHOLOGICAL ISSUES

Perception. Surprisingly, PE is not just about timing. Although most men diagnosed with PE ejaculate within four minutes, men with PE who are satisfied with their performance don't think of themselves as having PE. And on the other hand, there are men who last longer than that who are dissatisfied with their performance and consider themselves to have PE. The range of factors in the *experience* of PE can be surprisingly personal. Perceptions may also reflect the fantasy world of porn, cultural norms, or the level of satisfaction of one's partner.

Try Mind-Body Therapy. . . .

Psychotherapy alone or with medication can help identify relationship and personal issues (including anxiety and fear) that may contribute to premature ejaculation. A study conducted in Spain involving 157 patients compared treatment for PE using medication (dapoxetine) or psychotherapy or the two in combination. Initially, participants ejaculated in less than one minute. The medicine extended the time to ejaculation to about 3½ minutes. In contrast, psychotherapy extended the time to about 7½ minutes.

Tantric sex. The essence of tantric practice involves slowing down intimacy, coordinating your breathing with that of your partner, becoming exquisitely attuned to each other, and then experiencing your sexuality together at that slower pace. This approach heightens pleasure and intimacy, adding a spiritual dimension to the experience. Note that tantric and Taoist sexual practices also utilize specific training in breathing, sensory awareness, and relaxation, which enable voluntary control of the pelvic floor muscles in the pre-ejaculatory stage.

Please be sure to review chapter 88, "How to Please a Woman," which provides insight on both physical and emotional aspects of pleasuring your partner.

Lifelong PE	Acquired PE	Variable
Onset		
From first sexual experience on	Initially normal response; later onset	Normal but varied
Causes		

Genetics
  30% in twins' studies
  Confirmed association
  between PE and genes
  that code for
  serotonin; also link
  with COMT gene
Pelvic floor tone
  Strengthening and
  training resulted in
  cure of 54% of men
  with lifelong PE
  (Biofeedback and
  Kegel exercises)
Hypersensitivity
  On average, threefold
  increase in the
  number of dorsal
  nerve fibers, alleviated
  by surgery
	Aging
	  ED, low ibido
	Nerve function
	  Trauma, surgery
	  MS, Parkinson's
	  Neuropathies
	Body chemistry
	  High thyroid, low thyroid
	  Low serotonin function
	  High testosterone, low T
	  Low vitamin D, low B12
	  Low magnesium
	  Low nitric oxide
	  Low prolactin
	  High leptin levels
	Low pelvic floor tone
	Drugs
	  Dopaminergic drugs like Ritalin
	  Amphetamines and cocaine
	Hypersensitivity
	Psychological
	  Depression or anxiety
	  Performance anxiety
	  Porn addiction
	  Psychological factors
	  Relationship conflict
	Health Conditions
	  Diabetes (as many as 50%)
	  Diabetic hypoglycemia
	  Erectile dysfunction (30% –50%)
	  Prostatitis
	  Varicoles
		Normal at times, premature at other times
		
		Considered normal
		
		Also see Acquired PE

Treatment		
Medication: SSRIs Pelvic floor training Surgery (in China)	Resolve health issues Improve body chemistry Restore pelvic floor tone (Kegels, Emsella Chair) Sex therapy, couple's therapy, individual therapy, tantric yoga	Reassurance therapy Behavioral therapy

Figure 78.2. Therapies for sexual timing issues.

DELAYED ORGASM

As big a problem as premature ejaculation is, a surprising number of men suffer from the opposite problem: it takes them too long to reach orgasm. Some men aren't able to climax at all. This condition, called delayed climax or delayed ejaculation (DE), may be caused by several factors, including:

Biological issues:

- Age. As we get older, it takes longer to climax and ejaculate.

- Low testosterone or low thyroid hormone levels can delay ejaculation.

- Drinking alcohol before sex can delay orgasm.

- Medications can delay ejaculation. These can include 5-alpha-reductase inhibitors, alpha-blockers, anticholinergics, antidepressant drugs (including SSRIs), antiepileptics, antihistamines, antihypertensives, antipsychotics, anxiolytics, monoamine oxidase inhibitors, muscle relaxants, and opiates. Make sure you check the list of side effects of the medications that you take.

Physical health issues:

- Infections of the urethra, prostate, or testicles can delay ejaculation.

- Conditions that affect nerves or the nervous system, such as diabetes, multiple sclerosis, pelvic radiation, pelvic trauma, prostate surgery, or spinal cord injury, can delay or eliminate ejaculation.

- Physical or developmental abnormalities present from birth also can play a role.

- Lymph node surgery for testicular cancer spread

Psychological issues:

- Depression and other types of mental health disorders

- Unrealistic expectations. For many men, there's a disconnect between the reality of sex with a partner and their preferred sexual fantasy during masturbation.

- Concern about pregnancy, performance anxiety, fear of intimacy, sexual orientation conflicts, shame, or guilt can delay orgasm.

What You Can Do About It

There are several treatment options for men with delayed ejaculation.

Try This First. . . .

- *Strengthen the pelvic floor.* Kegel exercise programs (described earlier in the chapter) that strengthen the pelvic floor bolster the orgasm muscles. Privategym.com has specific instructions on how to do this.

- *Relaxation and breathing exercises* that enhance and coordinate mind-body responses may allow you to focus better on pleasure. Tantric yoga, which we described earlier, is an excellent example of this approach.

- *Male vibrators.* In the same way that women can be stimulated to orgasm by vibrations, male vibrators help men achieve climax. I remember one couple who came to see me because it typically took three hours for the gentleman to ejaculate. I referred them to us.funfactory.com to purchase a male vibrator. When they returned to my office a month later, the wife brought me flowers. With the help of a male vibrator, he was able to achieve orgasm in about 20 minutes. Us.funfactory.com has high-quality and effective male vibrators.

. . . If That Didn't Work

Make sure that your body chemistry is balanced:

- *Testosterone.* Check free and total testosterone levels and make sure that they are adequate. I prefer my patients to have levels of at least 400 or higher.

- *Thyroid.* Ask your doctor to check your thyroid levels and replace thyroid hormones as needed.

- *SSRIs.* As we described earlier, antidepressant medications delay ejaculation. If this is an issue for you, consider alternative therapy to SSRIs.

Medical approaches to strengthening core muscles and the pelvic floor:

The *Emsella Chair,* by BTL, uses powerful magnetic fields to contract muscles. The FDA approved the chair to help women with incontinence, and it has also been shown to improve sexual function in women. In addition, the manufacturer developed a protocol for men that strengthens the pelvic floor. I performed a clinical research study on men and their spouses that found an improvement in the intensity and duration of orgasm and presented this research at a major medical meeting.

Psychological therapies. Sometimes there are underlying psychological issues that prevent orgasm. Visiting a sex therapist can help a man address psychological issues that interfere with climax.

The effects of pornography. In some cases, unrealistic sexual fantasies and images can make it difficult for real sex to live up to expectations. Therefore, it is essential to readjust to "normal" and "typical" rather than the fantasy. Cognitive behavioral therapy or hypnosis can be helpful in dealing with an addiction to pornography.

The Final Climax

According to evolution, the primary purpose of the male orgasm is as a reward for battling other aggressive males for the right to reproduce. However, humans have evolved to achieve this pleasure strictly for the sake of enjoyment. As a result — and because, on average, men climax in 5 minutes whereas women climax in 17 minutes — reaching orgasm too quickly has become a liability. On the flip side, as men age (or for many other reasons), it can become difficult to achieve orgasm. If you suffer from either of those problems, I hope that the suggestions in this chapter will help you achieve an intimate life that brings both you and your partner great pleasure. I've discussed several solutions you can try at home and medical approaches and technologies available through your doctor. Please don't be ashamed to reach out or intimidated to try something new. As sports greats Wayne Gretzky and Michael Jordan both said, "You miss 100% of the shots you don't take."

For more information on issues raised in this chapter please see:

BrandeisMD.com

AFFIRMScience.com

Privategym.com

Us.funfactory.com

www.bodybybtl.com

Chapter 79
A Comprehensive Approach to Sexual Function
Judson Brandeis, MD, Urologist

Make each day your masterpiece.
— John Wooden

During my 25 years as a urologist, I have had the privilege of taking care of thousands of men. When you surgically remove a man's cancerous prostate or even perform a vasectomy on him, you get to know a man on a deeper level that goes beyond medicine. I realized that one of my strengths as a clinician is my comprehensive and personal approach to evaluating and treating sexual dysfunction. What follows is the discussion and thought process I use when evaluating a new patient.

The experience starts when patients enter my office. I create a relaxing and masculine environment where men feel comfortable opening up to me. The setting is critical because I can only help someone if they put all their cards on the table. For example, I recently met with a 55-year-old otherwise healthy and prosperous man with ED, but his story did not match his erectile function. I communicated that I was having a difficult time making sense of his overall picture. At that point in our relationship, he felt comfortable enough to tell me about his history of drug abuse in his twenties. Finally the pieces of the puzzle fell into place, and I could begin the process of helping him. It is essential to form a therapeutic relationship with your doctor and be honest about your medical history.

ASSESSING CARDIOVASCULAR HEALTH

Most erectile dysfunction is related to issues with blood vessels. Of course, any history of smoking, diabetes, high cholesterol, or high blood pressure must be addressed, and the ability to have physical intimacy is a strong motivator for change.

Loss of sexual function is often concrete proof that there is something physically wrong.

Going deeper, I look for a family history of cardiovascular disease in men with early erectile dysfunction since ED often precedes heart disease by five to ten years. I frequently send patients for heart scans, which can now predict early cardiovascular disease with great accuracy. I also send patients for vascular ultrasounds and find aneurysms and blood vessel blockages. If something does not make sense to me, I always try to find the underlying reason by ordering the appropriate tests.

I explain to men that blood pressure medications limit blood flow to the genitals. Nitric oxide boosters and stress reduction can reduce a man's dependence on blood pressure medications and improve erectile function.

Many of my patients have Kaiser as their insurance. The Kaiser system is excellent at taking care of a large population of Americans at a reasonable cost, but when I have a man sitting in front of me, my only concern is his wellbeing, not cost containment or the millions of other patients in the system. So, my approach is to optimize the performance of the individual I accept as my patient.

CONSERVING NERVE FUNCTION

Some men have erectile dysfunction because of nerve damage, especially those who have undergone prostate cancer surgery or radiation. Even when there is nerve-sparing surgery, men will rarely regain 100% of their presurgical potency. I put these patients immediately on a nitric oxide booster, a daily dose of Cialis, and daily treatment with a vacuum erection device to stretch and adequately oxygenate the penis. Early use of low-intensity shockwave therapy and PRP are also important therapies I use to restore erectile function in the post-surgical period. Without early intervention, there is little hope of regaining potency.

Another common but overlooked medical issue that causes ED is lumbar spine problems. The squeezing of the lower sacral nerves that causes back pain can also compromise the nerve signals to the penis. I had a 44-year-old patient with lumbar disc herniation who had ED that resolved after spine surgery.

OPTIMIZING PHYSICAL HEALTH

I put all my patients on an InBody body composition scale and discuss weight loss, nutrition, and muscle building. Excess fat can produce estrogen in men and limits a man's ability to exercise. I work with my patients to get their percentage of body fat under 20%. To do this, we need to restrict calories, and as a result, men need to make all of their calories count. I explain that the healthiest way to lose weight is by dropping one pound of fat per week, which is much harder than it sounds. Often this means significantly reducing alcohol consumption, because those calories come with no nutritional value.

Physical optimization requires determination and a long-term commitment. I do not shame or judge patients because everyone needs a different approach. My office is within an hour of the headquarters of Google, Facebook, Apple, Oracle, Tesla, and the Lawrence Livermore Lab. I attract engineers as patients, and they need data to change habits. Other men need a wake-up. For example, I had a 68-year-old man who was CEO of a successful company. I could sense that he and his younger wife were moving in different directions, and that he was occupying himself with work to avoid the discomfort of getting back into shape and reconnecting with her. I brought him into my office, looked him in the eyes, and sternly said, "What the FUCK are you doing! You are going to mess up the best thing you have going!" The next time I saw him, he told me that no one had ever talked to him like that before, but that was what he needed to make a shift. Within three months, he had lost 15 pounds of fat and had started taking his beautiful wife on hikes all over Northern California.

I also discuss physical fitness with my patients. Men over 40 need two or three days of cardio and two or three strength-building days every week. I especially like circuit training with lighter weights and more reps, reducing the risk of injury, and augmenting cardiovascular fitness. I discuss the importance of avoiding injury that will set men back and the need for consistency. Increased muscle mass will boost a man's basal metabolic rate, which is the number of calories a man burns every day just by being alive. Men also feel better about themselves when they are leaner and more muscular, and this boosts libido. I recommend the Emsculpt machine to men with financial resources to quickly increase muscle mass and get back into shape.

I need to rule out any unrecognized health issues, so my patients get lab work to check their kidneys, liver, blood count, vitamin D, B12, PSA, and electrolytes. Also, normal thyroid function is essential for erectile function. Then, of course, I check testosterone and free testosterone as well.

Testosterone is critical for libido and energy, concentration, sleep, athletic performance, muscle building, and fat burning. I used to be conservative about replacing testosterone, getting men back to "normal" levels, but I have discovered that men do much better when their testosterone levels are around 1000, and I have seen very few adverse effects. Of course, some men have their prostates grow and have difficulty urinating, while others complain about hair loss. However, optimizing testosterone plays a critical role in helping men get back into shape and regain their libido. For every one man with a complaint about testosterone replacement, I have 20 who swear by it.

OPTIMIZING RELATIONSHIPS

I always explore relationship issues with my patients. I see so many recently divorced men who have difficulties with erectile function, so much so that I joke with them and my staff that there is a divorce hex I need to break.

One aspect of relationships that needs to be addressed is the health of the partner's genitalia. I vividly remember the disappointment on my patient's face. We had worked together to restore his erectile function, and he was able to have penetrative intercourse with his 68-year-old wife. But unfortunately, she had a history of breast cancer and could not use estrogen, so her vagina was narrow and dry. Intercourse was painful for her and stirred up bleeding, so she refused to attempt intercourse again. As a result, I always supply my patients with a silicone-based lubricant such as UberLube and encourage them to discuss estrogen replacement with their spouses. Because of this patient, I enlisted a colleague to write the chapter on what men need to know about menopause.

Everyone has a story, whether they are a widower getting back into the dating pool (chapter 73), a monogamous couple getting older, or a couple rediscovering each other when the nest is finally empty. I believe it is essential to understand my patients' goals and give them realistic expectations.

Psychological issues certainly affect erectile function. For example, anxiety produces adrenaline which works against erections. Depression can dramatically reduce libido. Medications for depression, especially SSRIs such as Zoloft and Paxil, are also well-known to reduce erectile function and orgasm. Sometimes by changing antidepressants, the ED will resolve. This can be true of a surprising number of other medications as well. (See chapter 77 for a list of various classes of medications known to cause ED.)

SPECIFIC TREATMENTS

Many of my patients also have difficulty with clogged and narrow blood vessels. Fortunately, several regenerative treatments can help grow new blood vessels.

Shockwave therapy. I was an early adopter of shockwave therapy to treat erectile dysfunction. This technology uses pulsed high-pressure acoustic waves to stress the blood vessels in the penis. Mechanical stress in the body creates an injury response that activates stem cells and promotes the secretion of growth factors, leading to additional blood vessels that can increase blood flow to the penis. Using this technology, men with mild erectile dysfunction no longer need to rely on Viagra, men with moderate erectile dysfunction get better results from Viagra, and men with more severe erectile dysfunction are able to function without injection therapy. For more information on low intensity shockwave therapy, please see chapter 80.

Nitric oxide is a critically important and frequently overlooked solution to erectile dysfunction. As men age, their nitric oxide production slowly declines, affecting the delivery of blood throughout their bodies. Replacing nitric oxide improves circulation to the muscles, so many elite endurance athletes supplement with nitric oxide boosters. Studies have shown a small but noticeable improvement in athletic performance from supplementing with nitric oxide boosters. Furthermore, there are more nitric oxide receptors in the brain than any other organ in the body, so elevating nitric oxide levels improves mental sharpness. When I learned more about the effects of nitric oxide on erectile function, I created a supplement called AFFIRM, which utilizes both pathways in the body that boost nitric oxide. My patients and I have seen great results from supplementing nitric oxide.

PDE-5 inhibitors such as Viagra (sildenafil), Cialis (tadalafil), and Levitra (vardenafil) work together with nitric oxide boosters to improve the signals from nerves to dilate blood vessels. The PDE-5 enzyme is only present in the penis, which is why these medications are so effective in shunting blood specifically to the genitals. I put many of my patients on 5 mg of tadalafil every evening to improve their nighttime erections, which I feel are the key to long-term erectile health.

Trimix. Men with erectile dysfunction related to nerve problems or severe narrowing of blood vessels are candidates for injection of medication into the penis. This therapy is called Trimix because, typically, there are three medications, papaverine, phentolamine, and prostaglandin E-1. It is necessary to teach my patients how to inject the medication into the penis properly. We always start with a low trial dose because this medication can cause priapism (an erection that will not go away without medical attention). Injection therapy lacks spontaneity, but it is the only option for some patients. Information on the current range of medications and supplements available is in chapter 81.

Vacuum erection device. For men who are not experiencing nighttime erections, I recommend using a penis pump, also known as a vacuum erection device. Men are supposed to get 30 to 60 minutes of erections every night, which maintains the elasticity of the lining of the erectile bodies and oxygenation of the erectile tissue. When the body no longer does this naturally, men need to replace nighttime erections with artificial erections using a penis pump. I recommend a series of five 1-minute cycles in the morning and the evening. The pump is the least expensive, most effective intervention men can use to maintain size and function. Those men who are comfortable using a penis pump can apply a silicone ring on the base of the penis to maintain an erection for penetrative intercourse. You can learn more about penis pumps in chapter 82.

The P-Shot. At the end of a course of shockwave therapy, I will frequently recommend a P-Shot, which introduces platelet-rich plasma into the erectile bodies of the penis. Platelets have two functions in the body. The first is to form blood clots if we are bleeding, but the second and less well-known function is to release growth factors at the injury site. Therefore, injured tissue grows back more quickly than the surrounding tissue. Platelets contain 140 different growth factors, including vascular growth factors that stimulate the growth of blood vessels. To prepare a P-Shot, we draw blood and then spin the blood in a centrifuge. The red blood cells are heavy and gather at the bottom. Next, we extract the platelets and inject the platelets into the penis with a tiny needle using ultrasound guidance. PRP is like fertilizer for stem cells stimulated by shockwave therapy, and recent data demonstrate that P-Shots improve erectile function independently. In addition, I am conducting a clinical research study at BrandeisMD using a combination of PRP, penile traction, a penile suction device, and AFFIRM nitric oxide booster to improve both the length and girth of a man's penis. You can learn more about PRP in chapter 83.

An implant. Another option I discuss with my patients, especially younger men with a history of prostate cancer surgery or diabetes, is placing an inflatable penile prosthesis. This curative treatment for erectile dysfunction allows men to get an erection on demand and maintain an erection for as long as they desire. For many men, the idea of placing a synthetic implant is a substantial psychological hurdle that they need to overcome. However, once the implant is placed, it is all internal, and the quality-of-life questionnaires show a high satisfaction rate with penile implants. I refer all my patients desiring penile implants to Dr. Ed Karpman in San Jose, CA, who wrote about them in chapter 85. Ed taught the implant course that I took, and in his hands, this procedure typically takes 20 minutes and is done on an outpatient basis.

I now recommend pleasure aids, also known as sex toys, to my patients who need additional stimulation to reach climax. The reality is that as we age, our nerves are less sensitive, and we need extra stimulation. The Fun Factory was founded by an engineer who used his expertise to create high-quality sex toys manufactured in Germany. I encourage my patients, reminding them that there is no shame in getting a little help. Women very commonly use vibrators without any social stigma. Why not men? To learn more about sex toys, see chapter 86.

Creative Solutions. Not everyone can achieve an erection firm enough for penetrative intercourse. However, some of my happiest and most sexually satisfied patients have found ways to be creative. Susan Bratton has written a brilliant chapter on how to please a woman. Ms. Bratton's insights are found in chapter 88.

In summary, it is important to me that my patients feel good, look good, and have great physical intimacy. I try to create a comprehensive and long-term plan not only to restore erectile function, but to set men on a path for lifelong health and fitness that includes erectile fitness. By improving blood flow to the penis, we are improving the entire circulatory system. By helping men engage in physical intimacy, we boost their happiness and the strength of their intimate relationships. Happy, healthy men make great husbands, fathers, professionals, leaders, and neighbors.

Chapter 80
Wave Goodbye to ED
Judson Brandeis, MD, Urologist

If you're having a bad day, catch a wave.
— Frosty Hesson

When Viagra came out in 1998, it created a sexual revolution. Men who previously were unable to be physically intimate with their partner were now empowered. However, six hours after they took the pill, their powers disappeared.

PDE-5 inhibitors such as Viagra work by promoting signaling that opens blood vessels, increasing blood flow to the penis, which results in a rigid erection.

However, the other aspect of the equation is the health of the blood vessels through which the blood is pumped. If those blood vessels are clogged, the blood pressure generated in the penis will not be enough to prevent blood from leaving the penis through the veins. As a result, the pressure within the blood vessels will not be sufficient to achieve a firm erection or effective, pleasurable sex.

> *Shockwave therapy is the only treatment option currently available*
> *that focuses on improving tissue health to restore erectile function, as*
> *opposed to pills, pumps, or shots that have only a temporary effect.*
> *— Journal of Sexual Medicine, 2018*

The role of shockwave therapy in sexual health. Low-intensity shockwave therapy is a promising new technology that can stimulate the growth of new blood vessels to the penis. What we have learned is that shockwave therapy is potentially a curative treatment for erectile dysfunction caused by low blood flow to the penis. Shockwave therapy is an FDA cleared technology with investigational status for erectile dysfunction treatment. However, there is a significant body of literature on the efficacy of treatment of erectile dysfunction. Shockwave therapy is safe with minimal discomfort and does not interfere with physical or sexual activity. It is effective in more than 75% of men with mild to moderate ED but does require long-term maintenance, as would be expected, given the aging process.

Clinical improvement. Typically, shockwave therapy moves a man up a decade in terms of their level of sexual functionality. This means that a 55-year-old male who has to take Viagra typically will no longer need to do this after a course of shockwave therapy. A 65-year-old man for whom Viagra no longer works effectively will typically find that Viagra now works well. However, he is not likely to get to the point where he no longer requires Viagra. A 75-year-old man who no longer has success with Viagra will reach the point where Viagra works fairly well, but not very well.

Shockwave treatment is most effective when it is paired with synergistic treatments such as a nitric oxide booster, a PDE-5 inhibitor such as Viagra, use of a vacuum erection device, and PRP (platelet-rich plasma) injections to the penis.

Course of treatment. The advantage of shockwave therapy for erectile dysfunction is that the new blood vessels grown are semi-permanent. However, there is a certain amount of natural decline that occurs over time, so the blood vessels that grow eventually become less resilient. The duration of effect of shockwave therapy varies depending on a man's age and underlying health conditions. Some men need maintenance therapy every two to three months, and other men only require maintenance treatment once a year.

History of shockwave therapy. Shockwaves were discovered during World War II when depth charges were being used to blow up submarines. After the war, shockwave technology was harnessed by researchers in the field of urology to disperse kidney stones. Subsequently, orthopedists pioneered the use of *lower*-intensity shockwaves to stimulate growth of new blood vessels for soft tissue repair and wound healing. Based on these advances, in 2010 a group of researchers in Israel explored the use of shockwaves to stimulate growth of blood vessels in the penis. Their research showed improvement in erectile function.

Patients who benefit most. High responders to shockwave therapy tend to be younger, respond better to PDE-5 inhibitors such as Viagra, and benefit from repeated treatment with regular maintenance. The research found that shockwave therapy could be a preventative treatment for erectile dysfunction in high-risk patients such as type I diabetics and younger patients with coronary and vascular disease.

THE PATIENT EXPERIENCE

In a typical patient experience with shockwave therapy, a man will use a topical numbing cream 30 minutes prior to the treatment. A physician or a nurse then uses a device that resembles an ultrasound applicator, or a device that makes rapid tapping noises. (There are two types of devices. One operates on electromagnetic polarity changes and the other on pneumatic energy.) This generates waves of intense energy that are directly applied to the shaft of the penis on the left and right side and on either side of the base of the scrotum. The shockwave energy on the sides of the penis generates new blood vessels from the deep cavernosal artery. Shockwaves on either side of the scrotum improve blood flow through the internal pudendal artery, which feeds arteries in the penis. The head of the penis and the urethra have a separate blood supply and do not actively participate in the generation of an erection, and therefore are not typically treated. Treatment is uncomfortable, but not painful, and typically takes 15 to 20 minutes. Men can resume normal activity afterwards and can engage in physical intimacy that night.

A typical course of treatment is once or twice a week for 3 to 12 weeks with maintenance treatments every 3 to 6 months. Patients should not use anti-inflammatories such as aspirin, Motrin, or ibuprofen. In addition, steroids such as prednisone, Medrol, or epidurals will decrease the effectiveness of treatment. Otherwise, it seems to be safe to use shockwave therapy even while on blood thinners.

Patients typically begin to see results from treatment within four to six weeks. Sometimes men will see results after the first or second week, which typically occurs through the release of nitric oxide. In the third and fourth week these improvements will dissipate, but by the fifth week most men start seeing improvement again.

HOW IT WORKS

Shockwave technology (SWT) currently takes two forms: radial and focused.

- *Radial sound waves.* The radial sound waves that are used in shockwave therapy are lower in intensity, delivering a wider path with more diffuse energy. The purpose of radial waves is to stimulate tissue development and growth, not to destroy it.

- *Focused* waves. In contrast, focused waves aim the energy at a specific focal point. In medicine, focal waves are applied to disintegrate kidney stones using extracorporeal shockwave lithotripsy, for example.

To differentiate shockwaves from soundwaves, vibrations produced by sound are a type of energy that occurs in a consistent, linear, wavelike fashion. Examples include sonar from a dolphin, music from a guitar, or diagnostic sound waves from an ultrasound machine. In contrast, shockwaves carry more intense energy, so the waves rise more acutely and then drop off more dramatically. Shockwaves travel faster than sound waves.

There are numerous medical applications of shockwaves. In orthopedics, SWT is used to treat plantar fasciitis, tendonitis, and other ailments. SWT is also being investigated as a treatment for peripheral artery disease and heart issues.

In urology, shockwaves are used to treat erectile dysfunction, generated through spark gap technology to stimulate the blood vessels of the corpora cavernosa (the spongy tubes in the penis that create an erection).

Shockwave therapy produces a strong pulse of energy that creates cavitation bubbles that expand and then collapse. As these cavitation bubbles collapse, they break down calcification and other deposits. Cavitation bubbles affect the tissue and create a shear force that increases cell permeability and stimulates microcirculation and metabolism. A variety of cells are stimulated to grow, including stem cells, osteoblasts, and fibroblasts. Schwann nerve cells are also activated, and vascular endothelial growth factor is released, stimulating the growth of new blood vessels.

THE RESEARCH

Mechanisms of action. Tom Lue, MD, a researcher and a urologist at UCSF, has performed leading-edge work on the mechanisms of action that underlie this therapy, concluding:

- Shockwave therapy causes microtrauma that leads to the release of vascular endothelial growth factor or VEGF, stimulating the growth of healthy new tissue.

- The therapy also directly increases nitric oxide synthesis in tissues of the penis.

- Stimulation with shockwaves results in stem cell expansion.

Clinical studies. In clinical trials involving humans, the outcome of shockwave therapy is determined by evaluating erectile function or by measuring blood flow in the penis.

- *Erectile function.* The international index of erectile function (IIEF 5) or SHIM score is graded 5 through 25, with questions that directly relate to the strength of the erection.

- *Blood flow.* Penile duplex ultrasound is used to measure arterial blood flow. The limitation of this form of testing is that it requires direct injection of a vasoactive compound, which is uncomfortable and sometimes must be reversed.

Treatment of erectile dysfunction. The first randomized, sham-controlled study on shockwave therapy for ED was performed in 2012 on 67 men. The protocol involved a series of 2 treatments per week for 3 weeks, with a 3-week rest. The rest interval was followed by a second series of 2 treatments per week for another 3 weeks. The erectile function score increased by 6.7 on the evaluation compared with final scores of 3.0 for the sham group. Blood flow increased eightfold—8.2 mL/min versus 0.1 for the sham group.

Shockwave therapy plus a nutritional supplement. In a clinical trial by Judson Brandeis, MD, the protocol utilized low-intensity shock wave therapy plus a supplement, AFFIRM nitric oxide booster. Patients were treated once a week for 6 weeks. More than 70% of the patients responded with an average SHIM score increase of 5.2 at 5 weeks. This is the first paper in the literature to evaluate radial pressure wave therapy with a nitric oxide booster and shows more improvement in SHIM score than that found in studies looking at radial wave therapy alone.

Outcomes research. Two meta-analyses were published in 2017. The first looked at 14 studies on low-intensity shockwave therapy involving a total of 833 patients, showing average improvement in the erectile function score of 2.0. With shockwave therapy, there seemed to be a better response in patients with mild ED versus severe ED. Other meta-analyses looked at 7 randomized controlled trials with 602 patients. There was an increase in erectile function score of 4.17 over patient in the control group with high statistical significance.

An important paper on shockwave therapy published in the *Journal of Sexual Medicine* in 2018 reported that 6 or 12 treatments over a period of 6 weeks were efficacious with long-lasting effects that continue to be evident at 6 months. Twelve sessions yielded even more significant improvement in erectile function scores and also in duplex ultrasound evaluations, with an average increase of 5.0. Additional treatments at 6 months added another 2 points to the increase in erectile function score.

The Sexual Medicine Society of North America and the American Urologic Association position statement offer the perspective that the use of shockwaves or stem cells or platelet-rich plasma are safe but experimental and should be conducted under research protocols in compliance with institutional review board approval.

Triple Therapy

The data show that low-intensity shockwave therapy is a noninvasive treatment that semi-permanently improves blood flow to the penis in approximately three-quarters of carefully selected men with mild to moderate ED. It has no significant side effects. Patients with nerve-related issues or severe ED are unlikely to respond. We can resurrect a classic Thunderbird, but not a rusted-out Plymouth.

Shockwave therapy treats the corpora (the erectile bodies in the penis) distally and proximally and results in the growth of new blood vessels. At BrandeisMD we have developed a triple therapy protocol, using three interventions in tandem:

- *Nitric oxide booster.* Patients tend to respond earlier to treatment and have a longer lasting response. In addition, nitric oxide boosters provide general health benefits, naturally lowering blood pressure, improving cognition and athletic performance, and reducing the risk of heart disease.

- *PDE-5 inhibitor such as Viagra or Cialis.* Using a PDE-5 inhibitor enables more nitric oxide to stimulate the blood vessels.

- *Shockwave therapy.* The third aspect of triple therapy is the encouragement of blood vessel growth with low-intensity, broadly focused shockwave therapy.

Additional supplemental treatments complementing shockwave therapy include vacuum erection devices, platelet-rich plasma, and stem cell therapy.

For more information on erectile dysfuction, please see: www.BrandeisMD.com. To find a physician who provides shockwave therapy, please see: GAINSWave.com.

Chapter 81
Viagra and Beyond
Judson Brandeis, MD, Urologist

I am taking Viagra and drinking prune juice.
I don't know whether I am coming or going.
— Rodney Dangerfield

It is hard to remember life before iPhones, microwaves, and Viagra, but it was in 1998 that the FDA approved Viagra for the treatment of men with ED in the United States. Over the following 20 plus years, more than one hundred million men have taken Viagra and Cialis (termed PDE-5 inhibitors) to improve their sexual performance. Ironically, the researchers at Pfizer, who identified the erectile benefits of Viagra, were actually trying to develop a medication to treat heart problems. By blocking the PDE-5 enzyme, they hoped they would be able to open up the heart's blood vessels to some extent and and improve cardiovascular circulation.

Pfizer was disappointed with the results of the early clinical trials of Viagra, and by 1993, the pharmaceutical giant was ready to abandon the project. Then an observant nurse noticed that many of the men in the study were lying on their stomachs after receiving experimental sildenafil. It turns out that the men were embarrassed because they were getting erections. At that moment, Pfizer knew they were on to something HUGE!

In 1993, the NIH launched a campaign, reporting that impotence was a major public health problem and suggesting that the term "erectile dysfunction" replace the term impotence. Five years later, three medical researchers received the Nobel Prize in Medicine for discovering the role of nitric oxide in opening up blood vessels throughout the body, including the arteries that support penile erections, and the FDA approved Viagra for the treatment of men with ED in the United States. Following the release of Viagra, the FDA approved similar medications like Cialis and Levitra, all variations in a class of drugs described as PDE-5 inhibitors.

PDE-5 INHIBITORS

All PDE-5 inhibitors work essentially the same way, but there are slight differences between them. (Note that all medications are described by two names, their trade name, and their generic name.)

Viagra (sildenafil) has an onset of action of 30 minutes after the initial dose and a maximum duration of action of 4 to 6 hours. Visual disturbances like a bluish haze have been reported with sildenafil more often than with other PDE-5 inhibitors. The maximum dose of Viagra is 100 mg. Taking more than 100 mg doesn't improve Viagra's effectiveness, but it does increase the incidence of side effects, including headaches, facial flushing, visual changes, and reflux. The generic sildenafil is typically sold as 20 mg tablets, which allows the patient to escalate the dose as needed. Viagra should be taken on an empty stomach, or at least avoiding high-fat meals. Grapefruit juice can delay the onset of effect but can also increase blood levels of the drug.

Cialis (tadalafil) has an onset of 20 minutes and a duration of action of 24 to 36 hours. The maximum dose is 20 mg. Because of its long half-life, tadalafil 5 mg is sold as a daily dose. Cialis should ideally be taken on an empty stomach or at least avoiding high-fat meals. One unusual side effect of Cialis is muscle aches. Tadalafil is as effective as sildenafil and vardenafil but has a longer duration of action. The recommended starting dose for as-needed use is 10 mg, increasing to 20 mg if necessary. Lower doses of tadalafil of 2.5 or 5 mg are available for once-a-day administration.

Daily tadalafil has also been approved for treatment of lower urinary tract symptoms due to benign prostatic hypertrophy. Significant improvement in symptoms has been demonstrated. Men presenting with both erectile dysfunction and lower urinary tract symptoms may benefit from the convenience of taking one medication to treat both conditions.

Levitra (vardenafil) has the quickest onset of action at 10 minutes and lasts approximately 6 hours. The maximum dose is 20 mg. It has a side effect profile similar to Viagra and Cialis. There is a sublingual form of Levitra (taken under the tongue) called Staxyn, which supposedly has an even more rapid onset of activity.

Stendra (avanafil), which was approved in 2012, has a quick onset of action, and its effects last about 8 hours. It has a lower incidence of side effects. The dose options are 100 and 200 mg.

General recommendations. All four PDE-5 inhibitors (avanafil, sildenafil, vardenafil, and tadalafil) work to sustain levels of cyclic GMP within the penile erectile bodies to allow men with ED to achieve erections in response to appropriate sexual stimuli. Avanafil has the most rapid onset of action at 15 minutes. Sildenafil and vardenafil should be taken on an empty stomach, since high-fat meals and alcohol delay absorption. Food does not interfere with the absorption of tadalafil and avanafil.

Potential interactions:

Alpha blocking medications. These medications, commonly used for treatment of benign prostatic hypertrophy, may cause a decrease in blood pressure when taken in combination with PDE-5 inhibitors. Such alpha blocking drugs include doxazosin, terazosin, tamsulosin, and silodosin. Tamsulosin and silodosin are safer in terms of effects on blood pressure.

Nitrates. All PDE-5 inhibitors are contraindicated in men taking nitrates. None of the PDE-5 inhibitors can be taken with sublingual nitroglycerin or nitrate-containing medication in any form, whether taken regularly or intermittently. PDE-5 inhibitors are vasodilators that can lower blood pressure and interact with nitrates, so the combination can lead to a severe drop in blood pressure. If you have taken a PDE-5 inhibitor, you must wait 24 to 48 hours before nitrate treatment.

Grapefruit juice. Although our clinical information is incomplete, men who take Viagra should be aware that grapefruit juice can boost blood levels of the drug. That could be a good thing for some men with erectile dysfunction, but it could trigger headaches, flushing, or low blood pressure.

Common side effects. Like other subsequently developed PDE-5 inhibitors, Viagra's effect on the body is predominantly localized to the penis. but has been shown over the years to also target the blood vessels in other parts of the body. Resulting symptoms associated with PDE-5 inhibitors include:

- Nasal congestion 4%–7%
- Flushing in 12% of patients
- Headaches 11%
- Back Pain 9%
- Reflux 5%
- Blue vision due to a PDE-5 inhibitor cross reaction with a PDE-6 inhibitor, which occurs in 3% of patients, lasts 2 to 3 hours and disappears spontaneously
- Nonarteritic anterior ischemic optic neuropathy (NAION), a rare symptom that has occurred in 23 cases over a seven-year period (1998 to 2005) during a time period when millions of doses of the drug were consumed
- Extremely rare reports of effects on hearing.

OXYTOCIN

Oxytocin is a peptide hormone produced in the body. In both men and women, it is linked strongly to sexual behavior, orgasm, and bonding that is associated with sexual intercourse. However, oxytocin performs markedly different functions in men and women. In women it plays a key role in the induction of labor and in reducing bleeding after childbirth. Oxytocin also plays a key role in bonding between a mother and her newborn, in the letdown of milk when nursing an infant, and in the deepening of the mother's bond with her baby. In a man, oxytocin is released during arousal and promotes bonding between sexual partners associated with intercourse.

For men, taking an oxytocin supplement before or during sex has been shown to increase overall sexual satisfaction in a number of different parameters. Studies report a major effect on increased feelings of connection with a partner, as well as enhancement of the sensation of orgasm. In fact, a case study demonstrated restoration of orgasm in a gentleman suffering from acquired anorgasmia disorder (inability to achieve an orgasm). Oxytocin can now be obtained as a supplement in several different forms.

Drug delivery and timing of response:

Intranasal. The most common and quickest route is in the form of an intranasal spray. This method allows for rapid onset, with plasma oxytocin levels rising within 20 minutes, although most men feel the effects immediately. Studies show that oxytocin levels remain elevated for 60 minutes when applied intranasally. Researchers are unsure of why this occurs, given oxytocin's short half-life of 3 to 4 minutes. One conjecture is that oxytocin continues to be absorbed through the nasal mucosa in this time frame.

Oral drops. Another form is through oral drops, which are applied sublingually beneath the tongue. Some men prefer this method, taking 4 drops 10 to 20 minutes before intercourse.

Side effects. In current studies examining the effects of intranasal oxytocin on men's sexual health, no side effects have been reported. Intranasal oxytocin has been evaluated in numerous studies in women for different indications. Minor potential side effects that have been reported include stuffy nose, mild allergic reactions, or headache.

Given its ability to affect the central nervous system, patients with a history of psychosis should not take oxytocin. While there are many commercially available forms of oxytocin, this hormone has far-reaching effects throughout the body and thus should be taken under the care of a physician. As one of many potential boosters in men's sexual medicine, current research is ongoing.

APOMORPHINE

Apomorphine is a dopamine receptor activator in the brain. Due to its effects on the dopamine-2 receptor, it directly stimulates nerves that induce penile erection.

While apomorphine is derived from dehydration of the morphine molecule, there is no opiate activity associated with the medication. Unlike opiates, apomorphine is not a scheduled medication. This means that in a urine drug test, apomorphine will not show up as an opiate.

While apomorphine is more commonly used in treatment of Parkinson's disease, it was found that low doses were enough to stimulate erection with minimal unintentional effects. Another issue was finding the right dose and route of administration. Recently, studies have found efficacious and safe methods of using this medication for erectile enhancement.

Timeframe of use. Sublingual tablets of apomorphine are available for absorption underneath the tongue. The medication is absorbed within 7 minutes. Most men report effects within 20 minutes. Rarely this may take up to 50 minutes.

The effects typically last for hours, with plasma levels of apomorphine returning to normal after 8 hours. This means that no more than one (1) tablet should be used within an 8-hour period.

Effect in women. Studies have investigated apomorphine for treatment of low arousal and sexual dysfunction in women, with findings of increased sexual satisfaction scores.

Side effects. Adverse symptoms are uncommon, but include nausea, vomiting, headache, or dizziness.

Comparison with Viagra. PDE-5 inhibitors such as Viagra act locally, affecting the smooth muscles of the penis to enhance relaxation of penile blood vessels. This supplement results in increased blood flow to the penis, enhancing erection. In contrast, apomorphine acts directly in the brain to stimulate nerves that affect oxytocin-activated nerves in the spinal cord. These nerves trigger relaxation of the same smooth muscle tissue of the erectile bodies (corpora cavernosa), enhancing blood flow to the penis and thus erection. While the end result is the same, the pathway for enhanced erection is distinctly different. Viagra affects the blood vessels directly; apomorphine exerts its effects through the nervous system.

PT-141 (BREMELANOTIDE)

Bremelanotide is an FDA-approved medication for the treatment of hypoactive sexual desire disorder. In men it is classified as an experimental medication that has demonstrated efficacy in boosting erection and libido.

Timeframe and drug delivery:

Injection. Bremelanotide is injected subcutaneously into the fat under the skin, just 1/2 inch below the skin's surface, similar to an insulin injection. Onset to erection can be variable but typically occurs 30 to 60 minutes after injection and lasts for 1 to 2 hours. (Use the bremelanotide injection at least 45 minutes before sexual activity.) Libido increases in 30 to 60 minutes as well and can last 1 to 2 days.

Intranasal. In one study, it was found that intranasal administration of 20 mg of PT-141 resulted in an erection after 30 minutes and lasted for about 1 hour. Single doses were safely administered and well tolerated.

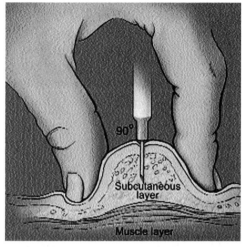

Figure 81.1. A subcutaneous injection into the fatty layer of tissue (pinched up to give the injection) under the skn.

Mechanism of action. Bremelanotide activates melanocortin receptors in the brain that directly innervate the penis. By activating these receptors, bremelanotide is purported to trigger erection as well as stimulate arousal in men.

Cautions. Do not use more than one bremelanotide injection every 24 hours. Do not use more than eight total injections within one month.

Side effects. Nausea is the most common side effect and can be treated with Pepcid OTC or Zofran 4 mg. Other common side effects include:

- Vomiting
- Hot flashes or flushing (sudden warmth, redness, or tingling)
- Cough, stuffy nose
- Headache, tiredness, dizziness
- Pain, bruising, redness, itching, bleeding, numbness, or tingling at injection site
- In very rare cases other severe side effects may occur. Bremelanotide may darken the color of mucous membranes or skin.

NATURAL NITRIC OXIDE BOOSTERS

When I was at UCLA, one of my professors, Louis Ignarro, PhD, won the Nobel Prize for discovering how nitric oxide and cGMP regulate blood flow by dilating arteries. Pfizer was the first pharmaceutical company to discover and formulate medication based on the new science of nitric oxide. Pfizer called these incredible little blue pills Viagra.

How it works. When an electrical impulse travels to the end of a nerve, the nerve releases nitric oxide onto the smooth muscle cells in the wall of an artery. This creates a chemical reaction that produces a molecule called cGMP. A rise in cGMP leads to a cascade of events that opens blood vessels.

The effects of aging on nitric oxide levels. As we age, the amount of nitric oxide that we produce can fall by as much as 10% every decade beginning in your early twenties. By age fifty, most men have nitric oxide levels below optimal levels, which results in a decrease in circulation throughout the body. If left untreated, we risk a decline in our athletic ability, short-term memory, and even erectile function. We know from decades of research on both nitric oxide and cGMP that they play a key role in a man's ability to be sexually intimate. Low levels of these raw materials underlie erectile dysfunction.

Nitric oxide from food. There are two pathways the body uses to increase nitric oxide:

- *Foods that contain the amino acid L-citrulline,* which is found in high quantities in watermelon, beans, nuts, meat, and leafy greens. Within the body, L-citrulline is converted to L-arginine in the kidneys. The L-arginine is then combined with oxygen to create nitric oxide. In the process, arginine is converted back to citrulline which then circulates back to the kidney where it is converted again to arginine.

- *Foods containing natural forms of nitrates that can be converted into nitric oxide.* Salad greens are a rich source of nitrates, as well as beets. Foods high in nitrate ($NO3$) can be converted by the saliva in the mouth into nitrite ($NO2$) and then into nitric oxide (NO) in the stomach.

The difference between nitric oxide boosters and sublingual nitroglycerine. When a man has chest pain from heart issues, one of the medications that is often given is nitroglycerin tablets, which dissolve under the tongue (sublingual form) and are fast acting. Nitroglycerine belongs to a class of drugs called vasodilators that work by converting into nitric oxide in the body. Excess nitric oxide relaxes blood vessels, so that your heart doesn't have to work as hard, which reduces chest pain.

When a man is taking PDE-5 inhibitors (e.g., sildenafil, vardenafil, or tadalafil), the use of nitroglycerine is absolutely contraindicated, because PDE-5 inhibitors combined with sublingual nitroglycerine can quickly drop blood pressure, which can cause fainting.

However, nitric oxide boosting supplements that are swallowed, instead of dissolved under the tongue, do not have the same rapid, short-term boost in nitric oxide levels. Oral nitric oxide boosters that are slow-release, like AFFIRM, can be taken at the same time you are taking a PDE-5 inhibitor.

The research on supplementation. Although there is no accurate method for measuring total nitric oxide in the body, clinical studies have provided tangible evidence of the benefits of supplementation:

- *Lowering blood pressure.* A study from the Hypertension Institute at Vanderbilt found that a single dose of a nitric oxide supplement reduced blood pressure within 20 minutes of ingestion. (The effect lowered systolic blood pressure by 4 mm Hg and diastolic blood pressure by 5 mm Hg.)

- *Weightlifters.* Recently, a study from Baylor University with weightlifters compared men in two similar groups over eight weeks. Those in the group using the nitric oxide boosters were able to improve their bench press max by 13 pounds over the control group.

- *Cyclists.* In a study involving nearly two dozen cyclists, participants took a supplement to boost nitric oxide production. The result was improvement in their track times of roughly 1.5% in just one week. Subjectively, participants reported feeling significantly less muscle fatigue after exercising.

Resource. I created a supplement called AFFIRM that uses both of the nitric oxide (NO) pathways to increase levels of NO in the body. Because nitric oxide is essential for the flexibility of the body's arteries, optimizing the available amount can help the body move blood more efficiently. I recommend that many of my patients take two AFFIRM tablets twice a day. I have heard from these men that it improves their erectile function and short-term memory, as well as athletic performance. Furthermore, I have been able to get many of my patients off their blood pressure medications.

For additional information on the supplements and medications discussed in this chapter, please see:
www.BrandeisMD.com and
AFFIRMScience.com.

Chapter 82
Penis Pumps
Joel Kaplan, PhD, Medical Device Inventor
Judson Brandeis, MD, Urologist

If you pump casually, you will pump forever.
Pump hard to begin with and keep it up until you get that water flowing.
Then a great deal will happen.
— Zig Ziggler

Since the dawn of humankind, men have been searching for the miracle product that will make their erections bigger and harder for sex. We've tried snake oils and other questionable (and sometimes dangerous) methods to achieve larger, rock-hard erections.

Finally, in 1874, Dr. John King designed an effective vacuum erection device (also referred to as a VED) and used it in the successful clinical treatment of erectile insufficiency. Since that time, manufacturers have created and modified a wide selection of vacuum devices also known as penis pumps. Originally intended to simply treat erectile dysfunction, today penis pumps are designed for several uses, including male enhancement, correcting mild penile curvature (Peyronie's disease), and masturbation. Penis pumping can be a very pleasurable experience. Many men enjoy the tension of the vacuum pressure and the increased sensation from the rush of blood flow.

ENHANCING SEXUAL HEALTH

Therapeutic uses. It is hypothesized that low blood levels of oxygen (hypoxia) result in the buildup of fibrosis of the spongy cylinders of the penis—the erectile bodies (the corpora cavernosa)—causing long-term erectile dysfunction. Use of a vacuum device can significantly increase oxygen concentration in the penis. Exercising the penis with a vacuum device improves blood inflow to the penis, which raises oxygen levels. This can prevent fibrosis of the erectile tissue within the penis, reducing the potential for scar formation and impaired sexual function.

Structural changes occur in the penis over time. As men age, nitric oxide levels decline in the cells that line their blood vessels (the endothelia). Arteries become thicker and inflammation and plaque can build up, eventually stiffening the wall of the arteries of the penis. Illnesses such as diabetes and cardiovascular disease hasten the process.

A healthy man typically gets three to six erections a night during sleep, each of which lasts 5 or 10 minutes, so that he gets 15 to 60 minutes of penile exercise every night. As a man's health deteriorates, the nighttime erections decline, which becomes the starting point for erectile dysfunction. Using a vacuum device may delay the onset of erectile dysfunction.

An article published in the Journal of Sexual Medicine *in 2014 reported that even a single application of a vacuum erection device increases oxygenation of the penis.*

Sexual enhancement in healthy men. Penis pumps are commonly used to enhance sexual function and erections. Healthy men without sexual dysfunction frequently use a penis pump before sex to increase the size and rigidity of their natural erection. These penis pumps are also commonly utilized as a regular form of physiological exercise to improve erection quality over time. There is a considerable volume of anecdotal evidence from male enhancement blogs, forums, and other social media that report long-term gains in both erection quality and overall penile volume. However, clinical studies show inconclusive data on the effects of penis pumping on long-term penis size.

Penis pumps use light vacuum pressure to attract blood-flow to the penis, resulting in a larger, harder erection. Depending on the use, the penis pump will also include different accessories to enhance the sexual experience. If used to achieve and maintain an erection for sex, the pump will likely include constriction rings (aka cock rings), to hold the erection for intercourse for up to 30 minutes.

Pleasure. As such, penis pumps have also evolved to be used as masturbation devices. These masturbation pumps include a variety of accessories and features, such as stroking sleeves, vibration, and flesh-like inserts for a more sensual feel.

HOW IT WORKS

Vacuum erection devices work in a fairly straightforward manner. They are painless with only rare side effects. A man places the cylinder over his penis and activates the pump to create a seal. Under pressure, blood is drawn from the pelvis into the penis causing an erection. To keep the blood in place, a man places a tensioning ring around the base of the penis, which can stay in place for 30 minutes. Vacuum devices are essentially made of three main components, which either plug into each other or come in an all-in-one-design.

- The pump mechanism, which creates vacuum pressure

- The vacuum chamber that surrounds the penis

- A pressure limiter or safety gauge.

Trim or shave your pubic hair for a better vacuum seal. Apply water-based lubricant at the base of the cylinder and on and around the base of the penis. Lubrication will assist in creating a vacuum seal and help avoid skin irritation. (We recommend water-based lubricant because it will not cause damage to the pump and is easy to clean.)

USING A VACUUM DEVICE

In order for a man to achieve an erection using a vacuum erection device, it is necessary to place a tensioning ring around the base of the penis. This prevents the blood from returning back into the circulation. It is acceptable to keep the ring in place for up to 30 minutes. After 30 minutes it would be advisable to remove the tensioning ring. Most tensioning rings are made of silicone, but some are made of hard plastic. There are some tensioning rings that are open on the bottom and are tightened by placing a rubber band around the base. For some men, this is an easier application.

Swelling, bruising, or discoloration may occur if the pressure in the vacuum chamber is too high or is increased too quickly. (These side effects are temporary and will go away after 1 to 3 days.) There is no benefit to pumping at a higher pressure. Use the least amount of pressure necessary to bring more blood flow into the penis. Wait for the blood flow to enter the penis and then slowly increase the pressure to bring more blood flow.

Some penis pumps come with automatic settings that may not allow the user to control the pressure, while others allow you to choose the exact pressure you desire. Never pump higher than -10 inHg (mercury inches of pressure). Most men find that a range from -1 to -6 inHg is ideal for erection enhancement.

Vacuum erection devices (VEDs) have become a staple in men's sexual health and vitality. Withstanding the test of time, they have proven to be one of the safest and most effective tools for male enhancement. Surgeries and other medical procedures are often too costly or have negative outcomes. Prescription drugs (such as Viagra or Cialis), while effective, often have side effects or can't be used due to a pre-existing condition. Penis pumps are a great, natural alternative that can be used whenever you want, as often as you want (even multiple times in the same day), giving the user great flexibility and control.

Possible contraindications. If you are taking blood-thinners, consult your physician before purchasing a VED, as you may face a higher risk of internal bleeding complications.

Purchase options. The two most common types of pumps are available in manual or automatic options. With a manual pump, you manually squeeze a pump handle, a pressure bulb, or some other form of pressure trigger. Automatic pumps can be operated by turning on a switch or clicking a button.

- Every penis pump should have a valve or button for control, to decrease or release the vacuum pressure.

- It is essential to purchase a VED with a pressure limiter or safety gauge to ensure proper and safe use.

- The cylinder can be plastic or a harder polycarbonate.

- Tensioning rings can be rubber or silicone, circular, or anatomic.

- Pumps can also be FDA compliant or not, which is related to the amount of testing they have undergone.

Lower-quality adult-store penile pumps are the least expensive option. However, these pumps have no pressure limiter, so they can cause deep bruising. They are difficult to operate and require both hands to work. There is usually no guarantee, warranty, or patient instructions and they are designed to be disposable.

Semi-medical-grade devices are of better quality and cost more. Sometimes these devices have pressure limiters, guarantees, or warranties. However, they tend to have low quality plastic which results in a mediocre seal. Operationally they tend to be adequate.

Medical-grade devices that are more reliable are higher priced. The pump is both manual and battery operated, extensively tested and 100% FDA compliant. They are easier to use, which is why there usually is a money-back guarantee and a three-year warranty. The taper-fit seal and anatomically correct tensioning rings result in a better patient experience.

KEY TAKE AWAYS

- It is beneficial for healthy men with mild ED to use a vacuum erection device.

- These devices improve oxygenation of the penis, which can delay and possibly reverse the destructive processes of aging.

- For a middle-aged man with ED, using a vacuum device once or twice a day will help prevent fibrosis and poor circulation.

- Using the device is safe and comfortable, with no known side effects.

- There are three grades of vacuum devices and using a higher-grade device will generally result in the highest satisfaction and success and justify the moderate increase in price.

For more information on penis pumps and vacuum erection devices, please see https://drjoelkaplan.com/.

Chapter 83

Platelet-Rich Plasma (PRP) for ED and More
Charles Runels, MD,
Physician of Regenerative Medicine

We must always change, renew, rejuvenate ourselves.
– Goethe

THE ORIGINS OF PRP THERAPY

If you want to see what works, what really works to help people in the terms of peak recovery and peak performance, see what's being done by those who care for elite athletes and multimillion-dollar racehorses. When someone's performance is worth millions of dollars for one day's work, people won't spare any expense to optimize that performance. Even a slight decrease in an elite athlete's output will be the difference between winning and losing—that is, in being worth millions or worth nothing.

That is how platelet-rich plasma developed as a tool to help people become stronger and faster and harder. The sports doctors and orthopedic surgeons who were trying to help football players (and professional golfers, and baseball players) recover were dealing with tissues that healed poorly because of poor blood flow.

For example, if you are a surgeon and you're working on a knee, you have a problem, because the cartilage of the knee contains very little blood flow. If you operate on the knee, it may not heal because there's no blood to promote the healing. If you don't operate on the knee and try to correct the problem with physical therapy, nutrition, and rest, again, the knee may never heal because whatever has been injured cannot receive enough blood flow for healing. The same problem of poor blood flow and slow healing occurs in dentistry.

Blood Flow is the Key

Given these challenges in healing avascular tissue, these two specialties, the dentists and the orthopedic surgeons (and the veterinarians caring for the joints of million-dollar racehorses), had to look for new ways to help tissue heal. They had a unique problem that other physicians did not have. For example, if you're a plastic surgeon, there's plenty of blood flow in the face. If you're a gynecologist, there's plenty of blood flow surrounding the ovaries and the vaginal tissue. So, you would not have the problem of trying to heal tissue or operate on tissue without enough blood supply.

The reason blood supply is so important is the thrombin cascade. The platelets in the blood that are activated during surgery cause clotting, but not just clotting of the blood. Importantly, the clotting factors also contain a platelet-rich fibrin matrix, and the activation of platelets brings growth factors to the area and creates healing.

In the history of platelet-rich plasma (PRP), health professionals who deal with hard-to-heal tissues started using PRP to enhance healing. They employed a range of experiments to determine how to concentrate the most growth factors in the smallest space, because they were working in small localized areas such as a joint or a tiny wound around a tooth. That has led to the development of the various devices that are now FDA-approved to prepare platelet-rich plasma. The orthopedic surgeons and the dentists who were attempting to deal with these problems worked out the science.

What is PRP?

Platelets are an aspect of our blood that have a dual function. The first and most well-known is to stop the bleeding when we are injured. The second, and less well-known, is to release growth factors so that the tissue that is injured will heal much more quickly. Platelets carry over 140 growth factors, and have been used to treat wounds and athletic injuries, and have many other regenerative applications. To create the PRP, the medical office draws a sample of the patient's blood and then spins the blood in a centrifuge. The red blood cells are heavy and go to the bottom, the plasma is light and floats to the top, and the platelets float to the middle, where the technician extracts them. Those concentrated healing factors are the PRP, which is then injected back into the patient, into the tissue in need of healing or rejuvenation. This eliminates any risk of rejection, since the PRP is taken from the patient's own blood.

Applying PRP Strategies to Other Dimensions

Pushing the envelope. In late 2009, someone got the idea of using the growth factors in facial plastic surgery, given their track record of success with knee surgery and dental surgery. A few forward-thinking plastic surgeons had already been using PRP to improve healing after surgery in the face, but, until 2009 or so, no one was injecting PRP as a stand-alone procedure for the face. Then, in early 2010, when I was doing many Juvederm facial injections, one of the salespersons for a PRP centrifuge visited my office and said, "Hey, you should try injecting PRP in the face. You get new blood flow, you get new volume, and there's never been a side effect." Once I began using PRP to rejuvenate facial skin, I developed the method now known as the Vampire Facelift.

At that point, no one had injected the penis with PRP, but as a man hearing about something that would give new volume and new blood flow, I thought, "If it works in the face, maybe it will work in the penis." Some were researching injecting stem cells into the penis of laboratory rats, but no one had injected PRP into the corpus cavernosum of a person.

I finally came up with a way to inject the penis and tried it first on my own. Yes, I was terrified. I was worried that the platelet-rich fibrin matrix might cause cell death (necrosis) or priapism, but it seemed to make my body healthier and more functional. It even looked younger. So, I started offering it to my patients, with excellent results, and then started selling the procedure and promoting research in the area.

I got the idea of using PRP in women (now referred to as the O-Shot) by watching how the matrix behaved in men. For every aspect of physiology that a man has, a woman has a corresponding organ, often of a different size or shape. Men have a glans; women have a glans. Men have two corpora cavernosa; women do as well. Men and women both have a corpus spongiosum. With women, the O-Shot improves sexual function, and it decreases urinary incontinence.

The Good News—and No Bad News

I do not know of anything else in medicine that has so many uses, with as much research, with so few serious side effects. Given the huge potential for use with a very safe record, scientists continue to look for new applications. PRP comes from a donor and is then used in the healing of that same person, so it could potentially be used in countries where monetary resources are low and drugs are difficult to purchase.

Let me confirm that this is not a cure-all. It's the same with every medical therapy, and this is true of all PRP therapies. Occasionally, I'll receive an email from someone who was injected with PRP without benefit, saying, "That P-Shot doesn't work. I had it two weeks ago, and nothing happened." Should we quit using antibiotics for everyone because they do not work 25% of the time with people who have pneumonia in the hospital?

Let's consider some of the documented, researched ways to use PRP to repair and to improve male health, function, and appearance: a man's hair, skin, joints, and more.

SEXUAL MEDICINE

When it comes to the penis, platelet-rich plasma works wonderfully well for some men for all of the following problems:

- Erectile dysfunction

- Peyronie's disease

- Genital mismatch

- Lichen sclerosus of the foreskin (BXO)

- Recovery after prostate surgery.

Erectile Dysfunction

Erectile dysfunction can be caused by decreased blood flow, venous leakage, or nerve dysfunction. PRP has been shown to help with increasing blood flow, decreasing venous leakage, and growing new nerve tissue.

With this procedure (which I developed), called the P-Shot, we use a numbing cream or a lidocaine injection to "put the penis to sleep." Then a very small needle is used to inject the man's own platelet-rich plasma into both the corpora cavernosa and the glans penis. We often combine that treatment with a vacuum device to fill the penis with blood and even overfill it so that there is room for the growth of the new tissue. This often leads to improved erectile function. Using the scale for grading ED (ranging from 5 to 25) a man's score will go up by 7 points on average.

The P-Shot will not help every man. Consider, for example, a man who has had type 2 diabetes for many years. He may have not only microvascular disease in the penis, but also atherosclerosis of the blood vessels that lead to the penis. In that case, the P-Shot procedure may be less likely to help.

A good rule of thumb to follow is that if a man has no signs of sexual arousal (tumescence) and nothing works, then, it's not likely that the P-Shot will help. For example, if he takes high dose Cialis or Viagra with no response, if he never has any sign of tumescence, or morning erection, or if he's tried Trimix and nothing helps. If the initial level of function is very low, or the nerves to the penis are severed or non-functional, PRP is not a good option, and these men potentially need a penile implant.

However, if he does have some responsiveness after the P-Shot, he may be able to cut the dose of his Viagra in half, or cut his Trimix injections in half; or, if he is on a low dose, he may be able to stop his erection medications completely or avoid starting them.

Peyronie's Disease

Peyronie's is the result of scarring of the penis, which causes the penis to be bent. The bend can be so severe that it can become mechanically impossible for a man to have penis-in-vagina sex. We know that PRP can help remodel scarred tissue into normal tissue, so it makes sense that the P-Shot (which uses PRP) may help Peyronie's (which is a very difficult problem to treat). We have had wonderful results for Peyronie's disease with the P-Shot procedure.

In sum, the P-Shot procedure, although not guaranteed, can be a wonderful help for Peyronie's disease, especially when combined with the penis pump.

Emerging Research on the Effect of PRP on Erectile Function

To date, PRP has been evaluated in more than 1,100 clinical trials, including 195 studies in the field of orthopedics. However, in the field of sexual medicine, the data has been scarce. In 2021, the Journal of Sexual Medicine published the first randomized, double-blind, placebo-controlled study on the use of PRP penile injections for the treatment of ED.

In the study, sixty patients each received two injections, one month apart, for the treatment of erectile dysfunction. That means half of the patients received actual PRP and half of participants received sham saline injections. Neither the subjects nor the doctors knew which patients received the actual PRP.

The study found that PRP injections improved erectile function in 69% of the men who received the PRP, while only 27% of the men improved who received the sham injections. The sexual health questionnaire score improved 20% at six months and no side effects were reported by any participant.

The PRP machine used in the study was a double-spin system with 60 ml of blood drawn, so make sure that if you get a P-Shot that your doctor draws 60 ml of blood and uses a double-spin PRP system.

Genital Mismatch

All sacred teachings can be summarized as Love God and Love each other. So, I want to say with absolute conviction that if men fall in love with men, or if women fall in love with women, love should be celebrated no matter what flavor genitals happen to be rubbing against each other. The Love counts more than the friction.

So, I gladly acknowledge that there are beautiful things to do with a penis other than insert it into a vagina; but, if a man is loving a woman, the way his penis fits his woman's vagina is more important than the size of his penis compared to that of other men. Ideally, a man's penis is large enough to push against the vaginal walls and massage the cliterourethral complex. Most of the pleasure that a woman receives from the penis happens not from the sensation of touch against the wall of the vagina, it's from pushing the vaginal wall outward to press against the urethra (not just the G-spot, the whole urethra), and against the inner part of the clitoris. If his penis is too large for her vagina, she may hurt and tear. I've examined women who would have great difficulty accommodating a penis that is over four inches long. Then, some women have a genetically larger vagina and need a larger penis to press against the walls of the vagina.

A not-so-funny trick is often played on humankind: you marry a most amazing woman, and you fit together perfectly. She vaginally delivers three babies, and her vagina now has a larger diameter. And, you (if you're like most men) will lose one half of the endothelium of your penis by the time you're 65 years old. Her vagina grows and your penis shrinks, so that now the genitals of two people in love no longer match.

In cases of genital mismatch, we now have ways to increase or decrease the size of the vagina (dilators, the O-Shot, surgery, radiofrequency, lasers). We can also increase the size of the penis using the P-Shot combined with a vacuum device, traction, and supplements.

If a man wants to grow his penis, often that can be done to such an extent that a woman can feel the difference, depending on individual response and the starting size. If you increase the girth of a six-inch penis by only one inch, you've doubled the volume! Usually, with the P-Shot, we see from a 10 to 20% increase in size. The P-Shot works best if combined with a vacuum device, supplements such as AFFIRM, good nutrition, and of course, no smoking. You can also combine it with traction devices and get some growth.

The guys with the biggest muscles have the easiest time growing more muscles when they lift weights. It's easier to grow a penis that's six or seven inches long than it is to grow a penis that's three or four inches long. But we have research showing that even with a smaller penis, there can be some growth, and we have more research underway to explore that idea (with Dr. Brandeis, the editor of this book).

If you're going to have the P-Shot procedure done, you should have it done by someone who is certified and licensed by the Cellular Medicine Association to do the procedure (see the directory on PriapusShot.com). Otherwise, you may be dealing with someone who is not using an FDA-approved kit and who perhaps is even doing an inferior procedure.

APPLICATIONS IN MEN'S HEALTH

Lichen sclerosus (BXO). If a man has lichen sclerosus of the foreskin (also called BXO), platelet-rich plasma can be used with great results just as PRP can help a woman with lichen sclerosus. The technique is simple and can be done by injecting PRP into the affected area by one of our licensed providers of the P-Shot procedure.

Prostate surgery recovery. We also use P-Shot to help the penis recover from prostate surgery. The normal protocol for recovering from prostate cancer surgery is to use a vacuum device twice a day and take low doses of Cialis and AFFIRM every day. Then, when the body recovers from the prostate surgery, the penis is in good health and is able to achieve tumescence (erections) again. These two modes of therapy maintain blood flow and keep the penis pliant, so it does not become contracted like a balloon that's never been blown up.

We recommend that same protocol, but enhance the process by providing the P-Shot once every eight weeks or so until the man recovers. However, if the man has had severe trauma from the surgery that's not recoverable, or has circulation problems through the iliac arteries, with poor blood flow to the penis in general, then helping blood flow within the penis will not help.

How to optimize the benefits of PRP. In some cases, there can be more than one aspect of the body that is below par. If a man has poor nutrition, if he is an alcoholic, if he's on high doses of cortisone, or has another disease that limits his anabolic capacity, then platelet-rich plasma would not work as well. Lifestyle factors that help healing such as vitamin C, good nutrition, and lots of rest, will enhance the effects of platelet-rich plasma. Adequate amounts of thyroid and growth hormone, either because you're producing it or because it's being corrected, also play a part in wound healing.

As usual, the whole organ system must be considered. Using the protocol of a P-Shot combined with low-dose daily Cialis, and a vacuum device twice a day, I've seen men who were years post-op with no erections recover good penile function following the protocol with the P-Shot. When it works (which is most of the time when done for the right reasons), PRP can do what nothing else does and can change a person's life.

How your partner may use PRP. In this chapter, we have discussed how platelet-rich plasma is used for men. Since many men have a woman they love, it is useful to know that it can help a woman with low sex drive, painful intercourse, or difficulty achieving orgasms. So when you have treatment, consider getting it for your lover as well.

Know that you don't have to wait until your erectile function declines. Even a Lamborghini needs regular tune-ups. I think eventually the research will show that having a P-Shot once a year could help prevent erectile dysfunction and keep men healthier than they would have been without it. It is possible that every woman should have an O-Shot immediately postpartum to help recover urinary and sexual function. If I could wave a magic wand and have had a P-Shot once a year, starting when I was about 17, I would certainly do so. Of course, I hadn't invented it when I was 17, but maybe your grandsons and granddaughters will do these procedures as part of a proactive health maintenance plan.

For more information on the work of Dr. Runels, please see:
Runels.com
CellularMedicineAssociation.org
PriapusShot.com
OShot.com
OrgasmSystem.com

Chapter 84
Stem Cell Medicine:
What Does the Future Hold?
Jeffrey Piccirillo, DO, Orthopedic Surgeon
& Doctor of Regenerative Medicine

Stem cells hold great promise to cure disease and reverse the aging process. Like any potentially miraculous new technology, they also create an opportunity for economic fraud, false promises, and unrealistic expectations. I asked Dr. Piccirillo to write a chapter on stem cells to help you separate truth from fiction. There are many devastating conditions, including erectile dysfunction, for which stem cells hold both promise and temptation. However, the science has not yet caught up with the marketing and widespread use. For this reason, the FDA has severely restricted the use of stem cells and stem cell products (which do not include PRP). I hope that this chapter serves as the basis for a deeper understanding of what stem cells are and how they work.

— Judson Brandeis, MD

"Code Blue, Trauma ICU. . . . Code Blue, Trauma ICU." Dr. Gregory Giamanco knows what this Monday is going to be like, as he walks through the doors. He's been in the hospital a total of 10 minutes, and the day is already going to hell in a handbag. His chief resident is waiting for him, in the Trauma ICU. He knows what awaits him on the other side of the automatic doors. . . . a 17-year-old kid who may never walk again. Last night he saw the story on the nightly news just before falling asleep — scenes of the ATV crash — and the rescue effort. He has already gotten a call from the resident, the details on the spine fracture and the paralysis. The thought crosses his mind that this young man's life is forever changed, unless his research can work a miracle. For now, it's through the doors, smile on his face, and coffee cup in hand.

He finishes his rounds and talks to the family; now it's time to walk across the street to "The Barn." This is no ordinary barn. It has all the same sounds and smells, but it's far from the quaint red wooden structures he remembers passing on the backroads of rural Iowa. This is a midrise in a high-tech industrial park, not more than 100 feet from the hospital complex, a top-tier trauma center. Lit with fluorescent lights and air conditioned, "The Barn" features the best chow and sanitation systems known to man. The workers, all with name tags and keycards, are in white clean-room jumpsuits. No single employee can enter the facility alone, given the required two-step verification.

Why? Because these are no ordinary farm animals. This is Building 14A, *the home of the* Mammalian Spinal Cord Research Program. *Some of the animals are Giamanco's special project. Severing the spinal cord of the animals. Injecting them with stem cells. Seeing if they can function normally again. He finds a researcher to get him into the secure area and is welcomed with screeches. The animals know who he is. They're climbing and swinging inside the massive cage, spines perfectly intact. It looks like all his years of research are finally paying off. Maybe, just maybe, that young man lying in the ICU will walk again.*

Science or science fiction? You decide. In 2003, Margaret Atwood wrote about transgenic knockout pigs that produced transplant kidneys, livers, and hearts. It was far-fetched science fiction. Today, not so much. We can actually help the human body repair tissues with the aid of stem cells.

Currently, scientists are working on "Knockout Pigs" to produce human-compatible tissues and organs in transgenic knockout pig hosts—organs that will transplant smoothly and avoid rejection. These transplant tissues and organs will also be able to fend off attacks by opportunistic microbes and viruses, just as Ms. Atwood so insightfully predicted. Additionally, a rapid-maturity gene is spliced into the kidneys, livers, and hearts of knockout pigs, so they can be ready sooner. What once read as fantasy has become a reality.

Today, many companies are using stem cells in conjunction with synthetic polymer scaffolding to recreate tissues in the laboratory. We can also repair tissues of the human body with the aid of exosomes, a form of stem cell derived from placenta tissue. So much for science fiction (which may not be fiction at all).

STEM CELLS: THE SHORT STORY

The best place to start is with a general understanding of what regenerative medicine means and how stem cells can play a role in slowing the aging process, allowing men to age with much less pain and degeneration.

Stem cells are specialized human cells that can differentiate into many different cell types (referred to as cell lines). The initial undifferentiated cell can divide to produce some offspring cells, which continue as stem cells, and some of those cells are destined to differentiate as various types of tissue throughout the body (220 different cell types). As a result, stem cells have the potential for use in therapies for replacing defective or damaged cells and tissue to address conditions ranging from traumatic injuries to Parkinson's disease, from heart disease to diabetes.

There are two major types of stem cells: embryonic stem cells and adult stem cells (which are also referred to as tissue stem cells).

- **Embryonic stem cells.** The cells that create the emerging life form are *totipotent*, meaning that they can divide into any other cell type within an animal, a process known as cellular differentiation. Embryonic stem cells are initially generalized, and must become more and more specific as they divide, a process that eventually creates the different organs, tissues, and systems of an organism.

- **Adult stem cells.** These undifferentiated cells found in adult humans were first identified in bone marrow. They are found everywhere in the body after embryonic development. These cells will divide to replenish dead, dying, or damaged cells. All adult stem cells feature self-renewal, while maintaining stem cell features and multipotency (the ability to differentiate into any cell in a particular tissue).

A snapshot of the science. Considering the story of stem cells from the point of conception provides deeper insight into how these cells can help us age with less pain and better healing. The act of conception occurs when the egg is fertilized by a sperm cell. The first cell formed is termed a zygote. This original embryologic cell is completely *totipotent* (the capacity to differentiate into any known cell type, as well as placenta tissue).

> *One single cell, the zygote, ultimately produces all the tissues in the human body.*

In the context of your own development, that first fertilized cell then developed into your cartilage, your hair, your heart, and your penis. Consider the capacity to heal and even reverse aging if we could harness the power of this type of cell when we are 50 years old.

The zygote continues to divide, and after seven cell division cycles, three distinctive cell layers form. Each of these layers is responsible for the formation of different tissue types and organs in the human body:

- Ectoderm (outer-most layer of cells)—skin, nervous system tissue, pituitary gland

- Mesoderm (middle layer)—cardiac muscle, skeletal muscles, smooth muscle in the digestive tract and kidneys, bone and cartilage, reproductive system

- Endoderm (inner-most cells)—digestive system, respiratory system, thyroid gland.

Ethical considerations. There has been an ever-increasing need in regenerative medicine over the past ten years to identify a plentiful, safe, and ethically acceptable source for stem cells to restore function in damaged or diseased organs and tissues.

We have discovered that full-term human placenta represents a prime candidate, as it is available in nearly unlimited supply, is ethically problem-free, and easily procured.

Placental cells display differentiation capacity toward all three types of tissue, and as a result, provide the ability to regenerate all tissue types throughout the human body.

These placental cells originate during the first stages of embryological development, so there is a possibility that these tissues may contain cells that have retained the growth potential of the early embryonic cells from which they derive, without harming a human embryo.

REGENERATIVE MEDICINE TODAY

If we have an injury or disease, or have begun to experience aging, and want to harness the power of regenerative medicine, what are our options in terms of current stem cell science? How do we acquire the cells, and what can we expect?

And what do men in my age group want to know when it comes to regenerative medicine and stem cells? The answer is obvious. What is currently available to me that will allow me to feel, act, and perform the way I did 20 years ago?

Enter platelet rich plasma (PRP). Over the past 20 years, science has developed the capacity to slow the aging process. The key to this emerging regenerative medicine is PRP (platelet rich plasma), which involves harvesting platelets from human whole blood, complete with all the associated growth factors.

I began using PRP in 2002 and have been involved in regenerative medicine ever since. PRP initially started in the hands of the dentists and was then researched and improved upon by orthopedists. Today it is used in dentistry, wound care, orthopedics, aesthetics, and sexual health. (To read more on the power of PRP, see the preceding chapter by Dr. Charles Runels.)

If PRP was the starting point of the journey to better immortality, then stem cells are the penultimate destination. But how do we get to that destination, and what are the many stops along the way? As physicians started using PRP with success in the early 2000s, forward-thinking physicians (like the authors of this book) began looking at how we could improve outcomes.

Donor and recipient: The same individual. PRP is derived from the blood of the specific patient who will be receiving the treatment, so that individual is both donor and recipient. We knew early on that PRP derived from a 20-year-old college athlete was different than PRP recovered in the same fashion from a 65-year-old grandfather with diabetes. So, the question was asked, "How can we improve PRP, and get the same results in the grandfather that we are able to get in the athlete?"

Making this type of inquiry, researchers and clinicians have refined techniques to improve on platelet-rich plasma. For example, we found that if the patient/donor performed 20 minutes of aerobic activity before drawing blood, that improved the quality of the PRP. We also learned that we can wash the platelets and freeze the blood plasma. While this research was occurring, others looked at what could be added to the PRP to make the final product more potent.

A NEW SOURCE OF STEM CELLS

The first stop, we came to realize, was the placenta. Imagine the scientific possibilities. Amniotic fluid is rich in growth factors, which can develop a human life from a single cell in just nine short months. It has an almost unlimited supply of multipotent stem cells and contains some pluripotent stem cells. The regenerative pathway was now more comprehensive. A search of the literature shows articles, published as early as 2006, that evaluated amniotic stem cells and the growth factors contained in the amniotic fluid to serve as a cellular matrix for tissue engineering. (Tissue engineering—You mean, like growing a new kidney for transplant? Margaret Atwood's novel *Oryx and Crake* is not so farfetched today.)

As science and technology developed in the regenerative space, researchers started to look deeper into placental tissue for sources of stem cells and growth factor peptides to aid in tissue regeneration. Consider: During every caesarean section, the obstetrician discards the placental tissues (e.g., placenta and umbilical cord). Both of these tissues are rich sources of stem cells that contain unique properties with enormous potential beyond those of adult stem cells. The following is a summary of what is *currently* available commercially, along with uses, reported benefits, pitfalls, and criticisms.

Wharton's Jelly — A Compound from the Umbilical Cord

Mesenchymal stem cells (MSC's) derived from Wharton's jelly are ideal for many reasons. They are recovered from healthy, screened, and tested umbilical cords donated after a scheduled caesarean section, so they are derived from procedures performed every day in hospitals across the U.S.

This compound is a gelatin-like substance found in the umbilical cords of placental mammals. It's primarily composed of hyaluronic acid and chondroitin sulfate, both of which are important in maintaining healthy joint cartilage. Wharton's jelly surrounds, insulates, supports, and protects the umbilical arteries and veins. It was first described more than three hundred years ago in 1656 by Dr. Thomas Wharton. Wharton's jelly found in humans is a unique form of connective tissue that contains only mesenchymal stem cells and no other cell types.

Wharton's jelly is one of the richest sources of mesenchymal stem cells that we know.

Looking at the concentration of stem cells to non-stem cells in Wharton's jelly, the range is from 1:300 cells to 1:1,700 cells. In contrast, the ratio of adult stem cells in a 60-year-old is 1:2,000,000.

■ MSCs from Wharton's jelly are "immune-privileged" and do not stimulate an immune response in the recipient, meaning they are unlikely to create an allergic or rejection reaction.

■ Tissue or blood typing is not required to receive these stem cells. Furthermore, they are non-tumorigenic, meaning they cannot produce tumors, as embryonic stem cells can.

■ Wharton's jelly derived MSCs are young and vibrant, and can multiply and divide at a rapid rate — one WJ-MSC can create up to one billion cells in 30 days, as opposed to the 200 cells that bone marrow-derived MSC from a 65-year-old person can produce.

■ WJ-MSC can differentiate into other cell types (such as bone, cartilage, etc.) as needed.

■ Finally, WJ-MSCs can release up to 300 bio-active molecules, growth factors, and cytokines, compared to the 100 to 200 that older adult stem cells are capable of producing. Ultimately, these substances have extensively contributed to the powerful healing, immunomodulatory, anti-inflammatory, and regenerative abilities of stem cell treatments.

Live Placental Stem Cells

The current investigation of these live placental stem cells has shown they can be given as IV therapy with a range of benefits that:

■ Reduce overall inflammation associated with an auto-immune disease.

■ Help battle early forms of neurodegenerative disease such as Parkinson's and Alzheimer's.

■ Can be given regularly to slow the aging process.

The human placenta is a rich source of stem cells. While adult stem cells need to be a match to the host (much like blood transfusions) to avoid rejection by the recipient's immune system, stem cells of the umbilical cord and of placental origin do not need to be matched.

Immune-privileged status. Young cells present in birth tissues have not fully developed the surface proteins ("HLA markers") found on the outer membranes of adult cells, and thus can "fly under the radar" of the recipient's immune system. This immune-privileged status makes the transplant a more straightforward task. Instead of harvesting the cells from the patient, which carries certain surgical risks, the doctor can now administer precise doses of stem cells that will be perceived as neutral by the patient's immune system.

Therapeutically active. Stem cells of birth tissue origin have another unique advantage. These cells are young and are therapeutically more active. While we do not yet know all of the mechanisms by which stem cells promote healing, we do know that these cells produce cytokines and growth factors and recruit local cells to perform the work of repair and regeneration. When birth tissue stem cells are compared to adult stem cells, they demonstrate a higher level of secretion of cytokines and growth factors, a faster speed of differentiation, slower cellular aging, stronger anti-inflammatory effects, and a greater number of future cell divisions before eventual cell death. Studies also have shown that umbilical cord stem cells have greater nerve-protective and nerve-restorative properties compared to adult bone marrow stem cells.

Exosomes — Potent Cells from Placenta Fluids

Exosomes are catalysts for whole-body health and regeneration with the capacity to:

- Alter inflammation

- Contribute to tissue and organ repair

- Support communication within the nervous system

- Enhance mitochondrial viability to support energy production at the level of the cell

- Participate in the transformation of aging cells

- Help regulate and normalize immune responses.

Exosomes are essentially placental stem cells with all the cellular material removed. These exosomes can target any damaged cell, whether in a joint (arthritis), the heart (heart failure), or the brain (Alzheimer's Disease). The use of exosomes in tissue regeneration is very new, but the future looks extraordinarily bright.

Lower risk. They have all the advantages of stem cell therapy, without the risk. And what are these risks? When a doctor injects stem cells into a host (your body), the DNA from that cell can mix with your DNA, exposing you to the other person's genetic material and the instructions it provides. This combination is called a Chimera. The most common "stem cell" treatment is a bone marrow transplant, and the company 23andMe, answered a consumer question as follows "If you have received a bone marrow transplant, we cannot recommend that you use the 23andMe Personal Genetic Service (Ancestry Service or

Health & Ancestry Service)." (The implication is that the genetic material in a transplant can skew the recipient's genome.)

Peptide therapy. Exosomes are recognized for cell-to-cell communication and provide instructions and resources to renew the receiving cells. These nano-sized extracellular vesicles contain specific peptides that send messages to the host's stem cells, allowing the body to respond to these signals with tissue regeneration.

Amniotic Tissue

This injectable biologic agent is derived from amniotic tissue, which can augment PRP or be used as a standalone product. The tissue has the capacity to create new blood vessels (described as *pro-vascular*) with the potential to reduce inflammation. Amniotic tissue also contains proteins that can signal the body's own stem cells to track to an area and promote tissue regeneration.

There are two distinct methods to derive these products. The original products were simply an aspiration from the amniotic sac (a common procedure in medicine termed amniocentesis) just before the delivery of the baby. The second method involves recovering amniotic cells from the lining of the placenta after a caesarean section, placing those cells in a growth medium, and then recovering the newly produced fluid, which is then packaged for delivery to physicians for use in treatment. Both products are robust in growth factors and anti-inflammatory cytokines.

However, the debate remains: Do these allografts contain pluripotent stem cells, with the capacity to develop into all 220 tissue types? This is hopeful, but not yet state-of-the-science. A study in 2019 by Alberto Panero, in the *American Journal of Sports Medicine*, showed live stem cells present in fresh amniotic fluid. However, when he looked at the prepared final product, he could not identify any live cells. Apparently, this is still a work in progress.

AUTOLOGOUS THERAPY: THE RECIPIENT IS THE DONOR

Currently we also have stem cell therapy that is autologous, derived from your own body. This all began with harnessing the healing power of our blood using platelet-rich plasma (PRP). Since our bone marrow produces our blood, the bone marrow is a rich source of stem cells.

Bone Marrow Concentrate (BMAC)

Under certain conditions, some stem cells can also create various types of new tissue, such as bone, cartilage, and fat, as well as blood vessels.

Bone marrow is the soft, spongy substance that fills the inner cavities of bones and produces blood. Bone marrow concentrate (BAMC) is made by first collecting bone marrow from a large bone (for example, the pelvic bone) through a minimally invasive procedure, such as a needle aspirate.

A doctor performs the procedure under local anesthesia, sedation, or general anesthesia. The aspirate is processed, spun in a centrifuge, similar to the way we separate PRP from the blood. Specific stem cells in the BAMC can help to create new tissue. Tiny spaces in the bone marrow hold blood; this blood contains stem cells, primitive cells that can grow into various types of blood cells.

Bone marrow processing methods vary widely and can affect the number and quality of cells, especially in terms of the useful stem and progenitor cells. Additionally, as we age, the number of stem cells in bone marrow declines. This is the ratio of stem cells to regular cells from birth to age 60:

Birth – 1:1500

Age 15 – 1:150,000

Age 40 – 1:500,000

Age 50 – 1:1,000,000

Age 60 – 1:2,000,000

Herein lies the reason for the significant research on placental-derived stem cells.

Micronized Fat

The evidence for the use of fat tissue in the field of cosmetic surgery is very promising, reflected in innovations such as the Vampire Facelift and various sexual health therapies (think tissue restoration, as well as plumper labia and thicker penises).

Fat is another tissue in the body that provides a source of stem cells. Fatty tissue removed through liposuction has a large amount of mesenchymal stem cells (MSCs). I have always felt that if the plastic/cosmetic surgeons can do this in facial rejuvenation, for breast enhancement, and Brazilian butt lifts, and get great results, why shouldn't it work for joint injections.

In the past, many orthopedic surgeons have used a technique called stromal vascular fraction in which fat stem cells, released from their surrounding collagen by an enzymatic process, are reinjected into a joint as a form of treatment for osteoarthritis. The results were quite promising. However, the FDA said that this was illegal and violated Section 127.

Since physicians were manipulating the tissues, the FDA classified this new product as a drug as a form of treatment for osteoarthritis.

Micronized fat aspirate can still be used at this point. There is some controversy as to whether the stem cells are released from the surrounding tissue or from the fat. A study out of Emory University, published in 2019, showed encouraging results using micronized fat in joint injections for arthritis, with less pain involved than a bone marrow aspirate. The study reviewed data collected from male and female patients approximately 60 years of age who received BMAC (bone marrow aspirate concentrate) or (micronized fat) MFAT injections for symptomatic knee osteoarthritis and completed both baseline and follow-up surveys at around six months to two years after treatment. Encouragingly, both BMAC and MFAT treatments led to significant improvements in pain and function according to all surveys, and there were no differences between BMAC and MFAT treatments.

THE FUTURE IS NOW

Every year, many Americans seek embryologic stem cell treatments across the U.S. and in foreign countries such as China, Germany, and Israel (for what is now referred to as stem-cell tourism).

Know that these treatments involve sophisticated protocols that only work in the hands of a qualified practitioner with specific training and skill. Whether you are looking to erase wrinkles, treat erectile dysfunction, enlarge your penis, or treat the wear and tear on your joints, you will want do the following:

- Find a qualified provider with a documented track record.
- Shop around to determine the best provider for you.
- Remember that cheapest is rarely the best.

And in the words of Mae West, "You are never too old to become younger!"

Stem Cell Uses and FDA Regulations

The FDA has the authority to regulate stem cell products in the United States.

Today, doctors routinely use stem cells that come from bone marrow or blood in transplant procedures to treat patients with cancer and disorders of the blood and immune system.

With limited exceptions, investigational products must also go through a thorough FDA review process as investigators prepare to determine the safety and effectiveness of products in well-controlled human studies, called clinical trials. The FDA has reviewed many stem cell products for use in these studies.

As part of the FDA's review, investigators must show how each product will be manufactured so the FDA can make sure appropriate steps are being taken to help ensure the product's safety, purity, and strength (potency). The FDA also requires sufficient data from animal studies to help evaluate any potential risks associated with product use.

That said, some clinics may inappropriately advertise stem-cell clinical trials without submitting an IND (an Investigational New Drug Application). Some clinics also may falsely advertise that FDA review and approval of the stem cell therapy is unnecessary. But when clinical trials are not conducted under an IND, it means that the FDA has not reviewed the experimental therapy to help make sure it is reasonably safe. So be cautious about these treatments.

Researchers hope stem cells will one day be effective in the treatment of many medical conditions and diseases. But unproven stem cell treatments can be unsafe—so get all of the facts if you're considering any treatment.

Stem cells have been called everything from cure-alls to miracle treatments. But don't believe the hype. Some unscrupulous providers offer stem cell products that are both unapproved and unproven. So beware of potentially dangerous procedures—and confirm what's really being offered before you consider any treatment.

The facts: Stem cell therapies may offer the potential to treat diseases or conditions for which few treatments exist. Sometimes called the body's "master cells," stem cells are the cells that develop into blood, brain, bones, and all of the body's organs. They have the potential to repair, restore, replace, and regenerate cells, and could possibly be used to treat many medical conditions and diseases.

But the U.S. Food and Drug Administration is concerned that some patients seeking cures and remedies are vulnerable to stem cell treatments that are illegal and potentially harmful. And the FDA is increasing its oversight and enforcement to protect people from dishonest and unscrupulous stem cell clinics, while continuing to encourage innovation so that the medical industry can properly harness the potential of stem cell products.

To do your part to stay safe, make sure that any stem cell treatment you are considering is either:

- FDA-approved, or

- Being studied under an Investigational New Drug Application (IND), which is a clinical investigation plan submitted and allowed to proceed by the FDA.

KEY TAKE AWAYS

All stem cells have the potential to develop into different types of cells, and this science can be quite fascinating. By understanding the science, you can become a better educated consumer, if and when the time comes that you desire a regenerative procedure.

- Totipotent: A stem cell that can develop into any and all of the 220 cell types within the human body, as well as extraembryonic cells or placental cells. Embryonic cells within the first few cell divisions after fertilization are the only cells that are totipotent.

- Pluripotent: A stem cell that can develop into all 220 tissue types, but not into placental tissue. Embryonic cells, after the first few cell divisions, fall into this category. It is the pluripotent stem cell that has the most promise in the field of regenerative medicine.

- Multipotent: Multipotent cells can develop into more than one tissue type, but are more limited than a pluripotent cell. Adult stem cells, such as those derived from fat or bone marrow, fall into this category, as do stem cells derived from both tissue and blood (placenta, umbilical cord, Wharton's jelly, and umbilical cord blood).

- Although PRP and stem cell therapies are gaining popularity in the medical community, there will always be practitioners who are jumping on the bandwagon for the wrong reason. Buyer beware: Before agreeing to a procedure, always do your own research, check out the physician, and if need be, seek a second opinion. If you feel the price is excessively high, or excessively low, or if you don't feel comfortable, it's never a bad idea to walk away and reassess.

Books

Jeffrey Piccirillo, DO. *Perfect PRP: How to achieve excellent outcomes with platelet-rich plasma from aesthetics to urology.* Ocala, FL: KDP Publishing, 2021.

Jeffrey Piccirillo. *The Journey to Perfect PRP: A patient's guide on how to get the optimal outcome from your PRP injection.* Ocala, FL: KDP Publishing, 2021.

For additional information on the work and services of Dr. Piccirillo, please see RegenMedicalGroup.com & www.perfectprpthebook.com

Chapter 85

When a Penile Implant Is the Best Option
Edward Karpman, MD, Urologist
Judson Brandeis, MD, Urologist

Patient satisfaction rates with penile prostheses are higher than 85%,
and sexual quality of life is improved in both patients and their partners.
— Dr. Gregory Barton, Sexual Medicine Reviews, 2019

Dale was 52. He remembered that day in the urologist office like it was yesterday. Gleason score 8, prostate cancer. He remembered his father's struggle with prostate cancer and also the day his father died. Dale went to the top prostate cancer surgeon in town and had his prostate removed. Fortunately, his cancer was cured. Unfortunately, the nerves on either side of the prostate that helped initiate an erection had to be removed as well.

At that point, Dale and his wife had been married for 25 years and had three beautiful children. He was professionally successful and committed to his community. However, the physical intimacy that Dale had enjoyed with his wife was missing. Two years after his prostatectomy, he worked up the courage to ask his urologist about a penile implant. Viagra had not worked for him, and Dale was reluctant to use shots every time he wanted to get an erection. He could tell that his wife was missing the physical connection as well, but he sensed that she felt badly about saying anything.

Dale's urologist put him in touch with another urologist who had expertise in performing penile implants. The actual operation took under an hour, and Dale went home the same day. He took pain medication for about 3 to 4 days, and he was pretty sore for a week. Fortunately, as an accountant, he could work from home. Six weeks after the surgery, he went back to his surgeon for the final check. Then he watched the videos and made it a point to learn exactly how the implant worked.

That night, Dale took his wife out and, as they relaxed over dinner, he opened up, confessing how difficult it had been for him over the past two years. His wife was understanding, but she also confided how much she missed their physical connection. Later on that night, they experimented together, inflating the implant for the first time. His penis was slightly shorter than they remembered, and the head of the penis was a little floppy, so they had to use the silicone-based lubricant the urologist had recommended. However, once he was inside, it felt just like the old days; in fact, it may have even been better. Before, he used to have issues with climaxing too early, but with the implant, it seemed he could go forever. After two years of waiting, Dale and his wife fully reconnected.

Penile implants are designed for men who cannot use oral medications to achieve an erection or do not find them effective. Penile prostheses have been used for the treatment of erectile dysfunction since the 1950s. These devices have a patient satisfaction rate of more than 90%.

These implants can also be used by men with Peyronie's disease to improve both erections and curvature. A man requesting a penile implant must have enough manual dexterity to operate the implant effectively.

The inflatable implant. Approximately 90% are inflatable penile prostheses designed to approximate the rigidity and flaccidity of the normally functioning penis. These devices consist of two hollow cylinders placed within the corpora cavernosa and the pump, which is placed in the scrotum like a third testicle.

Erection is achieved by repeatedly squeezing the pump. Each compression sends fluid from the reservoir to the intra-corporal cylinders achieving rigidity. Pressing the valve mechanism in the scrotal pump causes fluid to flow from the cylinders back to the reservoir.

The semirigid implant. These implants are available as a semirigid rod, which is easy to use, but results in a permanent erection. These devices represent less than 10% of all implanted prosthetics.

Minimal risk of infection. One of the risks of implants is infections. Men who have diabetes are at particular risk of bacterial infections. New implants utilize antibiotic coatings to minimize infection rates, which are typically less than 2%.

KEY TAKE AWAYS

Successful placement of a penile implant has the highest satisfaction rate of all treatment options for erectile dysfunction. Penile implants have allowed men to have effective, reliable, and cosmetically acceptable erections.

For more information on penile implants and the work of Dr. Karpman, please see www.elcaminourology.com.

Chapter 86
Sex Toys
Dirk Bauer, Engineer
Judson Brandeis, MD Urologist

Sex toys have long since graduated from the floppy rubber things you hide in your bedside table to beautiful works of interactive art.
— *Gwyneth Paltrow*

Have you ever wondered about pleasure aids, also known as sex toys? Believe it or not, in 2018, sex toys were a $25 billion dollar industry, and that is projected to double by 2026. Pleasure aids are widely recognized in popular culture for women. However, male sex toys receive far less attention. Pleasure aids bring new stimuli to the routine sexual practices performed by men for themselves or with a partner. These tools are capable of taking sensations to new and otherwise unreachable heights.

Unless you have been seeing a sex educator or counselor, the topic of male sex toys may seem entirely foreign. However, their popularity is increasing, especially after movies like *50 Shades of Grey*. Open discussion in mainstream women's magazines and television shows like *Sex and the City* have boosted the popularity and acceptance of sex toys for women. Currently, sex toys and their manufacturers have research labs, trade shows, and conventions to showcase and promote their products.

One particular stigma associated with toys is prostate-based stimulation. There is a misconception linking prostate massage to homosexuality, with the idea that enjoying anal stimulation may reflect one's sexual preference. Prostate massage has received significant attention in sexual medicine research. Prostatic-massage-induced orgasm is possible, and manipulation of the prostate can result in increased fluid expressed from the gland. This type of orgasm is a different type of ejaculation, as defined by both patient reports and more objective methods of measuring pelvic floor muscle contractions.

Internet advertisements often falsely advertise devices that promote various aspects of sexual behavior. It is not uncommon to see claims that a particular toy can help men last longer or grow the size of their penis. These invalid claims cast disbelief and discrimination on other products as well.

The popularity of male sex toys had lagged behind female sex toys. Retail stores that offer such devices still cater primarily to women. However, as interest among men increases, online sites like us.funfactory.com provide the opportunity for research and shopping in private.

Male sex toys are varied but can be organized into several basic categories:

- Sex simulators or masturbation sleeves, such as the Fleshlight or the Egg

- Tools for modifying penile sensation, such as vibrators, "cock rings," and stimulating topical agents. Some of the sex simulating devices vibrate as well

- Constriction bands such as "cock rings" that slow blood flow from an erect penis, producing a different type of sensation when stimulated

- Anal devices, such as anal vibrators, butt plugs, and other non-vibrating stimulatory agents

- "Pumps," which refer to the broad group of devices meant to draw blood to the penis for erection enhancement and increase penile size.

Sex toys offer a range of potential medical benefits, and the FDA has cleared several sexual aids. Sex toys have various uses for enhancement and stimulation, but much of their effectiveness depends on the user. For example, men can directly use vibrators for external stimulation of their genitals, either applied to the shaft or the head and frenulum. Vibrators can also be applied to sensitive areas such as the nipples, perineum, anus, and prostate.

Sex stimulators, or "sleeves," are devices intended to fit around the penile shaft. They are designed to create different sensations while masturbating. Studies have shown that penile sleeves may also be helpful for patients with premature ejaculation as they can help reduce sensitivity during intercourse. The primary use remains for masturbation, which can be performed by a man alone or with a partner. Based on sales analysis from Lovehoney, a prominent sex shop in England, these toys are the most popular among men who use sex toys alone. These devices are designed to look and feel similar to anatomic sites such as the vagina, anus, or oral cavity. A popular trend is for actors in the adult film industry to have sex toys modeled after their anatomy.

Vibrators are becoming increasingly popular. One study found that men who use vibrators are more likely to report engaging in health-promoting sexual behaviors and report higher levels of erectile function. The FDA has cleared penile vibrators for stimulating erections and facilitating ejaculation in men with spinal cord injury.

Constriction bands create prolonged erections by preventing blood outflow from the veins of the penis. Men who have venous leakage can achieve a longer-lasting erection. Constriction bands also help those men who lose their erection due to anxiety.

Anal devices include vibrating and non-vibrating tools used to stimulate the external and internal anus, focusing on prostate manipulation.

Vacuum erection devices function by enclosing the penis in a chamber that can generate negative pressure. These are often used in combination with constriction bands to draw blood into the penis and keep it there. Studies of vacuum devices have demonstrated benefit to sexual satisfaction outcomes for partners.

Interesting Observations

- Sexy lingerie is bought by attached men and women at the same rate.

- Women buy anal sex toys at the same rate regardless of their relationship status: 23%.

- Single men buy male sex toys more often than attached men, including anal stimulation toys.

The amount of rigorously developed research on sex toys is limited. We examined the current body of evidence from peer-reviewed journals to offer deeper insight into this topic:

- In 2003, a nationally representative study conducted in Australia reported 12% of men had used a sex toy in the preceding year.

- In 2006, a random-digit-dial survey of 1,114 sexually active adults between the ages of 18 and 39 in Seattle found that 20.3% of men used sex toys in a typical month.

- In 2009, a study in the U.S. sought to identify characteristics of vibrator use in men. Researchers found that 44.8% of men had used a vibrator during sexual activity at some point in their lives.

- One nationally representative study reported that approximately 40% of women had used a vibrator with their partners.

- Vibrators can be used by everyone; women and men, singles, and couples. According to a study by The Center for Sexual Health Promotion at Indiana University, 45% of men between the ages of 18 and 60 have used a vibrator during sexual interaction. A man can use it on his partner and enjoy giving her pleasure, or he can have his partner use it on him and experience the sensation firsthand.

KEY TAKE AWAYS

- Sex toys are a $25 billion global industry. Male sex toy use is rising in popularity and is more common than you would suspect.

- Devices can offer men sensations or stimuli that they would otherwise be unable to achieve on their own.

- There are many types of toys, and men should carefully research the benefits and potential harms when expanding their sexual repertoire.

For more information on sex toys, please see
https://us.funfactory.com.

Chapter 87
Everything You Need to Know About Condoms and Lubes
Judson Brandeis, MD, Urologist
Milla Impola, Sex Educator

Breaking a mirror is seven years of bad luck.
Breaking a condom is eighteen.
– Anonymous

Condoms are the only type of contraception that can both prevent pregnancy and protect against sexually transmitted infections. When used correctly every time you have sex, male condoms are 97% effective, which means that 3 out of 100 women will become pregnant in one year when men use condoms as contraception. However, many men do not use condoms correctly or consistently, so the actual effectiveness of condoms is around 86%. This chapter will help you understand how to have better results with condoms.

A BRIEF HISTORY

The first condom was first described by the Italian anatomist Gabriello Fallopio during the Italian Renaissance, which consisted of a linen sheet made to fit the glans to protect against syphilis. Colonel Quondam, a physician to King Charles I in the mid-1600s, invented the sheep gut condom. He provided the King with a means of preventing illegitimate offspring, and the word condom is probably a corruption of his name. The original condoms were made from the intestines of sheep, calves, and goats. The introduction of liquid latex in the mid-1930s made it possible to have higher tensile strength and a much longer shelf life. Today, condoms are made of natural materials (lamb intestine), latex rubber, or plastic (polyurethane).

> *Natural condoms are effective barriers against sperm and bacterial sexually transmitted diseases. However, they do not protect against viral organisms such as HIV, which are smaller than bacteria.*

The advantage of natural condoms is the transfer of body heat between partners. Latex condoms are less porous than natural condoms and form a more effective barrier that can block even viral organisms such as HIV. However, latex condoms reduce heat transfer that tends to contribute to sexual pleasure.

Oil-based products like moisturizers, lotions, and Vaseline can damage latex and reduce the efficacy of a condom. However, water-based lubricants are safe to use with all condoms. Condoms need to be stored in places that are neither too hot nor too cold. Keeping the same condom for several years in your wallet (as many a high school student has done) can reduce the effectiveness of the condom.

Condoms for oral and anal sex. Condoms are effective in protecting against pharyngeal gonorrhea during oral sex. Sex workers with inconsistent condom use during oral sex are 17 times more likely to develop oral gonorrhea than consistent condom users.

Approximately 5% to 10% of the world's population engages in anal sex. Men who have sex with men are 18 times more likely to be infected with HIV than the general population. Consistent condom use reduces the risk of HIV transmission during anal sex by 70% to 90%.

A study examining condom issues reported by men attending a sexually transmitted disease clinic found that 19% of cases of failure were associated with "fit and feel problems," 15% involved breakage, 14% were due to loss of erections, 9% resulted from the loss of erection while putting on the condom, 8% involved slippage during withdrawal, and 7% involved slippage during sex. Condoms are designed to fit a penis size of 7 inches, which is almost 2 inches larger than the average American male penis. For this reason, it is safer to have a custom-fitting condom. Customcondoms.com has a technology that can provide better fitting condoms that are less likely to fail.

Some men are allergic to latex. In extreme circumstances, men can develop breathing issues—anaphylaxis. More common is a delayed hypersensitivity reaction, resulting in itching, hives, cough, watery eyes, sneezing, and a runny nose.

ORGANISM	EFFICACY
HIV	>90% (for latex condoms)
Hepatitis B	>90%
Gonorrhea	>90%
Trichomonas	>90%
Chlamydia	50-90%
Haemophilus ducrei	10-50%
Herpes Type 2	10-50%
HPV	No efficacy

Figure 87.1. Effectiveness of condoms in preventing sexually- transmitted infection.

Instructions on how to properly use a condom. Make sure that the condom is not expired and has not been exposed to extreme heat or cold. Make sure that the packet has not been perforated or damaged in any way. Take the condom out of the package, careful not to tear it with jewelry or fingernails, and do not open the packet with your teeth.

Place the condom over the tip of the erect penis. Use your thumb and forefinger to squeeze the air out of the tip. Gently roll the condom down to the base of the penis. If the condom does not roll down, you may have put it on upside down. If this occurs, the condom may have sperm on it, so you should discard it and begin with a new one. Sperm can leave the penis before ejaculation.

If you use a latex condom, do not use oil-based lubricants such as lotion, body oil, or Vaseline because they can damage the condom and make it more likely to split. Some condoms have a layer of spermicide, which prevents pregnancy but does not protect against sexually transmitted infections. After ejaculation, withdraw the penis while it is still erect. Hold the condom on at the base of the penis. Remove the condom from the penis, being careful not to spill any semen. Throw the condom away in a trash bin, not the toilet.

KEY TAKE AWAYS

- *Natural condoms do not protect against viral organisms such as HIV, which are smaller than bacteria.*

- Natural condoms *are* effective barriers against sperm and bacterial sexually transmitted diseases.

- When used correctly every time you have sex, male condoms are 97% effective, which means that 3 out of 100 women will become pregnant in 1 year when men use condoms as contraception. However, many men do not use condoms correctly or consistently, and the actual effectiveness of condoms is around 86%.

- Oil-based products such as moisturizers, lotions, and Vaseline can damage latex and compromise the efficacy of a condom. However, water-based lubricants are safe to use with all condoms.

- Custom size and shape condoms are available from Internet sites such as www.customcondoms.com.

LUBRICANTS

Lubricants (lubes) make sex more enjoyable and less painful by reducing friction, chafing, and uncomfortable rubbing. This is especially true as we age, where lubrication can add to your sexual experience, so don't feel embarrassed about using them. Even if your partner produces ample amounts of vaginal fluids, lubrication can further increase your sexual pleasure.

Most post-menopausal women experience vaginal dryness and discomfort during sex. After menopause, the genitourinary area (including the vagina and vulva) has less blood flow due to declining estrogen levels. Vaginal tissues receive less blood flow and, as a result, become thinner, stiffer, and produce less natural vaginal fluids. Lubricants decrease the discomfort of sex by temporarily reducing friction. In younger women, using silicone or water-based lubricant reduces condom failure resulting in fewer unintended pregnancies and sexually transmitted infections.

According to an article in the *Journal of Sexual Medicine*, 70% of men have used lubrication during sex, but only one in four uses it routinely. Lubrication increases the pleasure of intercourse. According to a 2013 study from Indiana University's Center for Sexual Health Promotion, 50% of men reported that lubrication helped them achieve orgasm better. Interestingly, other researchers found that men who used a well-lubricated condom became just as aroused as men who did not use a condom.

Types of Lubricants

Water-based lube is helpful in all aspects of physical intimacy, including penetrative sex, masturbation, and sex toy play. Water-based lubes are also ideal for people with sensitive skin and women with potential vaginal irritation. Water-based lubricants are easily removed from sheets and clothing by laundering and do not leave a stain.

Water-based lubes do have some downsides, though. They wash away during water-play/shower sex. What's more, water-based lubricants get sticky and require frequent reapplication.

Silicone-based lube is slippery, long-lasting, and ideal for a more extended session. It requires less lube to be applied and needs reapplication less often. Silicone-based lubes are also great for shower sex or masturbation in the shower since they don't wash away so easily. The catch is that silicone-based lubes are more difficult to wash off and may stain sheets.

Silicone-based lubricants should not be used with silicone-based sex toys, as they can break down the devices over time. However, this doesn't mean all sex toys are off-limits with silicone-based lubricants—there are many toys made from other materials.

Oil-based lube provides a slippery sensation that lasts longer than water-based lube. These lubes are ideal for masturbation (with hands or toys), penetrative unprotected sex, water-play, and sensual massage.

Oil-based lubes (or any other oil-like products such as petroleum jelly or mineral oil) should not be used with latex condoms, as they can dissolve the latex of the condom and may cause latex condoms to break. Latex diaphragms and latex sex toys should also be kept away from oil-based lubricants. Another downside to oil-based lubes is that they can be more challenging to clean from sheets and from your body.

Lubes for anal sex. Personal lubrication is recommended for anal sex since the anal canal does not produce fluids to help ease penetration. In addition, the tight muscular sphincter at the entrance of the anus offers much more resistance than the vagina, which is full of folds and stretchable tissue. Using a personal lubricant can also make anal sex safer. A water-based lubricant decreases the chances of condom breakage while having anal sex, in contrast to oil-based lubricants or saliva, which both increase the chances of condom breakage during sex.

The chances of the condom slipping off during anal sex are also related to lubrication. Applying lubrication to the *outside* of the condom can decrease the chances of slippage, while using lube *inside* the condom can increase the chances of slippage.

Good to know before you buy. In general, avoid any lubricant that contains any artificial flavors, colors, sugars, essential oils, additional additives, or glycerin. It is unpredictable how you'll react to these additives. Especially if it is your first time using a personal lubricant—some of those extra features like "warming" or "tingling" can be more overwhelming than expected.

There is one brand of lubricant, called Pre-Seed, designed for couples who are trying to get pregnant. Researchers at the State University of New York (SUNY) in Syracuse found that Pre-Seed did not affect sperms' ability to swim.

Generally speaking, many studies have found that lubricants reduce the likelihood of pregnancy because they increase the pleasure experienced when using a condom and therefore increase the likelihood of use.

**For more information on condoms and lube, please see the website of:
Global Protection Corp. at globalprotection.com.**

Chapter 88
How to Please a Woman
Susan Bratton, Intimacy Wellness Expert

The real lover is the man who can thrill you by kissing your forehead.
– Marilyn Monroe

She looks up at you and says, "You're the best lover I've ever had."

She is always a yes to intimacy… even making "dates" with you so she can look forward to the next time you get your hands on her. The intensity and number of orgasms she has with you are legendary. And every woman you've been with feels this way about you. It's not them. It's you. Your skills.

It's true. Once you have the right set of skills, every woman you're with can achieve new levels of orgasmic ecstasy… Even the woman who believes she can't orgasm from penetration or she doesn't believe female ejaculation is possible for her. Of course she can! She just doesn't know how, yet. Which is where you come in, dear sir.

There are easily fifteen different kinds of orgasms a woman can experience. From clitoral, to G-spot to breastgasms to orgasms from intercourse… When you lead her, any woman can become more orgasmic and experience more kinds of orgasms, achieving levels of pleasure she couldn't imagine… until she met you.

Being a great lover is a learned skill. Sure, making babies requires only tab A into slot B. But legendary lovemaking? That requires soft and hard skills which determine the difference between the lover she ghosts and the one she can't stop seeing. Moreover, all these great sex skills can be learned easily and some in an instant.

A legendary lover understands how to strike the balance that good sex requires.

Women's bodies and minds all work within a relative range of similarity. The skill you want to develop is the ability to get into her world and understand how *her mind and body differ from yours*... And then give her what she needs to have hours of pleasure, connection and orgasms with you.

The Platinum Rule

Are you familiar with The Golden Rule? It's the principle of treating others the way you want to be treated. "Do unto others as you'd have them do unto you." However, in masculine/feminine sexuality, The Platinum Rule eclipses The Golden Rule.

Treat her the way she wants to be treated, not the way you want her to treat you. Why? Because her dominant hormone is estrogen. Yours is testosterone. The way we act behind closed doors is driven by our hormones and our cultural conditioning. Her approach to sexual pleasure is different than yours. Once you approach her mind and body the way she needs you to, you release a treasure trove of unbridled pleasure.

Both partners' desire occurs on a sexual spectrum, based on your life experience and cultural conditioning.

(A lover's libido is also impacted by how happy, well fed, and rested they are in the moment. Hence the breadth of this book, which includes not only a focus on male sexuality, but also on male health.)

Once you're aware of generalities between the way you approach sex and the way your lady does, you can play to these differences to increase your mutual sexual satisfaction. The magnetic attraction of your masculine and her feminine sexual energy works to your mutual benefit.

Here are some generalizations about the difference between you and your lady:

- Overall, most men are unduly confident in their sexual skills. Guys overestimate how good in bed they are. Even as you're reading this chapter, you may be telling yourself you already know all of this . . . Testosterone creates a level of certainty you have to consciously override to become a more masterful lover.

- Equally, a woman's estrogen dominance makes it hard for her to let go mentally to relax into her pleasure. A little secret: arousal begins with relaxation, not with stimulation.

- As a man, you feel relatively invincible and do not worry that you are going to get physically hurt from a sexual partner. It doesn't even enter your mind to worry about that.

- Yet, she craves security and protection because she may have had a lifetime of experiences of men trying to take advantage of her, or even invasive, inappropriate, or harmful experiences. Plus, the onus is on her to worry about conceiving a child or contracting an infection.

The differences continue right to our genitals.

- It's in the timing. You are hungry for sex and ready in a matter of seconds (30 seconds if you're in your 30's or 40's), while she benefits from being warmed up slowly. It will typically take her at least 20 minutes to be ready for sex, mentally and physically.

- And it's not always easy to tell. Half of your erectile tissue is external to your body. When you get an erection, it signals that you're ready. And it's obvious. But with only 5% of her erectile tissue visible when you peer under her clitoral hood, often she is rushed into sex before she's ready.

- She also wants to connect with you emotionally before connecting physically. (This makes sense. Since it's possible that she might conceive a child with you, her mind and body are primed to find out *who* you are before she makes love with you.)

The Banana Diagrams

The common wisdom that it takes 20 minutes of foreplay to get a woman aroused is a good rule of thumb, with one caveat. She needs significant direct genital stimulation for her clitoral structure (not just the tip of her clitoris) to become engorged (filled with blood).

Sex doesn't feel as pleasurable without a firm erection for any of us. The more blood that flows into the genital system, the more the erectile tissue expands. This expansion increases the surface area. The more surface area, the more pleasure that your brain processes. Foreplay requires manual and oral genital stimulation for her erectile tissue to become swollen. Kissing and breast play increase her engorgement and pleasure because her lips and breasts are part of her erectile system. (Remind yourself that the woman in your arms is unique. Great sex means exploring that uniqueness to discover what give her pleasure in this very moment, and when you're with her, what pleasures *you*.)

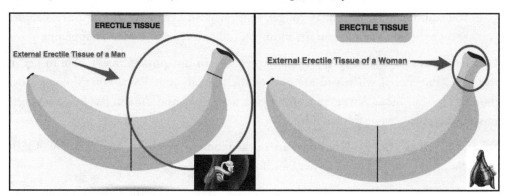

Figures 88.1. Male erectile tissue which is 50% visible and 88.2. Female erectile tissue is only 5% visible, making it difficult to tell when a woman is ready for sex.

So rushing penetration has the effect of undermining her ability to have orgasms from intercourse. And even if she says she enjoys being close to you… She's not going to want as much sex over time as you do if she isn't coming while you're inside her. Let's make sure that doesn't happen.

There are two categories of skills to master: the mental and physical. The overarching rule of thumb is that you go too fast for her. Both mentally and physically you feel ready to go long before she does (a researcher would point out that means 19 minutes before she's ready). Rushing leads to a poor sexual experience for her.

Physical Stimulation

The word to keep repeating to yourself to become a better lover is: SLOW. The primary mistake men make is to go too fast. She's not ready as fast as you are. You are ahead of her. You are ready to plunge inside her. She isn't even aroused yet. You offer sex and forget to romance and hold her. Testosterone makes you crazy ready for sex but estrogen makes her worried about what could go wrong before she even starts. If she's not even warmed up, she can't think about penetration.

When you slow down…

And then go *more slowly*….

You actually net more and better sex in the long run.

Slowing down has its advantages for you too.

At least 25% of men of every age from 20–90 struggle with premature ejaculation. Most stamina issues stem from performance anxiety. When you slow down and "get present" with her it keeps you from worrying about the past or projecting catastrophe into the future. Being present lowers your performance anxiety. Staying in the present moment gives you additional stamina to last longer. (Ultimately it heightens *your* pleasure, because you are more likely to be there in the moment, fully experiencing what's happening.)

Getting present means being emotionally present, not just physically available to her in real time. Presence is when you are paying attention to your lover, not thinking other thoughts in your head. A woman can feel your attention. And she can feel when it's gone missing. She craves your full attention.

When you release your goals and you are in the moment, you allow the interplay of intimacy to unfold, which lowers anxiety for both of you.

When lovers are in full orgasmic mutual pleasure, time stands still and deep connection can flourish. Only then can she begin to have not just one orgasm, but many. She can

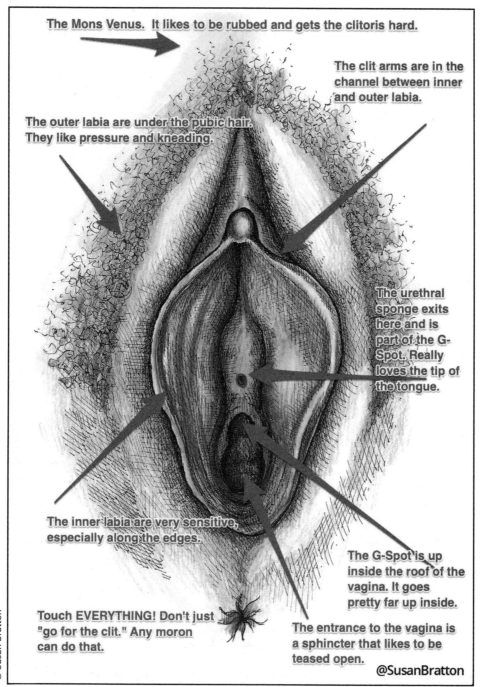

The Mons Venus. It likes to be rubbed and gets the clitoris hard.

The clit arms are in the channel between inner and outer labia.

The outer labia are under the pubic hair. They like pressure and kneading.

The urethral sponge exits here and is part of the G-Spot. Really loves the tip of the tongue.

The inner labia are very sensitive, especially along the edges.

The G-Spot is up inside the roof of the vagina. It goes pretty far up inside.

Touch EVERYTHING! Don't just "go for the clit." Any moron can do that.

The entrance to the vagina is a sphincter that likes to be teased open.

@SusanBratton

© Susan Bratton

Figure 88.3. Feminine sexual anatomy.

become multi-orgasmic. She can begin to have orgasms from many types of stimulation. This leads to her ability to stay in the moment of orgasm for longer periods of time. With practice, she can expand the moment of orgasm from milliseconds to minutes.

What does it take to put her in the zone, and what gets in the way? Overstimulation is actually a downer. Overstimulation of the tip (the glans) of her clitoris is the #1 reason she doesn't live up to her profoundly impressive orgasmic potential. When that tip is stimulated too fast and too hard, her clitoris becomes overly sensitive. She doesn't want any more touch. She's "one and done" instead of being able to stay in orgasmic bliss for extended periods of time. (So taking a mechanical approach to sex just doesn't work for her.)

Most women have no idea they have as much erectile tissue as you do. They don't know that rushing means they have less pleasure. They are unaware that erectile tissue surrounds their entire vaginal opening.

- *The feminine glans.* In the drawing, the button-shaped structure is the clitoral glans. *The crura or legs* are additional erectile tissue on each side of the clitoris that extend the entire length of the vaginal area.

- *Urethral sponge.* The small "flower-shaped" opening is her urethral sponge, mistakenly called a G-Spot. It's a tube of erectile tissue that starts at the outside top of her vaginal opening and travels inside the roof of her vagina.

- *Perineal sponge.* This bundle of erectile tissue, the perineal sponge, is between the bottom of her vaginal floor and her rectum.

The entrance to her vagina is a very sensitive sphincter muscle. All of this tissue responds beautifully to touch. The more you pleasure all of this tissue (slowly, gently, mindfully), the more intense her orgasmic pleasure.

The vagina does not have any glands that provide lubrication. Her "wetness" comes from her blood plasma seeping through the walls of her vaginal skin. The more blood flow she gets to her pelvis, the more lubricated she becomes. Great sex relies on blood flow and good hydration.

When you slow down and give her full body touch, then move on to stroking her entire vulva with organic oil, it will settle her nervous system and allow her to become engorged because you are getting her blood flowing. Understanding the importance of engorgement is the key to becoming your woman's ultimate lover.

Try beginning with massage. The single most powerful foreplay technique to ensure orgasmic sex is a sensual genital massage. Get good at pleasuring her "yoni." Yoni is a Tantric sex term for a woman's genitals. The vagina is simply the birth canal. Calling a

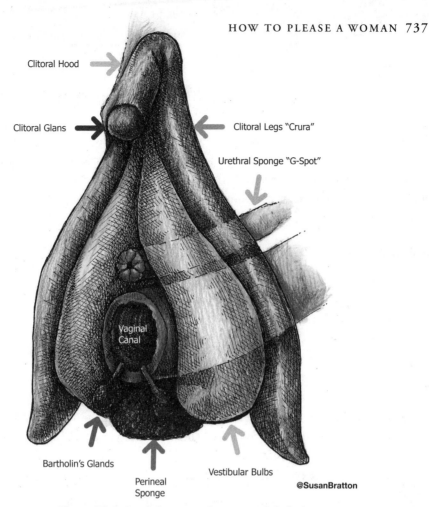

Figure 88.4. Feminine sexual anatomy labeled.

woman's genitals a vagina minimizes a woman's many wonderful parts. Yoni is a sweet word you can teach to your lady. She will feel honored that you speak reverentially about her feminine parts.

When you massage her and tell her what you're doing, it connects her brain to her Yoni. The blood flow and the neural connections you create improve her orgasmic response. (That is also a great way to get her feedback on how to give her the most pleasure. And it gives you tasteful language you can use every time you seek physical intimacy.)

I'm rubbing your mons.

Now I'm kneading your outer labia.

I'm running my finger along the edges of your pretty inner labia. They are turning dark rose under my touch and they look like a butterfly.

This is your G-Spot. It feels so soft.

This kind of verbal reassurance signals to her she's in good hands. Tell her to just relax and receive. Let her know it's your honor to love her in this way.

In sharing with you how to have great sex, I began by giving you an anatomy lesson and underscoring the importance of engorgement for her pleasure. But great sex starts long before you get your hands on her. Which leads me to the foundation of great sex, which is understanding how to seduce a woman respectfully. Seduction simply means moving her toward pleasure.

Seduction

She wonders…

Will it feel good for me?

Will I have an orgasm?

Will I be safe?

Will I be loved?

Being testosterone dominant, you hold the torch for frequent and pleasurable lovemaking. She wants to be transported by you into realms of pleasure. But she needs you to get things kick-started because she has less testosterone (T is the hormone of arousal) than you do. She loves and wants sex as much as you do, but it helps when you instigate.

For men, one of the most intimidating aspects of sex is knowing when she is "in the mood." When should you approach her? Will you get rejected? Couple this with the deep-seated shame for their desire that most men carry in their soul from societal programming. Is it any wonder that initiating sex can feel emotionally risky?

Anger and victimhood build over years of offering sex and being rejected. Many men wait for her signal. But her signals are so subtle that they go unnoticed. She won't out-and-out seduce you. And you don't know when she is open to your advances and when she's not. So a whole lot of great sex gets left on the table.

Often men stop offering, because they've been rejected too many times. They worry that this will be just one more rejection. What they don't realize is that they're making too big an offer. A big offer is, "Do you want to have sex?" She's not ready like you are. So she doesn't want sex. If you make smaller offers, which I'll explain further, you can move her more slowly up the arousal ladder at the pace she requires. More small offers net you more sex overall.

What I want you most to know is that your woman needs *you* to be the sexual torch carrier and the initiator of sex. Instead of becoming angry at rejection, I'll show you how to become a master seducer so you can keep the fires burning for both of you. I want you to consider "pleasure offerer" to be one of your "jobs" in the relationship. Don't expect her to initiate. If she does, great! But take that off the table. Assume she is not biologically wired nor socially programmed to initiate sex. That way you won't feel put upon by always being the one who sets the pleasure in motion. You are the sexual champion. You carry the torch for instigating physical intimacy. When you "own" the task, you can get really good at it. I'll show you how to master seduction in a way that removes any apprehension and creates joy every time.

I'm going to stack the deck in your favor with two gems of awareness. When you understand how to gently move her toward wanting sex and you know the most likely times she will be open to intimacy, you will drive your win rate through the roof.

I call the times when her body is more primed to want sex her 5-day desire window. When you track this window, you can increase the possibility of her being a yes to having sex with you. The slippery slide is knowing how to take her up the arousal ladder during this window by making her small offers instead of big offers for which you might get rejected.

Generally, being testosterone dominant means you'd gladly have sex every day. Whereas your lady, being estrogen dominant, means she's on a monthly cycle (even after menopause).

Every woman's desire runs in cycles, even after menopause. So, here's how you figure out the five days she's ovulating, which are the days she's most likely going to want sex:

Count nine days after the start of her period. Those next five days are her most lusty. If she doesn't have a period anymore or you're not sure WHEN she has her period, use the full moon as your guide.

Target the five days around the full moon to have a sexy date with her. Make a date with her in advance of the day in this five-day window you are targeting. For example, if her five-day window starts on a Monday, plan the date for Friday night.

Let's say her period starts on the 1st of the month and lasts about five days. Day 6, 7, and 8 are good days to make a date with her. Then day 9 is the beginning of her strongest arousal window and it lasts through days 10, 11, 12, 13, and 14.

Tease her with anticipation instead of just springing a date on her. That way she will have time to get turned on and excited, primp a little and "be ready" for your surprise. Even scheduling a couple of dates in that window stimulates her hormones further while giving her time to get fully turned on and experience incredible pleasure.

Remember, when a woman is ovulating — that's her strongest arousal window — typically around the fertile full moon, she's most open to sexual pleasure. Those are the days she may be most receptive, but they are in no way the only days she'd be open to a romp. This is how you leverage her natural libido cycles.

Next is understanding her arousal ladder. The trick is to initiate intimacy slowly. Remember, she's not ready to go but she could be at any time. She needs you to initiate. Making her a lot of offers, even outside her five-day arousal window, will create more overall sexual experiences. However, you cannot just offer her sex. She will say no. It's too much. Sex is too big an offer if she's not turned on. She doesn't walk around hungry for sex like you do. So you have to start small and work your way up. That is what seduction is… Seduction is the art of slowly moving a lover toward pleasure.

Instead of offering her sex outright, make a series of small offers that lead her toward sex. Or give her a menu of choices from which she can choose. On some days she may need the foot rub first. On other days she may be ready for a yoni massage.

Would you like a glass of wine and a foot rub?

Would you like me to hold you while you tell me about your day?

Can I give you a sensual massage?

Her response will inform what you offer next. The more you get your hands on her in a way that pleasures her physically and emotionally, the more you increase your chances of having sex. A foot rub is foreplay to her. Being held is foreplay to her as well. Listening can be foreplay. On a tough day, listening, *really listening*, and a neck massage may turn out to be incredible foreplay. Sometimes that will lead to kissing, which will lead to full body touch, which will lead to…

At other times, you want to be content knowing that as a result of the foot rub, her body is realizing that it loves your touch, that it is beginning to crave your touch. She is realizing that you love touching her (we all like to be appreciated.) Each time you touch her you are moving her toward more physical intimacy.

Offering frequent opportunities to touch her, to hold her, to massage her, to be physically close to her with no strings attached results in more overall sex in your relationship and raises the quality of your intimacy across the board. But if you only touch her to get sex, she will stop wanting your touch.

THE BULLSEYE TOUCH TECHNIQUE

There is one more important aspect to her arousal ladder you must know so you don't unwittingly shut her down or drive her away. Imagine a bullseye. You want to touch her "outer rings" before going for the center bullseye. Her arms, legs, and head are her outer rings. Her erogenous zones are her inner bullseye. Work from the outside in.

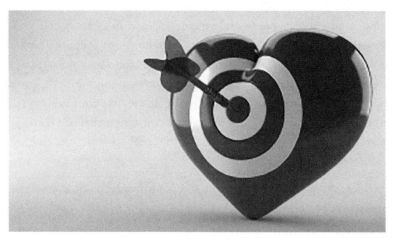

Figure 88.5. The bullseye touch technique. (Courtesy of Susan Bratton)

Providing full body touch, before ever reaching for her genitals, allows her to relax so the process of arousal can begin. Offering her sex is too goal oriented. First, she needs you to awaken her sensually, starting from the outside and working your way into her soft, creamy center.

In your case, you'd love her to handle your penis right from the start. In her case, she doesn't want you to go for her yoni first. You must fight your natural inclination to rush all these steps. Do all of this touch activity ten times more slowly than you want to. Your starter pistol has fired. But if you blast off and leave her behind, she will give up the race.

Hold her. Let her settle. Allow her to release any emotion. When you feel her body relax, pull her closer. You're creating a feeling of safety and relaxation. Next, begin by fondling her shoulders, her back, and her arms. Stroke her hair from the crown to the ends. Pet her like a kitten — always with, rather than against her fur.

Kiss her forehead, her eyelids, her neck, her collarbone… Then add in long, gentle caresses to her legs and back and belly. If she seems ready, peck little kisses on her lips. Warm her up before offering your tongue. Lightly touch her breasts before touching her nipples. You want to start with the outer erogenous zones and move to the inner zones, as she relaxes and melts into you.

Then you may move toward her genitals and follow the same bullseye touch technique. Start with her mons and outer labia before ever touching her clitoris or putting your fingers or tongue inside her. I recommend using organic avocado or sweet almond oil when you're warming up her genitals. That way it's easy to wipe off with a towel if you want to also pleasure her orally. Take time to make her comfortable and explore all the folds of her vulva.

See what kind of touch feels best—and where—in each moment. Each time you touch her, she will want different sensations because of her hormone cycling. Think about her as a kitty that on some days turns into a lioness. At times she wants the lightest of pressure. Then there are the days where she needs you to put your strength into the pressure of your touch. Making it safe for her to verbally guide you accelerates your skills as her best lover. Don't take her guidance as failure. Instead, consider it a sign that she trusts you with her most intimate secrets and that she is giving you the feedback you need to transport her to her orgasmic potential (and yours as well).

Explore! The more attuned you are to her, the more touch techniques you have, the better her pleasure and yours.

Driving Desire

The more variety of techniques you use, the more pleasure you create. Desire is created when there is a balance of novelty and safety. If you are safe, but do the same things all the time, sex gets boring. If you have a lot of variety, but it feels too dangerous, she can't get the safety she needs to surrender to pleasure. Toggling between excitement and calm takes her nervous system on a more pleasurable ride, escalating the pleasure each time you change the pace and surprise her body with a little more excitement...

Applying this same concept of a balance between stimulation and relaxation also encourages her to have more intensely pleasurable orgasms. If you constantly drive her stimulation hard, she won't last as long as if you alternate between stimulation and relaxation. These little adjustments of tempo and pressure will maximize her pleasure.

Just as you have a latent period after ejaculating that you need to wait out, she has one after a strong orgasm.

Think about giving her an orgasm and then allowing her nervous system to take a little break before stimulating her again.

There are four main kinds of orgasms:

1. Regular

2. Multiple

3. Extended

4. Expanded

You are most likely having Regular Orgasms. You get aroused, ejaculate when you climax and then you have to rest before you can go again. The latency period gets longer as you age.

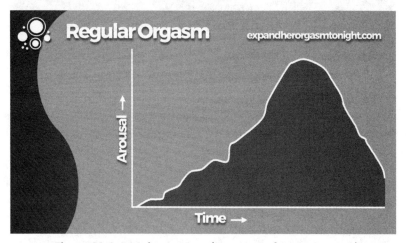

Figure 88.6. Regular orgasm. (Courtesy of Susan Bratton)

You can learn to become a multi-orgasmic man. Instead of ejaculating every time you orgasm, you can have full-body, non-ejaculatory orgasms. You can learn how to separate ejaculation from orgasm. Then you can come when you want to, which is what I call having "ejaculatory choice." This is a learnable skill that I teach using a technique called, "The ME Breath." You can discover more about this breath at https://personallifemedia.com/mol-tuning-fork-promo/. Becoming multi-orgasmic lets you have multiple orgasms while increasing your stamina. You last longer and are able to come repeatedly. Your pleasure increases her pleasure.

Most women also follow this model of one-and-done regular orgasms because they don't know all the erogenous zones of their body and they don't realize that there are several types of orgasms and numerous ways to orgasm.

Some women are able to have an orgasm, take a break, and have another orgasm. These multiple orgasms come from daisy-chaining multiple regular orgasms. As you can see, she needs a break from stimulation between climaxes. Even if she is multi-orgasmic already, she still has a latency period too, but it's much shorter than yours.

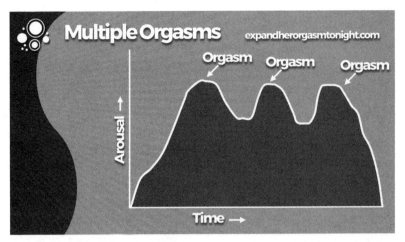

Figure 88.7. Multiple orgasms. (Courtesy of Susan Bratton)

An Extended Orgasm occurs when a woman can take the moment of climax and stretch time out like pulling taffy. Call the Extended Orgasm the time-warp orgasm. She can ride the sensation and stay in the peak.

Each of these Extended Orgasms allows her to prolong the ecstasy of climax. This comes with practice and requires a lover who is very tuned into her nervous system.

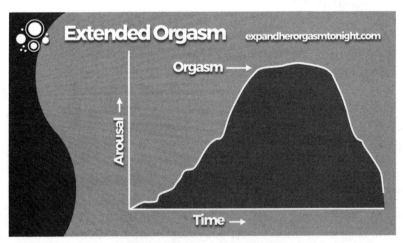

Figure 88.8. Extended orgasm. (Courtesy of Susan Bratton)

The final and penultimate orgasmic experience for a woman is the Expanded Orgasm. Expanded Orgasms are a series of stacking, increasingly intense and longer and longer moments of climactic pleasure.

The Expanded Orgasm practice is a learned technique that uses five unique strokes to give the clitoris the stimulation it needs without overstimulating and blowing her circuits.

Expanded Orgasms have been called many things from Extended Massive Orgasms, to Deliberate Orgasms or Orgasmic Meditation. They are all variations on the basic five strokes.

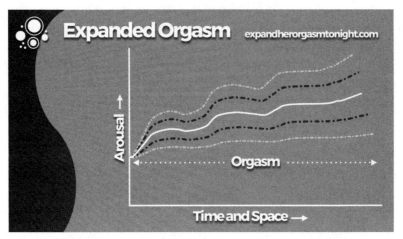

Figure 88.9. Expanded orgasm. (Courtesy of Susan Bratton)

This is a fantastic couples practice that keeps a woman eternally interested in intimacy. Expanded Orgasms are also one of the best ways to train a woman's body to come during penetration. The practice of Expanded Orgasm spills over into becoming orgasmic from intercourse. You can get three free pleasure reports at http://expandherorgasmtonight.com including, *What Is Expanded Orgasm?*, *The Power of Peaking*, and *Touching for Rapture*.

Spicy Sex

In addition to becoming a multi-orgasmic man with everlasting stamina and having an Expanded Orgasm practice with your lady love, you can continue to learn new skills together.

Couples that play together, stay together… especially in the bedroom.

When women don't want you for sex anymore, it's usually for two reasons. One, it's not that pleasurable for her. Two, she's bored by doing the same things.

Learning pleasuring skills will fix both issues. Couples can learn erotic genital massage skills, oral pleasuring skills, and intercourse techniques. My Steamy Sex Ed® Video Collection shows over 200 heart-connected techniques. It's made for couples to watch together.

Women can have clitoral, G-Spot, squirting, cervical, full body, anal, breastgasms, mouth-gasms, bellygasms, footgasms, orgasms from spanking, and even orgasms by verbal command. There are endless ways to stimulate the body to orgasm. Each of them is simply a learned skill.

You can also learn orgasm skills such as male-multiple orgasm with the ME Breath, giving her G-Spot orgasms or female ejaculatory orgasms (sometimes called squirting) from my http://femaleliquidorgasm.com program and Expanded Orgasms from http://expandherorgasmtonight.com.

When you move a woman's body, you move her emotionally. That's why sex positions are one of the best tools of the master lover. Sex positions in different locations add even more variety. The more you stimulate her entire body in any given sex position, the more pleasure you create. My favorite 7 Stimulating Sex Positions that incorporate manual stimulation as well as the use of toys to increase pleasure include: Discover Chingalinga, Headboard Daddy and the Lotus…

Very few couples are incorporating sex toys into their sex play. This is an untapped area of pleasure, rich with possibility… One for every day of the week!

Another pleasurable position is *Come Full Circle, a 360° double helix position.* It's an exciting one to try once and you get bragging rights!

If you have any trouble lasting as long as you want to or if your lady struggles to have orgasms from intercourse with or without external clitoral stimulation, try Thrust in Time. This is an intercourse technique that will have her coming without you even touching her clitoris… just from your penis inside her.

When you discover new ways of orgasming, new positions, new locations, and new toys you will have a sex life that just keeps getting better.

Using all your senses during sex also increases the pleasure. Look in her eyes. Let her know you love the way she smells. Make sounds that show your own pleasure, so she knows she's having a positive effect on you sexually.

Talk to her before, during, and after sex.

Women want verbal feedback during sex. They want to know they are doing a good job and that you find them sexy. Toggling between encouragement and appreciation helps lead her toward more pleasure. Alternate between adoration and sexual compliments. If you only tell her how hot she is, she feels objectified. If you only tell her what you find cute or sweet about her, she will worry that she is not sexy. Balancing the sexy and sweet verbal encouragement will help her blossom into her full sexuality.

Now you know that great sex requires balance:

- Masculine and feminine

- Relaxation and arousal

- Stimulation and recovery

- Novelty and safety

- Adoration and sexual desirability

Your sexual growth is a facet of your personal growth. If you have a growth mindset, you can continue to learn new sexual techniques and communication skills as you mature. The best lovers are those in their 50s, 60s, and beyond.

They are able to slow down and be present. They have empathy for their partner and they have accumulated a lifetime of skills. Sex can keep getting better with age. Sexual regenerative therapies like GAINSWave, platelet rich plasma, exosomes, stem cells, and vacuum erection devices can reverse atrophy. Nitric oxide supplementation and testosterone replacement therapy are easy, fundamental ways to keep your blood flowing and hormones pumping, and to stay healthy. Recent research on telomeres (genetic markers of aging) makes it clear that healthy sexual function also lengthens your life, measurably reducing your body's age.

Learning new sexual pleasuring techniques and bedroom communication skills keeps your sex life on an upward pleasure spiral your entire life. Great sex is a skill. Like any skill, mastery comes from practice. Here's to great sex!

For more exceptional insight and resources from Ms. Bratton, please see:
www.susanbratton.com/
www.personallifemedia.com/experts/susan-bratton/.
For more information on sexual medicine, please see:
www.BrandeisMD.com
www.TheTwenyFirstCenturyMan.com.

PART 12
SEXUAL MEDICINE
Introduction
Judson Brandeis, MD

The only victories which leave no regret are those
which are gained over ignorance.
— Napoleon Bonaparte

There has never been a time in world history in which information was so plentiful and accessible. Yet over the past 25 years in clinical practice as a urologist, thousands of men have come to see me who delayed seeking care until the problem was too uncomfortable to ignore.

Prostate cancer is a prime example. This silent killer is the second most common form of cancer-related death in men. Tragically, it is one of the most curable if it's diagnosed early. Men resist getting a PSA lab test or having the doctor stick a finger up their butt. Still, there is nothing sadder to me than diagnosing a man with prostate cancer that has metastasized and spread throughout his body. The treatment for metastatic prostate cancer is medical castration, which is devastating, given the emasculating effects of the absence of testosterone.

Peyronie's disease, or penile curvature caused by scarring, is a condition that should be treated early in the disease process. I feel empathy and frustration when I see men with severe curvature and penile shortening who can no longer have penetrative intercourse. In many cases, they either resisted acknowledging that this was a problem or didn't find an expert with the skillset to provide adequate care.

Testosterone is another example of an underutilized intervention. As men age, testosterone levels steadily decline. I have replaced testosterone in hundreds of men in their 60s and 70s with dramatic improvement. I know that millions of men would decide to boost this natural hormone if they were properly informed of the many beneficial health effects. These include conserving heart health, promoting mental function, and improving libido, all while retaining a man's muscle mass, vitality, and quality of life.

Even simple procedures like circumcision and vasectomy are underappreciated. I have circumcised dozens of men who went through their teens and twenties without being able to pull back their foreskin to enjoy sex. And I have performed vasectomies on dozens of men who had "martini babies." For a few of these men, their last child was younger than their grandchildren. Finally, sexually transmitted infections are entirely preventable through education and protection.

I hope that the chapters in this section will provide information and motivation for men who, for whatever reasons, did not seek help in a timely fashion. When I speak with my patients, I emphasize that there is no shame in having any of these conditions. Shit happens. For example, 80% of men with Peyronie's disease have no idea what caused their penis to start to bend. As the Dalai Lama has pointed out, "Although you may not always be able to avoid difficult situations, you can modify the extent to which you can suffer by how you choose to respond to the situation." A man is responsible to his partner, family, co-workers, and community, but most importantly, to himself. Men who are proactive about their health will continue to revel in their masculinity.

Chapter 89

Testosterone in Men: A Review
Gary S. Donovitz, MD, FACOG
Gynecologist & Hormone Expert

Testosterone to me is so important for a sense of well-being when you get older.
— *Sylvester Stallone*

You wake up one morning after another sleepless night. Who is that person in the mirror? He has less hair, more wrinkles, and a bigger waistline. He doesn't feel like going to work or going to the gym. His wife complains that he's irritable all the time. Sex has become a chore with fewer of the great outcomes he seems to remember.

How old is this guy? He may be 40—but he feels 50. Is this just a matter of getting old, or could it be something more serious? Is it andropause (male menopause)? Friends prefer to call it low T. The wife is on hormones. Is that the next step here?

Dropping hormones are a natural fact of aging. As men age, their blood levels of testosterone decrease. This decline after the age of 35 is gradual in most men, but can be accelerated in some. The premature decline in testosterone is a cause of the clinical syndrome termed testosterone insufficiency in younger men, associated with many of the classic symptoms associated with aging. Without treatment (supplementation), men experiencing testosterone insufficiency are at increased risk of dementia and Alzheimer's disease, cardiovascular disease, prostate cancer, diabetes, osteoporosis, and loss of muscle mass and strength. This clinical syndrome can affect a man's general health and wellbeing, because our hormones provide the basis of our health.

TESTOSTERONE INSUFFICIENCY

Testosterone levels decline 1% to 3% per year after the age of 30 according to data from the Massachusetts Male Aging Study. Researchers define low testosterone as a level of total testosterone less than 300 ng/dl. When levels drop that low, symptoms of premature aging are apparent and the aging process begins to accelerate. Low testosterone affects more than one third of males over 45 (as high as 38.7%). The actual incidence is much higher, according to the 2016 Consensus Paper by Abraham Morgentaler et al., the researchers who initially defined testosterone insufficiency as a clinical syndrome.

Although total blood serum testosterone is the most commonly used measurement of androgen activity, it is a poor indicator of tissue activity. What's more, symptoms do not always correlate with total testosterone. Given the need to identify men at risk, health assessment questionnaires should be utilized for screening as well.

Risks of low T. The symptoms of low testosterone can include:

- Low energy levels

- Insomnia

- Weight gain (especially around the midsection)

- Brain fog

- Loss of muscle mass

- Decreased libido

- Decreased sexual performance (erectile dysfunction)

- Joint pain

- Mood disturbances, including irritability and anxiety.

Unfortunately, only 5% of males who suffer from testosterone insufficiency receive testosterone replacement therapy (TRT). Even fewer are receiving testosterone optimization therapy.

History. The history of testosterone therapy is fascinating and unique. The Roman, Pliny the Elder, recommended the consumption of animal testes to treat symptoms of testosterone deficiency. The use of testicles grew exponentially towards the end of the nineteenth century when Charles E. Brown-Séquard (1817–1894) published a scientific paper on the results of his self-experiment in The Lancet. He gave himself daily 1-ml injections of a mixture of one-part testicular vein blood, one-part semen, and one-part juice extracted from dog or guinea pig testes, daily. Three weeks later, he was astonished and reported, "A radical change took place in me. I had regained at least all the strength I possessed a good many years ago. I was able to make experiments for several hours. My limbs, tested with a dynamometer, gained 6 to 7 kg in strength. The jet of urine and the power of defecation became stronger."

Nearly a half-century later, two scientists, Leopold Ruzicka and Adolf Butenandt, synthesized the hormone that is the most important hormone for men and, as it turns out, also useful for women. Both scientists received the Nobel Prize for their findings. Initially, testosterone was available for clinical use starting in the 1940s. Still, practitioners limited the therapy to those patients with the most severe cases of testosterone deficiency (TD) such as men with pituitary tumors or anorchia (a condition in which both testicles are absent at birth). It wasn't until the 1990s that physicians recognized a more expanded subset of patients who were symptomatic from prematurely low testosterone and would benefit from testosterone replacement therapy (TRT).

Controversy. Initially, there were concerns about testosterone and illicit performance enhancement in athletes and bodybuilders—the anabolic steroid craze. Even before that, physicians were concerned that testosterone "fueled the fire" of prostate cancer, proposing that testosterone therapy stimulated the progression of the disease and increased its severity. That has been shown to be a concern that does not have one shred of supporting evidence in the world literature.

In 2013, Vigen et al. reported an increase in heart attacks, strokes, and all-cause mortality in males taking testosterone, leading the Food and Drug Administration (FDA) to announce an investigation into cardiovascular (CV) risk in males using testosterone products. Subsequently, a black box warning was placed on all testosterone products.

> *On further analysis, the Vigen study actually showed that testosterone was protective of the heart, and there was less all-cause mortality among testosterone users. Subsequent scientific research has demonstrated that cardiovascular risk declines while on testosterone therapy.*

PREMATURE ANDROPAUSE

I believe that more men are slipping into premature andropause because of inadequate screening:

- If we rely solely on biologic tests like serum or saliva, which are still being perfected, we overlook opportunities to support our patients' health.

- With lab tests, normal ranges vary widely between laboratories and bear little correlation to clinical symptoms that our patients are experiencing.

- Free testosterone measurements are equally inaccurate in the clinical setting.

Health assessment questionnaires actually have a higher sensitivity in evaluating this clinical syndrome. Rather than medicating men with sleeping pills, weight loss pills, memory pills, and antianxiety meds (anxiolytics), hormone optimization guided by health questionnaires could expand our ability to improve the health and quality of life of males who would benefit from TRT.

Aside from the short-term biologic effects of low testosterone, the rationale for optimizing testosterone goes beyond feelings of well-being and cosmetic effects. Long-term low testosterone can affect the heart, brain, bones, and prostate.

Cardio and Vascular Concerns

Evidence from clinical studies suggests that patients with low testosterone levels are at increased cardiovascular disease risk. Low plasma testosterone has been shown to be associated with:

- High cholesterol

- Diabetes

- Inflammation

- Clogged blood vessels

Measures of risk:

- Excess abdominal fat

- Loss of insulin sensitivity causing type 2 diabetes

- Higher levels of C-reactive protein indicating inflammation

- Atherosclerosis indicating blockage of blood vessels

Furthermore, recent evidence suggests that testosterone deficiency has direct negative effects on the endothelium (the cells that line our blood vessels and heart, which supply nutrients and nitric oxide to our tissues, playing a role in both immunity and sexual function).

Damage to the lining of arteries can be repaired. However, without testosterone, there is an accumulation of damage to the vital endothelium, worsened by pro-inflammatory cytokines and an increased risk of cardiovascular disease.

BENEFITS OF TESTOSTERONE REPLACEMENT THERAPY

Testosterone replacement therapy is a safe and effective means of reducing the risk of clogged arteries and cardiovascular disease in men with low testosterone, because it:

- Reduces insulin resistance (the cause of diabetes)

- Reduces harmful cholesterol

- Reduces abdominal fat

- Reduces risk for coronary artery disease (CAD)

Documented improvements in men given aromatizable testosterone:

- Increased blood flow to the coronary arteries (even in patients with coronary artery disease)

- Decreased plaque in the coronary arteries

- Decreased inflammation in the coronary arteries.

Reduced cancer risk. Multiple studies have shown that low T is associated with high-grade prostate cancer (PCa), and a higher stage at diagnosis of their prostate cancer. Now that we know that testosterone does not "fuel the fire" of prostate cancer, the question: is the opposite true, that optimal levels of testosterone are indeed protective to the prostate? A pooled prospective study of 3000 men in Finland, Norway, and Sweden had testosterone blood levels evaluated. Eventually, 25% were diagnosed with prostate cancer afterward. There was a decreased risk of prostate cancer in the men with higher testosterone levels.

Osteoporosis. Decreased bone density is often thought of as a women's disease after menopause. The reality is, osteoporosis also affects men. Overall, one in five men over the age of 50 will have an osteoporosis-related fracture. Fractures from osteoporosis in males can be associated with higher rates of disability and death than in women. Given that men are currently developing low testosterone at younger and younger ages, we need to be aware that one of the biologic effects of low T is the loss of bone mass. Testosterone increases bone density in men with low levels of this male hormone.

Premature dementia. The number of Alzheimer's cases will triple by 2050 at a cost that will increase 500%, to $1.1 trillion per year. One of the biologic effects of low testosterone is an increase in cognitive decline, beginning in a man's mid-thirties, coincidentally with his drop in testosterone. This reduction in mental capability can progress to a decrease in verbal memory, possibly dementia, or even Alzheimer's disease. By the age of 85, one in three people will have Alzheimer's disease. As testosterone decreases, inflammation in the brain increases, causing damage to brain circulation, cells, and the mitochondria (the source of cellular energy production). Both estrogen and testosterone protect the brain by:

- Reducing cell death (apoptosis)

- Increasing blood flow to the brain

- Decreasing beta-amyloid deposits that result in Alzheimer's disease

- Decreasing inflammation-related cytokines

EVALUATING TESTOSTERONE

The clinical symptoms of male hypogonadism are well recognized and delineated earlier in this chapter. Aging is one of the most common and causes two critical changes. One, the testosterone levels of both total and free testosterone decrease. Two, sex hormone binding globulin (SHBG) increases, diminishing a male's free testosterone further.

Health assessment questionnaires and tests of the hypothalamic-pituitary-testicular axis are sufficiently accurate to permit the diagnosis in most patients.

- The patient is judged to have primary hypogonadism if the serum testosterone concentration is below normal and the serum luteinizing hormone (LH) and/or the follicle-stimulating hormone (FSH) concentrations are above normal.

- The patient has secondary hypogonadism if the serum testosterone concentration is below normal and the serum LH and/or the FSH concentrations are normal or low.

Testosterone testing. The initial test should be a blood draw to measure both serum total testosterone and free testosterone early in the morning.

- If the result is low, the doctor should repeat the test at least once.

- If hypogonadism is secondary and of moderate severity (e.g., <200 ng/dL) and/or associated with other hormonal deficiencies, test serum prolactin.

- If serum prolactin is elevated, a magnetic resonance imaging (MRI) of the brain should be ordered to rule out a pituitary tumor.

- For a man pursuing fertility semen analysis, an evaluation of testosterone insufficiency is also relevant if the patient is seeking fertility.

A man with low testosterone should be tested for:

- Estradiol, thyroid profile, and vitamin D levels

- Hemoglobin A1C (average blood sugar over the past two to three months, indicating risk of diabetes)

- CBC (complete blood count evaluating immune competence)

- CMP (complete metabolic panel).

TESTOSTERONE THERAPY

In Abraham Morgentaler, M.D.'s consensus report entitled, "Fundamental concepts regarding testosterone deficiency and treatment: International expert consensus resolutions," it was unanimously decided that "TD [testosterone deficiency] is a well-established, clinically significant medical condition that negatively affects male sexuality, reproduction, general health, and quality of life." It was also unanimously decided that, "…symptoms and signs of TD occur as a result of low levels of T and may benefit from treatment regardless of whether there is an identified underlying etiology [cause]," and that "there is no T concentration threshold that reliably distinguishes those who will respond to treatment from those who will not."

As reported, the initial starting concentration of testosterone predicts the magnitude and rapidity of response to treatment. The lower the baseline testosterone, the more substantial the increase in circulating testosterone values must be for the effect to be perceived by the subject, and the longer the duration of treatment to achieve an instrumentally noticeable effect. The timing and the range of impact of testosterone replacement shows considerable variation in terms of both measurable levels and desired outcomes.

Bioidentical vs. Synthetic Options

Many factors affect the choice of regimen, including patient preference, cost, convenience, and insurance coverage. The following are some of the more common options:

Bioidentical testosterone. A bioidentical hormone has the exact molecular structure of the testosterone that the body produces, confirmed by electron microscope. It tends to work synergistically with your hormone receptors. Utilizing soy and yams provides the raw material to produce testosterone identical in structure to human testosterone.

Synthetic testosterone has a different molecular structure than that the body produces, and so it can cause many more side effects and interfere with proper hormone function. It is usually administered as Testosterone cypionate, enanthate, or undecanoate.

There are a number of variables that contribute to the benefits and side effects of TRT. Understanding the pharmacokinetics is essential.

No oral supplements. There are no bioidentical testosterone preparations approved for oral administration because absorption is variable and often inadequate. Also, testosterone absorbed from the GI tract is rapidly metabolized in the liver and will not provide sustainable levels.

Transdermal administration—bioidenticals include Androgel, Testim, Axiron, Fortesta, and compounded testosterone cream. Most of these are administered twice a day, but absorption is not predictable. It is often difficult to achieve optimal hormone levels in the majority of patients.

Injectable testosterone—synthetics The esterified molecule of testosterone and its oil base extend the duration of efficacy. These forms (testosterone cypionate, enanthate, undecanoate) are administered twice weekly to every three months, depending on the product. The disadvantages are:

- The need for deep intramuscular (IM) administration of an oily solution 50 to 100 times per year

- Fluctuations in the serum testosterone concentration, which result in variations in symptom relief in many patients. Many patients have reported a roller coaster-like feeling with hormone levels varying significantly between injections.

On a positive note, this is the least expensive route of administration, and many insurance carriers will reimburse for these medications.

Bioidentical pellet. Finally, a doctor may place a bioidentical testosterone pellet under the skin of the buttock (Testopel or a compounded formulation such as BioTE). The benefit of this method is more consistent testosterone hormone levels. This method, however, does require an insertion procedure with local anesthesia. The literature reports more consistent blood serum levels of testosterone with this method. Adverse events include pellet extrusion, infection, or fibrosis, which today occur rarely.

SIDE EFFECTS

There are some side effects to testosterone administration for the clinical syndrome of testosterone deficiency. These include:

Suppression of sperm production (spermatogenesis). This has been especially prevalent in men receiving parenteral testosterone or sub-cutaneous pellets because of the extreme suppression of FSH as part of the normal feedback loop. This side effect is usually reversible in men who want to resume fertility. It is a good idea to get a semen analysis in younger males with testosterone deficiency who may desire pregnancy in the future.

Erythrocytosis (an elevation of red blood cell mass). Testosterone stimulates the production of red blood cells. The level of red blood cells (hematocrit) should be measured before initiating testosterone treatment. Less than 4% of patients receiving testosterone injections and fewer than 1% taking oral testosterone develop this symptom and occasionally will need to donate blood or have blood removed.

Obstructive sleep apnea (OSA). The estimated prevalence in North America is approximately 15% to 30% of males. Testosterone therapy can worsen the symptoms of sleep apnea in one-third of patients, especially if they are African American, older, obese, hypertensive, diabetic, have low thyroid levels, and/or are a smoker.

Reduction in testicular size. Occasionally there is a 10% to 15% reduction in the size of the testicle. This is thought to be due to a reduction in spermatogenesis in males on TRT. This side effect is reversible once therapy is stopped.

Liver damage. Non-oral testosterone preparations do not cause liver damage. Oral testosterone, particularly synthetic oral testosterone, has had reported cases. In the spirit of consistency, the FDA requires all testosterone preparations to carry this warning.

Fluid retention. A small percentage of patients will experience fluid retention while on TRT, but the degree of retention is generally mild. This is secondary to the early increase in muscle mass. This extracellular water weight usually resolves spontaneously.

Acne. TRT can increase oil production in the glands of the skin. As such, some men will experience an increase in acne that usually responds well to systemic therapy.

Skin rash. Skin irritation can occur with any of the topical testosterone preparations.

Allergic reaction. There have been reported cases of allergic reactions to the cottonseed oil in parenteral preparations.

Breast enlargement. Many men will have breast enlargement (gynecomastia) with low testosterone levels. After TRT, some men will develop gynecomastia from the conversion of testosterone to estradiol, causing breast growth. This side effect and its predecessor, nipple sensitivity, are fortunately rare. Treatment usually involves a reduction in testosterone.

KEY TAKE AWAYS

This chapter has focused on helping men who might have low testosterone recognize the symptoms characteristic of the clinical syndrome of testosterone deficiency/insufficiency.

The short-term benefits including symptom relief were discussed. Clearly most men feel better with TRT, which supports:

- More energy

- Better sexual performance

- Improved focus and cognition

- Better sleep

- Less anxiety or irritability.

Testosterone optimization can be of paramount importance in avoiding the side effects of using multiple medications to treat the symptoms of TD. In addition, there are long-term significant benefits for:

- The heart

- The brain

- Bones

- Prostate.

TRT can reduce the risks of cardiovascular disease, diabetes, Alzheimer's disease, osteoporosis, and prostate cancer.

The type of hormone (synthetic vs bioidentical) matters. The route of administration matters. Physiologic hormone replacement therapy or testosterone replacement therapy should mirror your hormone production when you felt your best in your 20s and 30s. It should be hassle free and be utilized with minimal side effects.

For males, optimizing your testosterone as you grow older provides the foundation for healthy aging. Feeling your best as you age provides the basis for pristine quality of life.

BOOKS

Gary Donovitz, MD. *Testosterone Matters ... More!: The Secret to Healthy Aging in Women.* Tucson, AZ: Wheatmark, 2020.

Gary Donovitz, MD. *Age Healthier Live Happier.* Celebrity Press, 2015.

For more information on testosterone therapy and the work of Dr. Donovitz, please see www.BioTEmedical.com.

Chapter 90
Prostate Health
Judson Brandeis, MD, Urologist
& David A. Miller, MD, Urologist

I am living proof that if you catch prostate cancer early, it can be reduced to a temporary inconvenience, and you can go back to a normal life.
— *General Norman Schwarzkopf*

The prostate is one of the most feared and misunderstood organs in the body. For men under 50, the prostate primarily brings us pleasure, unless it becomes infected (termed prostatitis). Once men reach 50, the prostate begins to enlarge in size and tends to bring more pain than pleasure, sometimes even becoming cancerous. This chapter will help you make sense of the complex world of prostate enlargement and prostate cancer.

Prostate function. Glands are the organs in the body that manufacture fluids containing hormones that have biological effects. The male prostate produces semen, providing about 20% of the seminal fluid that accompanies sperm during ejaculation. The rest of that fluid is produced by two small tubular glands, the seminal vesicles, located above the prostate. Sperm are produced in the testicles and then piped to the prostate through fine tubing, the *vas deferens*, which are approximately one foot (30 cm) in length, and just 1/10 of an inch (3–5 mm) in diameter. Given the astonishing delicacy of these organs, it is easy to see how this system can become compromised as we age.

The role of testosterone. The growth, differentiation, and activity of the prostate gland are primarily controlled by testosterone and its derivative, dihydrotestosterone (DHT) which act through testosterone receptors. The prostate glandular tissue is surrounded by a capsule which is a thin, but tough membrane similar to the skin of a plum.

BENIGN PROSTATE ENLARGEMENT (BPE)

BPE and BPH (benign prostatic hypertrophy) are similar terms describing a common urological issue that occurs in men after the age of 40. This involves *noncancerous* increase in prostate size.

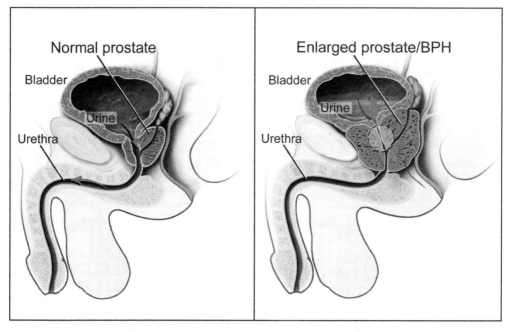

Figure 90.1. The normal size prostate allows the flow of urine out of the bladder. The enlarged prostate obstructs the flow of urine causing obstructive and irritative urinary symptoms.'

Prostate enlargement becomes increasingly common as men age. It is estimated that 50% of 50-year-olds, 60% of 60-year-olds, 70% of 70-year-olds, and 80% of 80-year-olds have some degree of prostate enlargement that leads to lower urinary tract symptoms.

The normal prostate in a younger man is approximately one inch in diameter (20-30 mm), about the size of a walnut. However, for reasons that are still not clear to scientists, the prostate tends to grow when men are in their 40s. The urethra, the tube that carries urine from the bladder through the penis, passes through the prostate. When the prostate becomes enlarged, it squeezes the urethra as it crosses through the prostate, reducing the stream of urine. As a result, it becomes difficult to fully empty the bladder, which results in the retention of urine. I like to describe the prostate as an apple with the core taken out. Men void through where the core used to be and, as the meat of the apple grows, it compresses the stream and leads to symptoms of obstruction.

Prevention. It is important to understand that there is a 30% placebo effect for any medication.

- *Herbal therapies.* Herbs are commonly used in the management of urinary symptoms. Saw palmetto is frequently taken for BPH, but a large review of 32 randomized trials comparing saw palmetto with placebo did not find any difference. Beta-sitosterol and *Pygeum africanum* do have studies showing some symptom improvement, although not at the level of medications currently in use.

- *Kegels.* The literature also suggests that Kegel exercises do not prevent prostate enlargement, but can help with controlling urinary leakage.

- *Nutrition.* New research has confirmed the value of reducing the intake of sugars, high carbs, and junk food. Gut health reflects the quality of our diet, and recent studies have linked gut flora with prostate outcomes. "Emerging studies indicate that the microbiome [gut bacteria] can influence prostate inflammation in relation to benign prostate conditions such as prostatitis/chronic pelvic pain syndrome and benign prostatic hyperplasia, as well as in prostate cancer."

There are certain over-the-counter medications that can exacerbate voiding difficulties in men and even lead to urinary retention. Antihistamines, decongestants, cough/cold, and allergy medications such as Benadryl and Sudafed should be used cautiously in men with underlying voiding difficulty. Usually, these types of medications have specific warnings on the labels regarding these potential side effects.

Early intervention. Growth of the prostate can lead to a range of obstructive symptoms such as a slow urinary stream, hesitancy, a stop-and-start pattern of urination, and/or retention of urine. It can also lead to urinary symptoms such as frequency, urgency, and nighttime urination.

Sphincter muscles above and below the prostate control the flow of urine. The sphincter above the prostate is controlled automatically by the brain. Although the sphincter below the gland can be controlled by intentionally contracting the muscle, once the prostate becomes enlarged, this condition requires medical intervention rather than will power. Eventually, men can develop urinary tract infections, bladder stones, and even kidney damage.

> *Treating an enlarged prostate early will help you avoid more involved surgeries later on—surgeries that can have significant negative side effects.*

Medications. First-line treatment for benign prostate enlargement causing urinary symptoms includes medical therapy:

- *Alpha-blocker medications.* This class of medication relaxes the smooth muscle in the prostate, opening up the urinary channel as it crosses through the prostate, but has no effect on prostate size. Terazosin and doxazosin are nonspecific blockers and can decrease blood pressure. Tamsulosin and silodosin (Rapaflo) have effects that are more specific to the prostate and have less blood pressure effect, but a higher incidence of retrograde or dry ejaculation. It is generally recommended to take these medications at bedtime so the blood pressure effects that result in fatigue and dizziness will primarily occur at night.

- *5 alpha-reductase inhibitors.* Medications like *finasteride* and *dutasteride* will shrink the prostate by about 20% over 6 months and artificially reduce PSA by about 50%. They are also used for androgenic alopecia (male pattern baldness). Side effects can include a decrease in libido.

- *Anticholinergic medications.* Some physicians will recommend anticholinergic medications to treat irritative symptoms like frequency, urgency, and incontinence. These medications include tolterodine, also known as Detrol, fesoterodine (Toviaz), and solifenacin (Vesicare).

- *Cautions.* One of the most commonly prescribed medications in this class is oxybutynin, also known as Ditropan. This drug crosses the blood-brain barrier and can cause cognitive issues. I strongly recommended against taking this medication. There is another medication, Myrbetriq, which also works well for irritative urinary symptoms and does not have the same side effects. I would recommend this as first-line treatment although for cost reasons, it is used less frequently. In addition, this class of medications can relax the bladder and lead to retention or worsening bladder emptying. A proper evaluation needs to be undertaken prior to starting these types of medication on men with difficulty urinating.

- *Combination therapy.* In patients with severe symptoms of benign prostatic enlargement, sometimes urologists use a combination of alpha-blockers and 5 alpha-reductase inhibitors. It is been shown that the combination of the two medications are better than either one alone.

- *Multiple benefits.* Another medication that is indicated for urinary symptoms is tadalafil (5 mg once a day), also known as Cialis. This medication has the added benefit of improving erectile function.

Procedures. For men who have symptoms that are not adequately treated by medication, many procedures can improve symptoms. It is critical to undergo a transrectal or transabdominal ultrasound of the prostate and bladder, as well as possibly cystoscopy and even an MRI of the prostate, before deciding as to which treatment is best suited for an individual. I would not proceed without this information. Treatment should be individualized based on prostate size, type of symptoms, and sexual function. A complete description of procedures is beyond the scope of this chapter. What I would recommend for a smaller prostate (less than 60 ccs) is either a Rezum procedure or a Uro-lift procedure.

- *Rezum procedure.* This procedure can be done in the office under sedation by injecting steam into the prostate through a cystoscope, which is placed through the urethra. The advantage of this procedure is that there is no foreign object permanently placed into the body, the actual procedure should take no more than 5 to 10 minutes, and there tends to be only a small amount of bleeding. The disadvantage is that obstructive urinary symptoms get worse for the first week. I like to put a Spanner stent in place immediately after the procedure and remove the stent three weeks later. I think the placement of a Spanner stent improves quality of life during the first week or two after the procedure. It typically takes several months for patients' urinary symptoms to improve significantly.

- *Uro-Lift procedure.* This intervention uses a small staple-like device to hold back the lateral lobes of the prostate that are causing obstruction. It is a quick outpatient procedure that is minimally invasive and the results are immediate. Its effectiveness is limited by the size of the prostate however, and an ultrasound is necessary to determine if the gland size is appropriate for a uro-lift. The advantage of this procedure is that there is no destruction or removal of prostate tissue, no catheter is necessary, and there is no deleterious effect on ejaculation. Postoperatively, one may experience frequency and urgency for up to 4-6 weeks .

Surgical interventions. There are other options for an enlarged prostate that are typically performed in a surgery center or outpatient surgery setting, including transurethral resection of the prostate (TURP), transurethral laser enucleation, bipolar TURP, greenlight laser TURP, and plasma vaporization. The decision on which way to go is typically based on the experience of the surgeon. Surgery on the prostate has significant effects on the amount of fluid released with ejaculation. The effects on erection tend to be mild.

For very large prostates, a simple open prostatectomy to remove part or all of the prostate is indicated. This can be done with the da Vinci surgical robot by an experienced robotic surgeon, but I would highly recommend finding an experienced urologist who can do this operation robotically. The recovery when this is done robotically is far superior to the procedure when it is done in an open fashion, and for very large prostates, the outcomes are far superior to a transurethral resection.

PROSTATE CANCER

The prostate also has the potential to become cancerous. Among cancers that affect men, prostate cancer is the most common (excluding nonmelanoma skin cancers), especially in the male population over 50. After lung cancer, prostate cancer is the most common cause of cancer-related death in men 50 or older.

Occurrence. Worldwide there are an estimated 1.3 million new cases of prostate cancer every year, making it the second most commonly diagnosed cancer in men. In the United States, it is the third leading cause of cancer with approximately 190,000 new diagnoses annually. For an American male, there is a 12% lifetime risk of being diagnosed with prostate cancer. Without screening, many cases of prostate cancer do not ever become clinically evident.

Most prostate cancers grow so slowly that the majority of men die of other causes before prostate cancer becomes clinically advanced. In autopsies of men who died of other causes, approximately 30% of men in their 50s and 70% of men in their 70s had evidence of prostate cancer. Worldwide there are an estimated 360,000 prostate cancer deaths every year, making it the fifth leading cause of male cancer death. In the United States, prostate cancer is the second leading cause of cancer death among men with 33,000 deaths every year. For an American male, the lifetime risk of dying of prostate cancer is 2.4%.

Higher risk? There are certain subsets of men who are at higher risk of prostate cancer including individuals with a family history of prostate cancer, those from families who carry the BRCA 1 or BRCA2 genetic mutation, and African-Americans. Studies suggest that PSA elevations may precede the clinical manifestations of prostate cancer by five to ten or more years. The diagnosis of prostate cancer is difficult because there are no symptoms until much later in the disease course.

Diagnosis—PSA level. Prostate-specific antigen, or PSA, is a protein synthesized by the epithelium of the prostate and secreted in seminal fluid. It is a diagnostic tool used as a tumor marker for early diagnosis, treatment, and monitoring of patients with prostate cancer. The exact value of normal for PSA varies with age.

- Some urologists use a cut-off point of PSA levels over 4 for all patients.

- Other doctors use an age-adjusted PSA scale.

- For men under 50, PSA should not be higher than 2.5.

- In men 50–60 the abnormal value is over 3.5.

- For men 60–70 the abnormal PSA value is over 4.5.

- Among men over 70, a PSA is concerning when it is over 6.5.

PSA binds to proteins and there is a correlation between the percentage of free (unbound) PSA and the statistical risk of prostate cancer.

- A lower percent-free PSA means that the chance of having prostate cancer is higher and you should probably have a biopsy. (When the percentage of free PSA is 10 or more, there is over 50% chance of prostate cancer.)

- Many doctors recommend a prostate biopsy for men whose percent-free PSA is 10% or less and advise that men consider a biopsy if it is between 10% and 25%. (When the percentage of free PSA is greater than 25, there is less than a 10% chance of cancer.) Prior to considering a prostate biopsy, it is essential to know your percentage of free PSA.

An enlarged prostate can result in an elevation of PSA, but testing for the level of percentage-free PSA and getting a prostate MRI can help to differentiate between benign and malignant reasons for the elevation.

Screening Recommendations

Per the American Urological Association, the greatest benefit of screening appears to be:

- In men ages 55 to 69 years;

- For high risk men—African American men and men with a first-degree relative with prostate cancer diagnosed before age 65.

Baseline PSA testing should begin in their 40s. It should be emphasized that PSA testing requires a candid discussion between the patient and physician and a full understanding of the pros and cons of testing. This shared decision-making is key, and there is no "one size fits all" regarding PSA testing.

- Screening is not routinely recommended in men age 70+ years unless the individual is in excellent health.

- In any man with less than a 10- to 15-year life expectancy PSA testing is not recommended.

It is acceptable to use a PSA cut off of 4.0 as a normal level. However, a PSA test should be repeated after the first abnormal value to confirm the validity of the lab test. It is important to understand the range of PSA. In men under 40, PSA is likely to be less than 1. It is rare for prostate cancer to spread unless the PSA is over 25. In men with widespread disease, PSA is typically in the hundreds or even the thousands.

Digital exam. Although there are many who would prefer to avoid the digital rectal exam, it remains an important part of the physical examination in men. There have been studies that revealed a diagnosis of prostate cancer in up to 18% of men with a normal PSA and an abnormal prostate exam. In addition, the size of the prostate can be assessed as well the presence of infection. Finally, in some cases anal cancers can be detected with the digital exam as well.

False positive PSA levels. Having an elevated PSA does not necessarily mean that you have cancer. There are certain times when the PSA will be elevated in the absence of cancer. If you check the PSA after these conditions, the PSA screening test will not be useful.

- Results can be skewed by the presence of infection in the urine or the prostate.

- Following a urologic procedure or intervention

- Following a digital prostate exam, which may also increase PSA up to 0.4 ng/m

- From activities that induce perineal trauma like ejaculation or bicycling (Abstain from this type of activity for 48 hours before a PSA blood draw.)

- Due to medication, notably 5 alpha-reductase inhibitors (finasteride or dutasteride), which will result in a PSA that is typically 50% of what the real measurement would be.

MRI technology in diagnosis. A multi-parametric 3 Tesla MRI of the prostate is very useful in detecting prostate cancer. This is especially true for men with an elevated blood serum PSA and a prior negative prostate biopsy, because some cancer can exist in the anterior prostate, which is not typically sampled in a standard prostate biopsy. However, many urologists will perform a 3 Tesla multi-parametric MRI of the prostate without first performing a standard biopsy if the patient has an elevated PSA and the urologist suspects prostate cancer. A 3 Tesla MRI is more accurate than imaging with a 1.5 Tesla machine.

A multi-parametric MRI-directed prostate biopsy requires technology that fuses the MRI image with the ultrasound image to guide a biopsy needle to cancer seen on the MRI. These biopsies are more sensitive than standard 12-core transrectal ultrasound biopsy techniques. Recent data show the benefit of combining both the targeted and 12-core template approach. Studies among men with an elevated PSA suggest that performing an MRI before performing a prostate biopsy offers potential benefits of increased detection in those with significantly higher risk of disease, while sparing men with benign prostates an uncomfortable procedure with potential morbidity. One study compared MRI with or without targeted biopsy to systematic biopsy alone and found a 57% improvement in the detection of clinically significant prostate cancer, a 77% reduction in the number of cores taken for procedure, and a 33% reduction in unnecessary biopsies.

I believe that a pre-biopsy MRI will eventually become standard protocol and that the majority of men will benefit from a 3 Tesla multi-parametric MRI of the prostate prior to a planned biopsy.

The hope is that "unnecessary" biopsies can be avoided in this way. Multiple studies are currently underway to determine if this will become the standard of care. Prostate MRIs are also useful for establishing the extent of local spread of prostate cancer. Additionally, for men who choose active surveillance of their prostate cancer, MRIs are a valuable method for following the progression of the cancer.

Comprehensive evaluation. The most important factors in selecting initial treatment for prostate cancer include PSA level, Gleason score (which is the estimated aggressiveness of prostate cancer), molecular characteristics of the tumor, the anatomic extent of the disease (including results of the prostate MRI, bone scan, staging CT scan) and an estimate of the patient's general medical condition and age. It is also important to consider a man's tolerance for loss of erectile function and continence.

Information that is often overlooked can be obtained from a tissue-based molecular assay such as Oncotype DX, Prolaris, Confirm MDX, or Decipher. Anyone with prostate cancer will want to discuss the benefits of sending the biopsy specimen for additional testing. Also, consider genetic screening for ATM germline mutation (a gene that plays a role in DNA damage response), as well as BRCA1 and BRCA2 (implicated in both female and male breast cancer) which are all associated with more lethal prostate cancer.

Active surveillance. Over the past 10 years, there has been a trend towards an increased number of men undergoing active surveillance. This entails tracking the PSA through periodic testing along with alternating MRI's and biopsies every few years, instead of immediately opting for aggressive treatment. For many low- to moderate-risk prostate cancers, this is an appropriate treatment approach because of the slow growth of prostate cancer. This also avoids the potential side effects of treatment, namely incontinence or erectile dysfunction.

Surgery. For a man who is considering prostate surgery, the best option is robotic prostatectomy. It is ideal to find a surgeon who performs at least 100 prostatectomies a year on the da Vinci robot made by Intuitive Surgical. It is perfectly appropriate to ask the surgeon his outcomes and, specifically, the rate of incontinence and erectile dysfunction. It would be similar to asking a baseball player his batting average, and your surgeon should not be offended by this question.

Radiation therapy. These interventions use an external beam source to destroy prostate cancer cells so that they do not grow. Older radiation therapy machines require approximately 40 treatments over 8 to 10 weeks. The newer CyberKnife requires only one week of treatment with similar outcomes, so this can be a beneficial approach.

Recent advances. The issue with earlier approaches to standard treatment for prostate cancer has been the effect on quality of life, including incontinence and erectile dysfunction. Newer treatment options include high-intensity focused ultrasound or HIFU, which has recently been FDA approved in the United States. In addition, using MRI guidance, focal laser therapy has been successful in curing selected prostate cancers without side effects.

In summary, for most men the prostate is involved in our best moments and our worst moments. It helps create the pleasure of orgasm and assists the sperm on their journey toward procreation. However, as we age the enlarged prostate impairs the ability to urinate, and a cancerous prostate has a deleterious effect on longevity. Furthermore, the treatment of a cancerous prostate can have effects on sexual function and urinary function. If you are among the many men confronted with these issues, work with a board-certified urologist to explore the new technologies that are improving treatment outcomes, but never be afraid to use the information in this chapter or that you find on the internet to advocate for yourself.

KEY TAKE AWAYS

- Check your PSA every other year from age 50 until age 75, unless you have a family history of prostate cancer or are African American, in which case you should begin checking it by age 40 and more frequently. Remember, testing is a shared decision-making process between you and your physician.

- An enlarged prostate that causes urinary symptoms is very common, and there are several medications you can take to improve those symptoms. Treating an enlarged prostate early will help you avoid more involved surgeries, which can have negative side effects.

- Cialis is a medication that can be used for both improving urination and boosting erections.

- If you have a new diagnosis of prostate cancer, make sure you have the option of genetic testing for prostate cancer, and get a second opinion on options for treatment.

If you have an elevated PSA, make sure you get an MRI of the prostate prior to prostate biopsy, and get an MRI-guided ultrasound fusion prostate biopsy instead of a standard prostate biopsy.

**For the medical practice of Dr. Brandeis, see www.BrandeisMD.com.
For the practice of Dr. Miller, please visit www.uro.com**

Chapter 91
Peyronie's Disease
Judson Brandeis, MD, Urologist

Love your curves and all your edges, all your perfect imperfections.
— John Legend

Peyronie's disease is an acquired disorder of scar tissue on the inner lining of the penis, resulting in penile deformity, pain, and in some men, erectile dysfunction. Peyronie's disease occurs in 5% of men over the age of 40. Peyronie's disease resolves spontaneously in little more than 10% of cases. Nearly half of patients will have worsening deformity. Peyronie's disease can be a physically and psychologically disabling disorder, leading to lower quality of life. Patients are encouraged to initiate treatment as soon as possible once diagnosis of Peyronie's disease is made. Surgical management should be considered in men with penile deformity that is compromising sexual function, if the deformity has lasted more than 12 months.

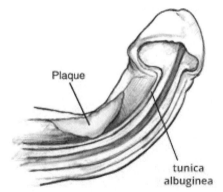

Figure 91.1. In Peyronie's disease, scar tissue on the shealth that wraps the erectile bodies (the tunica) causes curvature of the penis.

Approximately one of every twenty men above the age of 40 has Peyronie's disease. At least four of five men with this condition do not remember any specific event that led to the development of the disease. The underlying lesions of Peyronie's disease are the fibrous plaque of scar tissue that contains excessive collagen and fragmented elastic fibers that alter penile anatomy. Over time the plaques can become hardened and calcify.

Underlying causes. There is an association between Peyronie's disease and Dupuytren's contractures of the hand, which is a disease of collagen with a genetic origin. A history of genital trauma, prostate surgery, and/or diabetes have also been associated with the development of Peyronie's disease.

> *Caution—Risk of penile fracture: The tissue that encases the penis (the tunica albuginea) is tough, but in extreme circumstances, a man can actually suffer a penile fracture, which occurs when this lining tissue ruptures and blood oozes through the opening. Although rare, this unfortunate injury typically happens during aggressive intercourse when the woman is on top.*

Seek immediate treatment for a fracture of the penis. Sometimes a penile fracture requires surgery to repair the leak and frequently results in scar tissue that causes Peyronie's (shortening and curvature of the penis). If you are having aggressive sex, you hear a snap, and find that your erection has quickly gone away, you may have sustained a fracture. If this occurs and your penis swells and becomes black and blue, go to the nearest urologist or emergency room as soon as possible to avoid further damage.

Primary symptoms. Untreated Peyronie's disease improves in only 12% of men, with almost 50% of men demonstrating worsening of the curvature at 12 months. Presenting symptoms include penile pain and possibly a nodule or plaque, indentation, curvature, deformity, or shortening of the penis during erection. Sexual dysfunction may also occur. Peyronie's disease is most evident during an erection. Severe and complex curvature and compromised penile rigidity may make penetrative intercourse impossible.

Medication. Patients in the active phase of the disease experiencing pain with erection and changes in curvature may benefit from an oral medication, pentoxifylline 400 mg, 3 times a day. Pentoxifylline decreases fibrosis, prevents deposition of collagen, and reduces calcification in experimental animals. Studies show that oral medications like colchicine and tamoxifen are not helpful, nor are supplements such as vitamin E, PABA (para-aminobenzoic acid), or carnitine.

Injections. Injecting medication into penis plaque has shown some benefit. Verapamil and interferon have shown minimal benefit. Men with stable disease and curvature between 30 and 90 degrees have the option of Xiaflex injections. Xiaflex contains collagenase, which is an enzyme that degrades collagen. A typical course of treatment is 6 to 10 injections. A pair of injections are performed three days apart, and each pair is delivered six weeks apart. The downside is the cost of medication, and the fact that men are unable to undergo intercourse for four weeks after injection.

Therapies. Shockwave therapy is an investigational treatment that, in some patients, has shown improvement in the plaque size and curvature. Reduction in pain has also been documented with shockwave therapy. Penile traction therapy, in conjunction with medical management, Xiaflex, or shockwave therapy, has shown additional benefit.

Surgery. Surgical treatment for Peyronie's disease typically results in the straightening of the penis, but unfortunately results in a penis that is usually shorter due to the scar tissue. Patient satisfaction after surgery for Peyronie's disease is moderate.

KEY TAKE AWAYS

- Peyronie's disease is an acquired disorder that results in scar tissue on the inner lining of the penis, causing penile curvature, pain, and shortening.
- Peyronie's disease resolves spontaneously only about 10% of the time.
- The only oral medication that has shown some efficacy with Peyronie's disease is pentoxifylline 400 mg p.o., three times daily.
- Injection of Xiaflex is expensive and requires long periods of abstinence, but is FDA approved for the treatment of Peyronie's disease and does result in mild to moderate improvement. Make sure that you use a RestoreX device in conjunction with Xiaflex.
- Shockwave Therapy is a promising treatment with minimal side effects that seems to help a subset of patients with Peyronie's disease.

**For more information about Peyronie's disease
and the medical practice of Dr. Brandeis, please see:
www.BrandeisMD.com,
www.endo.com
and www.restorex.com.**

Chapter 92
Circumcision
Judson Brandeis, MD, Urologist

My wife told me that in the bible, Abraham circumcised himself...
Wow, I can't even get to the bank before it closes.
— *Jim Gaffigan*

Circumcision is the surgical removal of the foreskin of the penis and is the oldest surgical procedure in the world. Approximately one-third of the world's male population is circumcised. The incidence varies widely between countries. For example, the rate in England is only 6%, but in the United States it is 70%. In Africa the rate tends to be well over 80%. The reason for this is that HIV transmission is lower in men who are circumcised. Certain religions mandate circumcision, including Judaism and Islam.

BENEFITS OF CIRCUMCISION

The American Academy of Pediatrics recommends newborn circumcision, indicating that the preventive medical and public health benefits outweigh the risks. The most common reasons for circumcision later in life include:

- Release the trapping of the penis inside the foreskin (phimosis) or trapping of the foreskin behind the glans (paraphimosis)
- Reduce inflammation of the glans
- Lower incidence of genital warts (condyloma) caused by human papilloma virus (HPV). (Circumcision has been shown to also reduce the risk of this condition.)
- Reduced HIV transmission
- Lower rates of other sexually transmitted infections
- In boys, less incidence of urinary tract infections.
- Virtual elimination of the risk of penile cancer.

The goal of the procedure is a good cosmetic result with adequate removal of the outer and inner layers of the foreskin. Minimal bleeding (hemostasis) with no infection are essential. The procedure exposes the glans sufficiently to prevent phimosis and paraphimosis.

Complications of circumcision. One of the risks of circumcision is the possible loss of sensitivity. This is controversial and difficult to measure clinically. Other complications include bleeding, concealment of the penis under scar tissue, skin bridge or attachment of foreskin to the glans, infection, urinary retention, and damage to the urethral meatus (the opening of the urethra at the end of the penis, where urine and semen are discharged). Fortunately, most of these complications are rare.

TECHNIQUES OF CIRCUMCISION

There are several different techniques for foreskin removal, including dorsal slit, shields and clamps, and excision. The various techniques utilized for anesthesia including a penile ring block, dorsal nerve block, lidocaine spray injector, general anesthesia, and spinal anesthesia

A dorsal slit is used to expose the meatus of the urethra for urination. This sometimes is required in elderly men who are unable to urinate. It is not cosmetically appealing. Excision with suturing is usually done under deeper anesthesia and is a surgical procedure in which the excess foreskin is completely removed, and the penile skin is sutured in an interrupted fashion to the skin just below the glans and corona. This takes a few weeks to heal.

Shields and clamps. The Mogen clamp is the traditional tool used by the Mohl or Jewish Rabbi performing ceremonial circumcision. More commonly these days, pediatricians use the Plastibell which is a plastic collar placed around the penis. The foreskin is pulled over the collar, and a suture is tied around the skin causing the excess skin to fall off eventually. This is a safe procedure that is commonly performed.

Shang ring circumcision. A similar technique to a clamp has been developed for adult circumcision. The Shang Ring is a sterile device consisting of two concentric medical-grade plastic rings: an inner ring with a silicone band and an outer hinged ring. The inner ring fits inside the outer ring, which lock together. The technique seals the edges of the skin together so that suturing is not required.

To ensure that men do remove the device prematurely, a locking mechanism is included, which can only be opened using a special tool. The Shang Ring comes in multiple sizes based on penile measurement.

The advantage of the Shang Ring circumcision is that it is extremely quick, taking less than 15 minutes to apply, initially requires only local anesthesia, with minimal pain during the procedure and minimal pain afterward. It results in approximately one week of mild discomfort while the ring is in place.

Post-op instructions. After circumcision, patients may resume their usual sedentary activities but should not engage in strenuous activity that causes pain or discomfort. It is appropriate to take a shower two days after the procedure and then reapply a dressing. No swimming or beach trips for two weeks. No sexual activity or masturbation permitted for four weeks after circumcision. You will occasionally see a few drops of blood for the first two weeks. Some men experience pain with erections at night for the first week, but this typically resolves after the first week. If sutures are required, they are absorbed in a week or two and typically do not require removal.

KEY TAKE AWAYS

In summary, circumcisions are recommended because they reduce the risk of:

- Sexually transmitted diseases
- Urinary tract infections
- Penile cancer.

Circumcision is a safe procedure with minimal side effects and risks. The only downside would potentially be a mild loss of sensation in some men.

**For more information about circumcision
and the medical practice of Dr. Brandeis, please see
www.BrandeisMD.com.**

Chapter 93
Sexually Transmitted Infections
Judson Brandeis, MD, Urologist

It is bad enough that people are dying of AIDS.
No one should die of ignorance.
— Elizabeth Taylor

Sexually transmitted infections are an unfortunate consequence of an otherwise joyful activity. Since the emergence of HIV and the AIDS epidemic, awareness of sexually transmitted diseases has increased. However, it seems that society has again become complacent, and the incidence of sexually-transmitted diseases has been on the rise since 2014. The occurrence of gonorrhea and syphilis, two of the most serious conditions, has tripled in just five years:

- *Human papilloma virus.* 5.5 million new cases of HPV each year.

- *Chlamydia.* More than 1,800,000 new cases in 2018

- *Genital herpes.* 775,000 estimated cases of *Herpes simplex* virus 2 (HSV-2).

- *Gonorrhea.* Over 580,000 new cases in 2018

- *Syphilis.* In excess of 115,000 new cases in 2018, a 70% increase since 2014

- *HIV.* 37,000 new cases reported in 2019

- *Hepatitis B and C.* Almost 17,000 new cases in 2018.

Human Papilloma Virus

HPV is one of the most common sexually transmitted diseases in the United States. It is estimated by the Centers for Disease Control that almost 80 million Americans are infected with HPV. These infections result in 35,000 new cases of HPV-related cancers per year—cancers of the cervix, vagina, or anus.

There are multiple strains of this double-stranded DNA virus but two basic types. Some strains can potentially cause HPV warts and some do not. Warts commonly occur on the feet, hands, and/or genitalia.

Transmission. The initial infection occurs through microtrauma. The virus infects the basal cell layer and stimulates the growth of warts that are typically soft flesh-colored cauliflower-shaped clusters. The diagnosis is typically made through visual inspection. Biopsies are performed for pigmented lesions or a lesion that is hardened, fixed or not responding to treatment.

When there is exposure to the human papilloma virus through an opening in the skin, the DNA from the virus enters skin cells. The HPV causes infected skin cells to multiply and form warts. As the virus replicates, it sheds and is passed on to sexual partners.

The incubation from the time of exposure to the development of symptoms is approximately 6 to 10 months, but the range of incubation can be from 1 to 24 months. Genital HPV can be transient and subclinical (undetectable), and one in five cases of warts spontaneously regresses. However, the virus persists after treatment and recurrence after treatment is common, occurring in two out of every three cases.

- In patients who are immunosuppressed, there is an increased risk of infection and cancer.

- Among sexually active women, there is a major risk of potentially fatal cervical cancer. Of the women who develop this form of cancer, only two-thirds survive for five years.

Treatment. Topical medications tend to be a first-line treatment.

- Trichloroacetic acid or bichloracetic acid is applied once every 1 to 2 weeks and works to kill warts through coagulation of proteins.

- Podofilox 0.5% is applied twice a day for three days followed by four days off the medication for up to 4 cycles. Podofilox is a plant resin that works by arresting cell division, destroying the tissue of the wart. Clearance rates are around 50%.

- Sinacatech 50% ointment is used topically three times a day for up to 16 weeks. This is a water extract of leaves of green tea. The medication works by decreasing viral replication, while reducing the pro-inflammatory response to the infection.

Immune modulators. Another class of topical medication is immune modulators such as Imiquimod (Aldara), which work by stimulating immune responses, ultimately leading to cell death of the diseased tissue. There are two options: 3.75% cream used nightly or a higher dose of 5% cream applied 3 times a week. Both forms are used for 16 weeks. There is a 25% clearance rate at 16 weeks with side effects including pain, itching, irritation, redness, bleeding, or discharge. The cost of this medication tends to be significantly higher than the other medications.

Vaccines. A critically important tool in the prevention and treatment of HPV are vaccinations, currently Gardasil and Cervarix. Vaccination is recommended for females aged 13-26 and men aged 13-21. The research indicates that when vaccination was introduced in Australia, the rates of HPV declined significantly in women less than 30 years old who were given the vaccine, but did not decline in women over the age of 30 who did not receive the vaccine.

Cryotherapy. These treatments are an excellent tool for destroying genital warts by freezing them with liquid nitrogen. The tissue is allowed to thaw and then frozen again if necessary. The size and thickness of warts determine the number and length of the freeze/thaw cycles, and up to 3 treatments may be required. Cryotherapy is not painful, but patients may experience mild to moderate burning sensation during the treatment. Sometimes warts occur in the urethra (the fine tubing within the penis that carries urine and semen), and that requires more extensive treatment.

Recovery time from cryotherapy depends on the location and number of warts removed, but healing usually occurs in 1 to 3 weeks. After treatment, the penis may be irritated, sore, or mildly painful. There may be some swelling and shedding of dead tissue with resultant sores or blisters. It is important to call your physician for a fever over 101 degrees, significant bleeding, infectious discharge, or worsening pain. It is necessary to avoid intercourse until the treated area heals and the soreness is completely gone.

After treatment, patients should avoid sexual intercourse for approximately 1-3 weeks. Cryotherapy is ultimately successful in about 90% of cases, but more than one treatment may be required since the treatment may not cure or completely eradicate the human papilloma virus infection. The virus can remain in the body in an inactive state after the warts are removed. There are few complications after cryotherapy: however, in some cases, there is slight scarring, depending on the extent of the procedure.

Laser treatment. For patients who have failed cryotherapy and topical treatments, laser therapy can be effective. One of the dangers of using a laser is that the smoke plume can spread the virus, so it is important that both doctors and patients use a respirator/ventilator. Laser treatment, because of the cost of the laser, tends to be more expensive than other treatment methods. Also, there is concern that laser treatment may increase the risk of having warts return by destroying the local immune system which allows inactive viruses to become active. Once again, treating a wart does not cure the human papilloma virus, and the virus may remain in the body in an inactive state after the warts are removed. A person treated for warts may still be able to spread the infection; however, latex condoms may help reduce the risk of spread.

For large warts or when patients fail topical and local treatments, surgical excision with either electrocautery or a scalpel may be required. Laser therapy/electrocautery/surgical excision are considered third line interventions, because they tend to be more expensive and leave a scar.

Chlamydia

Chlamydia is a common STI that infects both men and women, with the potential to cause serious, permanent damage to a woman's reproductive system. This can make it difficult for her to become pregnant later and increases the risk of ectopic pregnancy, which can be life threatening.

In 2018 there were a total of 1.7 million cases of chlamydia in the United States with 50% of cases in the 20 to 24 age group. The susceptibility to chlamydia infections declines as an individual ages. Cases in people age 40 and beyond are only one-tenth of the number in younger populations.

Transmission. Chlamydia is transmitted by having vaginal, anal, or oral sex with someone who has the infection. The incubation period of symptomatic chlamydia ranges from 5 to 10 days following exposure. People who have had chlamydia and were treated in the past can still become infected again. The only way to totally avoid STDs is to not have vaginal, anal, or oral sex. A man can reduce his risk by using condoms every time he has intercourse.

Symptoms and diagnosis. The majority of infected persons have no symptoms (they are asymptomatic), which is how the virus persists. It is unclear how long those with no symptoms can carry the infection. Even when chlamydia causes no symptoms, it can cause a partner the risk of chronic pelvic pain, infertility, or ectopic pregnancy.

Symptoms of chlamydia in men may include a mucous-like or watery discharge from their penis, a burning sensation when urinating, and less commonly, pain and swelling of one or both testes. Men and women can also develop a chlamydia infection in the rectum, causing rectal pain, discharge, and bleeding.

A healthcare provider can diagnose chlamydia from a urine sample. Repeat infections with chlamydia tend to be frequent, so you should be tested again about three months after you are treated, even if your sex partner(s) was treated. You should not have sex again until you and your sex partner(s) have completed treatment. Whether your doctor prescribes a single dose of medication or seven doses, you should wait seven days after taking the medicine before having sex.

Risks if infection goes untreated. When chlamydia is untreated, although the initial damage that it causes may go unnoticed, it may spread to the eurethra, the tube that carries sperm from the testicles, causing pain and fever. Rarely, chlamydia can cause sterility in men, preventing them from being able to conceive children. It can cause serious reproductive issues in women, ranging from sterility to the injury or death of a fetus.

Genital Herpes

These sexually transmitted infections are caused by two types of viruses, but primarily by the herpes simplex virus 2 (HSV-2), which causes genital herpes symptoms. More than 50 million people have genital herpes in the United States (one of every six people aged 14 to 49 years). However, the frequency of outbreak varies greatly from once a month to once a decade or less.

Transmission. Genital herpes is transmitted during vaginal, anal, or oral sex with someone who has the disease. The virus is conveyed through herpes blisters, genital secretions, or on the skin in the genital area of the infected person. Herpes can be spread by a sex partner who does not have a visible sore or who may not know they are infected (termed asymptomatic shedding). Transmission can be decreased by:

- Taking a maintenance does of Acyclovir.

- Consistent condom use has been demonstrated to decrease the risk of HSV-2 transmission to an uninfected partner by up to 96%.

- Numerous studies suggest decreased risk of sexually transmitted infections in men who have been circumcised, which is evident of both HIV infection and herpes simplex virus type 2.

- It is important to avoid touching the sores or the fluids from the sores to minimize the risk of transmission, for example, causing an eye infection.

Symptoms. Most people who have genital herpes have mild symptoms or even none at all. Oftentimes, herpes blisters are misidentified as an ingrown hair or pimple. Because of this, the majority of people who carry the herpes virus are unaware that they have it. Herpes sores usually appear as one or more tiny blisters on or around the genitals, rectum, or mouth. The blisters break and leave painful sores that may take a week or more to heal. The first time someone has an outbreak they may also have flu-like symptoms such as mild fever, body aches, or swollen lymph nodes.

People who experience an initial outbreak of herpes can have repeated outbreaks. The repeated outbreaks tend to be shorter and less severe than the initial, primary outbreak.

Although the infection stays in the body for the rest of one's life, the frequency of outbreaks typically decrease over time.

Diagnosis and treatment. Medical providers can take a sample from the sore(s) and test it to confirm the diagnosis or order a blood test to look for herpes antibodies. The herpes blood test can help to determine if you have a herpes infection, but it does not reveal the source of the infection or how long you have been infected. It is important to notify all of your recent sexual partners to prevent additional spread.

The treatment for herpes simplex is Acyclovir 400 mg 3 times a day or Valacyclovir 1000 mg twice a day. (Valacyclovir is more convenient but also more expensive.)

Unfortunately, there is no cure for herpes. The virus exists in nerves and is reactivated periodically, especially when the immune system is weakened. However, Acyclovir or similar medications can prevent or shorten outbreaks. Men who take these medications daily can reduce the risk of transmission to their sexual partners. It is important not to have sex when the herpes infection is active.

Oral herpes. Infection due to the Herpes simplex virus 1 can result in cold sores or fever blisters on or around the mouth, especially during times of higher stress or lower immune function. Most of the time, people do not have symptoms. Usually people with oral herpes were infected during childhood or young adulthood from non-sexual contact with saliva. However, it is possible to contract genital herpes by receiving oral sex from a partner who has oral herpes. It is not possible to get herpes from toilet seats, bed sheets, swimming pools, or from touching objects around you such as silverware, soap, or towels.

Gonorrhea

Gonorrhea is a sexually transmitted disease (STD) that can infect both men and women. It can cause infections in the genitals, rectum, or throat. There are an estimated 1.1 million new cases of gonorrhea each year in the US. Like chlamydia, the peak age range is 20-24 and the incidence in men over 40 is about 20% of the incidence of men in their 20s.

Transmission. Men can contract gonorrhea by having vaginal, anal, or oral sex with someone who has gonorrhea, although transmission rates are higher from men to women than from women to men. The only way to avoid STDs is to not have vaginal, anal, or oral sex, but condoms can significantly reduce the risk of infection.

Some men with gonorrhea may have no symptoms at all. However, men who do have symptoms may have a burning sensation when urinating and a white, yellow, or green discharge from the penis. Rectal infections may either cause no symptoms or could cause rectal discharge, soreness, itching, or bleeding. Symptoms develop 2 to 7 days after exposure.

Diagnosis and treatment. Most of the time, urine can be used to test for gonorrhea. However, patients who have had oral and/or anal sex may need to collect samples from their throat, rectum, and/or urethra (urine canal).

If symptoms continue for more than a few days after receiving treatment, return to the healthcare provider to be checked again.

It is important to wait seven days after finishing all medications before having sex to avoid becoming infected with gonorrhea again or spreading gonorrhea to a partner(s). Despite having had gonorrhea and successful treatment, it is still possible to become infected again by having unprotected sex with a person who has gonorrhea.

> *Drug-resistant strains of gonorrhea are increasingly resistant to the antimicrobials most commonly used for therapy, including penicillin, tetracyclines, macrolides, fluoroquinolones, and even cephalosporins. There is the potential for the development of untreatable gonorrhea in the future.*

Risks if infection goes untreated. Untreated gonorrhea can cause serious and permanent health problems in men. Infection can result in a painful condition in the tubes attached to the testicles. In rare cases, this may cause a man to become sterile, preventing him from being able to father a child. Rarely, untreated gonorrhea can also spread to the bloodstream, causing a potentially life-threatening infection (sepsis) or can infect the joints. In a female partner, gonorrhea can cause severe pelvic infection that can result in infertility, miscarriage, premature birth, or intellectual injury or blindness to the unborn infant.

Syphilis

Syphilis is a sexually transmitted infection that can persist in the body causing serious health problems such a dementia if it is not treated. Once nearly eliminated in the U.S., syphilis is increasing, and over 115,000 new cases of syphilis were diagnosed in 2018. The majority of these cases involved gay and bisexual men having sex with men (MSM), primarily among younger men.

Transmission. Syphilis can be transmitted by direct contact with a syphilis sore during vaginal, anal, or oral sex, via sores on or around the penis, vagina, or anus, or in the rectum, on the lips, or in the mouth.

Symptoms. Syphilis is divided into stages indicating the level of severity (primary, secondary, latent, or tertiary; different signs and symptoms are associated with each stage.

Primary syphilis. A person with primary syphilis generally has a sore or sores at the original site of infection. These sores usually occur on or around the genitals, around the anus or in the rectum, or in or around the mouth. These sores are usually (but not always) firm, round, and painless.

Secondary syphilis. Symptoms of secondary syphilis include skin rash, swollen lymph nodes, and fever. The signs and symptoms of primary and secondary syphilis can be mild, and they might not be noticed.

Tertiary syphilis. Advanced syphilis is associated with severe medical problems which can affect the brain, heart, and other vital organs of the body.

Most of the time, a blood test is used to test for syphilis. Some healthcare providers will diagnose syphilis by testing fluid from a syphilis sore. Syphilis can be cured with an intramuscular injection of penicillin, but having syphilis once does not protect from getting it again. Even after successful treatment, it is still possible to become re-infected. Only laboratory tests can confirm whether a syphilis infection is present. Follow-up testing to confirm successful treatment is important.

Hepatitis

Hepatitis viruses A, B, and C infect the liver and cause inflammation that can damage the liver and destroy its function. Hepatitis A is a short-term infection. Hepatitis B and hepatitis C begin as short-term infections, but the virus remains in the body and causes chronic (long-term) infection in some people. There are vaccines to prevent hepatitis A and hepatitis B. Unfortunately, there are no vaccines to prevent hepatitis C.

Hepatitis A. Vaccination against hepatitis A virus is recommended for:

- Men who have sex with men
- Drug use, particularly intravenous drug injection
- Persons with chronic liver disease
- Persons with close contact with others who have hepatitis A
- Anyone traveling to countries where hepatitis A is endemic.

Hepatitis B. The primary risk factors associated with hepatitis B are unprotected sex with an infected partner and a history of other sexually transmitted infections. MSM and people who inject drugs are considered high-risk groups for HBV acquisition.

Hepatitis C. These infections manifest as liver disease, caused by contact with blood from an infected person, most often through injected drugs.

Symptoms. Approximately half of those who contract hepatitis C have a mild illness lasting a few weeks, but some develop a serious, long-term disorder. If left untreated, hepatitis C can cause serious health problems, including liver damage, cirrhosis (scarring of the liver), liver cancer, or even death.

There were more than 15,000 deaths related to the hepatitis C virus reported to the CDC in 2018. In addition, the U.S. added over 50,000 new cases to the estimated 2.4 million individuals living with hepatitis C.

Symptoms usually develop 2–12 weeks after exposure to the virus. Signs and symptoms can include yellow skin or eyes, poor appetite, upset stomach or stomach pain, vomiting, fever, dark urine, light-colored stool, joint pain, and/or fatigue.

It is fairly typical for people with hepatitis C to have no symptoms or to develop generalized symptoms such as chronic fatigue or depression. Many people eventually develop chronic liver disease, ranging from mild to severe conditions, including cirrhosis (scarring of the liver) and liver cancer. Chronic liver disease in people with hepatitis C usually develops slowly, without signs or symptoms, over several decades. As a result, chronic hepatitis C virus infection is often not diagnosed until the individual is screened for blood donation or during a routine doctor's visit.

Transmission. The hepatitis C virus is usually spread through contact with blood from an infected person. This infection most frequently occurs:

- When men share needles used to inject drugs

- Through sexual intercourse

- From getting tattoos or body piercings with non-sterile instruments.

Theoretically, people can become infected through contact with infected blood by sharing razors, nail clippers, glucose monitors, razors, nail clippers, toothbrushes, and other personal items, but this is rare.

Hepatitis C is not spread by sharing eating utensils, breastfeeding, hugging, kissing, holding hands, coughing, or sneezing. It is also not spread through food or water. However, if you are infected with the hepatitis C virus, you can spread it to others, even if you have no symptoms.

Testing. A blood test called an HCV antibody test is used to find out if someone has ever been infected with the hepatitis C virus. This test, sometimes called the anti-HCV test, looks for antibodies to hepatitis C. People with positive HCV antibody tests are given a follow-up HCV RNA test to learn whether they have an active infection.

After exposure to the hepatitis C virus, it can take 8–11 weeks for an HCV antibody test to be positive. A special kind of blood test called a nucleic acid test (NAT) that detects HCV RNA (also termed a PCR test, which looks for genetic evidence of the virus) can tell if a person is infected within 1–2 weeks of exposure.

HIV Prevention

I was growing up in New York when the AIDS epidemic first started. It was a terrifying time: healthy young men were dying from a mysterious disease. It took many years to even identify the virus and its modes of transmission, and decades to develop effective treatments. I still remember the shock of hearing that Magic Johnson had contracted HIV. It seemed like a death sentence for the basketball great, but now HIV/AIDS has become a controllable disease.

The HIV virus attacks the body's immune system. If untreated, HIV can lead to AIDS (acquired immunodeficiency syndrome). There is no effective cure, but with proper medical care, HIV can be controlled so people with the virus can live long, healthy lives and protect their partners.

In 2018, 37,968 people received an HIV diagnosis in the United States, adding to an estimated 1.2 million people in the U.S. who had already contracted the virus. Of those people, about 14%, or 1 in 7, did not know they had HIV. In 2018, gay, bisexual, and other men who have sex with men accounted for 69% of all new HIV diagnoses in the United States, and heterosexuals accounted for 24% of all HIV diagnoses. HIV is more prevalent in urban areas. In 2018, there were 15,820 deaths among adults and adolescents with diagnosed HIV in the United States, although many of these people died of other causes.

The CDC recommends that everyone between the ages of 13 and 64 get tested for HIV at least once as part of routine healthcare, and more often if your lifestyle increases your risk of contracting HIV. The CDC says that even if you are in a monogamous relationship, you should find out for sure whether you or your partner has HIV.

To reduce your risk of HIV transmission, choose sexual activities less risky than anal or vaginal sex. For example, there is little to no risk of getting HIV through oral sex. Sexual activities that don't involve contact with body fluids (semen, vaginal fluid, or blood) will not result in HIV infection.

If properly used, condoms are highly effective against HIV transmission and other sexually transmitted diseases (STDs), like gonorrhea and chlamydia. Condoms provide less protection against STDs that can be transmitted through sores or cuts on the skin, like human papillomavirus, genital herpes, and syphilis.

Condoms help prevent HIV for higher risk sexual activities like anal or vaginal sex, and for lower risk activities, like oral sex and sharing sex toys.

- Use water-based or silicone-based lubricants to help prevent condoms from breaking or slipping during sex.

- Latex condoms provide the best protection against HIV.

- Plastic (polyurethane) or synthetic rubber condoms are good for people with latex allergies. However, note that plastic condoms break more often than latex condoms.

- Natural membrane (such as lambskin) condoms have small holes in them and do not block viruses such as HIV or other STDs. These should not be used for HIV or STD prevention.

If you are having sex with someone with known HIV infection, you can take PrEP (pre-exposure prophylaxis), which is medication that significantly lowers the risk of HIV.

For more information about sexually transmitted infections and the medical practice of Dr. Brandeis, please see www.BrandeisMD.com

Chapter 94
Vasectomy
Judson Brandeis, MD, Urologist

Vasectomy means never having to say you are sorry.
—Anonymous

Vasectomy is one of the safest and most effective methods of permanent birth control available. It is much easier and less expensive for men to get a vasectomy than for their spouse to have a tubal ligation. Vasectomy is the contraception of choice of about 20% of couples in the U.S., Canada, and the U.K. Worldwide 50 million men undergo a vasectomy each year, including approximately 500,000 American men.

> *A vasectomy performed under local anesthesia is much less expensive and safer than a female tubal ligation.*

Benefits:

- Success rates are 99.9%.

- There is no risk of any health issues such as prostate or testicular cancer.

- There is no change in testosterone levels.

- Vasectomy does not affect erections.

- Vasectomy does not affect sensation, nor orgasm.

- Secretions are the same as before, so ejaculation looks and feels the same.

- Most men can return to a desk job the next day.

Urologists perform 80% of vasectomies, with the rest provided by family physicians and general surgeons. Doctors perform vasectomies in the office under local anesthesia.

ANATOMY OF A VASECTOMY

The testicle is an oval structure the size of a chestnut that produces sperm and testosterone. The sperm then migrates from a testicle into the epididymis (a highly convoluted duct behind the testicles, where the sperm mature). The mature sperm are then transported from the epididymis through fine tubing, the vas deferens, to the penis.

In a vasectomy, the vas deferens is surgically severed, blocking the release of any sperm in the ejaculate.

During ejaculation, the vas deferens contracts, and the mature sperm that originated in the testes and matured in the epididymis mix with fluid and are propelled through the urethra.

The Procedure

No scalpel vasectomy. Chinese physicians developed the no-scalpel vasectomy in 1974. A safer and less invasive method of vasectomy with less discomfort and faster recovery, its popularity spread quickly throughout the world. A no-scalpel vasectomy uses a small puncture in the scrotal skin rather than an incision.

Before the procedure:

- By law, a vasectomy consent form needs to be signed 72 hours before the procedure.

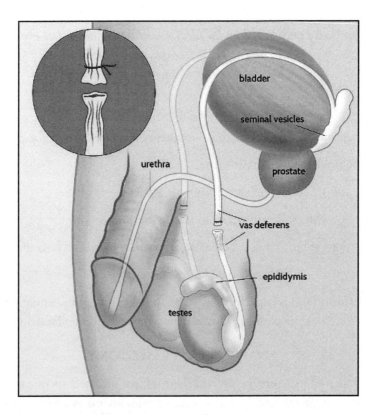

Figure 94.1 A vasectomy severs the tube carrying semen from the testicles to the urethera, the same tubing that carries urine for elimination.

- We ask that you do not take aspirin or other non-steroidal anti-inflammatories, such as Motrin, Advil, ibuprofen, or Aleve. for a week before the procedure. These medications will increase the chance of bleeding, which we try to avoid.

- The numbing portion of the procedure, comparable to anesthesia for dental work, can be uncomfortable. However, once the skin and vas deferens are numb, a man rarely feels any pain.

Course of Recovery

- Less than 1% of vasectomies induce bleeding following the procedure.

- Fewer than 2% have pain severe enough to impact quality of life.

- About 1% to 3% of men develop an infection that requires antibiotics.

- Fewer than 10% of men develop troublesome post-vasectomy pain.

In my hands, I have been fortunate to have only one patient out of 3,000 with a bleed requiring additional treatment. An infection that requires antibiotics occurs in about 1 out of every 100 patients. In my experience, vasectomy failures are extremely rare.

Post-vasectomy instructions:

- **Work.** Men should be able to work at a desk job the following day.

- **Sex.** Abstain from physical intimacy for 4 to 5 days.

- **Pain.** All most men need is Tylenol or nonsteroidal anti-inflammatories such as Motrin or ibuprofen for discomfort. It is unusual for anyone to require something more potent.

- **Exercise.** After the vasectomy, men can take part in mild exercise within 4 days. However, they should not engage in vigorous exercise, ride a bike, or do sit-ups or workouts involving abdominal muscles for at least a week.

- **Bathing.** It is okay to shower the night of the vasectomy, but no baths, Jacuzzis, or swimming pools for approximately four days.

Testing. Semen testing is required after approximately 20 ejaculations and eight weeks. For the next two months following the vasectomy, there are still millions of live, viable sperm in the vas deferens and in the ejaculate released during orgasm. It takes approximately 20 ejaculations to clear all the sperm from the vas tubing.

Therefore, after the procedure, when a man ejaculates, the ejaculate looks and feels the same. Once the vas is clear of sperm, the ejaculation will look and feel as it did before, but will not contain any sperm, which has been described as: "the whole swimming pool, but no swimmers."

Pain. It is unusual to have any patient with pain lasting more than a few weeks. Some patients initially complain of post-vasectomy pain syndrome, in most cases caused by chronic congestive epididymitis, and distinct from post-procedure pain. Following vasectomy, testicular fluid and sperm production remain constant. The majority of this fluid accumulates in the epididymis, which swells. While asymptomatic in most men, some will develop a chronic dull ache in the testicles, which is made worse by ejaculation.

First-line therapy is nonsteroidal anti-inflammatories and warm baths. Pain specialists can perform local nerve blocks or steroid injections in extreme cases.

Since I do not use clips to occlude the vas deferens, I rarely get patients with post-vasectomy syndrome. If there is some inflammation, I use a steroid pulse. That's enough to get patients feeling better. It is extremely rare, in my experience, to have any patient with pain lasting more than a few weeks.

Change Your Mind?

- Sperm banking

- Harvesting from the epididymis. The testicles continue to produce sperm, which can be harvested from the epididymis in the future if necessary.

- Vas reversal (please see the following sidebar for specifics).

Vasectomy Reversal

A change in life circumstances, for example, divorce or the death of a child can motivate a man to desire fertility again. The two principal options for male fertility include a vasectomy reversal or in vitro fertilization. Couples should consider the number of children desired, time commitment, financial resources, and maternal age. Vasectomy reversal is typically more cost-effective and is the favored approved for patients wanting multiple pregnancies with normal female partner fertility.

Reversing a vasectomy involves restoring the delicate tubing within the scrotum that carries sperm through the penis. The vas deferens has a tube diameter of 1/100th of an inch (0.3 to 0.5 mm) and the epididymal tube has an even smaller diameter of 1/150th of an inch (0.1 to 0.2 mm).

Putting together tubes the size of a paperclip wire requires specialized training and practice, even for an experienced surgeon. In fact, the medical literature shows a correlation between the surgeon's experience and the success rate of vasectomy reversal, so if you are seeking a reverse vas, you will want to choose your surgeon carefully.

Vasectomy reversal can be performed either under general anesthesia or local anesthesia through a small scrotal incision. The procedure typically takes between 2 and 4 hours. Also, the longer since the original vasectomy, the lower the likelihood of success in reopening the vas (patency). The other most important factor in transitioning from patency to pregnancy is the age of the female partner. With a female partner age 20 to 24, the pregnancy rate is 67%. With a female partner 25 to 40, the pregnancy rate is 54%, but over the age of 40, the pregnancy rate drops to 14%.

Technically, a vasectomy can be reversed. However, I do the vasectomy in a way that is more difficult to reverse because I do so many of them. Vasectomy performed in a way that is easier to reverse is also easier for mother nature to reverse.

Occasionally, I will have a patient ask me to do the vasectomy in a way that is possible to reverse. Typically, I will comply with a caveat that it is easier to recanalize in this situation. In addition, a vasectomy reversal is a three- or four-hour procedure that typically costs around $20,000 in 2021 dollars.

KEY TAKE AWAYS

- Vasectomy is one of the safest and most effective methods of permanent birth control available. Worldwide, 50 million men undergo a vasectomy each year.

- A vasectomy should be 99.9% effective in preventing pregnancy.

- Physicians performed vasectomies in the office under local anesthetic.

- Complications are rare after a vasectomy, occurring as bleeding or infection in 1% to 3% and as temporary discomfort in one man in ten.

- There are no long-term complications from the vasectomy.

- There are no sexual side effects from vasectomy. Sensation and orgasm remain the same, and there is no change in testosterone levels.

- Most men can return to work the following day.

- After a vasectomy, the testicle still makes sperm. If a man desires to have another child, sperm can be removed from the epididymis for in vitro fertilization, or vasectomy reversal is possible.

**For more information on vasectomy
and the medical practice of Dr. Brandeis, please see:
www.BrandeisMD.com**

Chapter 95
Staying Fertile
Philip E. Werthman, MD, MMH, FACS, Urologist

Difficult roads often lead to beautiful destinations.
— Zig Ziglar

Infertility is defined as the inability of a couple to become pregnant despite one year of unprotected intercourse. In studies of untreated couples pursuing pregnancy, 50% conceived within three months, 70% within six months, and 85% within 12 months. Of the 15% who did not conceive, half will become pregnant in the following 12 months with no specific treatment. In approximately one-third of couples with infertility, a male factor contributes to the failure to conceive. In the United States, approximately 12% of men between the ages of 15 and 44 have issues with infertility. Men as old as 80 have fathered children, but fertility rates seem to be lower in men over the age of 40. In all men, there are reports of declining sperm counts over the past several decades. However, the most critical determinant of a couple's reproductive potential is the age of the mother. Causes of male infertility include:

- Testicular issues (including genetic issues)—75%

- Hormonal issues—5%

- Sperm transport blockage—5%

- Unknown causes—15%

SPECIFIC CAUSES OF MALE INFERTILITY

Factors in a man's history that can affect fertility include lifestyle and habits such as cigarette smoking, drug use, environmental exposures, and heat exposure. The use of alcohol, tobacco, marijuana, opioids, radiation, or chemotherapy, or exposure to toxic chemicals can negatively impact a man's fertility potential. Prescription or illicit use of medications such as testosterone or other anabolic steroids has become commonplace and can act as a form of contraception, and can even lead to sterilization.

Varicoceles are the most common correctable cause of male infertility. The condition involves varicose testicular veins and is similar to varicose veins in the leg. Varicoceles can cause a reduction in sperm quality, sperm DNA damage, and low sperm production. In men with infertility and varicoceles, sperm quality and pregnancy rates improve after varicocele repair. A minor surgical or radiological procedure can resolve the problem.

Drugs such as opioids and other central nervous system-activating drugs, including cannabinoids, can cause low testosterone and infertility.

The administration of testosterone reduces sperm production such that most men stop making sperm temporarily while using anabolic steroids.

Obesity leads to low testosterone and high estrogen levels that can affect fertility. The metabolic syndrome that occurs with obesity and the insulating effect of fat can cause an increase in testicular temperature that creates infertility.

Environmental toxins. The pesticide dibromo-chloropropane is a well-known cause of infertility, as are lead, cadmium, and mercury, which are prevalent in our environment. Endocrine disrupters in the environment may play a role in the world-wide decline of sperm counts.

Cell phone usage. It is controversial as to whether cell phone usage has any detrimental effects on sperm parameters.

Smoking. There is data that cigarette smoking can affect sperm counts and increase levels of free radicals and lead to increased sperm DNA fragmentation.

Prolonged high testicular temperature from varicoceles or occupational exposure can affect fertility, in situations such as prolonged sitting, truck driving, welding, or baking. The heat from laptop use and exposure to Wi-Fi in the absence of heat have been found in lab research to affect male fertility adversely. Regular sauna or hot tub use can reduce sperm counts.

Aging. You've probably heard the phrase, "Sex is 90% mental." We know that normal testosterone and sperm production rely on the secretion of GnRH (gonadotrophin-releasing hormone) from the hypothalamus in the brain, as well as LH (luteinizing hormone) and FSH (follicle-stimulating hormone) secretion from the pituitary gland. Regulation of hormones of the hypothalamic-pituitary-gonadal (HPG) axis occurs primarily through negative feedback. As men age, their testosterone decreases because of irregularities in this HPG axis.

Azoospermia. The absence of any sperm in the ejaculatory fluid is termed azoospermia. In 1% of men, no sperm can be detected on a semen analysis. The lack of sperm is usually due to a blockage in the reproductive tract. Sperm production is normal, but the sperm are trapped inside. In other cases, the testicles fail to produce enough sperm for inclusion in the ejaculation. In actuality, most men with severe sperm production issues still produce a small quantity of sperm, enabling them to become fathers using advanced reproductive technologies. A lower number of men have no sperm production at all.

Genetic issues. Severe male factor infertility can be the result of a number of genetic issues such as:

- *Klinefelter's Syndrome*, (having an extra X chromosome) which is a fairly common condition affecting one in 400 men

- *Y-chromosome microdeletion*, in which some of the genes that control sperm production are absent

- *Congenital absence of the vas deferens*, a condition in which a portion of the vas is missing, resulting in a blockage.

Most men with these conditions can still father children with appropriate diagnosis and treatment.

Congenital issues. Cryptorchidism, or being born with an undescended testicle, is a common condition and is associated with fertility problems later in life. It is essential to recognize this condition early and have surgical correction by the age of two to preserve future fertility.

Sexually transmitted diseases. STDs are the most preventable cause of infertility. Diseases such as chlamydia or gonorrhea, if left untreated, can cause inflammation and scarring of the tiny sperm ducts, which can lead to a blockage or cause poor sperm quality.

VASECTOMY REVERSAL

Approximately 500,000 men each year will undergo vasectomy in the United States, and roughly 5% will change their minds and want to father more children. Options for having children include:

- Reversing the vasectomy

- Extracting sperm and injecting them into a woman's egg, a process described as In-Vitro Fertilization (IVF) with ICSI (intracytoplasmic sperm injection)

- Some men chose to freeze and store sperm in a sperm bank before having the vasectomy as an insurance policy, should they later change their mind.

FERTILITY TESTING

A healthy man produces 100 to 200 million viable sperm each day and trillions of sperm over a lifetime. Semen analysis is the crucial laboratory assessment of the male partner of an infertile couple. A man should obtain two samples after 2 to 7 days of ejaculatory abstinence. The samples are collected at least one week apart, since sperm numbers and concentration can vary significantly. It is important to note that a semen analysis is not a fertility test; it simply provides a rough idea of a man's fertility potential. A man with a normal sperm count can be infertile, and someone with an abnormal semen analysis may not have problems fathering children. The semen analysis is a good initial screening test, but is only one tool in assessing whether a couple has a fertility challenge.

The lab testing evaluates several factors in routine semen analysis:

- *Sperm shape.* Human sperm are notoriously abnormal in appearance. It is normal for the majority of the sperm to be abnormally shaped. However, if this number increases above 85%, a man's fertility may be reduced. On average, 85% of sperm are abnormal, and men can achieve fertilization with up to 96% of the sperm being abnormal. Motility is the least predictive factor of a man's fertility potential.

- *Movement.* More than 35% of sperm should move normally an hour after ejaculation. An average man will have 50% motility. Using a rating scale of 0-4, a score of 3 or 4 represents good movement and a high likelihood that sperm can travel the distance required to fertilize an egg.

- *The pH level* (acidity of the ejaculatory fluid) should be between 7.2 and 7.8 to achieve a normal result. A pH level higher than 8 could indicate the man has an infection, and values below 7.0 could indicate contamination or that a man's ejaculatory ducts are blocked.

- *Volume.* The volume of ejaculation should be greater than 2 mL (approximately ½ teaspoon), and an average ejaculation is less than 3.7 cc (1 teaspoon).

- *Liquefaction.* Semen is initially thick and it should take 15 to 30 minutes before the semen liquefies. The ability to maintain a watery consistency aids sperm motility. Poor motility reduces fertility.

- *Sperm concentration.* Healthy semen contains 20 to 200 million sperm per milliliter of the ejaculatory fluid, and the average is 70 million per cc.

- *Total motile count.* Multiplying the sperm concentration per cubic centimeter, by the number of ccs, by the percentage of motility provides a measure of the total number of motile sperm. Given the average of 20 to 200 million sperm in an ejaculation, there should be at least 20 million total motile sperm.

Advanced sperm testing. A semen analysis is not a particularly good fertility test and does not answer many questions that physicians and patients need to know to make treatment decisions. Advanced sperm testing or sperm DNA fragmentation analysis is now being used as an adjunct test. This test measures the amount of damage to the DNA inside the individual sperm cells and predicts how well the sperm will work. This has become valuable information for couples who have been undergoing unexplained infertility, recurrent miscarriages, or those planning on using assisted reproductive technologies.

Endocrine testing. Lab testing of a man with a sperm concentration less than 10,000,000/cc includes measurement of:

- Total serum testosterone.

- LH (luteinizing hormone)

- FSH (follicle-stimulating hormone)

- E2 (estradiol-estrogen hormone)

- PRL (prolactin-pituitary hormone).

Hormone abnormalities can sometimes be corrected by administering the appropriate medications.

Physiology Facts

- The coiled seminiferous tubes in the testis produce sperm. Uncoiled, these structures would extend to about 27 inches (70 centimeters) in length.

- Once sperm cells mature, they are transported to the epididymis. The epididymis is a delicate tube that extends from the testicles to the ejaculatory duct, the extraordinary length of approximately 12 feet (4 meters).

- Sperm continue to mature during the passage through the epididymis. The function of the epididymis is dependent on body temperature and testosterone levels. From the epididymis, the next stop is the vas deferens, which has the highest muscle to lumen ratio, 10-1, of any hollow organ in the body. Strong muscular contractions cause the sperm to be transported up through the system and deposited in the seminal fluid during an ejaculation. The epididymis and vas store a significant proportion of human sperm. It takes approximately 64-72 days from sperm production to maturation and release.

Considerations When Trying to Conceive

- Stop smoking.

- Avoid drugs and limit alcohol and caffeine consumption.

- No Jacuzzis, hot baths, or hot yoga. Hot showers are OK.

- Eliminate unnecessary medications such as Propecia.

- Absolutely NO TESTOSTERONE use. It is a contraceptive.

- Avoid petroleum-based lubricants and other lubricants not specifically designed for fertility.

- Avoid keeping a laptop computer on your lap or your cell phone in your front pocket.

- Abstain for several days before your partner's ovulation.

- However, also avoid periods of prolonged abstinence as sperm quality can deteriorate.

- Take a high-quality antioxidant supplement.

- Sperm production in the testicles function optimally at 2 to 4 °C below body temperature. In normal men, sperm production is constant at about 1200 sperm per second.

- During sexual stimulation, mature sperm mix with seminal fluid produced by the seminal vesicles and the prostate gland. Sperm cells and seminal fluid together are termed semen. The seminal vesicle fluid roughly makes up to 80% or more of the total semen volume, the vas deferens 5% to 10%, and the prostate gland another 10% to 20%. The ejaculate itself supports sperm metabolism and motility, and serves as an antioxidant that aids in protecting and activating the sperm.

ADVANCED REPRODUCTIVE TECHNOLGIES

The last 30 years has seen incredible advances in the field of reproductive medicine in general, and more specifically in male infertility. The advent of In-Vitro Fertilization (IVF) with Intracytoplasmic Sperm Injection (ICSI) means that a single sperm, taken from the ejaculate or harvested from inside the testicle, is capable of being injected into an egg to create an embryo and ultimately lead to the birth of a healthy child. Men who were unable to father genetic children because of low sperm count or motility, or azoospermia due to blockage, can all likely father their own children with this powerful technology. The most critical aspects when confronted with significant fertility challenges are to find expert physicians who can address both female and male factors.

KEY TAKE AWAYS

Male factor infertility is much more common than generally appreciated. Men share a significant role in the successes of conception, but also the problems. Lifestyle adjustments improve most sperm issues, but when that is not sufficient, it is important to get tested and consult with a specialist in male reproduction. The good news is that we live in a time in which technology enables many of the most severe cases of male infertility to be overcome and for most men to become fathers.

**For more information on fertility
and the medical practice of Dr. Werthman, please see
www.malereproduction.com.**

PART 13
NAVIGATING HEALTHCARE
Introduction
Judson Brandeis, MD

We have really good data that shows when you really patients
about their choices, they make more frugal choices.
They pick more efficient choices than the healthcare system does.
— Donald Berwick MD, Past Secretary of The Centers for
Medicare and Medicaid Services

The American healthcare system is bewildering. A Morning Consult survey of Americans in 2017 revealed that one-third of Americans did not know that *Obamacare* and *The Affordable Care Act* were two names for the same thing. Along similar lines, a 2016 Policy Genius survey found that just 4% of Americans can correctly define all four terms that determine how much they would personally have to pay for medical services and drugs they receive under their health insurance plans. (These are deductible, co-insurance, co-pay, and out-of-pocket maximum.)

America spent $4 trillion, or 20% of our GDP, on healthcare in 2020,
which works out to $12,000 for every person living in the United States.

According to the 2020 Commonwealth Fund report, the U.S. spends nearly twice as much on healthcare as the average industrialized country—yet has the lowest life expectancy and highest suicide rates among the 11 nations. The U.S. also has the highest chronic disease burden and an obesity rate two times higher than average.

The reasons for these massive expenditures and poor outcomes are complicated, but the complexity of the healthcare system and lack of consumer understanding certainly contribute to this. In writing the chapter on health insurance, we tried to craft something comprehensive and sophisticated, but not overly technical. I asked a high-ranking healthcare executive to read it, and his comments were, "I just wanted to follow up that I read your chapter on health insurance on my flight. It's great . . . very detailed AND highly approachable and understandable for the layperson. As I read it, I was struck by the fact that, even though you have laid out the basics with total clarity, the U.S. health insurance system is so byzantine that even a 40-year veteran of the industry can get confused. Congrats and thanks for helping me understand it a bit better."

If a 40-year healthcare executive may feel confused at times, how is a regular guy supposed to choose a health plan for his family or his employees? We hope that our efforts help to demystify how we pay for healthcare in America.

Once you have a better understanding of the healthcare system, this section offers insight on how to choose a doctor. In the same way that all baseball players are not equally skilled, physicians' training and abilities vary dramatically. However, while baseball players have easy-to-understand statistics that help you figure out who to pick for your fantasy baseball team, physicians' statistics are more complex and more challenging to find. This section will help you determine how to select your medical team.

It is helpful to understand the economics of medicine when you go to a doctor who accepts insurance as payment. Medicare and insurance companies have not significantly raised reimbursement for physicians in the 20 years I have been practicing. However, medical inflation increases about 4% a year. To pay the bills, physicians need to see more patients in the same amount of time. Doctors spend an average of 16 minutes per patient encounter, according to a study from Cerner that examined 100 million patient visits to 155,000 US physicians.

> *In an average visit with a doctor, chart review consumes five minutes, documentation takes four, and treatment planning takes three minutes, which leaves only four minutes for you.*

By becoming an educated and informed healthcare consumer, our hope is that you will be able to navigate our fragmented healthcare system better and form partnerships with your doctors, leading to improved outcomes for you and your family.

Chapter 96
Understanding Health Insurance
James G. Korkos, MD,
Health Insurance Medical Director
& Anesthesiologist,
Judson Brandeis, MD, Urologist,
Arthur Bookstein, MPH, Medical Student,
Michael Abassian, MPH, Researcher

Do something today that your future self will thank you for.
— *Anonymous*

INTRODUCTION

Healthcare is expensive in America. In 2018 the United States spent about $3.6 trillion on healthcare, which averages about $11,000 per person or 18% of the gross domestic product, whereas in 1960 spending on healthcare represented just 5% of the gross domestic product.

The Centers for Medicare and Medicaid Services projects that by 2028, medical costs will climb to $6.2 trillion (about $18,000 per person), which will represent about 20% of the gross domestic product, and this does not even factor in the impact of the COVID-19 pandemic. Contributing to the rising costs is the aging American population. Currently, individuals age 65 and over account for 16% of the United States population, but by 2030 this will be expected to exceed 20%, severely straining Medicare and Medicaid.

Medical cost inflation has grown faster than the overall rate of inflation (3.5% vs. 2.1%) over the past 20 years. As a result of these rising costs, medical bills are the leading cause of consumer debt and financial disaster for Americans. Over 137 million Americans in 2019 alone faced financial hardship related to medical care costs, including bankruptcy, foreclosure, or reliance on retirement savings.

No one wants to get sick or have to visit the hospital. However, most of us throughout our lives are going to require some form of medical care. If we want our lives characterized by physical and mental wellbeing, we must make an investment in our health. Health insurance protects us from financial uncertainty and mitigates risk. It does this by assisting with costs for services that are essential to maintain our health and treatment. These include wellness and preventive care programs at free to minimal cost, including vaccines, screenings, and check-ups. Consider that a three-day hospital stay can land a $30,000 bill on your desk. Or that a broken leg can run you up for $7,500. The management and treatment of chronic health conditions, including cancer and cardiovascular disease, can cost hundreds of thousands of dollars. Insurance plans approved in the marketplace cannot put yearly or lifetime limits on how much they spend on you to cover essentials benefits. Additionally, individuals without health insurance spend twice as much on healthcare than those with insurance, because insurance companies negotiate with providers to get discounted rates. It's clear that health insurance offers peace of mind.

KNOW WHAT YOU ARE PAYING FOR

Health insurance plans take in billions of dollars each year in premiums, but how much of those premium dollars are actually used to take care of their members? Medical Loss Ratio (MLR) is a financial measurement tool that assesses what percentage of every dollar an insurance company collects is actually spent on customer claims and activities that improve the quality of care for patients. The remaining percentage goes into marketing, profits, salaries, administrative costs, and agent commissions. For example, if MLR is equal to 80%, that means that 80% of money collected from insurance premiums is directly benefiting patients and their care, while 20% is used to keep the insurance company operating.

The Affordable Care Act (ACA) in 2012 established guidelines for the MLR. According to the ACA, in the large group market insurance companies must spend at least 85% of premiums on medical costs and healthcare quality improvements. That word "quality" is extremely important. Since quality programs are included in the MLR calculation, health plans are creating innovative programs to drive quality, and close gaps in care. In the individual and small group markets, this threshold is 80%. Individual states may increase the limit; for example, Massachusetts requires an MLR of at least 88%. If an insurance company fails to meet the applicable MLR standard in any given year, the insurance is expected to provide a rebate to its customers.

Health insurance costs are calculated based on the level of coverage, county of residence, family size, and, most importantly, the age of the covered person. Health insurance rates rise with age, with the most substantial increases after age 55, reflected in higher expected healthcare costs as the population of America continues to age.

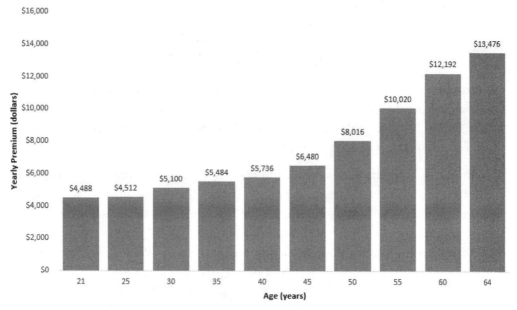

Figure 96.1. Annual insurance premiums by age.

Starting in 2014, health insurance companies were no longer able to refuse to cover individuals with a pre-existing condition.

Features That Determine How Much You Pay

Health insurance plans don't cover all of your health expenses. You must pitch in with your own finances until an out-of-pocket maximum is reached. This is known as cost sharing. The maximum out-of-pocket costs for 2020 were set at $8,200 for individual plans and $16,400 for family plans. This means if you have a family plan, the most you'll have to spend on healthcare is $16,400 throughout 2020. At that point, your insurance policy covers all costs.

Three concepts that dictate how you share costs with your insurance company include deductible, co-payment, and co-insurance. These three factors contribute to the yearly out-of-pocket maximum set by the plan.

A deductible is simply the amount you must spend before your policy begins to assist with costs. Say you need appendix surgery that is going to cost $15,000. If your deductible is $3,000, you will be required to spend that $3,000, and the remaining $12,000 will be covered in part or in total by insurance, depending on your policy. Deductibles are reset every year.

Co-payments are fixed prices you pay every time you receive some kind of medical service. For example, a primary care visit may have a co-pay of $15, the amount you are required to pay, while insurance covers the rest. Prescription medicines have copays, with specialty brands requiring higher co-pays than generic brands.

Co-insurance. Some plans share costs through percentage splits for remaining costs after a deductible has been met. This is known as co-insurance. Many plans have a 20/80 split, meaning you'll be responsible for 20% of costs after your deductible has been met, while your insurance policy will cover the rest.

The Affordable Care Act, also known as Obamacare, introduced many requirements that health insurance policies must meet in order to qualify as viable health coverage. This includes rules around cost and affordability, as well as essential services that are required at the federal level, but that also vary by state. In addition, the ACA introduced the individual mandate, which required that all American citizens have qualifying health coverage. In order for any health insurance pool to function properly, all citizens would be required to purchase insurance. This requirement is not enforced as of 2019. Plans that meet federal and state requirements, whether they are government plans or private plans, will be available on the health insurance exchange marketplace.

Family plans make the distinction between individual deductibles and a family deductible. It's important to keep this in mind. For example, if your partner meets their individual deductible, their insurance will kick in for them, but not for you. If a family deductible is met, then insurance will kick in for all members in your family. Ask your health plan about the distinction between individual deductibles and your family deductible.

Health insurance premiums can be tax-deductible. If you are insured through an employer-sponsored plan, you may not be eligible, as payroll deductions are made with pre-tax dollars. However, if you are self-employed, consult with your tax preparer to see if you are eligible to deduct your insurance premiums and health-related costs.

TYPES OF HEALTH COVERAGE

Health insurance in the United States can either be public or private. Public health insurance programs include Medicaid, Medicare, and the Children's Health Insurance Program (CHIP).

Public Coverage

Medicare is a public federal health insurance program for Americans over the age of 65. Those eligible receive free and subsidized healthcare, and the different parts of the program cover different health services. Part A covers inpatient hospital care. Part B covers necessary and preventive outpatient services and includes a monthly premium of $144.60 as of 2020. Part C is known as Medicare Advantage and allows you to buy into private health insurance, and add supplemental services such as vision or dental care. Lastly, Part D covers prescription drugs.

Medicaid is both a federal and state-run health insurance program that provides health coverage for low-income individuals and those most vulnerable.

Long-term care. The program covers long-term nursing home care, as well as rehabilitative care for recovery from injury for millions of seniors and people with disabilities, offering coverage for one in five Americans.

Individuals with disabilities. The federal-state joint program covers nearly 50% of children with special care needs and 45% of nonelderly adults who suffer from disabilities, such as mental illness or Alzheimer's disease.

As a result, Medicaid accounts for 20% of all healthcare spending. The federal government sets general eligibility requirements and benefits, while states tailor Medicaid to their populations with additional guidelines. For example, federal law requires that low-income

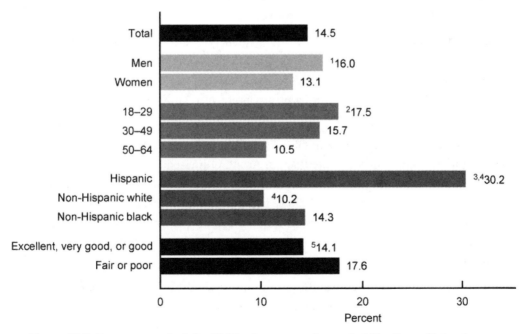

Figure 96.2. Percentage of adults 18-64 who were uninsured at the time of interview, by selected characteristics: United States, 2019

families, qualified pregnant women, children, and anyone who receives Supplemental Social Security Income (SSI) be eligible for Medicaid. Obamacare expanded Medicaid to
children in families with incomes of 133% of the federal poverty level in all states. States
have the option to expand these eligibility requirements and to cover additional groups of
people. Eligibility requirements are determined by the state you live in, and you can check
your eligibility through your state exchange.

Like Medicaid, the Children's Health Insurance Program (CHIP) is both a federal and
state program, but it is designed to cover children under 18 years of age.

Private Health Insurance

At least 67% of Americans have private health insurance either through their employer or
through the health insurance marketplace. Plans offered on a government exchange must
meet federal and state requirements, such as covering ten essential benefits. Private health
insurance not on the government exchange can be sold directly by insurance companies or
through a privately run insurance marketplace. These plans must also meet federal requirements, but insurers have more flexibility in the types of plans they offer.

Group plans offered by employers are considered private plans. These plans typically
include more people, so risk is spread across all the members of the plan, which makes
them more affordable than individual plans.

Capitated. Kaiser Permanente is the largest managed care organization in the United
States. Kaiser is unique because, although it is a nonprofit insurance plan, Kaiser also
provides patient services, and manages its own hospitals and clinics. Kaiser covers nearly
every aspect of a patient's care, from a primary care visit, an X-ray at one of its clinics, to
surgery in one of its hospitals.

Kaiser is an example of an Accountable Care Organization, a model of care that is becoming more popular in the United States. An ACO is essentially a group of physicians,
hospitals, and other specialty care providers who coordinate services to provide quality
patient care. Many of these ACOs follow "best practice" patterns. As healthcare spending
becomes more efficient and effective, and as contractual quality goals are met, the system
is rewarded for keeping patients healthy and limiting unnecessary spending, resulting in
lower out-of-pocket costs for patients.

In-network vs. out-of-network. In examining your health insurance policy, you will
come across terms like in-network and out-of-network. A health insurance network refers
to a group of physicians and service providers that have contracted with your health insurance company to provide health services. This helps insurance companies develop rela-

tionships with providers and set fixed costs. Some plans (like HMOs) will not cover your services if you get care outside the network. Other plans may charge you more for services you seek outside your network. Make sure to check your health insurance policy to see which providers and services are in-network for your plan, to avoid surprise costs or bills.

Capitation and fee-for-service. Capitation and fee-for-service are terms that describe how healthcare providers are paid. Capitation means that your physician is getting a fixed dollar amount for each patient they see, while fee-for-service means providers get paid for the type of services and procedures they utilize. Capitation is becoming the primary mode of payment as fee-for-service models are declining.

There are benefits and risks for each system. Capitation puts higher risk on physicians and hospitals because they get paid a fixed amount regardless of how costly treating a patient may be. However, it also incentivizes the healthcare system to keep us healthy. It is in the healthcare provider's interest to minimize unnecessary and preventable costs. Capitation increases financial risk for insurance companies, because they are financially responsible for whatever procedures and tests a patient may require. This increases the incentive to treat specific issues and illnesses, but puts less emphasis on overall wellbeing and prevention.

HMOs (health maintenance organizations) restrict your provider network in order to reduce costs. You will have to choose a primary care provider who is approved by your policy, and they will be responsible for coordinating your care. A referral will be required by your PCP to see a specialist as a form of quality and cost control. It is important to understand that HMO plans will not cover costs associated with out-of-network providers. This is often a source of confusion for some patients. If medical costs are incurred outside of your network (say if you're travelling), your out-of-pocket costs can rise substantially. Make sure you consult with your health insurance plan to see which providers you are allowed to consult to avoid unnecessary fees.

PPOs (preferred provider organizations) offer more flexibility in terms of which primary care provider and specialists you can see but have higher premiums. Your plan will have a list of in-network providers you can see at a reduced cost and out-of-network providers you can see at a higher cost. You do not need a referral from your PCP to see a specialist. Some states such as California do require that you have a primary care physician.

EPOs (exclusive provider organizations) are simply a combination of HMOs and PPOs. You do not need a referral to see a specialist, but you will not be covered for out-of-network providers. These plans have premiums that are mid-range between those of HMOs and PPOs.

Point-of-sale (POS) plans are another combination of HMO and PPO plans. You will have the option of in-network and out-of-network providers (out-of-network will be more costly) and a referral from your primary care provider is required to see a specialist. These plans are more expensive than HMOs, but less expensive than PPOs.

Supplemental Health Insurance Products

Standard health insurance packages may not include certain kinds of coverage that many Americans want. This additional insurance can be purchased separately as a supplement to one's primary health insurance plan.

Dental and vision insurance are two common types of supplemental insurance. Dental insurance is designed to pay for dental care, which can range from regular teeth cleanings to treatment of tooth and gum disease. Like health insurance plans, many dental plans are managed by HMOs and PPOs. Dental plans will rarely burn a hole in your wallet. It's important to note that dental insurance is often included in health insurance plans for children under the age of 18.

Vision insurance is designed to pay for eye care, such as vision exams, prescription glasses, and contact lenses. Most vision care plans will also provide discounts or full coverage for surgeries such as laser eye-correction surgery or cataract surgery. Vision care plans and the benefits they include can vary widely, but many plans are relatively inexpensive. Similar to dental insurance, vision insurance is usually included in health insurance plans for children under the age of 18.

Gap insurance is another type of supplemental health insurance that is meant to help patients cover the "gap" in coverage that is left by insurance plans with high deductibles. This type of insurance helps pay for out-of-pocket costs associated with healthcare. However, these plans are not regulated by the Affordable Care Act and do not emphasize consumer protection as much as qualifying health insurance plans do.

Critical illness insurance is a type of supplemental insurance for those with expensive illnesses that impact a patient's ability to financially support themselves for multiple years. Examples of diseases that critical illness insurance might cover include Alzheimer's disease, cancer, and stroke. Patients with one of these insurance plans may receive a lump sum cash payment after being diagnosed with a critical illness that their plan covers. If you have term life insurance, it's also possible to attach a critical illness "rider" to your life insurance policy, which essentially serves the same function as a critical illness insurance plan, but for less money.

BENEFITS AND COST

Ten Essential Benefits

The Affordable Care Act requires that all health insurance plans cover ten basic types of healthcare services, in addition to any other services they may cover. These required services are known as Essential Health Benefits (EHBs), and include the following:

- Ambulatory patient services—outpatient care that you can receive without being admitted to a hospital

- Emergency services

- Hospitalization for surgery and other procedures, as well as overnight stays

- Pregnancy, maternity, and newborn care

- Mental health and substance-use-disorder services

- Prescription drugs

- Rehabilitative and habilitative services and devices—treatment and devices that help people gain or recover mental and physical skills after an injury, disability, or onset of a chronic condition

- Laboratory services

- Preventive and wellness services, as well as chronic disease management

- Pediatric services, including dental and vision coverage for children.

Federal law requires health insurance plans to include coverage for these ten categories at the very least. However, federal law does not specify which specific services must be offered within each category. One key item that is not included in the ten EHBs is durable medical equipment (DME), such as wheelchairs and ventilators. Many people rely on DME equipment to survive and function on a daily basis, so it's important for patients to ensure that their unique health needs are covered when choosing a health plan. Usually, state laws will require health insurance plans to offer additional services beyond those that fall under the ten EHB categories required by the ACA. When applying for health insurance through a state, federal, or private exchanges, you will be provided with information on the services each plan covers before making a selection, so rest assured that you will know what you're paying for when purchasing a plan.

Preventive Care

Preventive healthcare services are included in all health insurance plans on government-run marketplaces. These plans allow members to access services such as vaccinations and screening tests at no cost, regardless of whether they have paid off their deductible. According to Healthcare.gov, there are 21 free preventive services that anyone with an ACA-qualifying health plan has access to as long as age requirements are met:

- Abdominal aortic aneurysm one-time screening
- Alcohol misuse screening and counseling
- Aspirin use to prevent cardiovascular disease
- Blood pressure screening
- Cholesterol screening
- Colorectal cancer screening
- Depression screening
- Diabetes (type 2) screening
- Diet counseling
- Fall prevention (for adults age 65 or older)
- Hepatitis B screening
- Hepatitis C screening
- HIV screening
- Immunization vaccines
- Lung cancer screening
- Obesity screening and counseling
- Sexually transmitted infection (STI) prevention counseling
- Statin preventive medication (for high-risk adults age 40 to 75)
- Syphilis screening
- Tobacco use screening and cessation interventions
- Tuberculosis (TB) screening (for certain high-risk adults).

Since some of these screenings are only free for people in certain age groups, it's important to check with your insurer to see which preventive services are available at no cost to you.

Cost Factors

The Affordable Care Act has determined that there are five factors that affect how much you have to pay in premiums for health insurance:

- Your age

- Your location

- Whether or not you use tobacco

- Individual vs. a family plan

- Your plan category (Bronze, Silver, Gold, Platinum, or Catastrophic)

Health insurance companies are not permitted to consider gender or past health history (also known as pre-existing conditions) when setting a patient's premium. Health insurance premiums can vary widely depending on the state and insurance market, but we all know that they have been rising. According to the Kaiser Family Foundation, health insurance premiums have doubled over the past 15 years.

When shopping for a health insurance plan, there are many important factors to consider. The monthly premium is a good starting point, but the true cost of health insurance goes far beyond just the premium. Over nine million people who received healthcare through governmental marketplaces in 2019 also received tax credit subsidies, which brings down the effective net cost of health insurance. Premium tax credits can be applied in advance of a tax return to reduce the cost of monthly premiums, or applied when filing a yearly tax return. These tax credits are only available to individuals and families with an income between 100% and 400% of the federal poverty line in their state. Premium tax credits are also limited to marketplace plans, so those with public health insurance plans, catastrophic health insurance plans, or off-exchange private health insurance plans cannot take advantage of them.

Prescription Plans

Many Americans rely on health insurance to access prescription drugs, which is based on the formulary of one's plan. A formulary is a list of generic and brand-name prescription drugs covered by the health plan. Your health plan may only help you pay for the drugs listed in its formulary.

You may be asked to pay a copay ranging from no cost to a specific amount. You may also be asked to pay a percentage of a brand-name drug listed on the formulary, making your out-of-pocket cost much higher. Your health plan's formulary is divided into three or four categories described as tiers. Drugs are placed in tiers based on the type of drug: Generic, preferred

PLAN	COST SPLIT BY INSURANCE PLAN %	
	Consumer	*Insurer*
Bronze	40	60
Silver	30	70
Gold	20	80
Platinum	10	90

Figure 96.3. Health plan tiers indicating the percentage of cost paid
by the consumer and insurer.

brand, non-preferred brand, and specialty. Drugs in lower tiers will cost less and those in higher tiers will cost more. Different insurance companies have different formularies.

Tiers. Insurance health plans split the cost between consumer and insurer based on tiers, which are categorized as bronze, silver, gold, and platinum tiers.

Bronze plans require consumers to pay higher co-pays and percentage of cost. Platinum plans are more expensive but require consumers to pay the least overall. Here is what typical formulary tiers look like:

- **Tier 1:** Tier 1 drugs are usually generics and have the lowest co-pays.

- **Tier 2:** Tier 2 drugs will cost you more than tier 1 medications. They include non-preferred generics and brand-name medications.

- **Tier 3:** Tier 3 includes generics, preferred brands, and non-preferred brands. Your out-of-pocket price for these drugs will be higher than tiers 1 and 2. Your health plan may place a drug in tier 3 if it's new or it if there's a similar drug on a lower tier.

- **Tier 4:** Tier 4 includes generics, preferred brands, non-preferred brands, and specialty drugs. Specialty medications treat conditions that are rare or serious.

Typically, a team of medical professionals approves the drugs on a health plan's formulary based on safety, quality, and cost-effectiveness. The team is made up of pharmacists and physicians who review new and existing medications. Health plans update their formularies every year, but they also make changes throughout the year. These changes occur when a new drug becomes available or when the FDA decides a drug is harmful.

When choosing your health insurance, you should also consider the medications you take. A formulary can help you with that. By reviewing different formularies, you can choose a health plan that covers your medications. Additionally, you can choose a plan that has your drugs listed in their lower tiers. The tier level for drugs varies from plan to plan and from insurance provider to insurance provider.

Ask your health plan about temporary coverage during the exceptions process. Your insurer may agree to cover the drug until they make a decision.

Pharmacy benefit managers (PBM) are large buying networks for drugs. They represent consumers from multiple employers and insurance companies. Some of the large PBM's—CVS, Express Scripts, Optum, and GoodRx.com—account for more than 70% of claims volume. PBMs started with the idea that their buying power would reduce healthcare costs, and these savings would be passed onto consumers. PBMs make money from fees from the supply chain, rebates from manufacturers, and the difference between what they pay for drugs from a pharmacy and what they get paid by insurance. Multiple sources have raised concerns that the PBMs are not passing on savings to consumers.

WHEN TO BUY HEALTH INSURANCE

Generally, if you want to shop for a new health insurance plan, you would do so on the Obamacare marketplace during the open enrollment period. This enrollment period can happen at any time of the year, however, it's usually in the autumn of the year before coverage begins. If you want to purchase a health insurance plan after the open enrollment period has already ended, there are two ways to do so. The first way is to be employed at a new job that provides group health insurance. The second way is to experience a qualifying event that allows you to enroll in a health plan during a special enrollment period. Qualifying events include turning 26 years old, getting married, having a baby, or moving to a new zip code. Some states consider other additional circumstances to be qualifying events as well.

KEY TAKE AWAYS

- In 2018 the United States spent about $3.6 trillion on healthcare, which averages about $11,000 per person or 18% of the gross domestic product.

- Health insurance costs are calculated based on the level of coverage, county of residence, family size, and, most importantly, the age of the covered person.

- Public health insurance includes Medicare and Medicaid.

- Private health insurance includes PPO, HMO, EPO, and POS plans.

- There are ten essential health benefits every health insurance plan must provide, as well as twenty-one free preventive care services.

- Each plan has its own network of doctors and formulary of drugs; it's important to check those aspects of service before buying insurance.

Chapter 97
Finding a Good Doctor
Alan Wang, Insurance Specialist

It is more important to know what sort of person has a disease
than to know what sort of disease a person has.
— *Hippocrates*

A good lawyer, a good plumber, and a good doctor are three professionals you need in life. One could make the argument that in today's world, it's relatively easy to find a good lawyer and a good plumber, but finding a good doctor can be challenging. If you're in search of a new physician, the internet provides resources that will make the task easier. You can use the algorithms available online to give you a snapshot of each of the providers you are considering. Just as you track the stats of your favorite players, you can use these resources in your decision making…

Imagine this, it's the bottom of the ninth in the World Series, seventh game, and your team is behind by one run, and the bases are loaded. You call for a pinch hitter. You have four players left on the bench. How do you decide which man? If you don't know whether they're right-or-left handed, their batting average, or their batting average *with men on base*, then you won't know who to choose. (A surprising number of statistics are necessary in good decision making.) Yet we put much more time and effort into figuring out baseball scores than we do in figuring out who will crack open our chest and repair our heart or saw open our skull and cut cancer out of our brain.

You need a strategy (or two) to find capable physicians and specialists. First, let's lay out a few definitions. For the purposes of this conversation, let's use the term "provider" so that it includes physicians, laboratories, imaging centers, hospitals, and pharmacies.

Let's also define good. When seeking the services of an attorney, for example, to help resolve a complicated legal matter, similar questions arise. How successful has this attorney been in addressing similar issues in the past? What was the outcome? Are they an expert in their field? Are they easy to work with? How and what did they charge for their services? These are all relatively quantitative means of determining and defining what is good.

When it comes to choosing a provider, most of the selection process becomes qualitative, based on experiential and fluctuating factors, rather than credible data that provides a fixed and measurable reality. When seeking a recommendation for a provider, people tend to ask friends, relatives, employers, co-workers, or other physicians. For some, it may be as random as just choosing a physician who is in the network of their health plan, and nothing more. Some, for example, have chosen to have a procedure at a particular hospital because it was close by and was recommended by their doctor, not knowing that the hospital had high mortality rates. Please note that this quandary applies regardless of what kind of insurance plan you have (HMO, narrow network, Kaiser Permanente, or the VA). Eventually, we all have to select a healthcare provider.

It is important to know that obtaining quantitative data on the performance of a provider can be extremely challenging and increases with complexity. Consider someone who is being admitted for cardiac surgery. Outcome measures can be difficult to translate for the consumer in a manner that is easy to understand. The type of surgery (single, double, or triple bypass?), patient experience, error rates, success rates, and the number of times a surgeon has performed a particular procedure are among the factors that need to be considered.

The other problem with selecting a provider has to do with cost. Not only is quality opaque at best, but most people do not know how much a provider charges until *after* they have obtained their medical service or prescription. This is not about deductibles, coinsurance, or co-payments. This refers to the actual cost of the MRI, office visit, surgical procedure, drug, etc. Think about when you last received medical services. When the doctor told you that you needed knee surgery, did he tell you how much it was going to cost? Probably not. What happened was that the insurance carrier pre-authorized the service, the knee surgery was performed, and then a few weeks later an explanation of benefits (EOB) was sent in the mail, indicating how much the surgery cost, what the discount was for using the network, and the patient responsibility (how much you owed). What is surprising to many is how much medical procedures cost in the final analysis. What is even more surprising to some is that every provider charges a different amount for the same procedure! Any one medical service can vary in cost by thousands of dollars.

FINDING A PHYSICIAN

So how does one go about finding the right doctor at the right price? Some tools exist, but most are only available for those who receive health insurance coverage through their employer. Unfortunately, these tools are simply not widely available to the average consumer with an individual plan. And even then, only certain very forward-thinking employers offer access to ratings and quality for price transparency. In a straightforward approach to solving this problem, healthcare consumers can use this four-step process to find a good doctor.

1. Establish the criteria most important to you in your choice of a provider. Vital information to consider in selecting a physician includes:

- Board certification

- Training and experience (length of time in practice)

- Expertise on your specific health issue

- Hospital affiliations

- Personality and ease of approach (Would you feel comfortable discussing their recommendations with them? Would you feel embarrassed if you told them that you wanted to get a second opinion?)

- Ease of access (Do they respond to e-mail? If you have a serious illness, is there someone available on call who is knowledgeable and accessible?)

- What are their staff like? Are they easy to work with, and do they demonstrate expertise and empathy?

- Does their approach to medicine (conventional, holistic, or a combination) fit your personal values?

- How much experience do they have in their specialty? (Does this surgeon conduct a few surgeries a year or hundreds? What are their outcomes?)

- Involvement in research.

2. Research the doctor's credentials to determine their level of competence in the type of treatment you require. There are a number of sites where you can find this type of information:

- The Federation of State Medical Boards (FSMB)

- Healthgrades

- Vitals

- US News & World Report

- Your insurance carrier's website, which gives information on the providers in their network

- Healthcare Bluebook

The Healthcare Bluebook can be searched by the name of the procedure, facility, or provider. The site enables consumers to search and compare different providers, allowing access to cost and quality data that may not be accessible elsewhere. The Bluebook supports price transparency, showing average costs for various procedures by the provider, while including information on quality transparency such as doctor-specific quality rankings. While there may be a cost associated with this platform, it is well worth the investment, as it could save a significant amount of money and result in a much better health outcome.

3. Speak with the new patient coordinator in the practice. In today's economy, most physicians no longer do free consults, but they may give online presentations, virtual Q & A sessions, or public talks.

The next step is to request an interview with the patient coordinator. Have a list of questions written out before your meeting. Do necessary research about your health conditions in advance so you can ask questions of greater depth to make the best use of their time.

Another essential aspect in selecting a physician is to determine if their approach is to "wait and see" or to be proactive in managing your health. Sometimes, good service provision involves asking uncomfortable questions and making recommendations that will help you change behaviors if you have a chronic health condition. Selecting a provider requires care and attention. After all, the relationship you have with your provider could save your life.

4. Be proactive. To the degree that you can, participate in managing your own health.

Being proactive in managing your health means you must not only research everything about your health condition, but that you are willing to ask questions of your doctor, and at times probe with deeper questions or seek a second opinion. Although highly trained and knowledgeable, physicians are still human. The more informed they are, the better they are equipped to treat your condition. However, this requires the patient to be an active participant in the total healthcare equation. Accepting what a physician says without any dialog could be dangerous. Asking intelligent questions provides everyone the opportunity to be more informed. If you don't know what to ask, or are hesitant to ask, or if you are ill or in pain, bring someone along who will serve as your advocate. You want someone who feels comfortable asking the doctor hard questions, yet who is sufficiently tactful that they will not damage your relationship with your doctor.

FINDING A GOOD HOSPITAL

When my son was born four years ago, the total cost of delivery was $35,000. No complications. No extra days in the hospital. No problems. Two years later, when our daughter was born, the cost was an astounding $55,000. It was the same number of nights at the hospital. No problems. No complications. Same delivery, but at a much higher cost. And of course, we didn't learn of the charges until *after* the children were born.

Why is this? When you have surgery, you get a charge for the hospital, the surgeon, the anesthesiologist, the pathologist, the assistant surgeon, and the Tylenol (which cost $1.50 for each capsule), and so on. The cost of surgery has multiple factors, and getting a figure upfront from most providers can be challenging.

Additionally, you will want to factor in specific aspects of care into your search. For example, hospitals may specialize. Are they skilled at saving trauma patients (gunshot wounds, knifings, domestic abuse), but not at treating cancer patients?

Hospital Ratings

When seeking information on hospital services, Leapfrog and Healthcare Bluebook are two additional resources to consider.

The Leapfrog Group. Leapfrog's hospital ratings look at process measures, structural measures, and outcome measures to produce a grade for almost every hospital in the country. The resulting Safety Grade utilizes up to 28 national performance measures of patient safety that are collected and publicly reported by the Centers for Medicare & Medicaid Services (CMS), The Leapfrog Group, and other data sources such as the American Hospital Association (AHA). These performance measures examine such issues as errors, injuries, accidents, and infection rates.

Healthcare Bluebook's quality ratings are designed to help patients understand each hospital's specific level of quality for a particular in-patient clinical procedure or specialty. Quality ratings are calculated for each clinical area by combining a hospital's performance in several areas—such as patient safety and compliance with standards of care. The calculations and ratings are based on a sample drawn from federal Medicare and Medicaid data.

In almost any other type of business transaction except healthcare, the seller posts the price for the item on sale, and the buyer is fully informed. The buyer can make an offer to accept that price, negotiate, or go to another seller who is selling the very same item, but at a lower price. In today's society, there are social engagement platforms that rate products and services so buyers can make an informed decision about quality and price.

Herein lies the problem in our 100-year-old healthcare payment system: There is no easy way for patients to compare the quality and cost of medical service. We call this the "black box" of healthcare. Some providers have inferior performance standards and charge an excessive amount, whereas others are high performing at a much more competitive price.

As a way around this dilemma, do your research and manage the process. More important than finding the right attorney is finding the right healthcare providers to help you when you need it. It takes effort and patience, but the return on investment is worth it. After all, what could be worth more than your health?

For more information on the work of Alan Wang, please see:
www.ubf.consulting.

PART 14
LEAVING A LEGACY
Introduction
Judson Brandeis, MD

The Peacemaker taught us about the Seven Generations. He said, when you sit in council for the welfare of the people, you must not think of yourself or of your family, not even of your generation. He said, make your decisions on behalf of the seven generations coming, so that they may enjoy what you have today.
— *Oren Lyons (Seneca), Faithkeeper, Onondaga Nation*

When you're nearing the end of your life and reflect back, how will you feel about your life? How will your family remember you? What will people say about you? What did you leave that was of enduring value? Did you maximize your potential? Were you a kind and generous person? Did you leave the world a better place than you found it?

The purpose of life is not to be happy. It is to be useful, to be honorable, to be compassionate, to have it make some difference that you have lived and lived well. – Ralph Waldo Emerson

The Judeo-Christian religions believe that you have one life to live on planet Earth. Other religions believe in reincarnation and envision each visit to Earth as a gift, a chance to improve upon the last. Regardless of your belief system, you have the opportunity to use your life/lives in service of something greater than yourself. Many of us have benefitted from the legacy of those who came before us. I feel gratitude for the people who helped me along the way: my family, friends, and teachers.

As Sir Isaac Newton famously declared, *If I have seen further than others, it is by standing on the shoulders of giants.*

Almost by definition, teachers create a legacy, but teachers come in many different forms. *The mediocre teacher tells. The good teacher explains. The superior teacher demonstrates. The great teacher inspires. – William Arthur Ward*

One such teacher for me was pediatric urologic surgeon Dr. Bernard Churchill. Dr. Churchill's reconstructive surgeries last as long as eight hours, and periodically throughout the entire surgical procedure, Dr. Churchill taught us anatomy, surgical technique, and life. He has the unique ability to explain subjects from the big picture down to the tiny details. Many of the chapters in this book that I wrote have benefitted from his broad insight and laser focus, the macro to micro approach. His perspective is reflected in the chapter on gratitude, and it's an honor for me to share his contribution here.

Consider *your* assets as opportunities to leave a legacy. Wherever you are, whatever your finances or gifts, it may be possible to amplify your impact. If you have knowledge, have you captured that knowledge for others, in books, through inventions, in public forums? If you have wealth, have you considered the best way to make a positive impact? We can use Warren Buffett as an example of intelligent philanthropy, but small sums can also make a difference. Perhaps you are the master at a craft or an avocation. Who could benefit from what you know?

Legacy is a selfless act. Lin-Manuel Miranda described it as "planting seeds in a garden you never get to see."

I hope that the time, effort, and care that I dedicated to this book will result in physically, emotionally, and mentally healthy men who will create their own positive legacies.

Chapter 98
Inspiration
Brian Banmiller, Broadcast Journalist

It always seems impossible until it's done.
— *Nelson Mandela*

When Dr. Judson Brandeis asked me to contribute a chapter for his well-timed and valuable medical self-help book for men my age, we discussed what topic would best fit into his overall narrative. Given my four decades of business news reporting locally, nationally, and internationally, he felt what I have learned from the thousands of characters I've interviewed might provide you, the reader, with some valuable insight into the human condition.

Initially titled "Humility," I told the doctor that after meeting so many of the good, bad, and terrible business leaders, politicians, and media personalities, I would be hard-pressed to find enough bigwigs with the true humility needed to fill out this chapter. Unfortunately, humility does not often lead to the skill sets required for success. As the comedian, Bob Hope once observed, "Sincerity is an important ingredient for success. If you can learn to fake that, you've got it made."

Instead, I thought "Inspiration" would be a more fitting way to impart what I have observed throughout my long career. There are so many stories that have genuinely inspired me that passing them on might prove valuable to readers. For simplicity, I have concentrated on just three disciplines: business leaders, politicians, and physicians.

BUSINESS LEADERS

Charles Schwab is a perfect example of the type of super-successful entrepreneur I most admire. His leadership has been an inspiration to millions. Chuck started with nothing and achieved everything, while providing a valuable service that helped change the world. His passion was to have Main Street participate in the growing economy as investors and owners. As he writes in his latest book, *Invested*, a year into his grand experiment in discount stock trading, living in a small Bay Area apartment with his wife Helen and new baby, he carried a six-figure debt and a pocketful of personal loans.

He also suffered from dyslexia, but managed to work around it to create one of the world's most admired companies, becoming an inspiration to thousands born with disabilities. But it was a rocky road. Customers flocked to Schwab. Yet his small team had scarce resources and no road map to manage the company's growth. So, he sold his company to Bank of America, a merger that almost doomed the company. He repurchased it in a cleverly leveraged buyout, then managed it through the stock market collapse of 1987 and the dot-com meltdown of 2000. Today his company is one of the leading financial services firms in the world, with more than three trillion dollars in client assets.

My own experience with Chuck Schwab is a personal one. Early in my journalism career, my home TV station in the Bay Area was promoting a new business show titled *Banmiller on Business*. The promotions department reached out to Schwab for a personal endorsement. Chuck readily agreed and cut a sixty-second radio commercial touting me as one of the best business reporters in the country. I found his kind words to be humbling and have been granted many insightful interviews over the years.

He often opened up to my audience about his battles with dyslexia, always an inspiration to anyone so afflicted who can learn to overcome such challenges. Chuck also encouraged young employees to get training in public speaking as a valuable tool for success. And he encouraged workers to take up a sport, as he did with tennis and golf, because they can be powerful confidence boosters. All through his long career, Schwab has always worked to give the younger generation the tools needed to succeed. His many books on investing have helped millions.

John Chen is best known as the chairman and CEO of Blackberry, once the world's leading cell phone maker, until a guy named Steve Jobs crushed the competition with the iPhone. John's expert skill in navigating Blackberry's competitive positioning came from his experience leading Sybase, a struggling company that he successfully revived and sold to SAP for $5.8 billion in 2010 in an all-cash offer. Chen has succeeded at Blackberry by focusing on the company's security software.

During an interview I did for *Banmiller on Business* on CBS News Radio, John shared his personal experience getting professional coaching on public speaking, which subsequently launched his career. Born in Hong Kong, John came to the U.S. at age 17, attended Brown University and Caltech, getting a master's in electrical engineering. His first job was design engineering at Unisys in L.A., where he watched other non-Asian engineers getting promoted while he did not.

Disturbed by this, John asked his boss why, only to be told his presentation skills were deficient in a job that required sales pitches. John decided he needed professional help if he was to have any chance of promotion. So, Chen hired a husband-and-wife team (she was an on-air talent and he a producer), who taped his pitch. He found his initial performance "alarming and embarrassing." So, he and his wife Sherry scraped together enough money to hire the team for six lessons costing $2,000, an entire month's salary he could hardly afford.

But with their coaching help, he turned his career around, getting the first of many promotions. The company was so impressed, it reimbursed John the entire cost of those lessons, proving that getting professional help does work. I smile every time I see John Chen interviewed on CNBC. He took the risk of investing in himself. And over the years Chen has inspired scores of immigrants to follow in his footsteps by polishing presentation and language skills so vital to success in today's global economy.

Chen has been an invited member of the Committee of 100, an organization of Extraordinary Chinese Americans, giving him an ideal platform to encourage young Asians to improve their communications skills. And he is a trustee of the charitable organization, The First Tee, a youth development organization impacting the lives of young people by providing educational programs that build character and instill life-enhancing values through the game of golf, a sport John loves. He has also been a major sponsor of the Ladies' Professional Golf Association, helping grow that organization into acceptance in the sports world.

Bill Gates became the worlds' youngest self-made billionaire at age 31. At just 17, he sold his first computer program, a timetable system, to his private high school for $4,200. This Harvard dropout's first job was as a computer programmer for TRW during his senior year in high school. Following his passion for tech, Gates and his childhood friend Paul Allen founded Microsoft in 1975.

Bill began his massive philanthropic efforts in 1994 when he created the William H. Gates Foundation, which focuses on global health. Three years later, he and his wife Melinda created the Gates Library Foundation, which worked to bring public access computers with internet connections to libraries in the United States. It became the Gates Learning Foundation to focus on ensuring that low-income minority students are prepared for college and have the means to attend. In 2000 the two groups merged into the Bill and Melinda Gates Foundation. Also inspirational is Gates pledge to give a considerable portion of his wealth to philanthropy.

In fact, his legacy goes far beyond co-founding Microsoft. Gates inspired another billionaire, Warren Buffet, to increase his own philanthropy. The two then founded the Giving Pledge, a movement encouraging other billionaires to donate most of their wealth to charity either during their lifetimes or after their deaths. Gates himself has already given more than $50 billion to charitable causes over his career. He has arguably changed the nature and responsibility of wealthy people worldwide, already inspiring more than 200 super-wealthy families to join the Giving Pledge.

I have interviewed Gates many times over his long career, so I have had the chance to watch firsthand how he grew in his professional and philanthropic lives. I first interviewed Bill in the mid-eighties in Seattle, where he was a guest speaker at an Urban Land Institute annual meeting. He seemed ill at ease, wore an "off the rack" dark suit with some dandruff on his shoulders. And he swayed in that first interview, making it a bit tough to keep the mike near his mouth.

When I last interviewed him, the clothes were impeccable. The dandruff was gone, and so was the nervous swaying. And he brought his camera crew, who set up the lighting to his taste. That gave me a "two-camera" shoot, incredibly beneficial when doing such high-power interviews. When I mentioned this dramatic change from my first interview to his longtime PR person, she smiled and replied, "It helps to become very rich and marry the right partner."

POLITICIANS

Two of my favorite political leaders passed away over the past few years, much to the detriment of civic discourse and political compromise.

Former two-term California Republican Governor George Deukmejian died of natural causes at his modest Long Beach home at age 89. With his passing, the nation's political class lost yet another of "the old guard"—those seasoned veterans who thought reaching across the aisle was a better way to move our country forward than the bitter partisan acrimony that now threatens to tear our nation apart.

USC Price School of Public Policy Professor Sherry Bebitch Jeffe perhaps said it best: "George Deukmejian was an extremely hard, conservative Republican. He was strong on law and order — but he could, and did, work across the aisle with Democrats when he felt it was right. I do not think we are ever going to see a political environment like that again, at least not soon. His passing underscores the drive away from being able to compromise and communicate between the two major parties." Unfortunately, the example he set is not being followed in today's increasingly hostile political environment.

For those who may not know the background of this son of Armenian immigrants, Deukmejian served 16 years in the California state legislature and one term as Attorney General before narrowly defeating Los Angeles Mayor Tom Bradley for Governor in 1982. Four years later, after helping recall three liberal state Supreme Court Justices, he won his second term in a landslide. His platform was a simple one: tough on crime and no new taxes.

Yet there was a side of George Deukmejian most voters never saw, but I had the good fortune of witnessing firsthand. Before embarking on a journalism career, I ran a political consulting firm in California, mostly helping businesses navigate the minefields of local politics. The legendary political consultant Bill Roberts asked me to help him run George's campaign for Attorney General in northern California. I readily accepted, knowing the best way to forge a successful career in journalism was to understand how the system worked in the rough and tumble world of politics.

I had many "learning" experiences working with George, but one stands out. One day during the campaign for attorney general, I showed George a sampling of calls from voters on various subjects, including questions about his hard-line stance on the death penalty. He randomly returned a constituent's call from my office, trying to explain his "law and order" stance to a woman who was not buying what he was selling. But George pushed on, despite the fact I had booked him on a popular radio program within the hour with hundreds of thousands of listeners. "George," I explained, "don't get worked up over one vote before a major appearance." We were late. George lost the lady's vote, but won the election in part because his brand of retail politics connected with voters. He employed a skill many new politicians fail to prioritize. He listened to the voters. Unfortunately, today's leaders listen to the pollsters and paid consultants.

Another member of "the old guard" was Arizona Republican Senator John McCain, war hero turned public servant. During his 31-year-long career in the U.S. Senate, he championed "the art of compromise." Finally, sidelined with brain cancer, his positive attitude toward his illness was the same trait that made him such a successful leader. His extraordinary life is well documented in the unofficial biography by Elaine Povich, apply titled: *John McCain: American Maverick.*

From Amazon book reviews: "This unofficial retrospective honors and pays homage to Senator McCain's astonishing journey—a story of courage, resilience, and leadership; irrepressibility, determination, and grit. . . . It covers his childhood as the son and grandson of admirals, his service as a naval aviator in Vietnam and subsequent harrowing five-year imprisonment in a POW camp, his congressional and senatorial careers, his family, his presidential campaigns, and perhaps his most important role yet, as an elder statesman willing to stand up for the nation."

His moral compass and bipartisan character are sorely missed in an increasingly polarized country with too few politicians taking inspiration from his leadership.

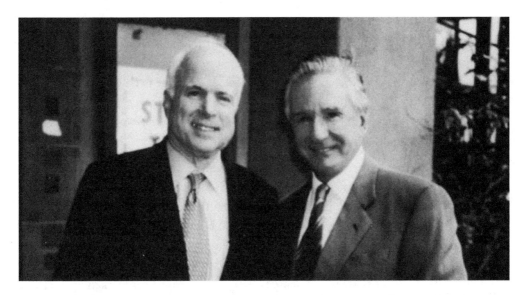

Figure 98.1. Republican Senator John McCain and Brian Banmiller. April 2003.

My own experience with Senator McCain showed me the depth of his character. During a one-on-one television interview some years ago, as we started the interview, my cameraman Sean Drummond suggested we change the shot from shooting his left side to shooting his right side. Afterward, I asked why? It turns out McCain had undergone treatment for skin cancer, and it showed in a dramatic scar on his left cheek. Most other politicians or celebrities I have interviewed over four decades would have asked us to shoot his or her "good side." Not so for Senator McCain. He cared more about the questions than how he looked. And cameraman Sean Drummond's sensitivity was indeed professional and impressive.

Having worked with Governor George Deukmejian and interviewed Senator McCain, I am reminded of a famous quote from another great statesman, Winston Churchill: "Courage is what it takes to stand up and speak. Courage is also what it takes to sit down and listen." That kind of courage is the building block of the "political compromise" that we so desperately need in America.

In 1978, both San Francisco Mayor George Moscone and Supervisor Harvey Milk were assassinated. Memories of the horror surrounding the killings and the fiery aftermath on the streets of San Francisco linger to this day.

As Mayor, George Moscone opened the door to create a city government that reflected the healthy diversity that is San Francisco. History will show that his strong leadership and compassion for those less fortunate sowed the seeds that helped the city grow to be a progressive beacon for all of America. As quoted in the *San Francisco Chronicle*, his son Christopher said, "My father was a strong leader, passionate. He stood for what he stood for, and that was that. And that's what we need a little more of now." On that point, liberals, moderates, and conservatives should hopefully all agree.

In commenting on his parents' relationship, son Jonathan reminisced, "My dad was the man who shook everybody's hand. He could get along with a tree." He said his mother often reminded her husband that others were not so magnanimous, but his larger than life personality helped him always see the bright side of politics.

My last memory of Mayor Moscone was sharing a beer with George and then Fire Chief Andy Casper at a Knights of Columbus Hall on Polk Street. He was fun to be around, and the city loved him for it. Tragically, he was shot a week later. But his brand of progressive politics did not die with that gunshot. With his inspiration, San Francisco has become a ray of hope for many of the disenfranchised in our fractured society. That is George Moscone's true legacy in the city he loved. And he inspired many young people to participate in the political process to make us all better citizens and leaders.

Harvey Milk went from running a camera shop on Castro Street to being elected San Francisco Supervisor in 1977, becoming one of the first openly gay government officials anywhere in America. After naval service, he returned to New York for a variety of jobs. He moved to San Francisco in late 1972, where he soon found his voice as a leader and

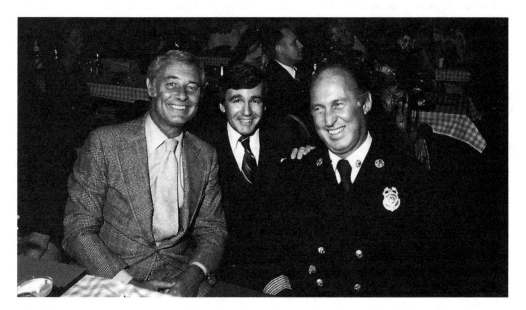

Figure 98.2. Mayor George Moscone, Brian Banmiller, and Fire Chief Andy Casper, November 1978.

activist in the gay community. After running and losing twice, he was ultimately elected Supervisor in 1977, broadening his appeal by working on issues from childcare to affordable housing to a civilian police review board.

My own experience with his outsized personality and broad appeal involved a Thursday Club luncheon held weekly in a slightly run-down building in the shadow of City Hall. This Thursday Club was an invitation-only event run by 25 of the city's more colorful characters, including well-known attorneys, politicians, firefighters, and police officers. Every Thursday, club organizers would invite a guest "speaker" who would not be informed that he/she was never going to be allowed to speak. Some would spend days preparing, only to be drowned out by clapping and booing.

Firefighter Leon Bruschera was famous for dropping the needle on a record played at high volume. His favorite was the sound of jet planes taking off. It was all great fun, except occasionally when the speaker did not get the joke and loudly complained, clearly to no avail.

Unfortunately, Harvey's soon-to-be killer did not get these jokes either. During one such raucous luncheon, Milk was invited to attend as a guest politician. I was also asked and sat directly across from Harvey at cafeteria-style tables complete with red checkerboard vinyl tablecloths. To my right sat Supervisor, former police officer and fireman Dan White. To my left sat Fire Fighter's Union President Jim Ferguson. Always the jokester, Bruschera loudly proclaimed that he was the chef for the day, and in honor of Harvey, he was not serving chicken, but meat instead. The audience (and Harvey) howled with laughter and banged the tables in salute. Supervisor Dan White stared ahead in cold silence with a scowl on his face.

Shocked by this, I asked Ferguson, "What's up with Dan?" Jim shrugged and said, "Dan is just screwed up—he's moody, and he doesn't really like Harvey." Dan, a conservative, was indeed frustrated with what he perceived as a breakdown in traditional values and a greater tolerance of homosexuality. In frustration, White eventually resigned as Supervisor. When the police union pushed him to return to the government, he went to City Hall to ask Mayor Moscone to re-appoint him. Slipping into an open window to avoid detection and armed with a 38 revolver, he confronted the Mayor who refused his request. In a rage, White shot Moscone four times, calmly re-loaded, and crossed the corridor to put five bullets into Harvey Milk's body before turning himself in at his old police station.

White's trial became known as the "Twinkie defense," as his lawyers claimed that their depressed client switched from a healthy diet to a high sugar one, causing his abnormal behavior and clouded thinking. The city reacted violently after the jury downgraded the crime from murder to manslaughter, rioting in the streets in what was called "The White Night Riots." Dan White served six years in prison, and after his 1985 release, he committed suicide.

Today Dan White is but an asterisk in history while George Moscone and Harvey Milk have the eternal love of the city, including high-profile buildings named after them, in particular, the new Terminal One at the San Francisco International airport, named after Harvey Milk. In July of 2016, the Navy announced it would name a yet-to-be constructed tanker the USNS Harvey Milk. In 2009 Sean Penn won an Academy Award as best actor for his portrayal of Harvey in the biopic "Milk."

Unfortunately, despite all the monuments and accolades honoring the sacrifice of these two dedicated public servants, as a nation, we seemingly continue to forget the lessons of our storied history, and violence against those who share different views continues to this day. Our educators need to motivate students with stories such as these if they are to step up and help heal our divided nation.

PHYSICIANS

I would be remiss not to mention my brush with death and how the medical community saved my life. I was suffering periodic attacks of acute gastritis, a painful stomach irritation that can mimic a heart attack. After a second episode, my gastroenterologist, Dr. Anderson Rowe, suggested he look down my esophagus while also performing his periodic colonoscopy. That decision saved my life, because he found cancer growing on my esophagus in time to cure the disease. I was fortunate to have world-renowned thoracic surgeon Dr. Wilson Tsai remove part of my esophagus and connected the rest to a shrunken stomach. What followed was months of chemotherapy, along with 11 related surgeries due to complications.

During this time, I kept my condition under wraps, although losing 40 pounds might have given friends some indication things were not all right on the health front. But I did not want to feed the rumor mill and take constant calls asking, "How are you feeling today?" With that behind me, I can now go public with a warning. Get tested. It can save your life. I am now cancer-free, thanks to some of the most dedicated doctors and nurses any patient could ever hope to have.

For more information about *Banmiller on Business* and the work of
Brian Banmiller, please see:
www.banmilleronbusiness.com.

Chapter 99
Gratitude
Bernard Churchill, MD, Pediatric Urologist

Gratitude is not only the greatest of virtues, but the parent of all others.
— *Cicero*

The purpose of this chapter is ambitious. We wish to convince you that adopting gratitude as your consistent attitude will improve every aspect of your health. This is, in essence, a prescription.

This commitment will require no added expense (you have already purchased this book), there are no contraindications, no complications, and you will see positive results soon after you begin. The long-term prognosis for your health is excellent, provided that your commitment remains consistent. One crucial caveat: Gratitude is only consistently effective with a lifelong pursuit of optimal health.

A life expectancy of 80 years is becoming more routine for most Americans, and during that time, your level of health will be challenged. At some point in your life, you may hear from your physician that you "have cancer," or "have suffered a pulmonary embolus," or "have experienced a minor stroke." It is at that precise moment that your years of gratitude practice will have the most significant value. Gratitude comes with a warning sticker, "This Condition is Quite Contagious."

WHY IS GRATITUDE SO IMPORTANT?

The term gratitude comes from the Latin word "gratus" meaning thankful or pleasing. Gratitude scholar Robert A. Emmonds explains, "All derivatives from this Latin root have to do with kindness, generousness, gifts, and the beauty of giving and receiving. Gratitude is pleasing. It feels good. Gratitude is also motivating. When we feel grateful, we are moved to share the goodness we have received from others." Gratitude is a three-step process:

1. Recognizing that one has obtained a positive outcome

2. Acknowledging that there is an external source responsible for this positive outcome

3. An appreciation of the motives of the donor.

The French summarize the same three-step process of gratitude in a slightly different way:

1. I recognize intellectually.

2. I acknowledge willingly.

3. I appreciate emotionally.

Only when all three steps come together is the appreciation of gratitude complete. Gratitude is different things to different people in different situations. Gratitude is an emotion, a mood, a moral virtue, a habit, a motive, a personality trait, and/or a coping mechanism. All of these definitions/mechanisms can play a valuable role in a positive approach to the ongoing challenges of life. Putting all this together, when you choose gratitude as the consistently dominant approach to life, you achieve the best personal benefit.

During the last 3,000 years of recorded history, there have been many memorable quotations that precisely define the nature, the power, and the significance of gratitude in interpersonal relationships, as well as its relevance and focus. The anonymous quote, "Gratitude turns what we have into enough," articulates the simplicity of gratitude. The power of gratitude to change individual lives is best characterized, in my opinion, by Willie Nelson, American musician and singer, activist, and folk philosopher, who stated, "When I started counting my blessings, my whole life turned around." The significance of gratitude in interpersonal relationships has been analyzed extensively by Summer Allen from the Templeton Foundation for Greater Good Science Center at the University of California, Berkeley. She concludes that gratitude is the "social glue that fortifies relationships between friends, families, and romantic partners and serves as the backbone of human society." The American author Cynthia Ozick found that, ironically. "We often take for granted the very things (or people) that most deserve our gratitude." So far, we have only discussed gratitude from the recipients' perspective. However, the donor perspective on gratitude is perhaps even more powerful. American poet, philosopher, and psychologist Eglin Arlington Robinson (1842–1910) articulated that, "There are two kinds of gratitude: the sudden kind we feel for what we take; the larger kind we feel for what we give."

Gratitude is inseparably joined to both "love" and "reverence." We are grateful for the people that we love (the memories and experiences). Gratitude is an essential ingredient of true love. Similarly, reverence and gratitude are inseparable. In my childhood, my parents both had great reverence for God, family, country, education, music, science, and basketball, which has given me an unwavering lifetime reverence and gratitude for these gifts.

Theological and Philosophical Wisdom of Gratitude

As long as people have believed in God, they have sought ways to express gratitude to God, the ultimate giver. Gratitude is the universal theological sentiment that almost all religions have tried to stimulate and maintain in their followers. Gratitude has been viewed as a prized human propensity for 4,000 years by Hindus, 3,000 years by Jews, for 2,500 years by Buddhists, for 2,000 years by Christians, for 1,400 years by Muslims, for 190 years by Mormons, and 176 years by the followers of the Baha'i faith. The common theme for prayer in almost all religions can be summarized in five words, "Thank You, God, for everything." The German theologian Karl Barth once said that the primary human response to God is not fear, not guilt, but thanksgiving. In Judaism, the crucial blessing in the central thrice-daily prayer, the "Amidah," is called "Modim," which translates to "We give thanks to You." Buddha presents a layered logical approach to theological gratitude: "Let us rise up and be thankful, for if we did not learn a lot today, at least we learned a little, and if we did not learn a little, at least we did not get sick, and if we got sick, at least we did not die, so let us all be thankful." Martin Luther referred to gratitude as "the basic Christian attitude." Others have referred to gratitude as "the heart of the gospel." The Eucharist, meaning "thanks" in Greek, is a Christian rite, which is a sacrament in the Catholic, Orthodox, and Anglican churches and an ordinance in others.

According to the New Testament, the rite was first performed by Jesus Christ at the Last Supper. Through the Eucharist, Christians remember and give thanks for Christ's sacrifice of himself on the Cross. The Pillar of Islam motivates believers to offer prayers of gratitude to God five times per day. Muslims also believe that fasting during the month of Ramadan puts themselves in a state of gratitude to God. Many theologians would agree with Cicero that gratitude is the parent of all other virtues. A "virtue" can be simply defined as "behavior of high moral standard." A list of virtues will vary somewhat with each religion, but the list generally includes humility, kindness, patience, diligence, charity, temperance, and chastity. A life inspired by gratitude will minimize sin as defined as a transgression of divine law. The seven deadly sins listed by Pope Gregory in 590 AD are just as detrimental to your health today as they were at that time. These include pride, greed, wrath (anger), envy, lust, gluttony, and sloth. All of these "sins" represent an irrational excess of normally healthy emotions and physiologic functions. Virtually all theologians agree we have free choice in these matters. For instance, substance and/or behavioral addiction is always preceded by inappropriate, excessive, and binge indulgence. Recent tabulations of global religious populations have listed younger "unaffiliated or areligious" as the third-largest group after Christianity and Islam. This group is also the fastest growing. The unaffiliated group subdivides into three smaller groups, including atheists, agnostics, and individuals who describe themselves as being "spiritual but not formally religious." This particular segment of the population generally embraces gratitude, especially the nondenominational American holiday of Thanksgiving, which is progressively growing in popularity. This group has been analyzed recently by author Tara Isabella Burton, who labels them as the

"Religiously Remixed." She comments that they "prioritize intuitional spirituality over institutional religion." She further describes their popularity as the "current craze for customized spirituality."

The study of gratitude and related virtues has long been a significant focus for philosophers. These very wise individuals have much to teach us about the pursuit of health. In 384 BC, Aristotle defined virtue as "a disposition to behave in the right manner, as a meeting between extreme deficiency and excess, both of which are vices." In other words, Aristotle strongly advocates moderation. Aristotle also felt that "we learn more moral virtue by habit and practice than by reasoning and instruction." His wisdom applies to our current use and abuse of food, alcohol, sex, drugs, and gambling. Confucius, the significant Chinese philosopher (551 BC–479 BC), had a unique version of the gratitude theme. He stressed two virtues as most important, which he called "Jen and Li." Jen translates as "benevolent concern for one's fellow men," and Li is a combination of manners, ritual, behavior, and etiquette. Scottish philosopher David Hume (1711–1776) stressed the negative aspects of ingratitude: "Of all the crimes that human creatures are capable of committing, the most horrid and unnatural is ingratitude." The American television fictional cartoon character Bart Simpson personified ingratitude when offering a Thanksgiving dinner blessing: "Dear God, we paid for all the stuff ourselves, so thanks for nothing." Professor Robert Emmons from the University of California, Davis, states that "Gratitude is an approach to life that can be freely chosen for oneself. It does not depend on objective life circumstances."

THE NEW SCIENCE OF GRATITUDE

Despite significant theological and philosophical acclaim, gratitude has only recently, in the last 30 to 40 years, been the subject of serious scientific study. Three developments have been responsible for this new scientific interest: the development of functional Magnetic Resonance Imaging (fMRI) to study brain function, the enlargement of the focus of psychology from negative subjects such as anxiety and depression to include "positive psychological" subjects such as gratitude, and the founding of innovative philanthropic funding agencies such as the John Templeton Foundation at the University of California, Berkeley.

Evolutionary biologists have also looked at gratitude and found that animals such as fish and birds engage in "reciprocal altruism" activities. The best example of this is the observation that chimpanzees are more likely to share food with a fellow chimpanzee who has previously groomed them. Studies comparing gratitude in fraternal and identical twins have shown that there is a genetic component to gratitude. The CD38 gene, which is involved in the excretion of the hormone oxytocin (the love hormone), is responsible.

Neurophysiologists using fMRI studies have shown increased brain activity in the prefrontal and anterior cingulate cortex in volunteer human subjects experiencing gratitude. More importantly, neurophysiologists have shown that gratitude changes the brain in a way that orientates people to feel even more rewarded when other people benefit. Psychologists have developed two methods to quantitate a level of gratitude: the Transpersonal Gratitude Scale (TGS) and the Multi-Component Gratitude Measure (MCGM). Relevant psychological studies have shown that there is an inverse relationship between gratitude on one hand and envy, materialism, narcissism, and cynicism on the other. As the negative parameters rise, gratitude is more difficult to establish, and conversely, as gratitude increases, these four negative psychological attributes diminish.

How Do I Improve My Personal Gratitude Skills?

The simple answer to this question is to utilize the "Carnegie Hall Methodology." This method was articulated by an unnamed New York City philosopher/cabdriver, who answered a passenger who asked him, "How do I get to Carnegie Hall?" with the following answer, "Commitment, practice, and more practice." This formula is the only way to master a musical instrument and is equally applicable to improving your gratitude skills. The key to practicing gratitude skills is to begin. Make a list of the five most important people in your life and think of ways that you can express your gratitude to them.

 "I love you" and "thank you" are always very useful, but "I am so grateful that we have had the last 20 years together" will also work. If you are religious, then "we feel very blessed to have your family as neighbors" solves many problems. Try to be sincerely grateful for someone or something daily. After you have decided on a particular focus for your gratitude, remember the words of William Arthur Ward, American columnist and writer, who stated that "Feeling gratitude and not expressing it is like wrapping a present and not giving it." Doing volunteer work is a beautiful, organized way of expressing gratitude. You will also meet many very nice people in "the volunteer environment." Charitable donations are, of course, a marvelous expression of gratitude. Contributions can be in the form of charity, which deals more with immediate needs, whereas philanthropy is a more strategic, long-term process. The United States is one of the most generous countries in the world, with total donations of $390 billion in 2016, which was approximately 2% of the gross domestic product.

I recommend the appreciation of flora, fauna, and the natural wonders of our beautiful planet to enhance gratitude. Music therapy, both playing and listening, is a multifaceted interpersonal process that is of proven value in improving health. Dance therapy also improves intellectual, emotional, and general fitness as well as motor function.

Healthy Living with Yourself

As a wise philosopher (my mother-in-law Rose Shandro) has pointed out, "Health is your greatest asset." Healthy living is a complex subject covered by libraries full of books. Seeking regular periodic times of serenity and tranquility is an excellent place to start living successfully with yourself. This involves slowing down the thought processes, letting go of negativity, and finding order in the face of chaos. Both religious prayer and mindful meditation are proven interventions in this area, and gratitude plays a central role in both processes. Combining serenity with regular outdoor exercise is of proven value. Melody Beattie, an American author of self-help books for codependent relationships, suggests that "Gratitude makes sense of our past, brings peace for today, and creates a vision for tomorrow." Scientific evidence suggests that the cultivation of gratitude is associated with increased life satisfaction, optimism, subjective well-being, positive affect, and happiness. Longitudinal studies have found that gratitude is associated over time with the growth of relatedness and autonomy, which are two basic psychological needs. Evidence suggests that gratitude may "broaden and build positive emotions and also that gratitude may combat the negative emotional processes that underpin depression, unhappiness, and burnout." Gratitude is a proven method of motivating self-improvement. Evidence also suggests that gratitude is important in preventing and treating substance and behavioral abuse. Gratitude may be the key ingredient in coping with major life challenges such as potentially lethal disease, major financial distress, and the demise of relatives and friends. Regular group gratitude practices, such as religious services, are a statistically proven method of reducing the incidence of suicide. Swiss Reform theologian Karl Barth explained how to become a contagious joy giver by stating that "Joy is the simplest form of gratitude."

Healthy Living with Your Family and Creating an Enduring Partnership

As a pediatric physician, I cannot overemphasize the importance of gratitude in establishing a healthy family environment. Gratitude within the family is optimally based on gratitude between partners. Gratitude scholars have developed a straightforward but very effective method of searching for a marital partner, building a relationship, and sustaining the bond together for a long duration called "find, remind, and bind."

- The "find" aspect means identifying people who are good candidates for a thoughtful, graceful relationship.

- It is beneficial to "remind" each other of the blessing and goodness of the existing relationship.

- Allow mutual gratitude to "bind" the partners together for a lifetime.

Maria Shriver had wise words to say about parenting: "At work, you are replaceable, but as a parent, you are irreplaceable." Parenting is improved by remembering words of William James, American philosopher, and psychologist, who said, "The deepest craving of human nature is to be appreciated." Successful incorporation of gratitude into daily life involves simplicity and consistency. A simple formula for implementing family gratitude, modified from John F. Kennedy's inaugural address: "Ask not what your loved ones can do for you, but what you can do for your loved ones." President Kennedy also stated that, "As we express our gratitude, we must never forget, the highest appreciation is not to utter words, but to live by them." As I was growing up my father was involved in two movements with similar slogan: "the family that prays together stays together" and "the family that plays together also stays together." This type of movement is even more critical in our time than it was in the 1950s.

Gratitude-Based Exercise

In the hunter-gatherer age, to survive, humans needed to be able to run fast, increase their cardiac output and tissue perfusion, significantly increase their oxygen consumption, increase muscle flexibility and strength, and increase mental alertness. In the 1800s between 80% and 90% of the U.S. population was directly involved in the robust personal physical activity of farming, without machine implements. The 1900s saw the progressive growth of tractors, automobiles, mass transit, elevators, television sets, and personal sloth. "Use it or lose it" is one of the essential maxims in maintaining and improving muscle, cardiovascular, respiratory, and cerebral efficiency. It is challenging to lose weight without combining diet *and* exercise. As stated 1,500 years ago, gluttony and slothfulness are truly "deadly" sins. Gratitude for physical ability at almost any level is the beginning point of any exercise program. You can develop a regular customized exercise plan for virtually any age and level of ability. Simple walking, hiking, cycling, resistance-band training, and simple stretching are all very inexpensive and highly effective in achieving optimal fitness.

Yoga is supported by 5,000 years of Indian Vedic spiritual and ascetic wisdom, which underlie a combination of simple meditation, breath control measures, and the adoption of specific body postures. Medical evidence and consensus have clearly confirmed that well-supervised yoga improves general wellness by relieving stress, promoting good health habits, enhancing flexibility, and improving mental and emotional status. Tai chi is an ancient Chinese art practiced as defense training known for its health benefits. It also combines meditation and physical activity and is highly recommended. Stretching is a simple, gentle activity that can be done by anyone, anywhere, anytime, and is particularly useful when it is combined with meditation or prayer.

Gratitude-Based Diet and Nutrition

Jamestown, the first English settlement in the United States, was established in 1607. Food supply was an immense problem right from the beginning, for three reasons: the landing in 1607 was too late to plant crops, most of the settlers had few agricultural skills, and the unbroken land presented unique challenges to cultivation. By 1610 about 80% of the settlers had died, primarily from starvation. The pilgrims of Plymouth, Massachusetts, celebrated the first Thanksgiving in 1621 to commemorate their first successful harvest in the New World. Both the Jamestown settlers and the Plymouth pilgrims had immense gratitude for an adequate supply of food. Fast forward to our era, when 36.2% American adults and 17% of American children are obese (2016 statistics). The American adult obesity rate is 5.8 times greater than China's, 7.7 times greater than South Korea's, and an almost unbelievable 8.8 times greater than Japan's. The National Institutes of Health estimates that obesity causes 300,000 preventable American deaths per year. Another startling statistic is that approximately one-third of the American food supply is wasted. Somehow in the last 400 years, our national sense of gratitude for a healthy balanced diet has been damaged. Eating moderate amounts of many different types of unprocessed fruits and vegetables, which are naturally composed of fiber and complex carbohydrates, is the best way of slowly, gently raising blood sugar and relieving hunger. Consuming water without added sugar and/or alcohol is the best way to satisfy thirst. Sustained weight loss is rarely achieved without the combination of diet and exercise. Portion sizes in many American restaurants are preposterously large. Often there is more than enough for two people to have a generous meal. Gratitude-based diet is perhaps best explained by a Native American prayer, "We thank the Great Spirit for the resources that made this food possible, We thank the Earth Mother for producing it, And we thank all those who labored to bring it to us, Made the wholesomeness of the food before us Bring out the wholesomeness of the spirit within us."

Gratitude and the Prevention of Bad Habits

Addiction is a brain disorder characterized by compulsive engagement in rewarding stimuli, despite adverse consequences. Addictions include substances such as food, nicotine, alcohol, cannabis, opioids, and psychostimulants, and behavior such as sex and gambling. The cumulative social consequences of addiction are catastrophic. The economic costs are higher than those of diabetes and cancer combined. Initiating addictive behavior in adolescence dramatically increases the likelihood of all types of addiction. For this reason, the recent widespread growth of vaping electronic cigarettes amongst teenage and preteen individuals is a particularly treacherous development.

In 1932 American theologian Reinhold Niebuhr composed a wonderful prayer, which subsequently became known as the "Serenity Prayer." It was later adopted and publicized by Alcoholics Anonymous who also incorporated it in their twelve-step recovery program. It reads like this:

"God, grant me the serenity to accept the things I cannot change, the courage to change the things I can, and the wisdom to know the difference."

This marvelous prayer, which is inspirational and instructive to a broad spectrum of society, has become a "nondenominational classic." It is not only a marvelous formula for the treatment of known addiction, but can also be used as a prescription for the prevention of addiction in susceptible individuals. This prayer incorporates three of the virtues we have been discussing: serenity, courage, and wisdom. The prayer also indicates that we can use these three virtues to freely choose the right course of behavior, the one that will give us the greatest source of future personal gratitude.

FINAL THOUGHTS

Develop a deeper appreciation for life; do not take things for granted. This is the philosophy that will best protect your health. Try the following simple 30-second exercise at least once a day. Sit quietly, in a relaxed fashion, and take three slow breaths in through your nose and out through your mouth. Then take three additional breaths, and with each exhalation whisper, "Thank you." Each day think of three people, things, or memories for which you are particularly grateful.

For information on the professional work and career of Dr. Churchill, please see:
www.uclahealth.org/urology/bernard-churchill.

Chapter 100
Leaving a Legacy
Larry Bienati, MBA, PhD,
Business Consultant & Professor

What you leave behind is not what is engraved in stone monuments,
but what is woven into the lives of others.
— Pericles

Defining your hero's journey. You have almost reached the final chapter in this journey of self-discovery. At this point, you may be wondering, where do I go from here? Is there a roadmap I can follow? How do I start my own personal transformation and write the next chapter of my hero's journey?

Given the pace of society and the information overload we all experience on a daily basis, it takes serious discipline to focus and translate ideas into action. However, this is not the kind of a book in which you will find a cookie-cutter formula to your future. Your discoveries are going to be personal and unique, requiring careful thought to develop an implementation strategy for the next phase of your life.

CHARTING YOUR ROADMAP

My goal is to provide a synthesis, ideas for developing your own plan, a vision that could serve as a catalyst for your continued personal exploration. It is time for action, time to write the next chapter in your journey.

There are so many examples in human history across cultures, races, and disciplines of individuals whose personal legacies have changed the world. These men have made tough choices, sacrificed a great deal, overcome enormous adversity, but never lost sight of a compelling vision to improve the quality and meaning of life for others and for generations to come. Siddhartha Gautama (who became known as the Buddha) walked away from his position as king, leaving behind power, wealth, his country, his young wife, and newly born child to find a way to alleviate human suffering, and founded Buddhism. Dr. Martin Luther King, Jr., lost his life in pursuit of his vision for racial equality. Dr. King reminded us that "the ultimate measure of a man is not where he stands in moments of comfort and convenience, but where he stands in times of challenge and controversy." The sacrifices of Nelson Mandela, the Kennedys, and so many others have improved the quality of life for generations to come. Steven Jobs overcame many personal life challenges to create one of the world's great companies, Apple, and inspired us to "Think different." The profound generosity that Bill and Melinda Gates have shown in the Gates Foundation by sharing their wealth for socially noble purposes has inspired others, including Warren Buffett and Mark Zuckerberg.

Yet there are those whose greed has been used for their own selfish pursuits and injured so many lives. I need not mention them, as you see their fall from grace daily in the media. Those legacies shall die with their personal self-interest at the detriment of others.

Let us also consider the legacy of ordinary people who are leaders in their own right. Success in life and personal achievement are never measured in money. The numbers of unhappy wealthy people are legion, also filling the nightly news. I have personally coached, mentored, and re-aligned a substantial number of affluent clients, people who chose a job for money, rather than for their passion or their skillset. As a result, in their quest for the almighty dollar, they lost relationships, impacted their family's wellbeing, and suffered lack of meaning and purpose in their life.

Ordinary heroes, however, can measure their legacy's success in many diverse ways—there is no one size that fits all. A life well lived can be achieved as a good parent, teacher, caregiver, essential worker, veteran, and in any of the other countless roles that our society needs in order to function well for all of us.

Often a true legacy is measured by showing up for work each day, working hard, striving to make a living, to better one's family and the greater society. It is time to praise and raise up the men who every day strive to do the right thing in service of others. These ordinary heroes have an unswerving commitment to maintain a sense of ethics, integrity, empathy, and altruism.

One of the heroes I have had the honor of working with is Bob Weiss, who grew up on a farm in rural Pennsylvania. Bob attended the University of Scranton, was called to serve our country in Vietnam, and was decorated for his service. He met the love of his life while in college, and they raised a wonderful family together. Bob was a CPA and worked hard, ascending to successful roles in a number of respected firms. When I met Bob, he was CEO of the Cooper Companies, Inc., a publicly held S & P 500 company, and he forever changed my life by his example.

Here was a CEO who believed that the most important asset in any organization are its people. He also believed that people and profit are not mutually exclusive, that both can exist in harmony through respectful, authentic, and engaged leadership. He led a company of more than 10,000 employees worldwide and over $2 billion in sales. He led from the front and always modeled the core values of the company in his personal actions. First in the office, and last to *leave each day, he would never ask anyone to perform a task that he himself would not do. He engaged his employees at all levels through personal attention and tireless effort, logging over two million air miles in his time as CEO. By serving as a role model, he inspired his employees to come to work each day and give their personal best.*

Bob believed that all employees deserved work-life balance and always emphasized the importance of balancing work responsibilities with quality time with our families, while giving back to the community where we live. He also modeled the path to wellness with his own personal transformation in mind, body, and spirit. The results in his health and wellbeing were profound. Building on what he had learned from personal experience, he became a pioneer in the employee wellness movement and invested millions of dollars in creating employee wellness programs across the globe. He would later be recognized as one of the most admired CEOs in the San Francisco Bay Area, among other accolades. He was known for his authentic, caring, and proven leadership, for his commitment to people, and for astounding financial success in his ten-year leadership at Cooper.

Bob was humble, engaging, a good listener, someone who always strived to bring out the best in people. He was selfless in his philanthropy to many noble institutions. Bob did it right. He balanced his scorecard of life by ensuring alignment with his profession, with his family, in his relationships, and through a personal commitment to improve the quality of life for others, with an impact on thousands of people. His goal was not to be CEO of one of the more admired companies in America. He simply strived to always do the right thing, and I had the honor of working side by side with this extraordinary hero.

Bob exemplifies a leader who was not driven by greed, but rather one who felt compelled to place the needs of others above self for the greater good of society. At their best, these men are also living role models of the personal transformation involved in optimizing personal health. These stories amplify what it means to ensure a balanced life, perpetuating an enduring legacy in service to others.

As we go to press, Bob is hiking the mountains and valleys around Donner Pass, first with one of his sons and then with the other, clocking five to six miles a day, and planning the development of a wilderness land trust in that area of northern California.

Every day I meet these extraordinary heroes who inspire me as well: the trash collector, the frontline worker, that toll collector at the Bay Bridge, our first responders, our front, line medical personnel, the field technician, the delivery driver, the single parent, that awesome father balancing his professional needs with time devoted to his children, and many others. Are you ready to identify the unique elements you contribute, as you define and perfect your own legacy? Let's build your roadmap!

PASSION AND PURPOSE

Wearing a number of hats over the years as professor, consultant, company leader, executive coach, and board member, I have noticed that certain unique qualities are characteristic of everyday heroes. Often these heroes are ordinary people doing extraordinary things. Passion and purpose are qualities that many of these heroes seem to share in some measure. As you ponder your own legacy statement, I encourage you to begin with a process of personal discovery.

Finding Your Passion. Nelson Mandela often referred to following one's passion as "oxygen for the soul." Yet most men do not land the job of their dreams from the start. Their initial career is often a means to an end. Looking back, you were probably willing to make some sacrifices in the short term towards a long-term vision of a position where all your talents could be unleashed, where you could find a greater depth of satisfaction in your work.

When we find our passion, we are in the harmonic flow of personal happiness. That positive energy spills into all aspects of our life and relationships. It also has profound health benefits.

Perhaps you are still working your way through your own personal discovery, or maybe you found your First Act and are now at a turning point, ready for the second. Think about the things you love to do and what interests you when you are in those moments, when you are in the zone of happiness and have everything in balance. I often suggest people seeking their passion to try this exercise. On a sheet of paper write down the five things you love to do that ignite your passion. Then, across the page write down the last time you did any of them. Sadly, many people cannot complete the exercise, so it becomes a wake-up call, a signal that they need to infuse more of their life with their passion, to better use their talents, and to act on pursuits that hold significance for them. At this point in your life, you may have choices and a level of understanding that you did not have in the past.

Finding Your Purpose. What is your "why" of existence? How do you wish to be remembered? It is time for you to create your own personal mission statement, your perspective on how you measure a life well-lived. I am often inspired by the vision expressed in *Man's Search for Meaning* by Victor Frankl, one of the greatest books every written. This is the account of a psychiatrist who survived the horror of the Nazi concentration camps by never losing site of a compelling vision for his future. He shares his story of how he survived the atrocities of Auschwitz and was compelled to learn from the experience. He realized that there is great power in hope, in believing that, in life, we "all have something significant yet to do."

Persistent Optimist. The power of hope can be inspiring and motivating. There is evidence that a compelling vision of the future, with a focus on overcoming obstacles to a greater purpose, has enabled many to survive and prevail over the toughest of life events.

Success is not a linear proposition. Consider yourself a survivor at this point. You have already encountered speed bumps along the way. Yet periodically we all need reminding that we must never lose sight of our sense of purpose. It is like a rope across a class four river that will enable you to balance the turbulence. There is great power in finding the good, in building on your strengths, and in seeking the higher ground in relationships and life challenges. This is where your emotional intelligence acumen will help you surmount adversity and stay true to your life vision.

Valuing People. Never lose sight of the power of being an authentic, open, honest, humble, and caring person. Learn from Dale Carnegie the importance of winning friends and building enduring relationships. My Sicilian mother raised me to live by core values in our family's legacy, and I consider the most important of these: "the heart that gives, gathers." We may also call this karma. The power of relationships and bringing out the best in people and in any situation is a rare and valuable quality in any hero's journey.

Perspective in Life. Perspective is an essential ingredient in creating a balanced life, the "secret sauce" that is central to how you are going to consciously define the next phase of your life. Your legacy statement is an opportunity to build perspective at this juncture. Life perspective is not only the way we see life, but also the way we live it, reflected in our personal experiences and our relationships. Allow your inner passion to define your continued purpose. Remain a persistent optimist in authentic service to others.

Ultimately it is your relationships with the people around you that define your quality of life. Albert Pine said, "What we do for ourselves dies within us; what we do for others' lives on forever." This is ultimately the mantra of everyday heroes.

WHAT IS YOUR LEGACY?

This idea of legacy is a term we often apply to a life well lived, a person who has served as the inspiration for change, who makes the world a better place by their presence and the impact they have on others.

At this moment, what would people say about you if they were writing you a testimonial for your retirement party (as you prepare to retire young, assume a role in a rising start-up, or take the job of your dreams). How would they describe your life and what it has meant to others, especially to the people you care about most deeply?

Would they say that you are a solid, authentic guy, someone who truly cares, who is willing to put service to others above self-interest, someone who loves his kids, is an excellent provider and a quality human being? Would they point out that you have integrity, that you're true to your word, the first one people turn to when they need someone they can count on, a stand-up guy they can rely on to always do the right thing?

THE FOUR QUADRANTS OF PERSONAL TRANSFORMATION

Quadrant One—Personal Health. The first quadrant begins with your health. You will not be worth much to your family, friends, or anyone else you care about if you do not get that "check-up from your neck-up." Without a commitment to your health and personal care your life cannot flourish. Start by asking vital questions. What steps do I need to take, starting today, to optimizing my own health? By now, you have identified some resources in the book that are relevant to you, and opportunities for improvement so you can flourish. The Key Take Aways at the end of each chapter and the algorithms available online offer templates for building you own personal optimization plan.

Quadrant Two—Spirituality or Faith. This quadrant may not apply to everyone, but I would be remiss to not call it out. Many men have defining core values that serve as a compass by which they wish to lead their lives. For some, faith is at the center of their guiding principles. Applying the tenets of faith or spirituality can provide the basis for a life well-lived. Affirm that connection as a gift. On the other hand, it is surprisingly easy to lose our way in the scheme of life events. If you feel that your faith or spirituality needs a reboot, this might be a good opportunity to revisit the question. This does not apply to everyone, so use what is relevant to you here.

Quadrant Three—Family and Relationships. As men, we are often tasked with being the breadwinner. In our quest to be the provider, we may lose sight of the importance of being there for our children and others who need our time, support, and authentic care.

Looking back, too many men feel misunderstood or unappreciated. Men felt they were making sacrifices to better the life of their families. They wanted to be more present and engaged, but work pressures, travel, and career advancement required tradeoffs. At the core, most men felt their efforts were always about service to others, above their own self-interest. Their needs, happiness, and aspirations often ended up on the back burner so others could have a better life. While it may not have been understood and appreciated, you knew you were giving your family and those important in your life "the roots and wings" for a better life. It is never too late. As you refine quadrant three, you need to have that conversation with your partner, with your children, and with others in important

Profile Questions

- What are your priorities in life at this time?

- What are your guiding principles?

- Describe two role models in your life. What characteristics and qualities do/did they hold? How have they impacted your life? These individuals can be from any time span during your life.

- Was there a time in your life when you were at your personal best and everything just seemed to be in a natural flow? What were you doing? What made it memorable?

- What do you like best (and least) about your job, if applicable? If you are retired, or semi-retired, what do you like best and least about how you spend your days?

- What talents do you have that you want to see unleashed again?

- At the present time, if you were to change one thing of significant impact in your professional career, or in your life, what would it be?

- What goals have you yet to achieve personally or professionally? How will they be measured?

- How can you best contribute to your community and to the world with your talents and interests?

- Where do you see yourself in three years? What will you be doing and where? Where do you see yourself in seven years? At that point, what will you be doing and where will you be?

Writing a powerful vision statement. An effective tool for building on the profile you have developed is to capture your vision in writing. Vision statements do not need to be long. In fact, most can be written in several sentences. Focusing on a few key words will help you transform your values into a succinct summary. The vision often extends into the future.

A solid vision creates commitment. It shows evidence of understanding, realism, and risk. A vision exudes hope and aspirations. Here, rather than focusing simply on what you have accomplished, create a vision of your next act.

relationships to retool this very important quadrant in your personal legacy statement (whether these issues are in the past, the present, or looming in the future for you).

Quadrant Four—Passion Unleashed. This quadrant emphasizes personal transformation, with an emphasis on meaning and, ultimately, on happiness. As Blum once said, "As long as you believe what you are doing is meaningful, you can cut through the fear and exhaustion and take the next step." For most of us, initially we were not working in the job or profession of our dreams. We may have pursued education, certification, employment, and life experiences as a means to end, working toward a distant personal mission, and deferring happiness. In the early days we needed to keep the lights on, pay the mortgage, ensure that the kids were getting a good education, provide for savings, and make sure we were comfortable and prepared for contingencies.

Quadrant four cannot be done alone, especially if you have a partner, children, or other close relationships. The conversation and questions you will need to address require debate, feedback, and a collaborative outcome. This is a way to hold everyone accountable for success.

Fast Forward: Are You Ready? Are you willing to embrace some of the ideas offered in the chapters, the algorithms, and the prescriptions provided by the thought leaders you have met in this book to build the blueprint for healthy, productive longevity? Are you willing to refine your personal vision statement? As Admiral William Halsey often stated when addressing his troops, "There are no great men; there are only great challenges, which ordinary men like you and me are forced by circumstances to meet."

So, it is your time to rise to the challenge of optimizing your manhood, seizing the profound words of the admiral? You have the blueprint for a better life. The next chapter belongs to you. Good luck on your journey as you leave an enduring legacy to better our world!

For more information on the teaching and consulting services of Larry Bienati, please see: www.Bienati.com.

Chapter 101
The Journey Continues
Judson Brandeis, MD, Author

You are the hero of your own story.
— Joseph Campbell

My call to adventure came in the form of an article in the *Urology Times* on new technology for erectile dysfunction. Always wanting to be on the leading edge of medical innovation and patient care, I left the comfort of my office in Walnut Creek, California, and flew to Miami to attend a weekend training. By the end of the second day, I was so excited that I purchased a Shockwave machine. And as soon as I returned to my office, I began using it to treat twenty of my most-trusted patients—and myself.

The results were so successful that my patients told their friends, who told their friends, and within a few months, I'd built a private-pay sexual medicine center right next to my urology group practice, complete with a masculine-themed office. Unfortunately, my professional partners were less-than-completely supportive of my new initiative. Whereas I had hoped that the additional income from the men's health center would help our group remain independent, they were hoping to be purchased by the local hospital and become employees. Although we continued the busy pace of private practice, tension continued to mount as our goals diverged.

A few months later, I discovered that my business email no longer worked. And the next morning, when I went in to work, the office manager handed me a one-page letter informing me that I had been terminated and demanding that I immediately leave the building (of which I was part owner!).

To say that I was stunned doesn't begin to describe what I felt. I had worked in this practice for seventeen years and attracted thousands of patients. It was the only job I'd had since finishing my residency at UCLA in 2001. My patients and the local medical community were my professional life. Yet literally overnight, I had nowhere to go, no patients to see, and no career.

Confused and furious, I weighed my options. I could leave the community and start from scratch in another location, but such a move would take my four children out of the schools where they were thriving. I could join Kaiser or another HMO, but those jobs are scarce, and I like being my own boss. Or I could start a solo practice. However, these days, practicing insurance-based urology requires a group of physicians to improve contracts and cover patients when you're unavailable. Being entrepreneurial (my wife and I had already started a supplement business called AFFIRM Science), I decided to take a chance and build out the private-pay, male sexual medicine and rejuvenation practice that I'd launched before my nightmare began.

But my former partners did everything they could to undermine my efforts. They blocked access to my patients (about 4,000 of them!), refused to pay me money they owed me, and more. Backed into a corner, I had no choice but to go to court. Thus began my hero's journey.

Over the next two years, I built a private-pay medical practice, expanded my men's health supplement company, and fought two David-vs.-Goliath lawsuits against my former partners' corporation, their insurance company, and their army of lawyers, all the while trying to be a good husband and father to four teenagers.

Renting a new medical office brought me into contact with Florence Fang former owner of the *San Francisco Examiner*. Florence is a self-made businesswoman, publisher, and philanthropist active in the San Francisco area. Her story of triumph over hardship inspired me to push forward on my own journey.

Just when things were starting to look up, COVID-19 hit, and I had to close my new medical practice for two months. Discouraged and still fighting two lawsuits, I read an article in the *Wall Street Journal* that advised, "If you don't emerge from COVID with a new skill or a new product, you will be behind when the pandemic ends." At that moment, I came up with the idea of writing a book to help men, especially those who work hard to support their families, their employees, and their community. Many of these men are reluctant to ask for help and behave as if they're indestructible, believing that it's a sign of weakness for men to go to the doctor or a therapist, reaching out only when something breaks. I wanted to write a book for men about prevention and early intervention to help men avoid burnout, premature aging, and premature death in their 40s, 50s, and 60s.

While I was writing and organizing this book, I was also building my medical practice (BrandeisMD), participating in clinical research trials, and growing AFFIRM Science. And, of course, the litigation was always present.

After two stressful years, I was victorious in both of my lawsuits! Feeling vindicated but bitter, I remembered the old quote: "A diamond is a chunk of coal that did well under pressure." I'd learned hard lessons about protecting myself and my family, and my children had endured the whole process and learned about facing adversity. And the result of all that pressure and pain was a unique medical practice where men can be comfortable talking about very uncomfortable things. I perform clinical research that improves men's quality of life, and I educate men on building healthier and more fulfilling lives.

This final chapter marks the end of a journey for me and the beginning of a new one. What I hope you take away from my journey is that everyone has problems and hardship, regardless of how things might look to others. I hope that *The 21st Century Man* has inspired you to take better care of your entire self. It's my gift to you, so that you can be of service to yourself and others.

A hero is someone who has given his or her life to something bigger than oneself.
— Joseph Campbell

For more information about the work and services of Dr. Brandeis, please see:
BrandeisMD.com
TheTwentyFirstCenturyMan.com
www.AFFIRMScience.com
www.mensmedicalstore.com.

Acknowledgements

All we have to decide is what to do with the time that is given to us

— JRR Tolkein

Our time on earth is finite, and our decisions on how to spend it show what we value. Writing a book like The 21ˢᵗ Century Man took an enormous amount of my time. Precious hours away from the people I truly care about, and sacrificing self-care to pursue a book that would help thousands of men I have never met.

My wife supported my vision during the writing process and helped me to create the time I needed to focus on the content and coordination. Our deep and personal conversations over our 20-year marriage helped to better define the emotional and spiritual aspects of my thinking on mid-life. I value our loving partnership and commitment to each other. She has also raised our four amazing children. I appreciate the sacrifices my children made while I was writing the book, and having a father whose specialty was sexual medicine. Helping them grow up has been an honor and an incredible learning experience.

I want to thank the thousands of patients I have cared for over the past 25 years, serving as their physician and in some cases, as their surgeon. I have learned so much from each of you and that has been an important part of my growth as a professional. It is truly a privilege to be a physician and play such a pivotal role in another person's life. I am especially grateful to the men at BrandeisMD who served in focus groups as informal advisors during this part of my personal journey.

My teachers along the way are too numerous to count. Among those who truly stand out:

- Don Scott, my high school track coach, biology teacher, and friend
- David Josephson, Music Professor at Brown University
- Dr. Mohamed Sayegh, Nephrology Professor, Harvard Medical School
- The outstanding Medical School faculty at Vanderbilt University
- The faculty of the Department of Urology at UCLA, especially Mark Litwin, Robert Reiter, Arie Belldegrun, Carrol Bennett, Shlomo Raz, R.B. Smith, Jean DeKernion, Bill Aronson, Rick Ehrlich, and Bernard Churchill
- Dan Horowitz, my attorney, friend and advisor

I also want to thank my parents for supporting my educational journey and my in-laws for being there for my children when being a doctor intruded on me spending time with my children.

> I greatly appreciate the input and fellowship of my managing and development editor, Nancy Faass and of Mark Weiman, our brilliant book designer, who were essential in assisting me in my first attempt at writing a book. Nancy, Mark, Armin Brott, Jerry Stine, Christopher Bernard, and George Foster have been the dream team to help me to make this book the best it could be.

Finally, I thank my chapter contributors, many of whom are friends and colleagues from medical school, residency, and private practice. I appreciate your expertise, fellowship, and support in making this an important contribution for men and the people who care about them.

Contributors

Judson Brandeis, MD, is a board-certified urologist who currently practices men's health and sexual medicine in Northern California. Dr. Brandeis attended Brown University, Vanderbilt Medical School, and received a Howard Hughes Medical Institute Research Award for his year of transplantation immunology research at Harvard Medical School. He completed two years of general surgical training and four years of urology residency at UCLA Medical Center and served as Chief of Urology at John Muir Hospital and at Hill Physicians from 2012 to 2018. Dr. Brandeis has been a pioneer in surgical robotics, Greenlight Laser, and MRI prostate biopsy.

At BrandeisMD, he performs clinical research using shockwave therapy, platelet-rich plasma, high-intensity focused electromagnetic waves, microvascular ultrasound, and nutritional supplements for conditions such as sexual dysfunction and Peyronie's disease. Dr. Brandeis is on the Board of Advisors for BioTE, GAINSWave, and BTL. He is the CEO of AFFIRM Science, which creates nutritional supplements based on current scientific data, formulating products that include AFFIRM, PreLONG, SupporT, and SPUNK. Dr. Brandeis is a member in good standing of the American Urologic Association, the Sexual Medicine Society of North America, and the International Society of Sexual Medicine. He has been voted Top Urologist in the Bay Area by *San Francisco Magazine* for eight consecutive years, 2014 to 2021, and has appeared on *The Doctors* TV show and numerous podcasts, including Ben Greenfield Fitness and Dr. Drew.   **BrandeisMD.com**
www.AFFIRMScience.com
www.TheTwentyFirstCenturyMan.com

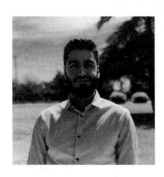

Michael Abassian, MPH, is a graduate of UC Berkeley's School of Public Health with a degree in epidemiology and biostatistics, and a degree in human biology from UCLA. As a Public Health Associate during his time with the Centers for Disease Control and Prevention, Michael conducted on-the-ground research and health impact assessments to influence health policy and improve population wellbeing. His passion for public health practice and research has developed his interest in the epidemiology of chronic disease, nutritional epidemiology, social epidemiology, and global health. He has participated in epidemiological research to identify and analyze health trends both in the United States and overseas and plans to pursue a career in clinical and epidemiologic research.

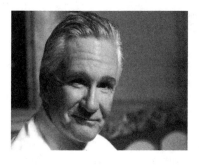

Brian Banmiller is a respected, well-known broadcast journalist who has spent more than 40 years in the news industry, covering business, politics, and the economy on television, radio, and in print. He was executive producer and anchor of the nationally syndicated television business news magazine *On The Money with Brian Banmiller*. He continues his four-decade-long career as a national business reporter for CBS News Radio where his *Banmiller on Business* reports are delivered to an audience of millions nationwide. Brian has reported on the rise, decline, and rebirth of Silicon Valley, the fall of communism in Russia, the rise of capitalism in China, the ongoing threat of war in Korea, the economic future of Hong Kong, political instability in the Philippines, Brexit in England, and the fractures in the European Union. He has also interviewed hundreds of well-known politicians and business leaders. **www.banmilleronbusiness.com**

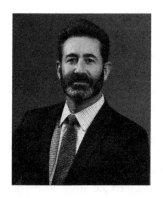

Russell Bartels, MD, is a gynecologist who has been in private practice in Scottsdale, Arizona, since 2002. With sexual health and wellness for men and women as his primary focus, Dr. Bartels combines the synergistic effects of hormone optimization, peptide therapy, and non-invasive procedures to help his patients feel better, function better, and look better. He is an expert on a number of innovative therapies, including FemiLift, Viveve, Cliovana, O-Shot for women, GAINSWave, Precision ED Solution, and P-Shot for men. In addition, Dr. Bartels lectures at conferences and trains physicians in vaginal rejuvenation, as well as treatments for erectile dysfunction and related symptoms, utilizing shockwave therapy, platelet-rich plasma, and hormone replacement therapy. He also offers a host of aesthetic services, including injectables, laser treatments, skincare, and CoolSculpting, as well as weight-loss programs. In addition, Dr. Bartels serves as a key opinion leader for several medical device manufacturers.

www.vitalitymds.com

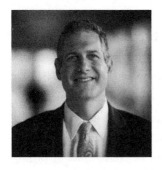

Ethan Basch, MD, is the chairman of the Medical Oncology Department at the University of North Carolina. He graduated from Brown University and Harvard Medical School, and did his internship and residency at Massachusetts General Hospital and fellowship at Memorial Sloan Kettering Cancer Center. Dr. Basch specializes in the treatment of prostate cancer and has been involved with setting national guidelines for the treatment of prostate cancer. He has served on the Board of Scientific Advisors of the National Cancer Institute and the Board of Directors of the American Society of Medical Oncology. Previously, he founded Natural Standard, a resource that presents scientific evidence on natural therapies.

unclineberger.org/directory/ethan-basch/

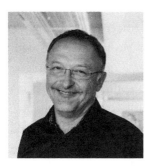

Dirk Bauer founded the FUN FACTORY at his kitchen table in 1995. He and his friend and fellow engineer Michael Pahl dreamed of creating colorful, high-quality erotic toys made of 100% medical-grade silicone. A year later, FUN FACTORY was launched. Bauer has now been at the helm of the company for 25 years. FUN FACTORY was the first sex toy brand to win a mainstream design award, the first to make waterproof toys, and the first to make rechargeable toys. In his spare time, Bauer enjoys biking along the banks of the Weser River.

www.us.funfactory.com.

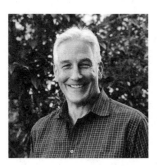

Brett Beaver, LMFT, is a licensed marriage and family therapist with more than 25 years of experience working with couples and families as well as individuals (adults, teenagers, and children). Brett brings a comprehensive range of best practices and processes to both individual therapy and group facilitation, based on his experience working in public health services and private consulting. The focus of his work includes life balance, stress reduction, and workplace communications. His approach encourages thought and self-examination to improve the quality of personal relationships and professional life. Brett holds a Master of Science degree from the University of Southern California (USC) in marriage and family therapy.

www.brettbeaver.com

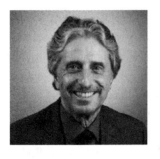

Lawrence Bienati, MBA, PhD, is a former senior leader in global medical device and healthcare companies. In addition, he is a management consultant to many world-renowned organizations in the public, private, and nonprofit sectors. Over the last 30 years, he has served as an associate professor of organizational strategy, executive leadership, strategic human resources, and organizational development at the graduate and doctoral levels playing a role in the development of our next generations of leaders. He has served at a number of universities in the San Francisco Bay Area, including Saint Mary's College, UC Berkeley, Cal-Maritime, Sacramento State, and California Northstate University. He is also the chief executive officer of Bienati Consulting Group, Inc. **www.bienati.com**

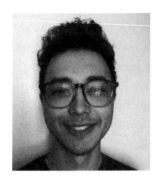

Arthur Bookstein, MPH, is a medical student at the University of Southern California Keck School of Medicine. He is a graduate of UC Berkeley with degrees in molecular and cell biology and public health and hopes to become a primary care physician who treats and empowers patients regardless of background. He plans to continue cancer epidemiology research, teaching, and social justice advocacy while pursues a medical career. In his free time, he loves cycling, tennis, piano, and traveling.

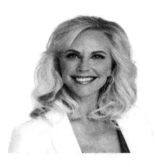

Susan Bratton, *Intimacy Expert to Millions*, is a champion and advocate for all those who desire lifelong intimacy and passion. She is co-founder and CEO of two organiza tions: Personal Life Media, Inc., a publisher of heart-connected lovemaking techniques and bedroom communication skills, and The20, LLC, a manufacturer of organic botanical supplements that enhance sexual vitality. In addition, Ms. Bratton is a best-selling author and publisher of 34 books and programs, including *Sexual Soulmates, Relationship Magic, Revive Her Drive, Ravish Him, Steamy Sex Ed, The Passion Patch*, and *Hormone Balancing*. She has been featured in the *New York Times* and on CNBC and the *TODAY Show* and has had frequent appearances on ABC, CBS, The CW, Fox, and NBC. You can find *The Susan Bratton Show* at betterlover.com, her personal shares on Instagram @susanbratton, and her lust-for-life supplements, FLOW, and DESIRE, at The20store.com. **www.betterlover.com**
www.the20store.com

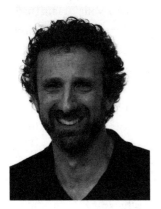

Armin Brott is a nationally recognized authority on men's health, and author of *Blueprint for Men's Health,* and *Your Head: An Owner's Manual,* as well as other books on the topic. He is co-founder of HealthyMen.org and creator of the nationally syndicated *Healthy Men* column. Armin is also a thought leader on the subject of fatherhood whose best-selling books include *The Expectant Father, The New Father, The Single Father,* and *Father for Life.* His columns, radio shows, public speaking, and media appearances have helped millions of men around the world become the fathers they want to be—and that their children need them to be.

www.MrDad.com
www.HealthyMen.org

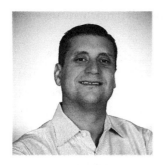

Robert J. Buonfiglio, PhD, is a licensed psychologist and executive coach in the San Francisco Bay Area. He is the current president of the California Psychological Association and is past President of the San Francisco Psychological Association. In addition, Dr. Buonfiglio is the chairperson of the Clinical Advisory Board at I V Y Labs, Inc., and is on the Advisory Board of Hive80.com.   **DrRobertJBuonfiglio.com**

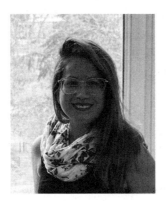

Adriana Bustamante, PhD, is a clinical psychologist in behavioral and cognitive therapy. She is currently writing a doctoral thesis entitled "E-health for addiction treatment: cognitive and behavioral therapies in mobile apps for smoking cessation in France" under Pr. Lucia Romo, assistant professor in psychopathology at the University Paris-Nanterre. Ms. Bustamante is a consultant and researcher for the mobile app for smoking cessation, Kwit SAS, under contract with the National Association of Research and Technology (ANRT).   **www.kwit.app**

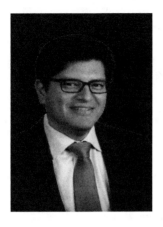

Miguel Canales, MD, founded the Silicon Valley Hair Institute to provide advanced treatments for hair transplantation. Dr. Canales attended Stanford University, received his MD from Harvard Medical School, and completed his surgical residency at Stanford. He is an internationally recognized specialist in robotic hair transplantation and an expert in diagnosing and treating hair loss. As the former medical director of Restoration Robotics, Inc. (the manufacturer robotic of a hair transplantation system), he pioneered the clinical development of the ARTAS Robotic Procedure. Dr. Canales led a team of principal investigators to achieve FDA clearance. He has trained plastic surgeons, hair restoration surgeons, and dermatologists in the ARTAS Robotic System throughout the U.S., Asia, Europe, and Latin America. In addition, Dr. Canales is a participant on more than eleven critical patents that are the basis for robotic hair transplantation.   **siliconvalleyhairinstitute.com**

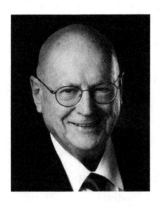

Bernard M. Churchill, MD, received his medical education at Harvard University and the Universities of Alberta and Toronto. He served as chief of the Department of Pediatric Urology at the Hospital for Sick Children in Toronto (1975–1995), as the director of the Clark Morrison Children's Urology Center, and as the Judith and Robert Winston Chair at the University of California at Los Angeles (1995–2015). He has authored 170 peer-reviewed papers, 21 book chapters, and holds eight patents relating to RNA antibiotic-susceptibility testing. His former residents and fellows have secured academic appointments in pediatric urology at 42 medical schools in 10 countries. Dr. Churchill is the founder of MicrobeDx, a biotech company whose mission is evidence-based antibiotic therapy. He is the 25th recipient of the American Academy of Pediatrics Urology Medal for career accomplishments. Dr. Churchill is married to Margaret Rose Shandro, and they have four sons and seven grandchildren.

www.uclahealth.org/urology/bernard-churchill

Mariève Cyr, MSc, is a medical student at McGill University. She specializes in bridging the gap between laboratory studies and real-world applications. Her research aims to reduce fatigue in shift workers and minimize adverse events in healthcare.

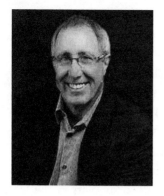

Gary Donovitz, MD, FACOG. With 30 years of clinical practice as a board-certified OB/GYN, Dr. Donovitz is an internationally recognized leader, speaker, educator, and advocate of hormone optimization. He is the founder and chairman of BioTE Medical, LLC, a leading innovator in subcutaneous hormone pellet therapy, and has personally performed more than 50,000 pellet insertions. The BioTE state-of-the-art facility trains physicians, healthcare providers, and medical staff members each month in BioTE Method Certification. Over 4,000 practitioners in more than 2,000 clinics nationwide have completed his rigorous curriculum and clinical training program, ensuring the highest safety, efficacy, and results for every patient. Collectively, these practitioners have performed more than 1.7 million pellet insertions to date. His commitment to the therapy constantly raises the bar for healthcare extends beyond hormone therapy, as Dr. Donovitz has been at the forefront of developments in robotic surgery and has trained physicians across the country on how to perform operations using these advances in technology. He is a fellow of the American College of Obstetrics and Gynecology, a fellow of the Royal Society of Medicine, chairman of the International Consensus Committee on Testosterone Use in Women, and founder of the Institute for Hormonal Balance. **www.bioTEmedical.com**

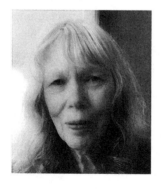

Nancy Faass, MSW, MPH, founder and director of HealthWritersGroup.com, is a writer and editor in San Francisco who has participated on more than 50 books for both consumers and professionals, by publishers that include Harper/Quill, McGraw-Hill, Jones & Bartlett, Healing Arts, New World Library, and others. For over two decades, she has worked collaboratively with clients to develop books, white papers, manuals, blogs, and web content on holistic health and integrative medicine. She has served as editor and coauthor for articles published in journals that range from *Pain Medicine* and *Spine* to the *Townsend Letter*. A graduate of UC Berkeley School of Public Health, Ms. Faass's services include nutritional consulting and health coaching.

www.HealthWritersGroup.com
www.TheNeverDietDiet.com

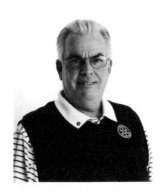

Jack Graham, in his first career, was a newspaper sportswriter and editor for 11 years. Subsequently, he owned and operated a large property and casualty insurance agency for 33 years before retiring in 2014. Jack is an active member of the Rotary Club in his community and has served as past president. He is also a director of the UC Berkeley Cal Men's Golf Committee, which helps oversee and manage one of the most successful golf programs in intercollegiate sports. On a personal level, Jack graduated with a BA from St. Martin's University in Olympia, WA, and served six years in the US Army Reserves. He and his wife, Shelley, have been happily married for nearly 50 years and have two children and three grandchildren.

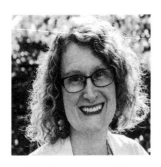

Heather Hannon MSN, RN CBCN, OCN, is a board-certified adult nurse practitioner specializing in oncology and advanced clinical genetics. She received her undergraduate degree in biology from Tufts University in Boston and her Master's Degree in Nursing from Massachusetts General Hospital Institute of Health Professions. She is currently pursuing her doctorate in nursing at Marymount University in Arlington, VA. Ms. Hannon has worked at multiple top-ten medical centers and has a wealth of experience in many aspects of cancer care, including medical and surgical oncology, cancer genetics, palliative care, and oncology nurse navigation. As a GI Oncology Nurse Navigator and Genetics Nurse at Bon Secours Cancer Institute in Richmond, VA, Ms. Hannon provides support and education to individuals and families throughout the cancer care continuum. Ms. Hannon is passionate about cancer survivorship, is interested in helping identify and manage the care of individuals who are at high risk for cancer, and assists patients with navigating long-term challenges related to treatment. She is a member of the Oncology Nursing Society, International Society of Nurses in Genetics, American Society of Clinical Oncology, and Academy of Oncology Nurse and Patient Navigators.

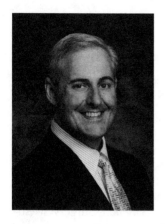

Toby Hill is the founder and president of Contra Costa Hearing Aid Center, Inc since 2008. Mr. Hill is certified by the American Conference of Audioprosthology and by the National Board of Certification in Hearing Instrument Sciences. He serves as a subject matter expert for the Speech Pathology Audiology Hearing Aid Dispensing Board and the National Board For Certification In Hearing Instrument Sciences. He began his career working for one of the major hearing aid manufacturers, but discovered that his real passion is working with people, helping them achieve the best hearing possible by carefully selecting and expertly fitting hearing aids. He has been a partner in one practice and now has a private practice with two locations to better serve the community. **https://www.contracostahearing.com**

HealthyMen.org is a national non-profit that seeks to foster an environment of health equity in which boys and men have the tools, resources, and support they need to take ownership of their health and wellness. Our mission is to optimize the quality of men's lives and enable them to be effective and productive members of their family and their communities through public communication, awareness, education, outreach, advocacy, and public policy. We do this by engaging and partnering with expert individuals and organizations to provide resources, support, training, and expertise that focuses on wellness and comprehensive health self-management as a core component of masculinity. **HealthyMen.org**

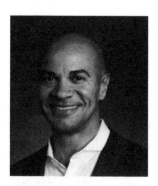

Greg Horner, MD, the Tri-Valley Orthopedic Specialists' hand surgery team leader, treats conditions affecting the bones, muscles, nerves, and tendons of the hand, and wrist, from fingertip to shoulder. After playing football at Northwestern University, he went on to medical school at Johns Hopkins, did an orthopedic residency at UCLA, and gained a hand fellowship at the New England Bone and Joint Institute. He performs arthroscopy and microvascular surgery for a wide range of problems from congenital disorders in infants to injuries in adults, including work-related disorders, fracture care, carpal tunnel syndrome, and sports-related conditions. **www.trivalleyorthopedics.com**

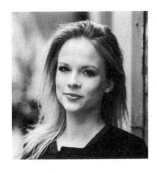

Milla Impola. After moving to Texas from Finland as a teenager and experiencing her first abstinence-only sex education class, Ms. Impola quickly developed an enthusiasm for comprehensive sex education as her life's calling. In her current role as marketing director at ONE Condoms, her favorite projects involve working with educators and artists to promote sexual health.

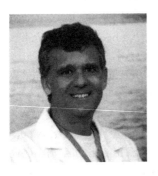

Michael Ingegno, MD, is an experienced, board-certified vascular surgeon practicing at the Vascular Surgery Medical Group in San Leandro and San Ramon, California. Dr. Ingegno is a graduate of Brown University and received his medical degree from the SUNY Downstate Health Sciences University in Brooklyn. He completed his internship and residency in general surgery at the University of California, Irvine, and completed a fellowship in vascular surgery at the University of Florida's Health Shands Hospital in Gainesville. Currently, Dr. Ingegno is chief of staff at San Leandro Hospital and the medical director of the Endovascular Suite and Noninvasive Vascular Laboratory at Vascular Surgery Medical Group. Dr. Ingegno has served as chairman of the Department of Surgery at San Leandro Hospital and as president of the Northern California Vascular Society.

www.vasculargroup.com

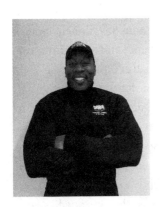

Johnny Jackson grew up in California and played football at the University of Arizona and graduated with a bachelor's in communications and in human development. Johnny played arena football from 2006 to 2008 and then played in the Canadian Football League. He began his career as a trainer at Crunch Fitness and has also worked at the University of California, Berkeley. Johnny has been the national trainer of the year at Crunch Gym for eight years in a row. He holds multiple certifications from the National Academy of Sports Medicine and Next College Student Athlete including nutrition, weight loss, and post rehab, as well as TRX certification.

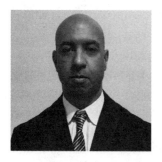

Malcolm Johnson, MD, is an emergency department physician, board-certified in emergency medicine, employed by Vituity, and the medical director of seven fire districts. He attended the University of Wisconsin, receiving a bachelor's degree in zoology, and completed medical school at the University of Wisconsin School of Medicine and Public Health. He completed his residency at Emory University School of Medicine and Morehouse School of Medicine in Atlanta.

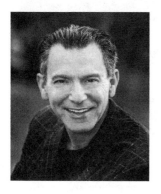

Joel Kahn, MD, FACC, is a practicing cardiologist and a clinical professor of medicine at Wayne State University School of Medicine in Detroit. He graduated Summa Cum Laude from the University of Michigan Medical School. Known as "America's Healthy Heart Doc," Dr. Kahn is triple board-certified in internal medicine, cardiovascular medicine, and interventional cardiology. He was the first physician in the world to be certified in metabolic cardiology with the University of South Florida. Dr. Kahn is founder of the Kahn Center for Cardiac Longevity in Bingham Farms, Michigan.

www.DrJoelKahn.com

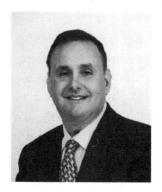

Joel Kaplan, PhD, received his doctorate in clinical psychology and human sexuality from the University of Chicago and from Saybrook Institute in San Francisco. Dr. Kaplan has diplomate status with the American Board of Sexology and is a sex researcher and certified sex therapist. Today Dr. Kaplan is known worldwide as the premier authority and pioneer in erection enhancement therapy. **www.drjoelkaplan.com**

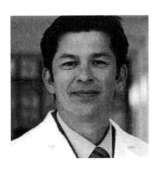

Edward Karpman, MD, is a board-certified urologist who is fellowship trained in male reproductive medicine and surgery, microsurgery, and male sexual dysfunction. He is the medical director of the Men's Health Center at El Camino Hospital in Los Gatos and at the California Vasectomy and Reversal Center. Dr. Karpman is a graduate of the University of California, Davis with honors, and the University of Vermont College of Medicine, where he scored in the top 5% of all medical school graduates in the nation on his medical board exams and was awarded the James Demeules Surgical Research Award. He completed his urologic surgery training at the University of California Davis Medical Center, where he received several awards for his research and publications and was the recipient of a prestigious fellowship to Baylor College of Medicine in Houston, Texas. He is currently involved in the development of new technologies for the treatment of prostate enlargement and serves as a proctor for penile implants, laser surgery of the prostate, and male incontinence operations, helping other physicians to perform these operations. Dr. Karpman has authored numerous articles and presented research at national meetings on penile implants and microsurgery. An expert in male infertility, he has been an invited lecturer, presented at national meetings, written articles, and authored a chapter on male infertility in the definitive textbook on the topic. Dr. Karpman has been interviewed by media that include NBC News, ABC News, Fox Radio, and NPR. **www.elcaminourology.com/**

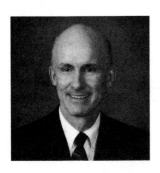

Brian M. Kinney, MD. Dr. Kinney's practice in Beverly Hills incorporates innovation with the latest technologies in surgery, utilizing minimally invasive and non-invasive techniques. Dr. Kinney is clinical associate professor of plastic surgery at the University of Southern California, where he teaches medical students and residents specialized surgical techniques and is the associate editor of *Aesthetic Plastic Surgery Journal* and the *Archives of Plastic Surgery*. He has served as president of the Plastic Surgery Educational Foundation (PSF), chairman of the board of trustees of the American Society of Plastic Surgeons (ASPS), board member of The Aesthetic Society, and board member of the International Society of Plastic Regenerative Surgery, of which he is the cofounder. An internationally recognized inventor and patent holder, he is a lead researcher for Thermi, Emsculpt, and Algeness: one of the original researchers on Emsculpt NEO; a researcher for Renuva, Renuvion, Motiva, and Intellifat; and is a co-developer of Algeness and Attenuate. He is also an expert teacher/trainer for

Thermi, Intellifat, Algeness, Motiva Implants, Renuvion, Emsculpt, and others. A recipient of awards for advanced breast augmentation techniques, he is actively involved in aesthetics research focused on fat injection and stem cell applications and has participated in FDA clinical trials for various injectables and implants. **www.drkinney.com**

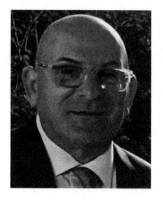

James Korkos, MD, is currently a senior medical director at Blue Shield of California. As an undergraduate, Dr. Korkos attended Vanderbilt University and the University of Wisconsin. He earned his doctor of medicine degree from the Medical College of Wisconsin, where he also completed a seven-year residency in anesthesiology. At John Muir Medical Center in Walnut Creek, California, he provided anesthesiology services for 15 years. He has also successfully secured venture capital for medical startups and developed an ambulatory surgical facility in Wisconsin. With more than 25 years of healthcare experience in total, before joining Blue Shield of California, Dr. Korkos served as the Northern California medical director for United Healthcare.

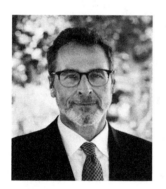

Jonathan Larose, Esq, MBA has extensive experience in all areas of family law. Jonathan earned his bachelor's at San Francisco State in political science and economics. He then earned his MBA, with an emphasis on finance, at the University of San Francisco and his law degree at New College of California School of Law. He creates pre-marriage, co-habitation, and post-marriage agreements. He also works on all issues related to paternity, divorce, annulment, and legal separation actions, including child and spousal support, community property, custody, breach of marital fiduciary duties, child relocations, asset tracing, international accounts and property, inter-state conflicts and jurisdiction, attorney fee reimbursement, domestic violence, and marital harassment. Jonathan is both a litigator and a mediator and is adept at forensic investigation. He works with a range of private experts, including accountants, appraisers, medical evaluators, vocational evaluators, bankers, human resources, estate and corporate attorneys, psychologists, international law firms, custody assessors, private judges, appellate experts, and private investigators. **www. jdlaroselaw.com**

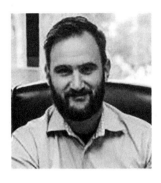

Max Lippman, DC, is a leader in the chiropractic community, serving the San Francisco Bay Area for the last decade. Working with professional athletes, tech CEOs, and weekend warriors, Dr. Lippman is a master of spinal manipulation, myofascial release, functional movement, and stress management. He studied at Oregon State University and received his doctorate from Life Chiropractic College West. Dr. Lippman is the past president of the Cal Chiro Contra Costa District, has served as president of the Danville Sycamore Valley Rotary Club, and is an active member of his community. Currently residing in Pleasanton with his wife and two kids, Dr. Lippman enjoys swimming, running, and catching an Oakland A's game on a sunny day.   **www.blackhawkchiropractor.com**

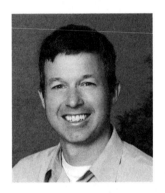

Matthew Lodewick, MD, is a University of California, Berkeley, graduate who studied molecular and cell biology, as well as comparative literature. He then studied medicine at the University of Alabama at Birmingham, and subsequently completed a pediatric residency and an adult and pediatric fellowship in allergy/immunology at Children's Hospital of Seattle and the University of Washington. He returned to the San Francisco Bay Area in 2004 to establish a practice in the treatment of allergies. Dr. Lodewick is a Fellow of the American Academy of Pediatrics, a member of the Allergy Association of Northern California, and a Fellow of the American Academy of Allergy, Asthma, and Immunology. In addition, he is a member of the Alpha Omega Alpha Honor Medical Society. His special interests include the management of asthma disorders and food allergies. When not in the office, you will find Dr. Lodewick enjoying time with his family, on a bike, on a trail, or with a book in hand.   **www.BayAreaAllergy.com**

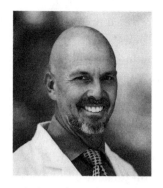

William Longton, MD, is a physician specializing in pain management and anesthesiology who treats patients at Pain Medicine Consultants in Pleasant Hill, California. Dr. Longton trained at Stanford University, where he participated in several studies related to the effects of pain on the human body. After completing his residency and fellowship in anesthesiology and pain medicine, Dr. Longton stayed on as a faculty member at Stanford Medical Center, attending the operating rooms and the pain clinic. He trained and taught side by side with some of the original leaders in the field of pain therapy. Dr. Longton has held leadership positions in pain management at Stanford University, Santa Clara Valley Medical Center, and John Muir Health Medical Center. He has almost 20 years of experience in his field and is board-certified in anesthesiology and pain medicine. His expertise includes multidisciplinary care and cancer pain management, with particular expertise in spinal cord stimulation and spinal medication delivery systems. Dr. Longton is an avid cyclist, skier, and windsurfer and is a previous world-class athlete and finalist in the U.S. Olympic Trials in swimming. **www.PainMedicineConsultants.com**

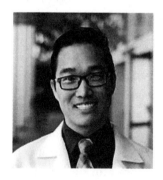

Scott Lu, MD, is currently completing a master's degree in the advanced study of clinical research with specialization in implementation sciences at the University of California, San Francisco. His research has focused on patient-reported outcomes among survivors of Kaposi's sarcoma in East Africa. In response to the tremendous need for highly developed research on SARS-CoV-2 infection, he is currently co-investigator on multiple UCSF studies, including: a CDC-funded study on the natural history and infectivity of SARS-CoV-2 infection to inform on policy and procedure for COVID-19 prevention and management and an NIH-funded study on the long term impact of SARS-CoV-2 infection.

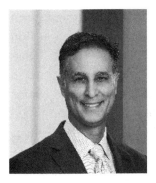

Ahad Mahootchi, MD, is a board-certified ophthalmologist and founder of The Eye Clinic of Florida, which provides world-class cataract and specialty ophthalmic surgery and care. Dr. Mahootchi is one of Florida's highest-rated cataract, glaucoma, and eyelid surgeons. PatientsChoice.org has recognized him as a Top Ten doctor in Florida, and he leads the region with best outcomes for eye and eyelid surgery. With 25 years of experience, he has performed more than 28,000 eye surgeries. In addition, he has more than two decades of experience in placing astigmatism-correcting implants and in laser vision correction. He is currently the most experienced surgeon in the country in placing XEN Gel Stent implants for glaucoma. Dr. Mahootchi was born in Carbondale, Illinois, and grew up in Tennessee. He attended Vanderbilt University School of Medicine in Nashville and performed his internship in internal medicine and residency in ophthalmology at Vanderbilt. He is board-certified by the American Board of Ophthalmology.

www.SeeBetterFlorida.com

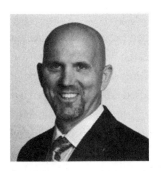

Eric Mariotti, MD, is a board-certified plastic surgeon, providing plastic and reconstructive surgery in the East Bay region of the San Francisco Bay Area. He is also the medical director of Premier Surgery Center where all of his procedures are performed. Dr. Mariotti's patients think of him as a down-to-earth guy who also happens to be a talented plastic surgeon. He served as chairman of the Plastic Surgery Division at John Muir Medical Center in Concord for more than 15 years. He has been in practice for over 20 years and is honored to serve the community where he grew up. **www.drmariotti.com**

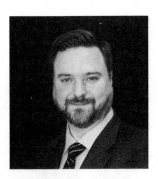

Bret McLaughlin, PhD, MBA, is a licensed psychologist and a specialist in forensic and clinical psychology. He earned a bachelor's degree in psychology, literature, and education from the University of California, Santa Cruz; a master's in British and American Literature from New York University; a masters and doctorate in psychology from The Wright Institute; and an MBA from California State University, Sacramento. At the Department of State Hospitals, Bret provided mental health evaluations and served as an expert witness in the California courts. At the Department of Corrections and Rehabilitation, he served as vice-chair of the Psychology Department at the California Medical Facility and as chief psychologist and chief of mental health at the California Healthcare Facility. He is currently the founding dean of the College of Psychology at California Northstate University and is a board member for the Sacramento Valley Psychological Association.

www.cnsu.edu

Men's Health Network is a national non-profit organization whose mission is to reach men, boys, and their families where they live, work, play, and pray with health awareness and disease prevention messages and tools, screening programs, educational materials, advocacy opportunities, and patient navigation. **www.MensHealthNetwork.org.**

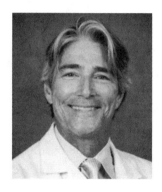

David Miller, MD, grew up in Georgia, where he received his medical degree from the Medical College of Georgia in Augusta in 1992. He completed his general surgery and urology residencies at Vanderbilt University Affiliated Hospitals in Nashville where he also served as chief resident of urology. Dr. Miller then completed a fellowship in urologic oncology at the Monash Medical Center in Melbourne, Australia. He is board-certified by the American Board of Urology and is an active member of the American Urological Association and the American Medical Association. In addition, David is an active member of the Richmond Academy of Medicine. His extensive research over the years has provided him the opportunity to present and publish his findings, for which he has received a number of accolades. **www.uro.com**

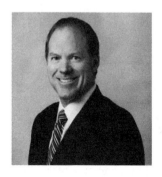

Michael Murphy, MD, MPH, is a board-certified head and neck surgeon whose practice encompasses a full range of services for patients of all ages. Dr. Murphy is also board certified in sleep medicine and treats sleep apnea and other sleep disorders. His dual board-certification as a sleep specialist and surgeon enables him to provide surgical and non-surgical treatment options for patients with sleep disorders. Laryngology (the study of voice and swallowing disorders) has also been an area of particular interest throughout his career. He works closely with a speech pathologist, and together they offer a comprehensive approach for patients with voice and swallowing disorders. Dr. Murphy grew up in Moraga, CA, and returned home to join Diablo Valley ENT in 2002. He is married with two children and enjoys golf, snow skiing, and running.

stanfordhealthcare.org/doctors/m/michael-murphy.html

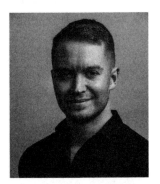

Jay A. Olson, PhD, is a postdoctoral fellow at Harvard University. He develops behavioral interventions targeting issues ranging from jet lag and shift work fatigue to smartphone addiction and behavioral disorders. His research has been featured on such media outlets as CNN, NBC, *Time Magazine*, and the *New York Times*.   **www.jayolson.org**

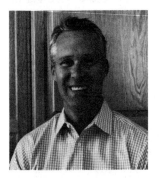

Joshua Perlroth, MD, was born in the San Francisco Bay Area and attended Duke University, earning a BA in history. He then attended USC Keck School of Medicine and completed his internal medicine residency and infectious diseases fellowship at Harbor-UCLA Medical Center. Since 2007 his practice in the San Francisco Bay Area has focused on the treatment and management of infectious diseases, and he is affiliated with four hospitals. He has served as chair of the Department of Medicine at John Muir Walnut Creek since 2015. In addition, he is the chair of the Antibiotic Stewardship Committee and serves on the Medical Executive, Pharmacy and Therapeutics, and Quality Improvement committees for John Muir Health.   **www.iddoctors.com**

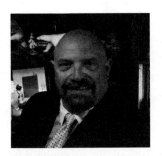

Jeffrey Piccirillo, DO, is a board-certified orthopedic surgeon who developed an interest in platelet-rich plasma in 2002. He did his undergraduate work at Penn State University and attended medical school at the Philadelphia College of Osteopathic Medicine, graduating as valedictorian in 1989. Jeff continued his training at the Chicago Osteopathic Medical Center in orthopedic surgery from 1989 to 2004. Then, he entered private practice, focusing on general orthopedics, with an interest in adult reconstructive surgery and sports medicine. In 2002, when a representative from one of the major joint replacement companies brought a centrifuge

into the operating room, his love for regenerative medicine and PRP began. In 2009, he switched from a surgical practice to one focusing on the regeneration of tissue. As his protocols and products evolved, Dr. Piccirillo started consulting for other practices, teaching them how to provide regenerative medicine. His recent book, Perfect PRP, covers his trademarked method for optimal use of PRP. **www.perfectprpthebook.com**
www.regenmedicalgroup.com

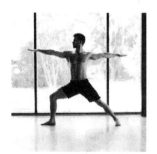

Dean Pohlman is an E-RYT 200 certified yoga instructor and the founder of Man Flow Yoga. An authority on yoga for men and for fitness, his workouts and programs have been used by professional and collegiate athletes, athletic trainers, personal trainers, and everyday guys who just want to be a little healthier. His website is one of the most popular training programs in yoga for men available on the Internet, with more than 20,000 trainees and customers. In addition, Dean is a successfully published author through DK Publishing (*Yoga Fitness for Men*), selling 35,000 copies worldwide in English, French, and German. He co-produced the *Body by Yoga* DVD series, which has sold more than 40,000 copies on Amazon.com since its release in 2016. Dean lives in Austin, Texas, with his wife, son, and two dogs, Flowtron and Kaya.

www.manflowyoga.com

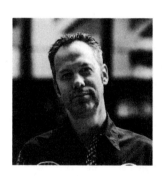

Brad Robinson is a sound and video engineer living in the San Francisco Bay Area. He studied electrical engineering at Vanderbilt University. As a 23-year veteran of the technology industry, he provides design and integration services for the residential, hospitality, commercial, government, and education markets. Brad started his career as co-DJ on Dr. Brandeis's Friday-night house-music radio show Club91 on WRVU in Nashville in 1995. Since that humble beginning, Brad has been a house music DJ performing at a wide variety of venues and a member of the Space Cowboys, a San Francisco-based music and art collective with ties to the Burning Man community. **www.djbradrobinson.com**

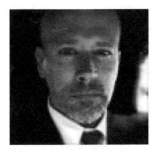

Charles Runels, MD, initially worked for three years as a research chemist at the Southern Research Institute. He then completed medical school at the University of Alabama in Birmingham, after which he completed his residency and became board-certified in internal medicine. During twelve years as an ER physician, he founded the largest group of emergency room physicians in his state, while also serving as medical director of a hyperbaric treatment service for wound care. He then began medical practice and initiated research in areas of wellness, endocrinology, cosmetic medicine, and sexual medicine. He has contributed to multiple peer-reviewed scientific publications in the areas of hypertension, hormone replacement, immunology, and dermatology. In cosmetic medicine, he is designer of a protocol using growth factors to rejuvenate the face, widely known as the Vampire Facelift, and founded the American Cosmetic Cellular Medicine Association. His recent work includes research on urinary incontinence and sexual function using platelet-rich plasma (PRP) in both men and women, resulting in the development of the O-Shot and P-Shot (Priapus Shot) procedures. Over the past 10 years, he has trained more than 2,000 physicians worldwide in these procedures. Dr. Runels is the father of three sons and lives in Fairhope, Alabama.

www.Runels.com
www.CellularMedicineAssociation.org

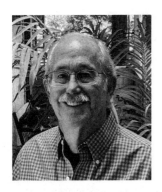

Paul C. Scholberg, DDS, is a graduate of University of the Pacific School of Dentistry and practiced dentistry for more than 40 years in Danville and Pleasanton, California. Dr. Scholberg has served as a clinical instructor and assistant professor at the University of the Pacific Dental School. He has extensive experience providing cosmetic dental reconstruction and "smile design" involving the use of high-tech digital software to create an optimal smile. Dr. Scholberg has participated in undergraduate, postgraduate, and continuing education and is currently happily retired.

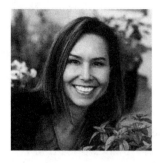

Angela Stanford is a sought-after nutrition and wellness expert focused on preventative and integrated health. For more than 20 years, she has been helping others learn how to eat mindfully and make lifestyle choices. She practices personalized nutrition and coaches clients through roadblocks to achieve their vision of vibrant health and wellness. From corporate wellness to her private practice in Danville, California, Angela counsels individuals, delivers corporate wellness programs, and teaches classes and workshops. Angela earned a BA in Nutrition from the University of Illinois, completed her dietetic internship at UW Hospital and Clinics in Madison, Wisconsin, and holds an MBA from the University of San Francisco. Angela is a credentialed registered dietitian nutritionist (RDN), a nationally board-certified health and wellness coach (NBC-HWC) accredited through the American College of Lifestyle Medicine and the American College of Sports Medicine, and a registered yoga teacher (RYT). **www.vitalandwell.com**

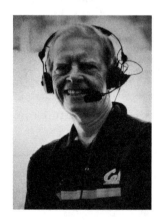

Joe Starkey began broadcasting sports on radio and television with the California Golden Seals of the National Hockey League. Since 1975 he has been calling games on radio for the California Golden Bears of the Pacific-12 conference. His call of the finish of the 1982 Big Game between UC Berkeley and Stanford is rated among the best of all time. From 1987 through 2008, he also called games on radio for the San Francisco 49ers, including three Super Bowls. He is a member of three halls of fame: the National Football Foundation for his distinguished career as a sports announcer for college football, the University of California Sports Hall of Fame, and the Bay Area Radio Hall of Fame.

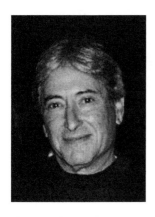

Jonathan Steinberg, DPM, has been practicing podiatric medicine and surgery in Walnut Creek and Concord, California for more than twenty years. He attended the Pennsylvania College of Podiatric Medicine and completed his surgical residency at Riverside Hospital in Wilmington, Delaware. Dr. Steinberg is a past chairman of the Podiatry Section at the John Muir Medical Center campuses in Walnut Creek and Concord. He is board-certified by the American Board of Podiatric Surgery, a fellow of the American College of Foot and Ankle Surgery, and an Expert Medical Reviewer for the Board of Podiatric Medicine. **www.muirfootandanklecenter.com**

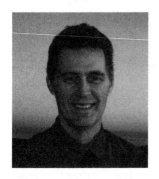

Jerry Stine is a nutritional consultant, longevity coach, and the director of the Lifespan Institute for Functional and Anti-aging Nutrition. The Lifespan Institute was founded in 1987 to develop advanced life-extension and performance enhancing programs. For the past 25 years, Jerry has been an independent nutritional counselor with an active private practice and has served as a consultant for several respected vitamin manufacturers. **www.LifespanInstitute.com**

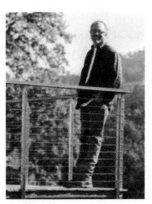

Michael Tebb is a graduate of Cal Poly at San Luis Obispo with a concentration in landscape design. He has served as a landscape designer for more than three decades in the San Francisco Bay Area, providing personalized services and creating exquisite landscapes for his clientele. Michael believes that "one's property should be an oasis that relaxes, soothes, and inspires. It must showcase, yet feel like home." He uses structure, space, path, and flow to create an experience as the viewer moves through the landscape. His work incorporates California native flora and hardscape, integrating the effect with the surrounding land. Michael Tebb works throughout California. **www.michaeltebbdesign.houzzsite.com**

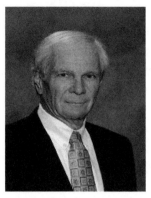

Peter D. Vash, MD, MPH, FACE, is an assistant clinical professor of medicine at UCLA Medical Center and a fellow of the American Association of Clinical Endocrinologists. He is also in the first cohort of scholars at UCLA who completed the program in 1978 and is a board-certified internist specializing in endocrinology and metabolism, with an emphasis on obesity and eating disorders. While a scholar, he trained in endocrinology, earned an MPH, and established an outpatient obesity study clinic at UCLA Medical Center. There Dr. Vash implemented randomized, controlled clinical trials to test the effects of a very low-calorie diet, in the form of either an amino acid solution or carbohydrate solution, on weight-loss results, cost, and safety. He is a past president of the American Society of Bariatric Physicians and served on the North American Society Board for the Study of Obesity (NASSO). Dr. Vash works in private practice with patients suffering from obesity and eating disorders and has lectured extensively, both nationally and internationally, on the medical management and treatment of obesity. In addition, he has been an invited expert witness to speak before a U.S. Senate sub-committee and the FTC concerning medical weight-loss issues and the safety and impact of commercial weight-loss programs. **www.attenuatepro.com**

www.petervashmd.com

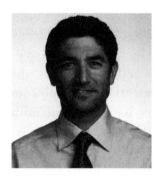

Adam Wallach, MD, attended New York University School of Medicine, performed his post-medical training in dermatology at Cornell Medical Center, and then attended NYU for his residency. He initially worked in private practice in New York City, where he was also an assistant professor at Saint Vincent's Hospital in Manhattan. In 2001 Adam relocated to Northern California, where he has since practiced medical, surgical, and cosmetic dermatology. He is an advising physician at John Muir Hospital in Walnut Creek, California, and currently practices in Danville and Truckee, California. Dr. Wallach actively participates in teaching students who rotate through his office, and he enjoys a stellar reputation among patients and doctors alike. Additionally, Dr. Wallach is known for his detailed performance of facial surgery for the treatment of skin cancer and his expert use of fillers and lasers. **www.wallachdermacenter.com**

Alan Wang is a health insurance expert, culture analyst, and consultant to leading organizations throughout the world. Mr. Wang has helped organizations change the way in which they view healthcare and support the healthy behaviors of employees within their own company culture. He advises corporate leaders on creating new dynamic areas within the health insurance continuum that contribute to stronger and more resilient organizations. He also champions the benefit of disruptive solutions that break the chain of conventional wisdom as a means of effective problem solving, and he applies historical and evidence-based means to develop new ways of creating change.   **www.ubf.consulting**

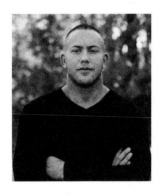

Adam Wenguer is the founder and CEO of Element Health, LLC, which provides full spectrum CBD, hemp-based products. An expert in the use of CBD and cannabis for peak wellness and performance, he is also highly trained and experienced in the utilization of botanical and mycological compounds for ceremonial/shamanic application. Adam holds a BA in applied physiology and kinesiology from the University of Florida. He is a lifelong martial artist and combat instructor, a four-stripe brown belt in Brazilian jiu-jitsu, Muay Thai/boxing, and armed combat. Adam is a mindfulness-based meditation practitioner/instructor and proponent of conscious hunting. He has more than 15 years' experience as a strength and conditioning specialist and health coach at a premier five-star wellness resort, working with a wide array of professional athletes, company executives, and individuals seeking optimal health. Many were suffering from a similar pattern—sleep issues, anxiety, inflammatory conditions, and a general emotional and spiritual disconnect—which led to his creation of Element Health.

www.ElementHealthSupply.com
IG: @ElementHealth

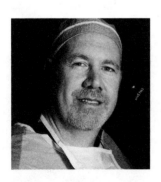

Philip Werthman, MD, is considered the top fertility specialist in Los Angeles by both his colleagues and his patients. Dr. Werthman began his medical career at Hahnemann University School of Medicine in Philadelphia, Pennsylvania, where he was the class valedictorian, having ranked first in his class for all four years of medical school. He was also awarded the Medical Staff Award for highest attainment on the National Boards medical examination. Dr. Werthman subsequently completed his seven-year residency and fellowship in urology at the University of California, Los Angeles. Issues of male infertility and microsurgery fascinated him, so he decided to further specialize in andrology (literally, the "study of man," a subspecialty within the discipline of urology) and completed his training with a visiting fellowship in male infertility and microsurgery at the Baylor College of Medicine in Houston. **www.malereproduction.com/about-cmrm/dr-philip-werthman/**

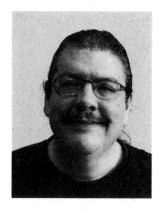

Kevin A. Wilson has been a freelance writer in aesthetic medicine since 1998. His portfolio includes collaboration on peer-reviewed scientific literature for physicians and white papers for leading companies around the globe. The bulk of his work has been with *The Aesthetic Guide,* for which he has written countless articles. Mr. Wilson is currently a data management specialist in Syracuse, NY, and he continues to write for *The Aesthetic Guide.* He also serves as a volunteer working with youth in addiction recovery services at the Sgt. Elisha Parker Community Youth Center in Syracuse.

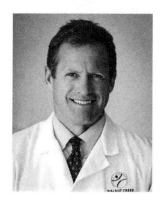

William Workman, MD, has a strong background in sports medicine, both as a practicing physician and an athlete. He was among the first orthopedic surgeons to obtain additional board certification in orthopedic sports medicine. As an athlete, he competed in baseball as a pitcher for the University of California Golden Bears and played professionally in the California Angels system. After completing a five-year orthopedic residency at Yale Medical School, Dr. Workman completed an orthopedic sports medicine fellowship at Harvard Medical School. While at Harvard, he served as a team physician and traveled with the New England Patriots (NFL). In addition, he has provided orthopedic sports medicine coverage for the Boston Bruins Hockey Club (NHL), New England Revolution Soccer team (MLS), the United States Women's Soccer Team, the women's professional tennis tour (USTA), and Harvard University Athletics. His extensive involvement with elite-level athletes has furthered his understanding of athletic injuries and treatment. Dr. Workman currently serves as team orthopedist for the Oakland Athletics (MLB). In addition to his work with the A's, Dr. Workman has gained national recognition for his arthroscopic approach to the treatment of injuries, which he teaches to orthopedic surgeons worldwide. He is a consultant to major international sports medicine corporations, conducts clinical research, and is actively involved in national and international sports medicine societies. **calsportsdoc.com**

References

Chapter 2—Smart Ways to Reduce Your Health Risks

Mineo L. Good genes are nice, but joy is better. *Harvard Gazette.* Harvard University Website. https://news.harvard.edu/gazette/story/2017/04/over-nearly-80-years-harvard-study-has-been-showing-how-to-live-a-healthy-and-happy-life/ Published April 2017. Accessed August 29, 2021.

Waldinger R. What makes a good life? Lessons from the longest study on happiness. YouTube Website. https://www.youtube.com/watch?time_continue=166&v=8KkKuTCFvzI&feature=emb_title Published Jan 2016. Accessed August 29, 2021.

Zajacova A, Lawrence E M. The relationship between education and health: reducing disparities through a contextual approach. *Annu Rev of Public Health.* 2018;39:273-89. doi: 10.1146/annurev-publhealth-031816-044628.

Chapter 5—Strengthening Your Heart

Inman BA, St. Sauver JL, Jacobson DJ, *et al.* A population-based, longitudinal study of erectile dysfunction and future coronary artery disease. Mayo Clin Proc. 2009;84(2):108-13. doi: 10.4065/84.2.108.

Nehra A, Jackson G, Miner M, *et al.* The Princeton III Consensus recommendations for the management of erectile dysfunction and cardiovascular disease. Mayo Clin Proc. 2012;87(8):766-778. PMID: 22862865. https://www.ncbi.nlm.nih.gov/pmc/articles/PMC3498391/pdf/main.pdf. Accessed August 29, 2021.

Chapter 7—Preventing Cancer

Cancer Facts and Figures 2018. American Cancer Society Website. https://www.cancer.org/research/cancer-facts-statistics/all-cancer-facts-figures/cancer-facts-figures-2018.html. Accessed August 29, 2021.

Cancers attributable to UV Radiation. International Agency for Research on Cancer Website. https://gco.iarc.fr/causes/uv/home Published 2012. Accessed August 29, 2021.

Occupational Cancer. National Institute for Occupational Safety and Health Website. https://www.cdc.gov/niosh/topics/cancer/default.html. Accessed August 29, 2021.

Chapter 8—Decoding Your Cancer Genes

Inherited thrombocytopenia. Platelet Disorder Support Association Website. https://pdsa.org/inherited-thrombocytopenia.html. Accessed September 1, 2021.

Support for patients and families. National Institute of Health Website. https://rarediseases.info.nih.gov/guides/pages/120/support-for-patients-and-families. Updated August 11, 2016. Accessed September 1, 2021.

Welcome to the Smart Patients Lynch Syndrome community. Smart Patients Website. https://www.smartpatients.com/communities/lynch-syndrome. Accessed September 1, 2021.

Women and heart disease. CardioSmart American College of Cardiology Website. https://www.cardiosmart.org/topics/women-and-heart-disease/overview Updated March 11, 2021. Accessed September 1, 2021.

Chapter 9—Avoiding Stupid Accidents

da Silva BA, Krishnamurthy M. The alarming reality of medication error: a patient case and review of Pennsylvania and national data. *J Community Hosp Intern Med Perspect.* 2016;6(4):31758. doi: 10.3402/jchimp.v6.31758.

Gholipour B. Men take more "idiotic risks," study finds. Live Science Website. https://www.livescience.com/49101-darwin-awards-are-men-idiots.html Published Dec 2014. Accessed August 29, 2021.

Hills T. The upside and downside of middle-aged risk taking. Psychology Today Website. https://www.psychologytoday.com/us/blog/statistical-life/201309/the-upside-and-downside-middle-aged-risk-taking. Published September 5, 2013. Accessed September 1, 2021.

Lendrem BAD, Lendrem DW, Gray A, Isaacs JD. The Darwin Awards: sex differences in idiotic behavior. *BMJ.* 2014;349:g7094. doi: 10.1136/bmj.g7094.

Risk-taking behavior rises until age 50. ScienceDaily. University of Oregon Website. https://www.sciencedaily.com/releases/2011/11/111110130102.htm Published Nov 2011. Accessed August 29, 2021.

Tamas V, Kocsor F, Gyuris P, *et al.* The young male syndrome—an analysis of sex, age, risk taking and mortality in patients with severe traumatic brain injuries. *Front Neurol.* 2019;10:366. doi: 10.3389/fneur.2019.00366.

Turbert D. Safety glasses and protective eyewear. American Academy of Ophthalmology Website. https://www.aao.org/eye-health/tips-prevention/injuries-protective-eyewear. Published March 23, 2019. Accessed September 1, 2021.

Williams RS. The 5 most common orthopedic injuries in people over 40. Coastal Orthopedics Website. https://www.coastalorthoteam.com/blog/the-5-most-common-orthopedic-injuries-in-people-over-40. Published February 23, 2017. Accessed September 1, 2021.

WISQARS—web-based injury statistics query and reporting system. Centers for Disease Control and Prevention Website. https://www.cdc.gov/injury/wisqars/ Accessed September 1, 2021.

Chapter 11—Coping with a Chronic Lung Condition

Consumer book on minimizing environmental toxins:

Cohen, Aly, vom Saal, Frederick S., and Weil, Andrew, eds. *Integrative Environmental Medicine*. Oxford, UK: Oxford University Press, 2017.

Journal articles and web pages:

Chuang HC, Ho KF, Lin LY, *et al.* Long-term indoor air conditioner filtration and cardiovascular health: a randomized crossover intervention study. Environ Int. 2017 Sep;106:91-96. doi: 10.1016/j.envint.2017.06.008. Epub 2017 Jun 15.

de Roos P, Lucas C, Strijbos JH, van Trijffel E. Effectiveness of a combined exercise training and home-based walking programme on physical activity compared with standard medical care in moderate COPD: A randomised controlled trial. *Physiotherapy.* 2018;105(1):116-121. doi: 10.1016/j.physio.2016.08.005.

Deering BM, Fullen B, Egan C, *et al.* Acupuncture as an adjunct to pulmonary rehabilitation. *J Cardiopulm Rehabil Prev.* 2011;31(6):392-9. doi: 10.1097/HCR.0b013e31822f0f61.

Feng J, Wang X, Li X, Zhao D, Xu J. Acupuncture for chronic obstructive pulmonary disease (COPD): a multicenter, randomized, sham-controlled trial. *Medicine (Baltimore).* 2016;95(40):e4879. doi: 10.1097/MD.0000000000004879.

Fulambarker A, Farooki B, Kheir F, Copur AS, Srinivasan L, Schultz S. Effect of yoga in chronic obstructive pulmonary disease. *Am J Ther.* 2012;19(2):96-100. doi: 10.1097/MJT.0b013e3181f2ab86.

Giorgini P, Di Giosia P, Grassi D, *et al.* Air pollution exposure and blood pressure: An updated review of the literature. *Curr Pharm Des.* 2016;22(1):28-51. doi: 10.2174/1381612822666151109111712.

Papp ME, Wändell PE, Petra Lindfors P, Nygren-Bonnier M. Effects of yogic exercises on functional capacity, lung function and quality of life in participants with obstructive pulmonary disease: a randomized controlled study. *Eur J Phys Rehabil Med.* 2017;53(3):447-461. doi: 10.23736/S1973-9087.16.04374-4.

Sinharay R, Gong J, Barratt B, *et al.* Respiratory and cardiovascular responses to walking down a traffic-polluted road compared with walking in a traffic-free area in participants aged 60 years and older with chronic lung or heart disease and age-matched healthy controls: a randomised, crossover study. *Lancet.* 2018;391(10118):339-349. doi: 10.1016/S0140-6736(17)32643-0.

Suzuki M, Namura K, Ohno Y, *et al.* Combined standard medication and acupuncture for COPD: a case series. *Acupunct Med.* 2012;30(2):96-102. doi: 10.1136/acupmed-2011-010112.

Tashkin DP. Does smoking marijuana increase the risk of chronic obstructive pulmonary disease? *CMAJ.* 2009;180(8):797-798. doi: 10.1503/cmaj.090142.

Chapter 14—Lowering the Risk of a Stroke

Boden WE, Miller MG, McBride R, *et al.* Testosterone concentrations and risk of cardiovascular events in androgen-deficient men with atherosclerotic cardiovascular disease. *Am Heart J.* 2020;224:65-76. doi: 10.1016/j.ahj.2020.03.016.

Sakakibara BM, Kim AJ, Eng JJ. A systematic review and meta-analysis on self-management for improving risk factor control in stroke patients. *Int J Behav Med.* 2017;24(1):42-53. doi: 10.1007/s12529-016-9582-7.

Stroke Facts. U.S. Centers for Disease Control and Prevention Website. https://www.cdc.gov/stroke/facts.htm. Accessed August 29, 2021.

Tong TYN, Appleby PN, Key TJ, *et al.* The associations of major foods and fibre with risks of ischaemic and haemorrhagic stroke: A prospective study of 418,329 participants in the EPIC cohort across nine European countries. *European Heart Journal.* 2020;41(28):2632–2640. doi: 10.1093/eurheartj/ehaa007.

Chapter 15—The Alzheimer's Tsunami

Ben Greenfield Fitness Website. https://bengreenfieldfitness.com/

Best foods for a healthy brain. Northwestern Medicine Website. https://www.nm.org/healthbeat/healthy-tips/nutrition/best-food-for-a-healthy-brain. Accessed August 29, 2021.

Facts and Figures. Alzheimer's Association Website. https://www.alz.org/alzheimers-dementia/facts-figures and https://www.alz.org/alzheimers-dementia/what-is-dementia/related_conditions/mild-cognitive-impairment. Accessed August 29, 2021.

Free Online Self-Assessment. Cleveland Clinic Website. https://healthybrains.org/brain-check-up/ Accessed August 29, 2021.

What are the signs of Alzheimer's disease? National Institute of Aging Website. https://www.nia.nih.gov/health/what-are-signs-alzheimers-disease. Accessed September 8, 2021.

Chapter 16—Reversing Early Dementia

Bredesen DE. Reversal of cognitive decline: a novel therapeutic program. *Aging (Albany NY).* 2014;6(9):707-17. doi: 10.18632/aging.100690.

Bredesen DE, Sharlin K, Jenkins D, *et al.* Reversal of cognitive decline: 100 patients. *J Alzheimers Dis Parkinsonism.* 2018;8(5):450. doi: 10.4172/2161-0460.1000450.

Chapter 25—Preserving Your Hearing

Bagai A, Thavendiranathan P, Detsky AS. Does this patient have hearing impairment? *JAMA.* 2006;295(4):416-28. doi: 10.1001/jama.295.4.416.

Burkey JM, Lippy WH, Schuring AG, Rizer FM. Clinical utility of the 512-Hz Rinne tuning fork test. *Am J Otol.* 1998;19(1):59-62. PMID: 9455950.

Carroll YI, Eichwald J, Scinicariello F, *et al.* Vital signs: noise-induced hearing loss among adults—United States 2011-2012. *MMWR Morb Mortal Wkly Rep.* 2017;66:139-144. doi: 10.15585/mmwr.mm6605e3.

Chole RA, Cook GB. The Rinne test for conductive deafness. A critical appraisal. *Arch Otolaryngol Head Neck Surg.* 1988;114(4):399-403. doi:10.1001/archotol.1988.01860160043018.

Curhan SG, Eavey R, Shargorodsky J, Curhan GC. Analgesic use and the risk of hearing loss in men. *Am J Med.* 2010;123(3):231-237. doi: 10.1016/j.amjmed.2009.08.006.

Eichwald J, Scinicariello F, Telfer JL, Carroll YI. Use of personal hearing protection devices at loud athletic or entertainment events among adults—United States, 2018. *MMWR Morb Mortal Wkly Rep.* 2018;67(41):1151-1155. doi: 10.15585/mmwr.mm6741a4.

Memel D, Langley C, Watkins C, *et al.* Effectiveness of ear syringing in general practice: a randomized controlled trial and patients' experiences. *Br J Gen Pract.* 2002;52(484):906-911. PMID: 12434959.

Recommendations for a noise standard. Occupational Noise Exposure. NIOSH Publication Number 98-126/CDC/NIOSH. Centers for Disease Control and Prevention Website. https://www.cdc.gov/niosh/docs/98-126/pdfs/98-126.pdf?id=10.26616/NIOSHPUB98126. Accessed August 29, 2021.

Roeser RJ, Ballachanda BB. Physiology, pathophysiology, and anthropology/epidemiology of human ear canal secretions. *J Am Acad Audiol.* 1997;8(6):391-400. PMID: 9433685.

Rosenfeld RM, Schwartz SR, Cannon CR, *et al.* Clinical Practice Guideline: Acute Otitis Exerna. *Otolaryngol Head Neck Surg.* 2014;150 (1_suppl):S2. doi: 10.1177/0194599813517083.

Schwartz SR, Magit AE, Rosenfeld RM, *et al.* Clinical Practice Guideline (Update) Earwax (Cerumen Impaction). *Otolaryngol Head Neck Surg.* 2017;156(1_suppl):S19. doi: 10.1177/0194599816671491.

Schwartz SR, Magit AE, Rosenfeld RM, *et al.* Clinical Practice Guideline (Update) Earwax (Cerumen Impaction). *Otolaryngol Head Neck Surg.* 2017;156(1_suppl):S20. doi: 10.1177/0194599816671491.

Sharp JF, Wilson JA, Ross L, Barr-Hamilton RM. Earwax removal: a survey of current practice. *BMJ.* 1990;301:1251. doi: 10.1136/bmj.301.6763.1251.

Chapter 29—Sleep

Consensus Conference Panel. Watson NF, Badr MS, *et al.* Recommended amount of sleep for a healthy adult: A joint consensus statement of the American Academy of Sleep Medicine and Sleep Research Society. *Sleep.* 2015;38(6):843-4. doi: 10.5665/sleep.4716

Cheng P, Drake CL. Sleep-wake disturbances in shift workers, page 1. UpToDate Website. https://www.uptodate.com/contents/sleep-wake-disturbances-in-shift-workers. Updated August 7, 2020. Accessed September 8, 2021.

Goldstein CA. Jet Lag, page 8. UpToDate Website. https://www.uptodate.com/contents/jet-lag. Updated February 12, 2020. Accessed September 8, 2021.

Gray SL, Anderson ML, Dublin S, *et al.* Cumulative use of strong anticholinergics and incident dementia: a prospective cohort study. *JAMA Intern Med.* 2015;175(3):401-7. doi: 10.1001/jamainternmed.2014.7663.

Harbourt K, Nevo ON, Zhang R, *et al.* Association of eszopiclone, zaleplon, or zolpidem with complex sleep behaviors resulting in serious injuries, including death. *Pharmacoepidemiol Drug Saf.* 2020;29(6):684-691. doi: 10.1002/pds.5004.

Hirschkowitz M, Whiton K, Albert SM, *et al.* National Sleep Foundation's updated sleep duration recommendations: final report. *Sleep Health.* 2015;1(4):233-243. doi: 10.1016/j.sleh.2015.10.004.

Ker K, Edwards PJ, Felix LM, *et al.* Caffeine for the prevention of injuries and errors in shift workers. *Cochrane Database Syst Rev.* 2010;2010(5):CD008508. doi: 10.1002/14651858.CD008508.

Liira J, Verbeek JH, Costa G, *et al.* Pharmacological interventions for sleepiness and sleep disturbances caused by shift work. *Cochrane Database Syst Rev.* 2014;(8):CD009776. doi: 10.1002/14651858.CD009776.pub2.

Maruyama T, Sato S, Matsumura M, *et al.* Evaluations of effects of sleep surfaces on athletic performance in youth. *Sci Rep.* 2020;10(1):11805. doi: 10.1038/s41598-020-68795-5.

Maski K. Insufficient sleep: Evaluation and Management, page 2. UpToDate Website. https://www.uptodate.com/contents/insufficient-sleep-evaluation-and-management. Updated February 19, 2021. Accessed September 8, 2021.

Maski K. Insufficient sleep: Evaluation and Management, pages 3-4. UpToDate Website. https://www.uptodate.com/contents/insufficient-sleep-evaluation-and-management. Updated February 19, 2021. Accessed September 8, 2021.

McDonnell B, Newcomb P. Trial of essential oils to improve sleep for patients in cardiac rehabilitation. *J Altern Complement Med.* 2019;25(12):1193-1199. doi: 10.1089/acm.2019.0222.

Ozkaraman A, Dügüm Ö, Özen Yılmaz H, Usta Yesilbalkan Ö. Aromatherapy: The effect of lavender on anxiety and sleep quality in patients treated With chemotherapy. *Clin J Oncol Nurs.* 2018;22(2):203-210. doi: 10.1188/18. CJON.203-210.

Rafique N, Ibrahim Al-Asoom L, Abdulrahman Alsunni A, *et al.* Effects of mobile use on subjective sleep quality. *Nat Sci Sleep.* 2020;12:357-364. doi: 10.2147/NSS.S253375.

Son J, Jung Sungwook, Song Haseung, *et al.* A survey of Koreans on sleep habits and sleeping symptoms relating to pillow comfort and support. *Int J Environ Res Public Health.* 2020;17(1):302. doi: 10.3390/ijerph17010302.

Chapter 30—Coping with Jet Lag

Ambesh P, Shetty V, Ambesh S, Gupta SS, Kamholz S, Wolf L. Jet lag: heuristics and therapeutics. *J Family Med Prim Care.* 2018;7(3):507-510. doi: 10.4103/jfmpc. jfmpc_220_17.

Arendt J. Managing jet lag: some of the problems and possible new solutions. *Sleep Med Rev.* 2009;13(4):249–56. doi: 10.1016/j.smrv.2008.07.011.

Herxheimer A, Petrie KJ. Melatonin for the prevention and treatment of jet lag. *Cochrane Database of Systematic Reviews* Website. 2002;2:CD001520. https://www.cochrane.org/CD001520/DEPRESSN_melatonin-for-the-prevention-and-treatment-of-jet-lag. Accessed August 29, 2021.

Leatherwood WE, Dragoo JL. Effect of airline travel on performance: a review of the literature. *Br J Sports Med.* 2013;47(9):561–67. doi: 10.1136/bjsports-2012-091449.

McHill AW, Smith BJ, Wright KP Jr. Effects of caffeine on skin and core temperatures, alertness, and recovery sleep during circadian misalignment. *J Biol Rhythms.* 2014;29(2):131–43. doi: 10.1177/0748730414523078.

McKenna H, Wilkes M. Optimising sleep for night shifts. *BMJ.* 2018;360:j5637. doi: 10.1136/bmj.j5637.

Sack RL, Auckley D, Auger RR, *et al.* Circadian rhythm sleep disorders: part I, basic principles, shift work and jet lag disorders. *Sleep.* 2007;30(11):1460–83. doi: 10.1093/sleep/30.11.1460.

Waterhouse J, Reilly T, Atkinson G, Edwards B. Jet lag: trends and coping strategies. *Lancet.* 2017;369(9567):1117–29. doi: 10.1016/S0140-6736(07)60529-7.

Chapter 38—Joint Health is the Key to Staying Active

Buddhachat K, Siengdee P, Chomdej S, Soontornvipart K, Nganvongpanit K. Effects of different omega-3 sources, fish oil, krill oil, and green-lipped mussel against cytokine-mediated canine cartilage degradation. *In Vitro Cell Dev Biol: Anim.* 2017;53(5):448-457. doi: 10.1007/s11626-016-0125-y.

Denning WM, Winward JG, Pardo MB, Hopkins JT, Seeley MK. Body weight independently affects articular cartilage catabolism. *J Sports Sci Med.* 2015;14(2):290–296. PMID: 25983577. https://www.jssm.org/volume14/iss2/cap/jssm-14-290.pdf. Accessed August 29, 2021.

Kaneko Y, Tanigawa N, Sato Y, *et al.* Oral administration of N-acetyl cysteine prevents osteoarthritis development and progression in a rat model. *Sci Rep.* 2019;9(1):18741. doi: 10.1038/s41598-019-55297-2.

Majeed M, Majeed S, Narayanan NK, Nagabhushanam K. A pilot, double-blind, placebo-controlled trial to assess the safety and efficacy of a novel *Boswellia serrata* extract in the management of osteoarthritis of the knee. *Phytother Res.* 2019;33(5):1457-1468. doi: 10.1002/ptr.6338.

O'Driscoll SW, Keeley FW, Salter RB. The chondrogenic potential of free autogenous periosteal grafts for biological resurfacing of major full-thickness defects in joint surfaces under the influence of continuous passive motion. An experimental investigation in the rabbit. *J Bone Joint Surg Am.* 1986;68(7):1017-35. PMID: 3745239.

Park MH, Jung JC, Hill S, *et al.* FlexPro MD, a combination of krill oil, astaxanthin and hyaluronic acid, reduces pain behavior and inhibits inflammatory response in monosodium iodoacetate-induced osteoarthritis in rats. *Nutrients.* 2020;12(4):956. doi: 10.3390/nu12040956.

Reeves ND, Maganaris CN, Narici MV. Effect of strength training on human patella tendon mechanical properties of older individuals. *J Physiol.* 2003;548(Pt 3):971–981. doi: 10.1113/jphysiol.2002.035576.

Shep D, Khanwelkar C, Gade P, Karad S. Safety and efficacy of curcumin versus diclofenac in knee osteoarthritis: a randomized open-label parallel-arm study. *Trials.* 2019;20(1):214. doi: 10.1186/s13063-019-3327-2.

Chapter 42— Emsculpt: High-Tech Muscle Building

Kinney BM, Lozanova P. High intensity focused electromagnetic therapy evaluated by magnetic resonance imaging: safety and efficacy study of a dual tissue effect based non-invasive abdominal body shaping. *Lasers Surg Med.* 2019;51(1):40-46. doi: 10.1002/lsm.23024.

Chapter 45—How to Quit Smoking

Consumer books:

Hilliard ME, Riekert KA, Ockene JK, Pbert L, eds. *The Handbook of Health Behavior Change.* 5th ed. New York, NY: Springer Publishing Company, 2018.

West, Robert, and Shiffman, Saul. *Smoking cessation (fast facts).* 2nd ed. Basel, Switzerland: Karger Publishers, 2007.

Journal articles:

Abbot NC, Stead LF, White A, Barnes J, Ernst E. Hypnotherapy for smoking cessation. *Cochrane Database of Systematic Reviews.* 1998;2(2).

Caponnetto P, Campagna D, Cibella F, *et al.* ECLAT (acronym for efficiency and safety of an electronic cigarette) as tobacco cigarettes substitute: a prospective 12-month randomized control design study. *PloS One.* 2013;8(6):e66317. doi: 10.1371/journal.pone.0066317.

Caponnetto P, Polosa R, Russo C, Leotta C, Campagna D. Successful smoking cessation with electronic cigarettes in smokers with a documented history of recurring relapses: a case series. *J Med Case Rep.* 2011;5:585. doi: 10.1186/1752-1947-5-585.

Diefenbach LJ, Smith PO, Nashelsky J, Lindbloom E. Clinical inquiries. What is the most effective nicotine replacement therapy? *J Fam Pract.* 2003;52(6):492-494. PMID: 12791233.

Fiore MC, Novotny TE, Pierce JP, *et al.* Methods used to quit smoking in the United States. Do cessation programs help? *JAMA.* 1990;263(20):2760–2765. PMID: 2271019.

Hajek P, Phillips-Waller A, Przulj D, *et al.* A randomized trial of e-cigarettes versus nicotine-replacement therapy. *N Engl J Med.* 2019;380(7):629-637. doi: 10.1056/NEJMoa1808779.

Hartmann-Boyce J, Stead LF, Cahill K, Lancaster T. Efficacy of interventions to combat tobacco addiction: Cochrane update of 2012 reviews. *Addiction.* 2013;108(10):1711–1721. doi: 10.1111/add.12291.

Regmi K, Kassim N, Ahmad N, Tuah N. Effectiveness of mobile apps for smoking cessation: a review. *Tob Prev Cessat.* 2017;3:12. PMID: 32432186. doi: 10.18332/tpc/70088.

Valentine GW, Hefner K, Jatlow PI, *et al.* Impact of e-cigarettes on smoking and related outcomes in veteran smokers with psychiatric comorbidity. *J Dual Diagn.* 2018;14(1):2–13. doi: 10.1080/15504263.2017.1384877.

West R, Walia A, Hyder N, Shahab L, Michie S. Behavior change techniques used by the English Stop Smoking Services and their associations with short-term quit outcomes. *Nicotine Tob Res.* 2010;12(7):742–747. doi: 10.1093/ntr/ntq074.

Whittaker R, McRobbie H, Bullen C, *et al.* Mobile phone text messaging and app-based interventions for smoking cessation. *Cochrane Database of Syst Rev.* 2019;10(10):CD006611. PMID: 31638271. doi: 10.1002/14651858.CD006611.pub

Chapter 47—Cocaine is Not Your Friend

Alcohol and drug abuse statistics. American Addiction Centers Website. https://americanaddictioncenters.org/rehab-guide/addiction-statistics. Accessed August 29, 2021.

Bogunovic O. Substance abuse in aging and elderly adults. *Psychiatric Times.* 2012;29(8). Psychiatric Times Website. https://www.psychiatrictimes.com/geriatric-psychiatry/substance-abuse-aging-and-elderly-adults. Accessed August 29, 2021.

Cheng YC, Ryan KA, Qadwai SA, *et al.* Cocaine use and risk of ischemic stroke in young adults. *Stroke.* 2016;47(4):918–922. PMID: 26965853. doi: 10.1161/STROKEAHA.115.011417.

Results from the 2017 National Survey on Drug Use and Health: Detailed Tables. Substance Abuse and Mental Health Services Administration Website. https://www.samhsa.gov/data/sites/default/files/cbhsq-reports/NSDUHDetailedTabs2017/NSDUHDetailedTabs2017.pdf Published 2018. Accessed August 29, 2021.

Chapter 48—The Dark Side of Cannabis

Brands B, Mann RE, Wickens CM, *et al.* Acute and residual effects of smoked cannabis: impact on driving speed and lateral control, heart rate, and self-reported drug effects. *Drug Alcohol Depend.* 2019;205:107641. doi: 10.1016/j.drugalcdep.2019.107641.

Hartley S, Simon N, Larabi A, *et al.* Effect of smoked cannabis on vigilance and accident risk using simulated driving in occasional and chronic users and the pharmacokinetic-pharmacodynamic relationship. *Clin Chem.* 2019;65(5):684-693. doi: 10.1373/clinchem.2018.299727.

Hartman RL, Brown TL, Milavetz G, *et al.* Cannabis effects on driving lateral control with and without alcohol. *Drug Alcohol Depend.* 2015;154:25-37. doi: 10.1016/j.drugalcdep.2015.06.015.

McClure EA, Lydiard JB, Goddard SD, Gray KM. Objective and subjective memory ratings in cannabis-dependent adolescents. *Am J Addict.* 2015;24(1):47-52. PMID: 25823635. doi: 10.1111/ajad.12171.

Minică CC, Verweij KJH, van der Most PJ, *et al.* Genome-wide association meta-analysis of age at first cannabis use. *Addiction.* 2018;113(11):2073-2086. doi: 10.1111/add.14368.

Rogeberg O. A meta-analysis of the crash risk of cannabis-positive drivers in culpability studies-avoiding interpretational bias. *Accid Anal Prev.* 2019;123:69-78. doi: 10.1016/j.aap.2018.11.011.

Rogeberg O, Elvik R. The effects of cannabis intoxication on motor vehicle collision revisited and revised. *Addiction.* 2016;111(8):1348-59. doi: 10.1111/add.13347.

Sewell RA, Poling J, Sofuoglu M. The effect of cannabis compared with alcohol on driving. *Am J Addict.* 2009;18(3):185–193. doi: 10.1080/10550490902786934.

Chapter 49—Health Benefits of CBD

Scherma M, Fadda P, Le Foll B, *et al.* The endocannabinoid system: a new molecular target for the treatment of tobacco addiction. *CNS Neurol Disord Drug Targets.* 2008;7(5):468-81. doi: 10.2174/187152708786927859.

Scherma M, Medalie J, Fratta W, *et al.* The endogenous cannabinoid anandamide has effects on motivation and anxiety that are revealed by fatty acid amide hydrolase (FAAH) inhibition. *Neuropharmacology.* 2008;54(1):129-40. doi: 10.1016/j.neuropharm.2007.08.011.

Chapter 50—Electronic Addiction

Chen KH, Oliffe JL, Kelly MT. Internet gaming disorder: an emergent health issue for men. *Am J Mens Health.* 2018;12(4):1151–1159. PMID: 29606034. doi: 10.1177/1557988318766950.

Grubbs JB, Wilt JA, Exline JJ, Pargament KI, Kraus SW. Moral disapproval and perceived addiction to internet pornography: a longitudinal examination. *Addiction.* 2018;113(3):496-506. doi: 10.1111/add.14007.

Laconi S, Andréoletti A, Chauchard E, Rodgers RF, Chabrol H. Problematic Internet use, time spent online and personality traits. *L'Encéphale.* 2016;42(3):214–218. PMID: 26827120. doi: 10.1016/j.encep.2015.12.017.

Northrup JC, Shumway S. Gamer widow: a phenomenological study of spouses of online video game addicts. *The American Journal of Family Therapy.* 2014;42(4):269–281. doi:10.1080/01926187.2013.847705.

Shensa A, Escobar-Viera CG, Sidani JE, Bowman ND, Marshall MP, Primack BA. Problematic social media use and depressive symptoms among U.S. young adults: a nationally-representative study. *Soc Si Med.* 2017;182:150-157. doi: 10.1016/j.socscimed.2017.03.061.

Vollmer C, Randler C, Horzum MB, Ayas T. Computer game addiction in adolescents and its relationship to chronotype and personality. *SAGE Open.* 2014;4(1):1–9. doi: 10.1177/2158244013518054.

Chapter 51—Pornography

Consumer books:

Barna Group and McDowell, Josh. *The Porn Phenomenon: The Impact of Pornography in the Digital Age.* Ventura, CA: Barna Group, 2016.

Brooks, Gary R. *The Centerfold Syndrome: How Men Can Overcome Objectification and Achieve Intimacy with Women.* Hoboken, NJ: Jossey-Bass Publications, 1995.

Journal articles and web pages:

2014 Pornography Survey and Statistics. Barna Group. Proven Men Website. https://www.provenmen.org/pornography-survey-statistics-2014/ Accessed September 1, 2021.

Pornography statistics. Covenant Eyes Website. https://www.covenanteyes.com/pornstats/ Accessed September 1, 2021.

Primary sources for this chapter:

A few research-based facts about pornography. Sex and Relationship Healing Website. https://sexandrelationshiphealing.com/blog/research-based-facts-pornography/ Published November 19, 2018. Accessed September 1, 2021.

How to deal with premature ejaculation. Innovative Men's Health Website. https://innovativemen.com/blog/how-to-deal-with-premature-ejaculation/ Accessed September 1, 2021.

Hull, Megan, ed. Porn addiction. The Recovery Village Website. https://www.therecoveryvillage.com/process-addiction/porn-addiction/related/pornography-statistics/ Updated July 13, 2021. Accessed September 1, 2021.

Chapter 52—Aesthetics and Grooming

Ludden D. Do women really prefer men with money over looks? Psychology Today Website. https://www.psychologytoday.com/us/blog/talking-apes/201907/do-women-really-prefer-men-money-over-looks. Published 2019. Accessed August 29, 2021.

Chapter 54—Protecting Your Skin

Akamatsu H, Hasegawa S, Yamada T, *et al.* Age-related decrease in CD271(+) cells in human skin. *J Dermatol.* 2016;43(3):311-313. doi: 10.1111/1346-8138.13048.

Imadojemu S, Sarwer DB, Percec I, *et al.* Influence of surgical and minimally invasive facial cosmetic procedures on psychosocial outcomes: a systematic review. *JAMA Dermatol.* 2013;149(11):1325-1333. doi: 10.1001/jamadermatol.2013.6812.

Lim HW, Arellano-Mendoza MI, Stengel F. Current challenges in photoprotection. *J Am Acad Dermatol.* 2017;76(351):S91-9. doi: 10.1016/j.jaad.2016.09.040.

Murad A, Tung R. Injection technique in neurotoxins and fillers: Planning and basic technique. *J Am Acad Dermatol.* 2018;79(3):407-19. doi: 10.1016/j.jaad.2018.01.034.

Chapter 56—Restoring the Hair on Your Head

Adil A, Godwin M. The effectiveness of treatments for androgenetic alopecia: A systematic review and meta-analysis. *J Am Acad Dermatol.* 2017;77(1):136-141.e5. doi: 10.1016/j.jaad.2017.02.054.

Badran KW, Sand JP. Platelet-rich plasma for hair loss: review of methods and results. *Facial Plast Surg Clin North Am.* 2018;26(4):469-485. doi: 10.1016/j.fsc.2018.06.008.

Olsen EA, Whiting D, Bergfeld W, *et al.* A multicenter, randomized, placebo-controlled, double blind clinical trial of a novel formulation of 5% minoxidil topical foam vs placebo in the treatment of androgenetic alopecia in men. *J Am Acad Dermatol.* 2007;57(5):767-774. doi: 10.1016/j.jaad.2007.04.012.

Chapter 59—Listen to the Music

Finn S, Fancourt D. The biological impact of listening to music in clinical and nonclinical settings: a systematic review. *Prog Brain Res.* 2018;237:173-200. doi: 10.1016/bs.pbr.2018.03.007.

Heshmat S. Why are we moved by music? Psychology Today Website. https://www.psychologytoday.com/us/blog/science-choice/201807/why-are-we-moved-music. Published 2018. Accessed August 29, 2021.

Lenc T, Keller PE, Varlet M, Nozaradan S. Neural tracking of the musical beat is enhanced by low-frequency sounds. *Proc Natl Acad Sci USA.* 2018;115(32):8221-6. doi: 10.1073/pnas.1801421115.

Sugaya K, Yonetani A. Your brain on music. *Pegasus, the Magazine of the University of Central Florida.* University of Central Florida Website. https://www.ucf.edu/pegasus/your-brain-on-music/ Accessed August 29, 2021.

Thoma MV, La Marca R, Brönnimann R, *et al.* The effect of music on the human stress response. *PloS One.* 2013;8(8):e70156. doi: 10.1371/journal.pone.0070156.

Chapter 65—Diseases of Despair

Age-adjusted death rates for selected causes of death, by sex, race, and Hispanic origin: United States, selected years 1950-2017. Poisoning of males going up. Centers for Disease Control and Prevention Website. https://www.cdc.gov/nchs/data/hus/2018/005.pdf. Accessed September 1, 2021.

Healthy life years lost to drug use disorders in the U.S. from 1990 to 2017. American Addiction Centers Website. https://americanaddictioncenters.org/learn/years-lost-to-drugs/ Accessed September 1, 2021.

Long-terms trends in deaths of despair. United States Congress, Joint Economic Committee, Social Capital Project. SCP Report no. 4-19. U.S. Senate Website. https://www.jec.senate.gov/public/_cache/files/0f2d3dba-9fdc-41e5-9bd1-9c13f4204e35/jec-report-deaths-of-despair.pdf. Published 2019. Accessed August 29, 2021.

Meara E, Skinner J. Losing ground at midlife in America. *Proc Natl Acad Sci USA.* 2015;112(49):15006-15007. doi: 10.1073/pnas.1519763112.

Opioid overdose deaths by age group. Kaiser Family Foundation Website. https://www. kff.org/other/state-indicator/opioid-overdose-deaths-by-age-group/?dataView=1& activeTab=graph&currentTimeframe=0&startTimeframe=19&selectedDistributio ns=35-44--45-54--55&selectedRows=%7B%22wrapups%22:%7B%22united-state s%22:%7D%7D%7D&sortModel=%7B%22colId%22:%22Location%22,% 22sort%22:%22asc%22%7D. Accessed September 1, 2021.

Santhanam L. American life expectancy has dropped again. Here's why. PBS NewsHour Website. https://www.pbs.org/newshour/health/american-life-expectancy-has-dropped-again-heres-why. Published November 29, 2018. Accessed September 1, 2021.

Suicide facts. Suicide Awareness Voices of Education (SAVE) Website. https://save.org/ about-suicide/suicide-facts/ Accessed September 1, 2021.

Suicide statistics. American Foundation for Suicide Prevention Website. https://afsp.org/ suicide-statistics/ Published February 2021. Accessed September 1, 2021.

Suicide warning signs. American Psychological Association Website. https://www.apa. org/topics/suicide/signs. Published November 2019. Accessed September 1, 2021.

U.S. Life Expectancy 1950-2021. Macrotrends LLC Website. https://www.macrotrends. net/countries/USA/united-states/life-expectancy. Accessed September 1, 2021.

Why are middle-aged white men more likely to die by suicide? SSM Health Website. https://www.ssmhealth.com/blogs/ssm-health-matters/october-2019/middle-aged-men-more-likely-to-die-by-suicide. Published October 14, 2019. Accessed September 1, 2021.

Chapter 66—Anxiety

Americans Feel Good About Counseling. Barna Group Website. https://www.barna. com/research/americans-feel-good-counseling/ Accessed September 8, 2021.

Any anxiety disorder. National Institute of Mental Health Website. https://www.nimh. nih.gov/health/statistics/any-anxiety-disorder.shtml. Accessed September 8, 2021.

Benson H, Beary JF, Carol MP. The Relaxation Response. *Psychiatry.* 1974;37(1): 37-46. doi: 10.1080/00332747.1974.11023785.

Jacobson, Edmund. *Progressive Relaxation.* Chicago, IL: University of Chicago Press, 1929.

McKay, Matthew. *Thoughts and Feelings: Taking Control of Your Moods and Your Life.* 4th ed. Oakland, CA: New Harbinger Publications, 2011.

McKay, Matthew and White, John. *Overcoming Generalized Anxiety Disorder: A Relaxation, Cognitive Restructuring, and Exposure-Based Protocol for the Treatment of GAD.* Oakland, CA: New Harbinger Publications, 1999.

Sapolsky, Robert M. *Why Zebras Don't Get Ulcers.* 3rd ed. New York, NY: Holt Paperbacks, 2004.

Chapter 67—Depression

American Psychiatric Association. *Diagnostic and Statistical Manual of Mental Disorders*. 5th ed. Washington, DC: American Psychiatric Publishing, 2013.

Fournier JC, DeRubeis RJ, Hollon SD, *et al*. Antidepressant drug effects and depression severity: a patient-level meta-analysis. *JAMA*. 2010;303(1):47-53. doi: 10.1001/jama.2009.1943.

Hall-Flavin, DK. Clinical Depression: What does it mean? Mayo Clinic Website. https://www.mayoclinic.org/diseases-conditions/depression/expert-answers/clinical-depression/faq-20057770. Accessed September 8, 2021.

Higuera V. Situational depression or clinical depression? Medical News Today Website. https://www.medicalnewstoday.com/articles/314698. Published September 28, 2018. Accessed September 8, 2021.

Hofmann, Stefan and Asmundson, Gordon J.G., eds. *The Science of Cognitive Behavioral Therapy*. Cambridge, MA: Academic Press, 2017.

Liberman JA. "Minimizing Risk: The Importance of Safety and Tolerability When Treating Patients with Depression or Anxiety" (Presentation, Renaissance Hotel, Washington, DC, September 28, 2006)

McKay, Matthew and Fanning, Patrick. *Prisoners of Belief*. Oakland, CA: New Harbinger Publications, 1991.

Chapter 68—Living with Vitality

May, Rollo. *Freedom and Destiny*. New York, NY: W. W. Norton, 1981.

Schneider, Kirk. *Rediscovery of Awe: Splendor, mystery and the fluid center of life*. St. Paul, MN: Paragon House, 2004.

Schneider, Kirk J. *Existential-Integrative Psychotherapy*. New York, NY: Routledge, 2015.

Schneider, Kirk J. and Krug, Orah T. *Existential-Humanistic Therapy*. Washington, DC: American Psychological Association, 2009.

Chapter 69—Find Yourself a Partner Who Can Be Your Best Friend

Breuning, Loretta Graziano. *Habits of a Happy Brain*. Avon, MA: Adams Media, 2015.

Fisher, Helen. *Why Him? Why Her? Finding Real Love by Understanding Your Personality Type*. New York, NY: Henry Holt and Company, 2009.

Hirsch Sandra Krebs, Kummerow Jean M. *Life Types, 3rd edition*. New York, NY: Grand Central Publishing; 1989.

Widerstrom, Jen. *Diet Right for Your Personality Type*. New York, NY: Harmony Books, 2017.

Chapter 75—Fatherhood

Cole S. What high-profile working fathers leaving their jobs means for the rest of us. Fast Company Website. https://www.fastcompany.com/3043595/what-high-profile-working-fathers-leaving-their-jobs-means-for-the-rest-of-us. Published March 13, 2015. Accessed August 27, 2021.

Lamb, Michael E, ed. *The Role of the Father in Child Development.* 3rd ed. New York, NY: Wiley, 1997.

Levine, Suzanne Braun. *Father Courage: What Happens When Men Put Family First.* New York, NY: Harcourt, 2000.

Lewis, Robert A. and Roberts, Craig L. "Postparental Fathers in Distress," pages 199-204 in *Men in Transition*, ed. Solomon, Kenneth and Levy, N.B. New York, NY: Plenum Press, 1982. doi: 10.1007/978-1-4684-4211-3_11.

Mehren E. Not having it all in Washington/leaving work for family is no longer unthinkable, even in the powerful profession of government. Greensboro News & Record Website. https://greensboro.com/not-having-it-all-in-washington-leaving-work-for-family/article_730a4bf6-bdba-5f3f-ada1-31f4a2086241.html. Published December 22, 1996. Updated January 25, 2015. Accessed September 1, 2021.

Pruett, Kyle. *Fatherneed: Why Father Care Is as Essential as Mother Care for Your Child.* New York, NY: Free Press, 2000.

Pruett KD. How men and children affect each other's development. Zero to Three Website. https://www.zerotothree.org/resources/1075-how-men-and-children-affect-each-other-s-development. Published April 18, 1997. Accessed August 22, 2021.

Chapter 78—Orgasm: Too Fast, Too Slow, or Just Right

Aversa A, Pili M, Francomano D, *et al.* Effects of vardenafil administration on intravaginal ejaculatory latency time in men with lifelong premature ejaculation. *Int J Impot Res.* 2009;21(4):221-7. doi: 10.1038/ijir.2009.21.

Canat L, Degirmentepe RB, Atalay HA, *et al.* Low serum vitamin D is associated with an increased likelihood of acquired premature ejaculation. *Int Braz J Urol.* 2019;45(3):621-628. doi: 10.1590/S1677-5538.IBJU.2018.0887.

Carani C, Isidori AM, Granata A, *et al.* Multicenter study on the prevalence of sexual symptoms in male hypo- and hyperthyroid patients. *J Clin Endocrinol Metab.* 2005;90(12):6472-9. doi: 10.1210/jc.2005-1135.

El-Hamd MA, Saleh R, Majzoub A. Premature ejaculation: an update on definition and pathophysiology. *Asian J Androl.* 2019;21(5):425-432. doi: 10.4103/aja.aja_122_18.

Jern P, Johansson A, Strohmaier J, Treutlein J, Piha J, Rietschel M. Preliminary evidence for an association between variants of the catechol-o-methyltransferase (COMT) gene and premature ejaculation. *J Sex Med.* 2017;14(2):1558-65. doi: 10.1016/j.jsxm.2017.11.002.

La Pera G. Awareness and timing of pelvic floor muscle contraction, pelvic exercises and rehabilitation of pelvic floor in lifelong premature ejaculation: 5 years experience. *Arch Ital Urol Androl.* 2014;86(2):123-5. doi: 10.4081/aiua.2014.2.123.

Mirone V, Arcaniolo D, Rivas D, *et al.* Results from a prospective observational study of men with premature ejaculation treated with dapoxetine or alternative care: the PAUSE study. *Eur Urol.* 2014;65(4):733-9. doi: 10.1016/j.eururo.2013.08.018.

Raveendran AV, Agarwal A. Premature ejaculation - current concepts in the management: a narrative review. *Int J Reprod Biomed.* 2021;19(1):5-22. doi: 10.18502/ijrm.v19i1.8176.

Waldinger MD. The pathophysiology of lifelong premature ejaculation. *Transl Androl Urol.* 2016;5(4):424-433. doi: 10.21037/tau.2016.06.04.

Chapter 80—Wave Goodbye to ED

COVID may lead to erectile dysfunction in men long after recovery. The Tribune (Chandigarh) Website. https://www.tribuneindia.com/news/health/covid-may-lead-to-erectile-dysfunction-in-men-long-after-recovery-251842. Published May 12, 2021. Accessed August 19, 2021.

Huang V, Munarriz R, Goldstein I. Bicycle riding and erectile dysfunction: an increase in interest (and concern). *J Sex Med.* 2005;2(5):596–604. doi: 10.1111/j.1743-6109.2005.00099.x.

Landripet I, Štulhofer A. Is pornography use associated with sexual difficulties and dysfunctions among younger heterosexual men? *J Sex Med.* 2015;12(5):1136–39. doi: 10.1111/jsm.12853.

Sommer F, Goldstein I, Korda JB. Bicycle riding and erectile dysfunction: a review. *J Sex Med.* 2010;7(7):2346-58. doi:10.1111/j.1743-6109.2009.01664.x.

Chapter 81—Viagra and Beyond

Diamond LE, Earle DC, Rosen RC, Willett MS, Molinoff PB. Double-blind, placebo-controlled evaluation of the safety, pharmacokinetic properties and pharmacodynamic effects of intranasal PT-141, a melanocortin receptor agonist, in healthy males and patients with mild-to-moderate erectile dysfunction. *Int J Impot Res.* 2004;16(1):51-59. doi: 10.1038/sj.ijir.3901139.

Krapf, Jill M., Buster, John E., and Goldstein, Andrew T. "Management of Hypoactive Sexual Desire Disorder (HSDD)," pages 233-249 in *Management of Sexual Dysfunction in Men and Women*, ed. Lipshultz, Larry I., Pastuszak, Alexander W., Goldstein, Andrew T., Giraldi, Annamaria, and Perelman, Michael A. New York: Springer, 2016. doi: 10.1007/978-1-4939-3100-2_21.

Molinoff PB, Shadiak AM, Earle DC, Diamond LE, Quon CY. PT-141: A melanocortin agonist for the treatment of sexual dysfunction. *Ann NY Acad Sci.* 2003;994:96-102. doi: 10.1111/j.1749-6632.2003.tb03167.x.

Chapter 83—Platelet Rich Plasma (PRP) for ED and More

Lifestyle:

Runels, Charles. *Savage Factors™: Peak Physical, Mental, and Sexual Performance through the Practices of Ancient Civilizations.* Fairhope, AL: KDP, 2019.

Pruimboorn L, Muskiet FAJ. Intermittent living; the use of ancient challenges as a vaccine against the deleterious effects of modern life-A hypothesis. *Med Hypotheses.* 2018;120:28-42. doi: 10.1016/j.mehy.2018.08.002.

Journal articles:

Alser OH, Goutos I. The evidence behind the use of platelet-rich plasma (PRP) in scar management: a literature review. *Scars Burn Heal.* 2018;4:2059513118808773. doi: 10.1177/2059513118808773.

Casabona F, Gambelli I, Casabona F, Santi P, Santori G, Baldelli I. Autologous platelet-rich plasma (PRP) in chronic penile lichen sclerosus: the impact on tissue repair and patient quality of life. Note: study by Goldstein and I (Charles Runels) showing it works for lichen. *Int Urol Nephrol.* 2017;49(3):573-580. doi: 10.1007/s11255-017-1523-0.

Cervelli V, Lucarini L, Spallone D, *et al.* Use of platelet-rich plasma and hyaluronic acid in the loss of substance with bone exposure. *Adv Skin Wound Care.* 2011;24(4):176-181. doi: 10.1097/01.ASW.0000396302.05959.d3.

Goldstein AT, King M, Runels C, Gloth M, Pfau R. Intradermal injection of autologous platelet-rich plasma for the treatment of vulvar lichen sclerosus. *J Am Acad Dermatol.* 2017;76(1):158-160. doi: 10.1016/j.jaad.2016.07.037.

Ibrahim MK, Ibrahim SM, Salem AM. Skin microneedling plus platelet-rich plasma versus skin microneedling alone in the treatment of atrophic post acne scars: a split face comparative study. *J Dermatolog Treat.* 2018;29(3):281-286. doi: 10.1080/09546634.2017.1365111.

Kumar CS. 265 Combined treatment of injecting platelet rich plasma with vacuum pump for penile enlargement. *J Sex Med.* 2017;14(1,suppl_1):S78. doi: 10.1016/j.jsxm.2016.11.174. https://www.jsm.jsexmed.org/article/S1743-6095(16)30656-7/fulltext. Accessed 8/29/2021.

Sanchez M, Anitua E, Delgado D, *et al.* Platelet-rich plasma, a source of autologous growth factors and biomimetic scaffold for peripheral nerve regeneration. *Expert Opin Biol Ther.* 2017;17(2):197-212. doi: 10.1080/14712598.2017.1259409.

Virag R, Sussman H, Lamboin S, de Fourmestraux V. Evaluation of the benefit of using a combination of autologous platelet rich-plasma and hyaluronic acid for the treatment of Peyronie's disease. *OAT Sex Health Issues.* 2017;1(1):1-8. doi: 10.15761/SHI.1000102.

Websites on the work of Dr. Runels:

Professional websites of Dr. Runels: CellularMedicineAssociation.org and www.Runels.com

Platelet-Rich Plasma (PRP): PriapusShot.com, OShot.info, OrgasmSystem.com, LichenSclerosusTreatment.com, and ILSVH.org

Vampire Facelift: VampireFacelift.com, VampireFacial.com, VampireSkinTherapy.com, and VampireHair.com

Lifestyle: www.SavageFactors.com

Chapter 84—Stem Cell Therapy

Consumer books:

Piccirillo, Jeffrey. *The Journey to Perfect PRP: a patient's guide on how to get the optimal outcome from your PRP injection.* Self-published, 2021.

Piccirillo, Jeffrey and Runels, Charles. *Perfect PRP: How to achieve excellent outcomes with platelet-rich plasma from aesthetics to urology.* Self-published, 2021.

Journal articles and web pages:

Davies JE, Walker JT, Keating A. Concise review: Wharton's jelly: the rich, but enigmatic, source of mesenchymal stromal cells. *Stem Cells Transl Med.* 2017;6(7):1620-1630. doi:10.1002/sctm.16-0492.

Kearl M. Dickey-Wicker Amendment, 1996. *Embryo Project Encyclopedia* (2010-08-27). ISSN: 1940-5030. Arizona State University Website. https://embryo.asu.edu/handle/10776/2050. Accessed September 1, 2021.

Mautner K, Bowers R, Easley K, *et al.* Functional outcomes following microfragmented adipose tissue versus bone marrow aspirate concentrate injections for symptomatic knee osteoarthritis. *Stem Cells Transl Med.* 2019;8(11):1149-1156. doi: 10.1002/sctm.18-0285.

Panero AJ, Hirahara AM, Anderson WJ, *et al.* Are amniotic fluid products stem cell therapies? A study of amniotic fluid preparations for mesenchymal stem cells with bone marrow comparison. *Am J Sports Med.* 2019;47(5):1230-1235. doi: 10.1177/0363546519829034.

What is a stem cell? Definition, uses & research facts. Study.com Website. https://study.com/academy/lesson/what-is-a-stem-cell-definition-uses-research-facts.html. Published September 19, 2017. Accessed August 29, 2021.

Chapter 89—Optimizing Testosterone

Abate N, Haffner SM, Garg A, *et al.* Sex steroid hormones, upper body obesity, and insulin resistance. *J Clin Endocrinol Metab.* 2002;87(10):4522-7. doi: 10.1210/jc.2002-020567.

Antonopoulous AS, Antoniades C. Mechanisms of testosterone deficiency-related endothelial dysfunction: invited commentary for the Hellenic Journal of Cardiology on Tsikas et al. "Associations between asymmetric dimethylarginine, nitrite-dependent renal carbonic anhydrase activity and plasma testosterone levels in hypogonadal men." *Hellenic J Cardiol.* 2018;59(4):207-208. doi: 10.1016/j.hjc.2018.06.001.

Baillargeon J, Urban RJ, Ottenbacher KJ, *et al.* Trends in androgen prescribing in the United States, 2001 to 2011. *JAMA Intern Med.* 2013;173(15):1465-1466. doi:10.1001/jamainternmed.2013.6895.

Baillargeon J, Urban RJ, Ottenbacher KJ, *et al.* Errors in percentages. *JAMA Intern Med.* 2013;173(15):1477. doi:10.1001/jamainternmed.2013.9183.

Brown-Séquard CE. Note on the effects produced on man by subcutaneous injections of a liquid obtained from the testicles of animals. *Lancet.* 1889;134(3438):105–7. doi: 10.1016/S0140-6736(00)64118-1.

Carruthers M, Trinick TR, Wheeler MJ. The validity of androgen assays. *Aging Male.* 2007;10(3):165-72. doi: 10.1080/13685530701483738.

Cervi A, Balitsky AK. Testosterone use causing erythrocytosis. *CMAJ.* 2017;189(41):E1286–E1288. doi: 10.1503/cmaj.170683.

Grossmann M, Thomas MC, Panagiotopoulos S, *et al.* Low testosterone levels are common and associated with insulin resistance in men with diabetes. *J Clin Endocrinol Metab.* 2008;93(5):1834-40. doi: 10.1210/jc.2007-2177.

Hak AE, Witteman JCM, de Jong FH, *et al.* Low levels of endogenous androgens increase the risk of atherosclerosis in elderly men: the Rotterdam study. *J Clin Endocrinol Metab.* 2002;87(8):3632-9. doi: 10.1210/jcem.87.8.8762.

Leopold Ruzicka produced androsterone from cholesterol and demonstrated that testosterone can be produced from cholesterol. Nobel Prize Website. https://www.nobelprize.org/prizes/chemistry/1939/ruzicka/facts. Accessed August 29, 2021.

Morgantaler A, Zitzmann M, Traish AM, *et al.* Fundamental concepts regarding testosterone deficiency and treatment: international expert consensus resolutions. *Mayo Clin Proc.* 2016;91(7):881-896. doi: 10.1016/j.mayocp.2016.04.007.

Mulligan T, Frick MF, Zuraw QC, *et al.* Prevalence of hypogonadism in males aged at least 45 years: the HIM study. *Int J Clin Pract.* 2006;60(7):762-9. doi: 10.1111/j.1742-1241.2006.00992.x.

Osterberg EC, Bernie AM, Ramasamy R. Risks of testosterone replacement therapy in men. *Indian J Urol.* 2014;30(1):2–7. doi: 10.4103/0970-1591.124197.

Traish AM, Saad F, Guay A. The dark side of testosterone deficiency: II. Type 2 diabetes and insulin resistance. *J Androl.* 2009;30(1):23-32, the Rotterdam study. doi: 10.2164/jandrol.108.005751.

Vigen R, O'Donnell CI, Barón AE, *et al.* Association of testosterone therapy with mortality, myocardial infarction, and stroke in men with low testosterone levels. *JAMA.* 2013;310(17):1829-1836. doi: 10.1001/jama.2013.280386.

Webb CM, McNeill JG, Hayward CS, *et al.* Effects of testosterone on coronary vasomotor regulation in men with coronary heart disease. *Circulation.* 1999;100(16):1690-1696. doi: 10.1161/01.cir.100.16.1690.

Wheeler MJ, Barnes SC. Measurement of testosterone in the diagnosis of hypogonadism in the ageing male. *Clin Endocrinol (Oxf).* 2008;69(4):515-25. doi: 10.1111/j.1365-2265.2008.03325.x.

Zmuda JM, Bausserman LL, Maceroni D, Thompson PD. The effect of supraphysiologic doses of testosterone on fasting total homocysteine levels in normal men. *Atherosclerosis.* 1997;130(1-2):199-202. doi: 10.1016/s0021-9150(96)06057-1.

Zmuda JM, Thompson PD, Dickenson R, Bausserman LL. Testosterone decreases lipoprotein(a) in men. *Amer J Cardiol.* 1996;77(14):1244-1247. doi: 10.1016/s0002-9149(96)00174-9.

Chapter 90—Prostate Health

Porter CM, Shrestha E, Peiffer LB, Sfanos KS. The microbiome in prostate inflammation and prostate cancer. *Prostate Cancer Prostatic Dis.* 2018;21(3):345-354. doi: 10.1038/s41391-018-0041-1.

Richie JP, Catalona WJ, Ahmann FR, *et al.* Effect of patient age on early detection of prostate cancer with serum prostate-specific antigen and digital rectal examination. *Urology.* 1993;42(4):365-74. doi: 10.1016/0090-4295(93)90359-i.

Shrestha E, White JR, Yu SH, *et al.* Profiling the urinary microbiome in men with positive versus negative biopsies for prostate cancer. *J Urol.* 2018;199(1):161-171. doi: 10.1016/j.juro.2017.08.001.

Wu P, Zhang G, Zhao J, *et al.* Profiling the urinary microbiota in male patients with bladder cancer in China. *Front Cell Infect Microbiol.* 2018;8:167. doi: 10.3389/fcimb.2018.00167.

Chapter 96—Understanding Health Insurance

Congressional Budget Office. Federal Subsidies for Health Insurance for People Under Age 65: 2019 to 2029. Congress of the United States, Congressional

Budget Office Website. https://www.cbo.gov/system/files/2019-05/55085-HealthCoverageSubsidies_0.pdf. Published May 2019. Accessed August 29, 2021.

Fontinelle A. Is vision insurance worth it? What you should know. Investopedia Website. https://www.investopedia.com/articles/pf/11/vision-care-insurance.asp. Updated June 15, 2021. Accessed August 29, 2021.

Health Insurance Coverage in the United States 2018. Report Number P60-267 (RV). U.S. Census Bureau Website. https://www.census.gov/library/publications/2019/demo/p60-267.html. Published November 2019. Accessed August 29, 2021.

Suh E. Health insurance basics: your 101 guide to health insurance. Polygenius Website. https://www.policygenius.com/health-insurance/learn/health-insurance-basics-and-guide/#the-different-types-of-private-health-insurance. Updated April 21, 2021. Accessed August 29, 2021.

U.S. Centers for Medicare & Medicaid Services Website. https://www.cms.gov/Research-Statistics-Data-and-Systems/Statistics-Trends-and-Reports/NationalHealthExpendData/NationalHealthAccountsProjected. Accessed August 29, 2021.

U.S. private health insurance-statistics & facts. Statista Research Department. Statistca Website. https://www.statista.com/topics/1530/health-insurance-in-the-us/ Published February 11, 2021. Accessed August 29, 2021.

U.S. Sources of Healthcare Coverage 2019. Wikipedia Website. https://en.wikipedia.org/wiki/Health_insurance_coverage_in_the_United_States#/media/File:Health_Insurance_Coverage_in_the_U.S._2016_-_v1.png. Accessed August 29, 2021.

Walton J. How does dental insurance work? Investopedia Website. https://www.investopedia.com/articles/personal-finance/111715/how-does-dental-insurance-work.asp. Updated Aug. 28, 2020. Accessed August 29, 2021.

Why health insurance is important. Protection from high medical costs. HealthCare.gov Website. https://www.healthcare.gov/why-coverage-is-important/protection-from-high-medical-costs/ Accessed August 29, 2021.

Yabroff KR, Zhao JX, Han XS, Zheng AY. Prevalence and correlates of medical financial hardship in the USA. *J Gen Intern Med.* 2019;34(8):1494-1502. doi: 10.1007/s11606-019-05002-w.

Chapter 99—Gratitude

Allen S. *The Science of Gratitude: A White Paper.* Berkeley, CA: University of California, John Templeton Foundation, Greater Good Science Center, 2018. UC Berkeley Website. https://ggsc.berkeley.edu/images/uploads/GGSC-JTF_White_Paper-Gratitude-FINAL.pdf. Published May 2018. Accessed September 9, 2021. This is an excellent compilation on the science of gratitude and the list of references is encyclopedic.

Breathnach, Sarah Ban. *The Simple Abundance Journal of Gratitude.* New York, NY: Grand Central Publishing, 2019. Ms. Breathnach wrote 13 books on the subject of gratitude, many of which were massive bestsellers. She was a master communicator and her books, which are highly readable and very helpful, are very much applicable in 2020.

Emmons, Robert A. *Thanks!: How the New Science of Gratitude can Make You Happier.* Boston, MA: Houghton Mifflin Company, 2007.

Sheen, Fulton J. *Life is Worth Living;* revised edition. San Francisco, CA: Ignatius Press, 1999. Many of the thoughts expressed in this chapter were inspired by Dr. Sheen. He was a brilliant communicator, his books are widely available on amazon.com, and all of his television shows are available on Netflix. The television and printed messages are timeless.

wikipedia.org. All the theologians, philosophers, psychologists, and self-help authors quoted in the chapter on gratitude have extensive biographies available online, which include their significant works and an assessment of their contributions.

Figure Credits

Figure 1.1. The hero's journey. (Art by Paul Veres, RegentPress.net; figure of the young hero, istockphoto.com/msan10)

Figure 2.1 Life expectancy. (By Max Roser, Martin School, Oxford, UK. Available at https://ourworldindata.org/life-expectancy and Wikimedia.org, public domain)

Figure 2.2. Estimated deaths from all causes in males, U.S., 2019. (Art by Mark Weiman, RegentPress.net; data from the Centers for Disease Control, CDC.gov)

Figure, Part 2. The effects of aging on performance. Data on 100 meter sprint world records (World Masters Athletics) available at https://world-masters-athletics.com/records/. Data on 50 meter freestyle and butterfly qualifying times (U.S. Masters Swimming) available at https://www.usms.org/content/scnats00nqt. Both sites accessed September 22, 2021.

Figure 5.1 Artery structure showing the epithelium. (Image: istockphoto.com/urfinguss)

Figure 6.1 Coronary circulation (Anterior). (By Blausen Medical Communications, Inc. donated via OTRS, Wikimedia.org, public domain)

Figure 6.2 Measuring blood pressure levels in adults. (Data: https://www.CDC.gov/bloodpressure/facts.htm)

Figure 7.1. Estimated new diagnoses and deaths from cancer in males, U.S. 2020. (Art by Mark Weiman, RegentPress.net; data from CDC.gov)

Figure 7.2 New cancers and number of cases per 100,000 American men, 2021. (Graphics from BrandeisMD; data from cancerstatisticscenter.cancer.org)

Figure 7.3. Depiction of a testicular self-examination. (Illustration by Bruce Blaus, Wikipedia, public domain)

Figure 10.1 Pain in America. (Art courtesy of BrandeisMD; data from CDC.gov)

Figure 10.2 Why Americans Take Opioids. (Art courtesy of BrandeisMD; data from CDC.gov)

Figure 10.3 Osteoarthritis. (By Bruce Blaus, Wikimedia.org, public domain).

Figure 11.1. The lung and airways, with a close-up of the alveoli where oxygen is infused into the bloodstream via minute blood vessels. (National Heart Lung and Blood Institute, Public domain, via Wikimedia Commons)

Figure 11.2 Potentially Damaging Exposures (Information courtesy of BrandeisMD)

Figure 12.1 Recognition by IgE antibodies drives the release of histamine and the rapid development of symptoms. (istock.com/ttsz)

Figure 13.1 The structure of an artery wall, showing the multiple layers of muscle that enable the arteries to effectively pump blood throughout the body. (BruceBlaus: Blausen.com staff (2014). "Medical gallery of Blausen Medical 2014". WikiJournal of Medicine 1 (2). DOI:10.15347/wjm/2014.010. ISSN 2002-4436., CC BY 3.0 via Wikimedia Commons)

Figure 13.2 Veins of the leg. (By Henry Vandyke Carter - Henry Gray (1918) Anatomy of the Human Body. Bartleby.com: Gray's Anatomy, Plate 582, Public Domain, https://commons.wikimedia.org/w/index.php?curid=560936)

Figure 13.3. How the muscles of the leg move blood up veins toward the heart, against gravity. (By OpenStax College - Anatomy & Physiology, Connexions Web site. http://cnx.org/content/col11496/1.6/, Jun 19, 2013., CC BY 3.0, https://commons.wikimedia.org/w/index.php?curid=30148264)

Figure 13.4. An illustration of the one-way valves in the veins and the risks of poor circulation when the valves and the veins become impaired. (By Jmarchn, modified from Varicose veins.jpg of National Heart Lung and Blood Institute (NIH) - Own work, CC BY-SA 3.0, https://commons.wikimedia.org/w/index.php?curid=62387372)

Figure 16.1. Aspects of health with the potential to cause memory loss. (Bredensen Dale, MD. The End of Alzheimer's, New York, NY: Avery, 2017.

Figure 18.1 Symptoms of prediabetes. (Courtesy of Jerry Stine, www.LifespanInstitute.com)

Figure 18.2. Symptoms of hypoglycemia. (Courtesy of Jerry Stine, www.LifespanInstitute.com)

Figure 20.1 Reductions in infectious disease and the rise of chronic, fatal disorders. (Isabel A. Cáceres. Massachusetts Deaths 2006. Massachusetts Department of Public Health. Available at: http://www.mass.gov/dph/resep. Accessed 09-07-2021.)

Figure 20.2 Protection against bacteria, mold, parasites, viruses, budding malignancies, and management of the immune response. (By BruceBlaus. Blausen.com staff (2014). Medical gallery of Blausen Medical 2014. WikiJournal of Medicine 1 (2). DOI:10.15347/wjm/2014.010. ISSN 2002-4436. - Own work, CC BY 3.0 https://commons.wikimedia.org/w/index.php?curid=28223981)

Figure 22.1. The majority of back injuries involve some type of disc event. (Art: istockphoto.com/wildpixel)

Figure 23.1. The magnificent spine. (Henry Vandyke Carter. Gray's Anatomy, public domain)

Figure 24.1. Anatomy of the eye. (By BruceBlaus. Blausen.com staff (2014). Medical gallery of Blausen Medical 2014. WikiJournal of Medicine 1 (2). DOI:10.15347/wjm/2014.010. ISSN 2002-4436. - Own work, CC BY 3.0, https://commons.wikimedia.org/w/index.php?curid=29025014)

Figure 65.5. Suicide rates by age and gender, U.S. (Source: CDC.gov)

Figure 68.1. Factors that promote or deter living with vitality. (Courtesy of Robert Buonfiglio, PhD, DrRobertJBuonfiglio.com)

Figure 69.1. The Four Temperaments. (Source: © 2021 Nancy Faass, HealthWritersGroup. com with thanks to a number of innovators in temperament theory)

Figure 76.1. Cross section of the penis. (Mcstrother, CC BY 3.0 <https://creativecommons. org/licenses/by/3.0>, via Wikimedia Commons)

Figure 76.2. Anatomy of the penis. (CFCF, CC BY-SA 3.0 <https://creativecommons.org/ licenses/by-sa/3.0>, via Wikimedia Commons)

Figure 77.1. Arteries of the penis. (By Henry Vandyke Carter – Henry Gray (1918) Anatomy of the Human Body (Bartleby.com: Gray's Anatomy, Plate 1158, Public Domain https://commons.wikimedia.org/w/index.php?curid=35171260)

Figure 77.2. Cross section of the penis, which increases in size as much as five times during an erection. (Qbrains, CC BY-SA 4.0 <https://creativecommons.org/licenses/by-sa/4.0>, via Wikimedia Commons)

Figure 77.3 Close up of the artery structure showing the epithelium. (Art: istockphoto. com/urfinguss)

Figure 77.4. Basic components of a nerve cell (neuron). (Source: Dhp1080 – "Anatomy and Physiology"; by the US National Cancer Institute #039; Surveillance, Epidemiology and End Results (SEER) Program ., CC BY-SA 3.0, https://commons.wikimedia. org/w/index.php?curid=1474927)

Figure 78.1. Zebras fighting for supremacy in the herd and the right to father the offspring of the group. (By Kore - Own work, CC BY-SA 3.0, https://commons.wikimedia. org/w/index.php?curid=30058235)

Figure 78.2. Causes of lifelong and acquired PE. (Information courtesy of BrandeisMD)

Figure 81.1. Subcutaneous injection. (en.wikibooks.org/wiki/Structural_Biochemistry/ Subcutaneous)

Figure 87.1. Effectiveness of condoms in preventing sexually- transmitted infection. (Data: CDC.gov)

Figures 88.1. Male erectile tissue which is 50% visible.

88.2. Female erectile tissue, which is only 5% visible, making it difficult to tell when a woman is ready for sex. (Courtesy of Susan Bratton)

Figure 88.3. Feminine sexual anatomy. (Courtesy of Susan Bratton)

Figure 88.4. Feminine sexual anatomy labeled. (Courtesy of Susan Bratton)

Figure 88.5. The bullseye touch technique. (Courtesy of Susan Bratton)

Figure 88.6. Regular orgasm. (Courtesy of Susan Bratton)

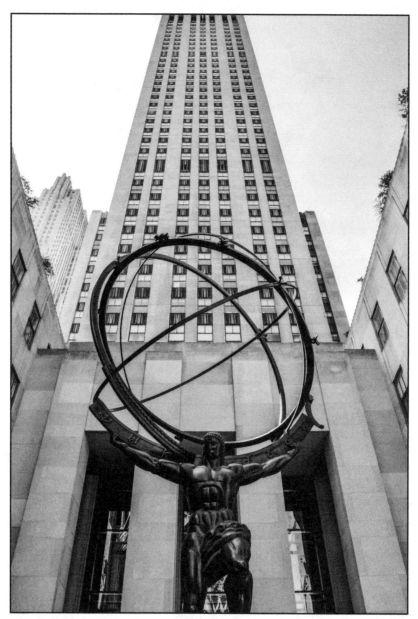

Atlas was given the task of holding up the heavens as punishment from Zeus for leading the Titans in their battle with the Olympian Gods for control of the heavens. Growing up in New York, I passed this statue frequently and always marveled at the power and awesome responsibility of Atlas. In the same way, I see good men, pillars of their community, providing support to their family, their profession, and their society.